Intimate Partner Violence

Intimate Partner Violence

A Health-Based Perspective

Edited by

Connie Mitchell, Editor-in-Chief
Deirdre Anglin, Associate Editor

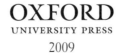

OXFORD

UNIVERSITY PRESS

2009

OXFORD
UNIVERSITY PRESS

Oxford University Press, Inc., publishes works that further
Oxford University's objective of excellence in
research, scholarship, and education.

Oxford New York
Auckland   Cape Town   Dar es Salaam   Hong Kong   Karachi
Kuala Lumpur   Madrid   Melbourne   Mexico City   Nairobi
New Delhi   Shanghai   Taipei   Toronto

With offices in
Argentina   Austria   Brazil   Chile   Czech Republic   France   Greece
Guatemala   Hungary   Italy   Japan   Poland   Portugal   Singapore
South Korea   Switzerland   Thailand   Turkey   Ukraine   Vietnam

Published by Oxford University Press, Inc.
198 Madison Avenue, New York, New York 10016
www.oup.com

Oxford is a registered trademark of Oxford University Press

Intimate partner violence : a health-based perspective / Connie Mitchell,
editor-in-chief ; Deirdre Anglin, associate editor.
p. ; cm.
Includes bibliographical references and index.
ISBN: 978-0-19-517932-3
1. Family violence—Psychological aspects. 2. Abused wives—Rehabilitation. 3. Victims of family
violence—Rehabilitation. 4. Spousal abuse. I. Mitchell, Connie. II. Anglin, Deirdre.
[DNLM: 1. Spouse Abuse. WA 308 I615 2009]
RC569.5.F3I579 2009
362.82'92—dc22   2008041764

Printed in the United States of America
on acid-free paper

1 3 5 7 9 10 8 6 4 2

In memory of Linda E. Saltzman, PhD (1949–2005)

For her legacy in public health investigation in
the field of intimate partner violence
and her commitment to health
and liberty for all.

Contents

I. Background

II. Identification

V. Important Related Topics

Foreword

Intimate partner violence has long been a source of profound human suffering. The injuries and humiliation associated with it have devastating effects on the health and well-being of its victims as well as its witnesses. Among these effects are included deaths due to homicide and suicide, physical injuries, long-lasting emotional and psychological problems, sexual and reproductive diseases and complications (including HIV), and a host of stress-related physical ailments. The magnitude of this problem and its consequences are slowly, but surely, being recognized. A new day is dawning as policy-makers and health authorities are realizing the enormous cost that we pay in suffering, productivity, and the basic quality of our lives by failing to prevent and respond to intimate partner violence.

Intimate Partner Violence: A Health-Based Perspective is a clear milestone in the efforts of the past 50 years to make the toll of intimate partner violence visible and its perpetration unacceptable. This volume demonstrates the myriad of ways that a health perspective on this problem complements the law enforcement and social perspectives that have provided the primary lens through which many people have viewed and addressed this problem. The chapters of this book span the key realms of health policy, public health prevention, acute and chronic care, as well as the legal, social, political, and economic issues that impinge on these systems and their response to the problem. The accumulated knowledge and insight contained within this volume provides good cause to celebrate how far we have come in understanding this problem and how best to address it. From its chapters a coherent picture emerges of the potential power that an integrated health systems response, addressing both prevention and care, can make to reduce the consequences of intimate partner violence.

One of the strengths of this book is its focus on the ways in which intimate partner violence impacts mental and physical health and the implications of this impact for how healthcare providers care for their patients. Because they promote healing, most health professionals are respected and trusted. They often are the first person that a victim confides in and asks for help. Consequently physicians and other health professionals are key gatekeepers in efforts to monitor, identify, treat, and intervene in cases of intimate partner violence, and some studies show that more cases of interpersonal violence come to the attention of healthcare providers than to police. The role of healthcare providers in addressing intimate partner violence needs to be better understood and institutional and educational barriers that limit the effectiveness of even committed providers reduced. Programs to educate healthcare providers are an essential step in this process. This book provides the first comprehensive text to address the intersection between intimate partner violence and health and is, therefore, a valuable educational tool and reference for healthcare and social service professionals. The role of healthcare providers is not limited, however, to intervening through clinical practices and referrals. As leaders and respected members of our communities, healthcare providers are among our most effective advocates for broad programs and policies that can contribute to prevention. As the nation embarks on a period of healthcare reform, the leadership of healthcare providers will be critical for ensuring that the healthcare system of the future is one that is responsive to the needs of victims and witnesses to this problem and that is clearly linked to community prevention strategies.

Parallel to creating a responsive healthcare system is the need to prevent intimate partner violence from occurring in the first place by reducing the creation of future perpetrators. Another important strength of this book is the attention it gives to public health prevention and the science that underlies it. In essence what is required is an array of programs and policies that are effective in creating a societal ethos that promotes respectful, nonviolent intimate relationships. The promotion of this ethos is not just the responsibility of individuals and partners, but also of our communities and our nation. Societal and community norms, policies, and structures create environments that can support respectful, nonviolent relationships. Developing and maintaining respectful relationships is difficult even under the best of circumstances. This is especially true because we don't always have good role models for these skills, in part because there are few systematic attempts in our society to teach, model, and support the skills that foster these relationships. What do respectful, nonviolent relationships look like? The literature on the causes of intimate partner violence suggests that these relationships would be characterized by shared decision-making, mutual trust, the mutual belief in a partner's right to autonomy, the mutual belief in nonviolent conflict resolution, the presence of effective communication skills, and the ability to negotiate and adjust to stress. What programs and policies will be effective in creating a society in which these relationship characteristics are widely held and practiced? This is the challenge we now face—how do we create such a society? The chapters of this book give us important insights into what such a society might look like—that is, the way healthcare providers would care for victims, the features of its healthcare system, and the outlines of the prevention strategies that might be most effective. Despite the fact that there is still a long way to go in eliminating intimate partner violence, this book inspires a clear sense of hope that we will find a way.

Socrates taught that, "Without proper knowledge right action is impossible, but with proper knowledge right action is inevitable." This volume provides the proper knowledge, which is knowledge that's based on science in the service of humanity. As we move forward in efforts to prevent intimate partner violence this book will be a valuable resource for researchers, policymakers, physicians, nurses, and other healthcare providers, public health workers, students, and, in fact, everyone concerned with the problem of intimate partner violence.

James A. Mercy, PhD
Special Advisor for Strategic Directions
Division of Violence Prevention
National Center for Injury Prevention and Control
Centers for Disease Prevention and Control

Preface

In my nine years as Director of Domestic Violence Education for a California-wide program to educate health professionals on family violence and sexual assault, I was humbled by the rapidly expanding body of research in the field of health and intimate partner violence (IPV). It was during my tenure as Director that I met Deirdre Anglin, my Associate Editor; I was also fortunate to establish close collegial ties to many experts around the state and the country, some of whom have generously provided chapters for this text. In 2001, the Institute of Medicine asked me to present testimony regarding the California curriculum as part of their investigation that was later published as the book entitled *Confronting Chronic Neglect: The Education and Training of Health Professionals on Family Violence*. One of the conclusions of the report was that the field was lacking in defined core competencies, academic curricula, and major academic health texts.

I believe my authors and I have written the first comprehensive text to combine health policy, public health prevention, acute care, chronic care models, and individual- and system-based interventions, regarding intimate partner violence. The text is multidisciplinary and should have appeal across several traditional health silos—trauma and chronic care medicine; psychiatry; and adolescent, obstetric and geriatric medicine—while integrating the social, political, economic, and legal issues that have an impact on health intervention.

Despite our efforts, there are a few gaps in this text. The natural history of intimate partner violence is not described. We know how intimate partner violence commonly presents in the health setting, but we don't know much about the natural history of the problem, namely victims who have experienced IPV yet did not seek out health, criminal justice, or community services. Likewise, our understanding of the etiology and dynamics of intimate partner violence continues to evolve, and there are distinct areas that need further elaboration such as the dynamics of heterosexual male victimization and intimate partner violence in lesbian, gay, trans-gendered, and bisexual relationships. Finally, there are very few well designed studies to test intervention strategies that are currently published, but many are on-going and will contribute to more precise standards of care for child, adult, and elder victims as well as perpetrators of IPV.

In this book we have elected to primarily use the term "intimate partner violence" as per the guidelines of the Centers for Disease Control and Prevention. However, other terms such as domestic violence or partner abuse may occasionally be used within the text.

While IPV tends to be a gendered health issue, meaning more victims appear to be women and more perpetrators appear to be men, we recognize the reverse is also true, and IPV occurs in same-sex relationships. We trust the reader will keep this in mind, as we avoided cumbersome joint pronoun use (she/he or her/him) throughout the text. In addition, the reader should be advised that most of the text refers to IPV victims as "patients" and less often as "victims" or "survivors." As a health text, the term "patients" seemed most appropriate, while recognizing that our patients may be primary victims, secondary victims, abusers, perpetrators, or perhaps some combination of all of these. Survivor is a term

of empowerment but not one in common use in the health setting.

Dr. Anglin and I share a philosophy as educators, health policy advisors, and now text editors, to promote evidence-based practice but to also recognize the value of practice-based evidence. This is not a book of clinical guidelines, of which there are many. Rather, it is intended to describe the current state of the field referencing the existing literature in the field, with appropriate attribution to consensus expert opinion, and clear delineation of issues needing further investigation. If the authors have inadvertently inserted non-corroborated dogma, or committed errors of omission or commission, despite our vigilance and the assistance of expert reviewers, these should be communicated to us. This text will only serve the field better through our collegial vigor to seek truth.

It is our sincere hope that this text will be used by students, clinicians, researchers, and policy makers in health care, public health, and social sciences to establish a solid foundation upon which we can all continue to build.

Connie Mitchell and Deirdre Anglin

Contributors

Elaine J. Alpert, MD, MPH
Associate Professor of Public Health and Medicine
Department of Social and Behavioral Science
Boston University School of Public Health
Boston, MA

Deirdre Anglin, MD, MPH
Professor of Clinical Emergency Medicine
Department of Emergency Medicine
Keck School of Medicine
University of Southern California
Los Angeles, CA

Phyllis Brashler, PhD
National Center on Domestic Violence,
Trauma & Mental Health
Chicago, IL

Sarah Buehl, JD
Clinical Professor of Law
University of Texas School of Law
Austin, TX

Jacquelyn Campbell, PhD, RN
Anna D. Wolf Chair in Nursing
Johns Hopkins University School of Nursing
Baltimore, MD

Ann L. Coker, PhD, MPH
Professor of Obstetrics and Gynecology
Verizon Wireless Endowed Chair
Center for Research on Violence Against Women
University of Kentucky
Lexington, KY

Phaedra S. Corso, PhD
Associate Professor of Health Policy and Management
University of Georgia College of Public Health
Athens, GA

Carol B. Cunradi, PhD, MPH
Senior Research Scientist
Prevention Research Center
Pacific Institute for Research & Evaluation
Berkeley, CA

KEITH DAVIS, PhD
Distinguished Professor Emeritus of Psychology
Barnwell College
University of South Carolina
Columbia, SC

THOMAS B. DODSON, DMD, MPH
Associate Professor of Oral and Maxillofacial
    Surgery
Harvard School of Dental Medicine
Cambridge, MA

LYNNE FAUERBACH, RN
Johns Hopkins University School of Nursing
Baltimore, MD

JESSICA GIL, PhD
National Institute of Health
Bethesda, MD

LINDA J. GOMBERG, JD, MA
Consultant in Private Practice
Seal Beach, CA

PEGGY E. GOODMAN, MD, MS
Associate Professor of Emergency Medicine
Director, Violence Prevention Resources
Brody School of Medicine
East Carolina University
Greenville, NC

DIANE M. HALL, PhD
Division of Violence Prevention
National Center for Injury Prevention
    and Control
Centers for Disease Control and
    Prevention
Atlanta, GA

LESLIE R. HALPERN, MD, DDS
Assistant Clinical Professor
Department of Oral and Maxillofacial Surgery
Harvard School of Dental Medicine
Boston, MA

ELIZA HIRST, JD
Staff Attorney
Disabilities Law Program
Community Legal Aid Society
Wilmington, DE

NANCY GLASS, PhD, RN
Associate Professor of Community Public Health
Associate Director, Johns Hopkins Center
    for Global Health
Johns Hopkins University School of Nursing
Baltimore, MD

L. KEVIN HAMBERGER, PhD
Professor of Family and Community Medicine
Racine Family Medicine Center
Medical College of Wisconsin
Racine, WI

DEAN HAWLEY, MD
Forensic Pathologist
Director of Autopsy Services
Department of Pathology and Laboratory
    Medicine
Indiana University School of Medicine
Indianapolis, IN

SHERYL L. HERON, MD, MPH
Associate Professor of Emergency Medicine
Emory University School of Medicine
Atlanta, GA

DEBRA HOURY, MD, MPH
Vice Chair for Research, Department of Emergency
    Medicine
Director, Center for Injury Control
Emory University
Atlanta, GA

MEGHAN E. HOWE, MPH
Senior Project Manager
Crime and Justice Institute
School of Public Health
Boston University
Boston, MA

LISA JAMES, MA
Director of Health
Family Violence Prevention Fund
San Francisco, CA

LYNDEE KNOX, PhD
Assistant Professor of Family Medicine
University of Southern California
Alhambra, CA

DIANA KOIN, MD
Eldersafe Training and Consultation to
    Prevent Abuse and Neglect
Napa, California
Associate Clinical Professor of
    Internal Medicine
University of California, San Francisco
San Francisco, CA

KRISTA KOTZ, PhD, MPH
Program Director
Family Violence Prevention Program
Kaiser Permanente Northern California
Oakland, CA

CYNTHIA KUELBS, MD
Assistant Clinical Professor of Pediatrics
University of California, San Diego
Medical Director
Chadwick Center for Children
    and Families
Rady Children's Hospital
San Diego, CA

GREGORY LUKE LARKIN, MD, MS,
    MSPH, MA, FACEP
Professor, Department of Surgery
Associate Chief, Emergency Medicine
Yale University School of Medicine
New Haven, CT

JANE LIEBSCHUTZ, MD, MPH
Associate Professor of Medicine and Social
    and Behavioral Sciences
Schools of Medicine and Public
    Health
Boston University
Boston, MA

KAREN LLOYD, PhD
Senior Director
Behavioral Health Strategy and Operations
HealthPartners
Bloomington, MN

JEFFREY M. LOHR, PhD
Professor of Psychology
University of Arkansas, Fayetteville
Fayetteville, AR

CARMELA LOMONACO, MA
Assistant Director, LA Net
Department of Family Medicine
University of Southern California
Los Angeles, CA

BRIGID McCAW, MD, MPH
Medical Director
Family Violence Prevention Program
Kaiser Permanente Northern California
Oakland, CA

GEORGE McCLANE, MD
Emergency Physician
Sharp Hospital
Clinical Faculty in Preventive & Primary Care
    Medicine
University of California San Diego, School
    of Medicine
San Diego, CA

MINDY MECHANIC, PhD
Associate Professor of Psychology
California State University Fullerton
Fullerton, CA

CONNIE MITCHELL, MD, MPH
Assistant Clinical Professor of
    Internal Medicine
University of California, Davis
Public Health Medical Officer
Maternal, Child and Adolescent Health
California Department of Public Health
Sacramento, CA

STEPHEN C. MORRIS, MD
Resident
Department of Surgery
Section of Emergency Medicine
Yale University School of Medicine
New Haven, CT

KATHERINE R. NASH, RN
Death Investigator and Forensic
    Nurse Examiner
Montgomery County, MD
Johns Hopkins University School
    of Nursing
Baltimore, MD

CHRISTINA NICOLAIDIS, MD, MPH
Associate Professor of Medicine, Public
  Health & Preventive Medicine
Oregon Health and Science University
Portland, OR

ANURADHA PARANJAPE, MD, MPH
Associate Professor of Medicine and Public
  Health Temple University School
  of Medicine
Philadelphia, PA

LISA M. PARKER, PhD
Instructor in Psychology
Department of Psychiatry
Harvard Medical School
Staff Psychologist
Klarman Eating Disorders Center
McLean Hospital
Belmont, MA

JENNIFER PARKS, MPH
Instructor in Emergency Medicine
Parkland Memorial Hospital
The University of Texas
Southwestern Medical Center at Dallas
Dallas, TX

KERRY PARSONS, RN
Johns Hopkins University School
  of Nursing
Baltimore, MD

CHRISTINE A. POULOS, RN
Johns Hopkins University School of Nursing
Baltimore, MD

CAROLYN SACHS, MD, MPH
Associate Professor
Emergency Medicine Center
University of California, Los Angeles
Los Angeles, CA

LINDA E. SALTZMAN, PhD
Centers for Disease Control
Atlanta, GA

PHYLLIS SHARPS, PhD, RN
Professor and Chair
Johns Hopkins University School of Nursing
Baltimore, MD

DANIEL J. SHERIDAN, PhD, RN
Associate Professor
Johns Hopkins University School of Nursing
Baltimore, MD

SUSAN SORENSON, PhD
Professor of Social Policy and Practice
Senior Fellow in Public Health
University of Pennsylvania
Philadelphia, PA

GAEL STRACK, JD
Chief Executive Officer
National Family Justice Center Alliance
San Diego, CA

ELLEN TALIAFERRO, MD
Medical Director
Keller Center for Family Violence Intervention
San Mateo Medical Center
San Mateo, CA

MAGDELENA VANYA, PhD
Associate Research Scientist
Prevention Research Center
Berkeley, CA

SUJATA WARRIER, PhD
Director, Health Care Bureau
New York State Office for the Prevention of
  Domestic Violence
Bloomfield, NJ

CAROLE WARSHAW, MD
Executive Director, Domestic Violence & Mental
  Health Policy Initiative
Director, National Center on Domestic Violence,
  Trauma & Mental Health
Chicago, IL

SANDRA WATT, RN
Johns Hopkins University School of Nursing
Baltimore, MD

DANIEL J. WHITAKER, PhD
Director, National SafeCare® Training and Research
  Center
Visiting Professor, Institute of Public Health
College of Health and Human Sciences
Georgia State University
Atlanta, GA

SHARON R. WILSON, MD
Associate Professor of Emergency
   Medicine
University of California, Davis Medical
   Center
Sacramento, CA

TRICIA WITTE, PhD
Assistant Professor of Psychology
Birmingham-Southern College
Birmingham, AL

THERESE ZINK, MD, MPH
Professor of Family Medicine and Community
   Health
University of Minnesota
Minneapolis, MN

Acknowledgments

Drs. Mitchell and Anglin would like to recognize the many people who have inspired or directly contributed to the writing or production of this text. We must first and foremost acknowledge the voices of survivors and advocates who understood the devastating impact of this shame-based disease and made us all pay attention. We recognize the prolific researchers from the nursing field who not only advanced the science but modeled collaboration, partnered with community groups, and demonstrated utmost respect for the safety of victims. We also appreciate the foundation laid by experts in child abuse and sexual assault and the published research from other fields, such as social science and criminal justice, which inform aspects of a health-based perspective.

We would like to recognize the following persons who have made particular contributions to our professional development in this field:

- Our patients who honored us with their trust when they disclosed intimate partner violence and taught us something with each encounter;

- Linda Saltzman for reminding us to always put dogma to the test and never aggrandize the truth;
- Jackie Campbell for being an impossible role model to emulate, but a beacon of light to follow;
- Lisa James and Debbie Lee at the Family Violence Prevention Fund, who constantly prod us to advocate for change and to exercise patient persistence;
- Barbara Falcon, our assistant who helped to "kick-off" the project;
- Sharl Talan, who pitched in, without question, to offer assistance when we needed it most;
- Many other colleagues who not only gave of their time and wisdom but with whom we enjoy working in respectful and collegial ways.

In addition, Connie Mitchell would like to recognize:

- Cindy Kuelbs for patiently teaching me about child abuse so I could see the corollaries in intimate partner violence;

- John McCann for giving me a chance to build a program from a blank slate at the University of California Davis;
- Colleagues in Sacramento on the Domestic Violence Death Review Team and the Health Domestic Violence Network for opportunities to put ideas into practice;
- Jody Rhodes, my literary agent and Joan Bossert, Abby Gross, and Jennifer Bossert who patiently guided me through the book production process;
- Deirdre Anglin, my associate editor and my best friend, without whom this book might never have been finished;
- My parents, Jerry and Dorothy Mitchell, who always made me feel safe and loved, and my sisters who keep me grounded;
- My husband, David Tai and sons, Mitch and Zack, with whom I live and experience relationship equity and mutual regard, and from whom I learn what masculinity is and isn't.

Deirdre Anglin would like to recognize:

- Connie Mitchell, my best friend, for her always insightful words of support and encouragement, and her unselfish sharing of opportunities to learn and further develop my knowledge and skills;
- My parents, Mary and Douglas Anglin, for teaching me, by their example, about respect and equality for all people;
- My children, Alexander, Sarah and Trevor, who are daily reminders about the importance of never giving up on efforts to create a safer, more equitable world for all.

Finally, both Drs. Mitchell and Anglin thank all their authors who remained committed to this project despite unanticipated delays and always ended their correspondence with words of encouragement and acknowledgment of the value of the text.

Reviewers

The following experts gave of their time and wisdom to critically review the chapters and ensure the integrity of the work:

Deirdre Anglin, MD, MPH
University of Southern California

Julia C. Babcock, PhD
University of Houston

Loraine Bacchus, MD
London School of Hygiene and Tropical Medicine
London, England

Jennifer Bennice, PhD
Medical University of South Carolina

Jeffrey H. Coben, MD
West Virginia University

Margaret Drew, JD
University of Cincinnati

Mary Ann Dutton, PhD
Georgetown University

Carmel Dyer, MD
University of Texas

Xiangming Fang, PhD
Centers for Disease Control
   and Prevention

Nancy Glass, PhD, RN
Johns Hopkins University

Henrica A.F.M. Jansen, PhD
World Health Organization
Geneva, Switzerland

Leigh Kimberg, MD
University of California San Francisco

Julie Kunce Field, JD
Private Practice, Fort Collins, Colorado

Chapter 1

Evolving Health Policy on Intimate Partner Violence

Connie Mitchell and Lisa James

KEY CONCEPTS

- Violence is a health risk, it is widely prevalent, and its costs in terms of economics and human suffering make it a major health problem.
- Historically, in terms of national policy, interpersonal violence has been framed as a criminal justice issue and only recently have the health consequences for individuals, families, and communities been defined, measured, or addressed.
- A national public health approach to interpersonal violence would better address the multifactorial nature of violence and the multidisciplinary approach to intervention than a criminal justice approach alone.

INTRODUCTION AND BACKGROUND

Violence is one of the leading causes of death worldwide for persons aged 15–44 years (1). Exposure to violence and/or abuse is a major health risk for human beings; it is widely prevalent, and its costs in terms of economics and human suffering make it a major health problem. About 26% of women and 16% of men in the United States report a lifetime occurrence of IPV defined as threatened, attempted or completed physical assault or unwanted sex by a current or former intimate partner (2,3). Women who have experienced partner violence are at significantly greater risk for heart disease, stroke, asthma, arthritis, heavy drinking, and high-risk sexual practices, than are women who have not experienced partner violence (3).

Sociologist Herbert Blumer stated: "A social problem does not exist for a society unless it is recognized by that society to exist . . . social conditions may be ignored at one time yet, without change in their makeup, become matters of grave concern at another time" (4). Medicine, like sociology, is influenced by the rise and decline of issues in the public eye. This chapter addresses the emergence of intimate partner violence (IPV) as a public health problem and the subsequent evolution of health policy, as well as key considerations for assessing or improving current IPV health policy.

DEFINING VIOLENCE

According to the World Health Organization (WHO), violence is defined as "the intentional use of force or power, intentional or actual, against oneself, another person, a group, or community that results in or has the high likelihood of resulting in injury, death, or psychological harm, maldevelopment or deprivation" (1). The inclusion of the use of power as a form of violence is particularly relevant to IPV. Abuse of power includes the use of threats, intimidation, or acts of omission or commission to reinforce the inequality of the relationship. According to the WHO, IPV is a form of interpersonal violence, one of three typologies that also include self-violence and collective violence (1) (see Figure 1.1). Self-violence includes personal abuse and suicide; interpersonal violence includes family and community violence; and collective violence includes social, political, and economic violence.

HISTORICAL PERSPECTIVE

In 1985, the United States Surgeon General, C. Everett Koop, focused the public health lens on violence behind closed doors—the violence that occurs in homes, predominantly against women and children (5). The American health community did not universally rise to his call to action. In 1996, the 49th World Health Assembly declared violence a growing and major health threat throughout the world and called upon policy makers, academicians, public health professionals, and healthcare workers to address its causes and consequences. Still, healthcare responses have been slow to evolve.

Historically, policy efforts addressing IPV have been focused on: (a) making the invisible visible, (b) providing community-based support for victims, (c) creating legal remedies and judicial reforms, (d) deterrence, (e) treatment, and (f) changing cultural norms and institutional cultures and reframing political issues. An outline of some of the achievements in each area (social, legal, and health) is provided in Table 1.1. As the table indicates, although slow to start, progress in the health arena has been surging in recent years. Both social scientists and legal professionals welcome and appreciate the public health model for addressing IPV since, by nature, it is multidisciplinary, evidence-based, and relies upon measurement of desired outcomes. A public health approach to IPV is discussed in further detail elsewhere in this textbook.

FORCES THAT SHAPE INTIMATE PARTNER VIOLENCE HEALTH POLICY

Health policy is shaped by a collection of events: expanding scientific literature, published expert consensus opinion, legislative or court decisions, and

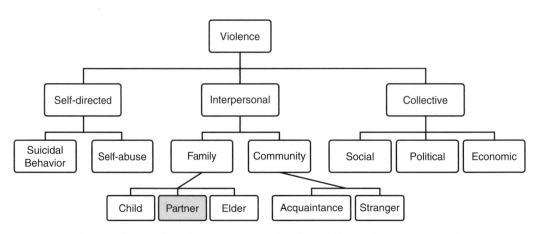

Figure 1.1 A typology of violence. *Source:* The World Health Organization, 2002.

Table 1.1 Social, Political, and Health Policy History of Intimate Partner Violence			
	Major Social/Cultural Event	Major Legislation or Court Decision	Advances in Health Policy or Health Science
1700s	**Late 1600s:** Puritans and Pilgrims promote that the family patriarch had not only the responsibility but the duty to enforce conduct, and moderate force might be necessary to ensure path to salvation **1776:** There are no "mothers" of the American Revolution.	**1641:** First American law prohibiting beating female spouses enacted in the Massachusetts Bay Colony, but Puritans still uphold "legitimate" use of physical force by parents, masters, or husbands	Tertiary care of violent injuries advances while treating wounds of war
1800s	**Civil War:** Fear of crime and perceived threat to public order leads to laws against domestic violence with stiff penalties, although rarely invoked **1848:** Seneca Falls Convention – Declaration of Sentiments **1870s:** A period of activism to stop wife beating and other forms of family violence coupled with a child protection movement	**1824** *Bradley v. State:* Husband can be convicted of assault and battery on his wife **1866:** Civil Rights Act declares Blacks as citizens and 14th Amendment gives Black men the right to vote **1871:** Alabama is first state to rescind a husband's legal right to beat his wife **1874:** *State v. Oliver* in North Carolina; a husband no longer had right to chastise his wife **1874:** The case of Mary Ellen in New York leads to the founding of Society for the Prevention of Cruelty to Children	Tertiary care of violent injuries advances while treating wounds of war
Early 1900s	**1910:** Suffrage movement and "feminism" enters popular vocabulary. Suffragettes organized activities designed to generally help women by getting the right to vote, own property, and not be considered legal chattel of their husbands **1913:** Sanger initiates birth control movement **1929:** Wall Street Great Crash and the Great Depression begins World War II	**1918:** Jeannette Rankin is the first woman elected to Congress; she introduces the constitutional suffrage amendment **1920:** Women receive the right to vote	Tertiary care of violent injuries advances while treating wounds of war
1950s	**1952:** Publication of *The Second Sex* by Simone de Beauvoir Communism and the Cold War emphasis on fear of outside forces, not fear within the home		Tertiary care of violent injuries advances while treating wounds of war
1960s	**Vietnam War** challenged as an unjust, unwinable war. Other dogma challenged **1963:** Publication of *The Feminine Mystique* by Betty Friedan **Public Violence:** John F. Kennedy, Martin Luther King, Robert Kennedy assassinated, race riots and protests foster public apprehension about violence **1966:** 300 charter members form the National Organization of Women (NOW)	**1960:** John F. Kennedy forms the Commission on the Status of Women chaired by Eleanor Roosevelt **1964:** Civil Rights Act prohibits discrimination based on race and sex President's Commission on the Causes and Prevention of Violence	**1960s:** Tertiary care of violent injuries advances while treating wounds of war **1962:** Kempe publishes landmark research describing child abuse

(Continued)

Table 1.1 *(Continued)*		
	Major Social/Cultural Event	Major Legislation or Court Decision	Advances in Health Policy or Health Science
1970s	**1970s:** Victim support becomes an important component of political activism; the emergence of sociobiology as a field that seeks to explain cultural patterns as a product of biological causes; both sociology and psychology embrace learning theory as a means of explaining behavior **1971:** Chiswick Center, first shelter for battered women, opens in London **1974:** Errin Pizzey writes first book on domestic violence (DV) *Scream Quietly or the Neighbors Will Hear* **1975:** NOW created a task force to examine wife battering **1976:** First shelter for battered women opens in US **1977:** "MS" magazine cover story: "Battered Wives: Help for the Secret Victim Next Door"	**1970s:** Increased emphasis on victimization in criminal justice research and practice; family violence identified as an important problem confronting police **1973:** *Roe v. Wade* makes it unconstitutional for states to prohibit abortion in first trimester **1978:** US Commission on Civil Rights identifies the use of physical force in a family as a means of intimidation and coercion	**1976:** Dr. Ann Flitcraft, researches domestic violence (DV) as a cause of injuries of women in the emergency department **1977:** Ambulatory nursing program at Brigham & Women's Hospital in Boston develops first DV Response Protocol **1978-1986:** Flitcraft and Evan Stark conduct a series of studies in healthcare setting regarding prevalence of DV **1979:** Lenore Walker publishes first work describing the cyclical nature of IPV and introduces the concept of "Battered Woman Syndrome." **1979:** International Classification of Diseases version 9 introduces ICD Code 995.8_ to be used for Adult Maltreatment. Subcodes include physical, sexual, and psychological abuse.
1980s	**1980s:** HIV-AIDS epidemic begins "**Pro-life**" movement gains momentum; **feminists** grassroots' organizations define and provide a wide range of services for DV victims and build upon model developed for rape victims **1980:** Family Violence Prevention Fund is founded	**1980s:** Deterrence approaches emphasized with implementation of mandatory arrest and more aggressive prosecution **1982:** US Commission on Civil Rights publishes: "Under the Rule of Thumb: Battered Women and the Administration of Justice" National Domestic Violence Prevention and Treatment Act is passed **1984:** U.S. Attorney General's Task Force on Family Violence holds hearings across the country **1984:** *Thurman v. city of Torrington* – damages awarded to DV victim for law enforcement's failure to respond appropriately to DV call **1984:** Minneapolis study concludes mandatory arrest reduces DV recidivism **1989:** *Webster v. Reproductive Health Services*, Supreme Court ruling gives states expanded authority to limit abortion rights	**1980:** Federal Office of Domestic Violence publishes and distributes a DV protocol and monograph **1981:** Jacquelyn Campbell publishes study showing that a major risk factor for femicide is DV **1982:** Susan Schecter authors text on *Women and Male Violence* **1984:** *Domestic Violence: A Guide for Health Care Professionals* published in New Jersey **1984:** Walker publishes first information on posttraumatic stress disorder (PTSD) or battered woman syndrome **1985:** C. Everett Koop convenes Surgeon General's Workshop on Violence and Public Health **1985:** *Injury in America* published by the Institute of Medicine; it identified a lack of trained scholars, health professionals, and other professionals with expertise in injury control **1985:** Despite protest of feminist therapists, "self-defeating personality disorder" becomes a DSM diagnosis **1985:** Jacquelyn Campbell publishes Danger Assessment screen of factors associated with DV homicide **1985:** Nursing Network on Violence Against Women founded

Table 1.1 *(Continued)*		
Major Social/Cultural Event	Major Legislation or Court Decision	Advances in Health Policy or Health Science
		1986: CDC established the Division of Injury, Epidemiology and Control **1986:** "Womankind," the first formal hospital-based program in the country establishes in Minneapolis, and "AWAKE" identifies battered women of abused children at Children's Hospital in Boston **1987:** *Protocol of Care for the Battered Woman* published by the March of Dimes Birth Defect Foundation **1989:** The American College of Obstetricians and Gynecologists issues a technical bulletin on DV
1990s	**1990s:** Explosion in microprocessor technology; bull market economy; rise of Christian fundamentalism and declining support for nontraditional families Film "Defending our Lives" about women incarcerated for the homicide of their abusive husbands wins Academy Award for best documentary **1994:** Nicole Brown Simpson and Ron Goldman murdered, and football athelete/celebrity OJ Simpson charged and later acquitted of the murders	**1994:** Violent Crime Control and Law Enforcement Act includes VAWA I, which authorizes $120 million in grants to states for DV and directs the National Research Council to develop a research agenda on violence against women **1994:** National Research Council publishes Understanding Violence Against Women and the four-volume book *Understanding and Preventing Violence* **1996:** National Domestic Violence Hotline established and national public awareness campaign titled "No Excuse for Domestic Violence" is launched by the FVPF in conjunction with the Advertising Council Welfare Reform Act Victims of Crime Act	**1990:** New York becomes first state to require that all licensed hospitals establish protocols and training programs to identify and treat DV **1991:** American College of Obstetricians-Gynecologists develops and distributes informational packet on DV to their membership **1990:** "Violent and Abusive Behavior" included as one of the public health priorities in Healthy People 2000 **1991:** The American Nurses Association issues a Position Statement on Physical Violence Against Women **1992:** American Medical Association (AMA) Council on Ethical and Judicial Affairs declares that physicians have "duty" to be aware of societal myths about DV and to prevent these misconceptions from affecting diagnosis and management **1992:** AMA Diagnostic and Treatment Guidelines on Domestic Violence are released and *Journal of the American Medical Association* (JAMA) publishes entire volume dedicated to the issue of violence **1992:** The American Public Health Association issues a position paper on domestic violence **1992:** Joint Commission on Accreditation of Healthcare Organizations (JCAHO) issues standards for the identification and management of DV patients

(Continued)

	Table 1.1 *(Continued)*		
	Major Social/Cultural Event	Major Legislation or Court Decision	Advances in Health Policy or Health Science
			1993: The National Center for Injury Prevention and Control at the Centers for Disease Control (CDC) established the Family and Intimate Violence Prevention Team
			1993: *Injury Control in the 1990s: A National Plan for Action* is published by the CDC
			1994: VAWA I directs CDC to study DV
			1994: AMA President Robert McAfee decries DV "a major health problem"
			1995: The Association of American Medical Colleges strengthened the curriculum on family violence
			1995: A Physician's Guide to Domestic Violence by Salber and Talliafero published by Volcano Press
			1995: California becomes first state to mandate that hospitals and clinics have protocols to screen for DV
			1999: CDC publishes guidelines for research that defined and promotes the phrase "intimate partner violence" that is now dominant in the medical literature but still used interchangeably with domestic violence elsewhere
			1996: National Research Council publishes research agenda for violence against women
			1995: AMA issues statement that: "Physicians may be held liable for failure to recognize abuse and respond to the patient's complaint."
			1996: National Health Resource Center established
2000s	**September 11, 2001:** Terrorist attack in NYC kills over 3,000 people **2002:** U.S. goes to war in Afghanistan **2003:** U.S. goes to war in Iraq **Office of Homeland Security** established and the country adopts a fearful and suspicious attitude. Focus on collective violence related to both war and terrorism.	**2000:** *U.S. v. Morrison* decides that Congress exceeded its power when enacting VAWA and rejects arguments that violence against women impacted interstate commerce. **2000:** VAWA II reauthorized **2004:** *Crawford v. Washington* Supreme Court decision requires DV victim to appear in court so that the accused may confront the accuser **2006:** VAWA III reauthorized	**2000:** The WHO creates the Department for Injuries and Violence Prevention **2000:** National Health Objectives released 18 or 40 objectives related to injury concern violence **2000:** First National Conference on Health and Domestic Violence by FVPF **2001:** Institute of Medicine report "Confronting Chronic Neglect: The Education and Training of Health Professionals on Family Violence," is released

Table 1.1 *(Continued)*		
Major Social/Cultural Event	Major Legislation or Court Decision	Advances in Health Policy or Health Science
		2002: World Health Organization issues "World Report on Violence and Health," which recognizes violence as a global public health problem and declares it preventable
		2004: National Violent Death Reporting System initiated through National Violent Injury Statistics System
		2006: CDC launches "Choose Respect," a national communication initiative designed to prevent abuse in dating relationships
		2005: VAWA III is reauthorized and includes the Health Title, but funding is not appropriated for health-related activities
		2007: CDC publishes study that estimated cost of violence in U.S. to exceed $70 billion each year

Gelles RJ. *Intimate violence in families.* Thousand Oaks, CA: Sage Publications, 1997; Buzawa ES, Busaza CG. *Domestic violence: The criminal justice response.* Thousand Oaks, CA: Sage Publications, 1996; Hampton RL, Jenkins P, and Cullotta TP, eds. *Preventing violence in America.* Thousand Oaks, CA: Sage Publications, 1996; Schornstein SL. *Domestic violence and health care: What every professional needs to know.* Thousand Oaks, CA: Sage Publications, 1997; Reiss AJ, Roth JA, eds. National research council. *Understanding and preventing violence.* Washington DC: National Academy Press, 1993; and Crowell NA, Burgess AW, eds. National research council. *Understanding violence against women.* Washington DC: National Academy Press, 1996.

active community advocacy or a demanding constituency. All of these issues have played a part in influencing the emergence and evolution of IPV health policy over the last 20 years.

Community Advocacy Efforts

The victim advocacy and feminist activist movements collaborated to advance the issue of IPV both publicly and politically. The foundation of their success has rested on a shared passion, the ability to create grassroots services and supports for victims of abuse, to raise funds, and to focus the attention of public figures and legislators on this critical issue. Intimate partner violence has been effectively framed as a classless issue, thus allowing both politicians and corporations to support efforts to address the problem.

Feminist and community advocates relied upon empowerment theory, defined as a process through which individuals, communities, and organizations can gain increased control of issues and problems. The principle aim of the empowerment movement is to enable the less powerful to take proactive actions to prevent threats to their well-being and achieve a higher quality of life (6–9). Kar, in his meta-analysis of empowerment of women for health promotion, outlined seven methods of the EMPOWER framework that have been embraced by the IPV advocacy community: (a) *E*ducation, training, and leadership development; (b) *M*edia events, campaigns, and press releases; (c) *P*ublic awareness, education, and participation; (d) *O*rganizing partnerships, associations, and coalitions; (e) *W*ork/job training to promote economic self-reliance and employable skills; (f) *E*nabling services such as medical/legal/financial/psychological; and (g) Rights protection and social reform.

The advocacy movement successfully evolved as the field, as a whole, matured. As information about the health impact of IPV on children emerged, strategies were created to identify and address the needs of all the victims in an IPV home. In addition, men wanted to participate in the advocacy movement in a proactive, preventative way, so advocates across the country started to work with men as allies. For example, in 2000, the Family Violence Prevention Fund surveyed men about domestic violence and found that men supported antiviolence activities but had never been actively asked to contribute to them. In 2001, the Family Violence Prevention Fund launched a series of public services announcements that targeted men and boys as allies and in 2004 created a successful male-led national campaign that folded primary prevention, masculine development, and sports enrichment into one package. This program, "Coaching Boys into Men." reached out into communities to athletic coaches (and fathers) and provided guidelines and strategies for modeling, teaching, and reinforcing healthy interpersonal relationships in male youth. Since the initial survey, initiatives like Coaching Boys into Men and others across the country have helped foster the leap from just 29% of American men talking to kids about violence to 68% percent of men talking to their sons (and 63% of men talking to their daughters) about healthy, violence-free relationships and 55% of all men talking to boys who are not their sons (and 47% talking to girls who are not their daughters) about healthy nonviolent relationships (10).

Professional Health Organization Policy

Nearly every major healthcare organization recognizes violence and abuse as a health issue and has issued policy statements on the topic (11). The American Medical Association (AMA), through its National Advisory Council on Violence and Abuse, has developed detailed policy and educational materials that address domestic, family, and intimate partner violence in terms of physicians' overall training and practice. The AMA policy supports routine inquiry about patients' histories of family violence and states that physicians "have a major role in lessening the prevalence, scope, and severity of child maltreatment, intimate partner violence, and elder abuse,

all of which fall under the rubric of family violence." In November 2007, the AMA revised its policy regarding the identification of violence-exposed patients and initial intervention (see Sidebar 1.1).

The American Academy of Family Physicians (AAFP) has advised its members that "family physicians are in an ideal position to diagnose and treat victims of family violence and are compelled to do so by the sheer magnitude of the problem." In a position paper on adolescent health care, the AAFP also advises that open and confidential communication with adolescent patients, along with careful clinical assessment, can identify many cases of sexual abuse (www.aafp.org). The American College of Obstetricians and Gynecologists (www.acog.org) recommends universal screening of women patients for signs of abuse by using a few simple, direct questions and has provided extensive clinical guidelines and resources for clinicians. Policies of the American Academy of Nurse Practitioners (www.aanp.org) encourage its members to identify, treat, and properly refer all victims of partner abuse and sexual assault, and to advocate for the use of national guidelines to assess, identify, and refer victims of violence. The American College of Emergency Physicians (www.acep.org) views the identification of domestic violence victims as a specialized area in the evaluation of emergency patients and encourages hospitals to develop multidisciplinary approaches toward the identification, treatment, and referral of domestic violence patients who present in the emergency department. Other health professional organizations addressing IPV include the American Nurses Association, the American Psychological Association, the American Public Health Association, and the American Dental Association among many others.

Legislation and Funding for Health Initiatives

Health policy is also shaped by funding, research, and legislation at the federal and state levels. According to an Institute of Medicine (IOM) report, family violence rarely emerges as a federal funding priority according to the National Institutes of Health (NIH) (11). A 2001 search of the NIH Health Information index for family violence research by NIH-funded or -supported scientists revealed no entries for "family violence," "spouse abuse," "domestic violence," or "child abuse." There was a single entry for elder abuse

Sidebar 1.1: American Medical Association Policy E-2.02. Physicians' Obligations in Preventing, Identifying, and Treating Violence and Abuse (adopted November 2007)

Interpersonal violence and abuse were once thought to primarily affect specific high-risk patient populations, but it is now understood that all patients may be at risk. The complexity of the issues arising in this area requires three distinct sets of guidelines for physicians. The following guidelines address assessment, prevention, and reporting of interpersonal violence and abuse.

1. *When seeking to identify and diagnose past or current experiences with violence and abuse, physicians should adhere to the following guidelines:*

   A. Physicians should routinely inquire about physical, sexual, and psychological abuse as part of the medical history. Physicians should also consider abuse as a factor in the presentation of medical complaints, because patients' experiences with interpersonal violence or abuse may adversely affect their health status or ability to adhere to medical recommendations.

   B. Physicians should familiarize themselves with the detection of violence or abuse, the community and healthcare resources available to abused or vulnerable persons, and the legal requirements for reporting violence or abuse.

   C. Physicians should not be influenced in the diagnosis and management of abuse by such misconceptions as the beliefs that abuse is a rare occurrence, does not occur in "normal" families, is a private problem best resolved without outside interference, or is caused by the victims own actions.

2. *The following guidelines are intended to guide physicians' efforts to address acts of violence and abuse:*

   A. Physicians must treat the immediate symptoms and sequelae of violence and abuse, while also providing ongoing care for patients so as to address any long-term health consequences that may arise as the result of exposure.

   B. Physicians should be familiar with current information about cultural variations in response to abuse, public health measures that are effective in preventing violence and abuse, and how to work cooperatively with relevant community services. Physicians should help in developing educational resources for identifying and caring for victims. Comprehensive training in matters pertaining to violence and abuse should be required in medical school curricula and in postgraduate training programs.

   C. Physicians should also provide leadership in raising awareness regarding the need to assess and identify signs of abuse. By establishing guidelines and institutional policies, it may be possible to reduce the volume of abuse cases that go unidentified, and consequently, help to ensure that all patients receive the benefit of appropriate assessment regardless of their age, gender, ethnicity, or social circumstances. The establishment of appropriate mechanisms should also direct physicians to external community or private resources that might be available to aid patients.

   D. Physicians should support research in the prevention of violence and abuse and seek collaboration with relevant public health authorities and community organizations.

3. *Physicians should comply with the following guidelines when reporting evidence of violence or abuse:*

   A. Physicians should familiarize themselves with any relevant reporting requirements within the jurisdiction in which they practice.

   B. When a jurisdiction mandates reporting suspicion of violence and abuse, physicians should comply. However, physicians should only disclose minimal information, in order to safeguard patients' privacy. Moreover, if available evidence suggests that mandatory reporting requirements are not in the best interests of patients, physicians should advocate for changes in such laws.

   C. In jurisdictions where reporting suspected violence and abuse is not legally mandated, physicians should discuss the issue sensitively with the patient by first suggesting the possibility of abuse, followed by describing available safety mechanisms. Reporting when not required by law requires the informed consent of the patient. However, exceptions can be made if a physician reasonably believes that a patient's refusal to authorize reporting is coerced and therefore does not constitute a valid informed treatment decision.

that was linked to the National Institute on Aging. The Computer Retrieval of Information on Scientific Projects (CRISP) database revealed 63 projects with the phrase "spouse abuse" and 38 with the phrase "domestic violence." Funding for these projects is not disclosed. While the Centers for Disease Control have invested funds to research this issue as a public health concern, clearly more federal investments in research would inform policy and practice.

Beyond research and support for some pilot programs out of the U.S. Department of Health and Human Services on health and domestic violence, the Violence Against Women Act (VAWA) — specifically the VAWA Prevent (Title IV) and VAWA Health (Title V)—are among the first legislation to address a healthcare response or public health approach to violence at the federal level. VAWA was first passed in 1994 and most recently reauthorized in 2005. Funding for VAWA programs is administered through the U.S. Departments of Justice and Health and Human Services, with the majority of funds being distributed to states for law enforcement and some community-based services. Funding for health-related projects under VAWA was first included in the 2005 reauthorization of the legislation (P.L. 109–162). At this point, however, no VAWA funds have been appropriated for health-related research or health professional training.

The purpose of VAWA Health is to improve the healthcare system's responses to domestic and sexual violence by:

- Allocating resources to train health professionals to identify and respond to domestic and sexual violence victimization; in this case, funds would go to medical schools working in collaboration with other health professional schools, including schools of nursing, public health, and dentistry. These funds may be used to offer specialized training for rural areas and to provide stipends to students underrepresented in the health professions
- Providing grants to foster public health response to domestic and sexual violence, which is intended to promote collaboration at the state and local level between HCPs, public health departments, and domestic and sexual violence programs
- Funding research to identify effective interventions in the healthcare settings that prevent and

address domestic and sexual violence, including the impact health interventions have on the health outcomes of patient exposed to abuse

The goal of VAWA Prevent is to break the often intergenerational cycle of violence by focusing on effective prevention programs targeting children who have been exposed to violence, young families at risk for violence, and men and boys. This would be accomplished by:

- Providing grants to assist children and youth exposed to violence
- Enhancing training for home visitation programs, which work with pregnant women and new parents in their homes, on how to recognize and address domestic and sexual violence and link women and children experiencing violence with community resources that can help them be safe; home visitation programs have been shown to successfully reduce child abuse but often are not as successful in homes where domestic violence already exists
- Offering a competitive grant program to engage men and youth in the prevention of domestic and sexual violence. Funds would go toward programs that help young people develop mutually respectful and nonviolent relationships, and engage men as allies and role models for younger men through public education and community-based programs.
- Directing the Centers for Disease Control Prevention to study best practices for reducing and preventing violence against women and children and to evaluate the effectiveness of interventions
- Making grants to states to carry out a campaign to increase public awareness of issues regarding domestic violence and pregnancy

Although both the VAWA Health and VAWA Prevent titles have been authorized, no funds have been appropriated to date. Some sections addressing children exposed to abuse and engaging men and boys each received funding in 2006 but as of 2008 no funds had been distributed due to budget delays in Congress during 2007. The IOM report concluded that until funding is proportionate to the magnitude of the problem, progress in addressing family violence as a health issue is likely to be limited (11).

Considerable legislation has also been enacted at the state level to tighten criminal justice responses, allocate resources for victim services and training, and improve surveillance and community coordination efforts. A number of states have enacted policies to improve healthcare responses to violence, as discussed later. In addition, many states also have reporting requirements for healthcare providers who treat victims of violence. These requirements range from general reporting requirements for any crimes involving weapons to requirements specific to IPV-related injuries. These reporting mandates engender controversy (see discussion below).

CORE COMPONENTS OF INTIMATE PARTNER VIOLENCE HEALTH POLICY

The Family Violence Prevention Fund (FVPF) has suggested six core components for consideration in developing a comprehensive health policy to address violence and abuse at the state level. In 2001, The FVPF created a state-by-state report card on health policy responses to IPV that provides details about actual legislative language. (The report card is available at the Family Violence Prevention Fund 's website: http://www.endabuse.org/statereport/list.php3.)

Core Component: Education for Health Care Professionals

Health policy advocates should support health departments, professional associations, or others responsible for educating healthcare professionals to develop training on IPV that includes information regarding prevalence, the dynamics of domestic violence, the health effects, routine inquiry, assessment, intervention, documentation, coding procedures, and reporting requirements. Training programs that include administrators should also include education on how to set up health systems to best respond to victims, such as training on ensuring health records confidentiality, model protocols for addressing domestic violence, policies to ensure ongoing training for providers, and strategies to provide referrals to culturally appropriate community resources for victims, abusers, and their children. The curriculum can stand alone or could be integrated into education

about the impact of IPV on specific health areas or issues, including HIV/AIDS, reproductive and prenatal care, mental health, and substance abuse. California legislateda training center to develop and implement standardized training regarding the care of victims of violence and published state guidelines (12). Some states, such as Florida, require that providers individually seek out continuing education on IPV on a periodic basis, although no universal support exists for such mandates (11).

Core Component: Protocols and Policies That Support Health Care Assessments for Intimate Partner Violence

Clinical protocols and regulations provide guidelines for patient care, increase patient safety, and direct quality improvement programs. Some states, such as California, have required that health clinics and hospitals have policies and procedures in place that require providers to routinely assess for IPV. Ideally, any policy should include a body that is responsible for periodically monitoring compliance with the IPV protocol, including monitoring the implementation of screening guidelines at healthcare facilities, the frequency with which patients are screened, the effects and impact screening has on identification of persons who are victims of domestic violence, services rendered to such persons by HCPs, and any other relevant information.

Core Component: Insurance Discrimination Against Victims of Domestic Violence

In 1994, domestic violence advocates learned that insurance companies throughout the United States discriminated against victims of domestic violence by using domestic violence as a basis for determining whether to issue insurance, how much to charge for it, and whether to pay a claim. This discrimination puts victims at risk, not only by denying them the benefits that insurance provides, but also by discouraging them from seeking protection. Using records of help-seeking activities, such as medical records and public legal records, insurers are able to learn about the history of domestic violence. Insurers are not required by law to tell applicants the reasons for rejection or other adverse actions, so victims may not know that domestic violence is a consideration. In response to voluntary surveys, approximately 50% of responding health, life, and disability insurers acknowledged considering domestic violence when determining whether to issue insurance policies. State legislation is necessary to prohibit insurers from using domestic violence as a basis for underwriting or refusing to insure someone or charging a higher premium due to domestic violence (known as "rating"). Most states have implemented these policies.

Core Component: Funding/Grants to Address Domestic Violence in the Healthcare Setting

Policies that provide general budget funding, grants, and resources to strengthen state and local health response to domestic violence can build the capacity of health professionals and staff to identify, address, document, and prevent domestic violence. These grants can promote local programs that improve response in hospitals, clinics, managed-care settings, and in public health using strategies such as:

- Developing, adapting, implementing, and disseminating clinical practice guidelines
- Providing training and follow-up technical assistance to healthcare professionals and staff to assess for domestic violence, and then to appropriately treat and refer patients who are victims of domestic violence to domestic violence services
- Developing and implementing policies, protocols, and strategies to ensure that the health and personal information of a patient who identifies or is identified as a victim of abuse is collected and held in a manner that protects the patient's privacy and safety
- Developing on-site access to services to address the safety, medical, mental health, and economic needs of patients by increasing the capacity of existing healthcare professionals, developing a specialized consulting service, or contracting with community service agencies

Pennsylvania is probably the best example of the success of this type of funding; through legislation, it has established a statewide medical advocacy project. Pennsylvania's HB 2268, originally passed in 1998, established the Domestic Violence Health Care Response Act. This act prescribes how certain "medical advocacy project sites" will be chosen and details how each will provide comprehensive training, universal screening, and domestic violence educational materials. Pennsylvania's governor Tom Ridge announced in February 2001 that an additional $1,000,000 would be allocated for medical advocacy projects in fiscal year 2001/2002. These medical advocacy projects are collaborative efforts, linking programs and healthcare systems, that include assessment for and identification of domestic violence victims seeking medical treatment and the provision of support, information, resources, and follow-up services within the healthcare setting. The Act also includes the development and implementation of policies and procedures to enhance the healthcare response to victims of domestic violence, and to provide for the ongoing training of healthcare personnel. Nineteen new projects were funded, bringing the number of medical advocacy projects to 36; these projects provide services to victims in 85 Pennsylvania healthcare systems.

Core Component: Intimate Partner Violence Prevention

A growing body of clinical experience and research evidence suggests that child abuse, domestic violence, and youth violence often occur in the same families, with devastating effects on children, families, and communities. Abuse and violence are highly associated with social and economic factors that put families at further risk of exposure to and perpetration of violence. Despite these connections, programs usually offer interventions that address only one form of violence or abuse, thus fragmenting responses to families. In addition, service-based responses to families that compartmentalize problems and offer single-issue interventions generally fail to include measures to prevent future violence or abuse. The time is ripe for strong collaborative prevention and early intervention activities that bridge the fields of child abuse, domestic violence, and youth violence and that focus on changing social norms that accept violence in our society.

A new public health approach must integrate creative prevention approaches and large-scale public education campaigns that begin to change cultural attitudes and norms. Policies should be considered to plan, coordinate, evaluate, and fund integrated, collaborative, and comprehensive public health and public safety approaches to violence prevention. Activities might include:

- Developing a statewide plan and coordinating statewide violence prevention efforts that incorporate public health and public safety approaches to address the interrelated problems of child abuse, domestic violence, youth violence, and community violence
- Launching large-scale multimedia public education campaigns that address violence prevention including domestic violence, sexual assault, youth violence, and child abuse
- Initiating programs that provide early support to young families, such as parenting support programs, early childhood intervention programs, and home visitation services to at risk families
- Creating supports, services, and prevention campaigns targeted at young men, which challenge the acceptability of violence and engage men as allies in prevention
- Providing support and services to children exposed to violence
- Promoting public education programs and wellness programs by community health centers and other community-based health projects
- Sponsoring community-based youth violence prevention programs, such as mentoring programs, after-school programs, and job training or development
- Integrating violence prevention initiatives into alcohol and substance abuse, HIV, unintended and teen pregnancy, sexually transmitted infection (STI) prevention efforts
- Providing technical assistance and training to help build the capacity of communities, organizations, and systems to develop, implement, and evaluate violence prevention programs.

The Illinois Violence Prevention Act of 1995 (P.A. 89–353, eff. 8–17–95) achieved some of this work at a state level, generating funds for its program from the sale of specially designed "Prevent Violence" license plates. Over $3.5 million in revenue was generated in the first year, with over 70,000 Illinois motorists having purchased the license plates. The Illinois Act also created a nongovernmental Commission/Authority that was both the policy making and administering agency.

Core Component: Domestic Violence Data Collection, Surveillance, and Research

Data collection and evaluation must also be a part of any major public health and prevention strategy.

States should support efforts to collect data, increase surveillance activity, and conduct research on domestic violence and health issues. States can also add domestic violence into existing data collection, planning, and research efforts. For instance, having a pregnancy question on death certificates can help identify violence-related deaths that remain difficult to detect because of data linkage problems. Domestic violence fatality review teams can review female homicides and suicides for evidence of domestic violence and perform safety audits looking for missed opportunities to prevent IPV-associated fatalities.

Other options to consider are adding questions relating to IPV to current federal and state healthcare data collection and surveillance activities, such as the Behavior Risk Factor Surveillance System (BRFSS); the Youth Risk Behavior Survey; Centers for Disease Control (CDC)-funded state Injury Prevention Research; the Pregnancy Risk Assessment and Monitoring Systems (PRAMS); current data collection mechanisms in state health benefit programs, such as healthy mother/health baby screening tools, prenatal screening, family planning, and HIV/STI screening; healthcare system provider and patient surveys; emergency department surveillance; state department of health comprehensive planning efforts, such as agency strategic plans and state public health plans; and Healthy People 2020 planning efforts. Policies can support county-level data collection efforts and encourage local programs to network with community domestic violence providers to collect and cross-reference data collection efforts.

Controversies and Concerns About Health Care Responses to Domestic Violence

As discussed above, some states have laws that require healthcare providers to report IPV, which has caused some controversy, primarily revolving around two questions:

- Are some victims of domestic violence under such coercion and in such danger that all victims should be regarded as members of a "vulnerable population," therefore triggering a reporting/responding chain of events to mobilize all possible resources to assist in their safety?
- Unless incapable of medical decision making, aren't domestic violence victims able to act autonomously in regard to healthcare decisions about their self-care and, therefore, shouldn't they be

the best judges for deciding among the options that address their health and safety needs?

Given the lack of evidence in the field that such laws do indeed improve the safety of IPV patients (due to inconsistent criminal justice responses and possible negative impact on help-seeking behaviors of women not ready to involve the police), many call for an immediate moratorium until further evidence of safety is provided. In an ironic twist, mandating health professional behavior may have actually improved health services, but it is a structure built on sand if the underlying premise of mandatory reporting—that it is a mechanism for providing safety—is indeed false (13). For a summary of state reporting laws, see the Family Violence Prevention Fund's website at www.endabuse.org; for more discussion, see the chapter on legal and forensic issues in this book.

Finally, although many advocacy organizations have developed strong partnerships with healthcare providers (HCPs), others have expressed reservations about the ability of the healthcare system to meet victims' needs. Their concerns include (a) the potential for the system to blame the victim and further traumatize the patient; (b) "medicalization" of the problem, so that the identified patient now bears the burden of a stigmatizing diagnosis; (c) a disease-model approach that treats the victim without accounting for the perpetrator as the vector of injury or illness; and (d) reductionist approaches to health research that fail to appreciate the influence of societal norms and systems. As health policy on IPV evolves, these concerns need to be continually reviewed and addressed.

FRAMEWORKS FOR ADVANCING HEALTH POLICY ON INTIMATE PARTNER VIOLENCE

The WHO has published recommendations for advancing health policy regarding violence in general that can also be applied to IPV (14) (Table 1.2). The WHO encourages policy makers to address interpersonal violence as a whole, rather than focusing on subtypes such as IPV, in light of evidence increasingly linking different subtypes with a set of common causes and cross-cutting risk factors. The WHO also advocates use of an ecological model for understanding the causes and consequences of interpersonal violence. Evidence increasingly shows that no single

Table 1.2: World Health Organization Recommendations Regarding Heath Policy to Prevent Violence
1. Create, implement, and monitor a national action plan.
2. Enhance capacity for collecting data on violence and abuse.
3. Define priorities for and produce research on causes, consequences, costs, and prevention of violence.
4. Promote primary prevention responses.
5. Strengthen responses for victims of violence.
6. Integrate violence prevention into social and educational policies and thereby promote gender and social equality.
7. Increase collaboration and exchange of information on violence prevention.
8. Promote and monitor adherence to international treaties, laws, and other mechanisms to protect human rights.
9. Seek practical and internationally agreed upon responses to the global drug trade and the global arms trade.

Source: World Health Organization, 2004.

factor can explain why some people are at higher risk for interpersonal violence while others are protected from it; clearly, there exists an interaction of factors at individual, relationship, community, and societal levels. The WHO advocates a public health approach to violence based on the findings of numerous empirical reviews on strategies to reduce crime and interpersonal violence. The conclusions were convergent in that interpersonal violence can be significantly reduced through "well-planned and multi-sectoral strategies that tackle multiple causes using frameworks such as the public health approach." This same research also concludes that policing and correctional approaches are expensive and that increasing expenditures will result in minimal returns.

Based upon the Core Functions of Public Health as defined by the CDC in 1993 (15,16), the following recommendations are made to further improve health policy in IPV:

- *Monitor health status.* Improve current health surveillance procedures to include an improved OSHPD database and regular administration of the Women's Health Survey.
- *Diagnose and investigate health problems.* Test the effectiveness of programs, interventions, and services. The National Research Council specified that attention should focus on (a) identification,

(b) health services, and (c) home visitation services for families at risk (17). Federal funding for health programs and education has been included for the first time in the Violence Against Women Act (III) signed by the President George W. Bush in December 2005, but the health education and research centers in VAWA III did not receive a fiscal appropriation by Congress.

- *Inform, educate, and empower people about health issues.* Early parent education and maternal and child welfare screening practices could constitute a major prevention effort. Education programs within the Women, Infant, and Child (WIC) program, family planning, and other programs directed at young families should be expanded. Preventive interventions targeting males, such as school-based programs like Safe Dates and public awareness campaigns like Coaching Boys into Men can be expanded.
- *Mobilize community partnerships to identify and solve health problems.* Expand community intervention services, as recent research shows victims who receive advocacy intervention after a shelter stay experienced less physical abuse, increased quality of life, and utilized more community resources compared to the control group (18). Research has shown that using the telephone to counsel victims of IPV has resulted in the increased adoption of safety behaviors that remained even 2 years after counseling ended (19).
- *Assure a competent public health and healthcare workforce.* One of Turncock's recommendations for improved public health law is to create uniform structures for similar programs and services (20). It is time to "decompartmentalize" interventions and "de-siloize" violence issues that have been divided according to victim gender and/or age. Grouping efforts to prevent violence into a single agency may increase efficiency and decrease costs, but will also foster a cross-fertilization of knowledge, skills, and sensitivities that could lead to a more comprehensive approach to care and prevention.
- *Evaluate effectiveness, accessibility, and quality of health services.* In light of the new findings from the U.S. Preventative Services Task Force (21) indicating insufficient evidence for or against screens for IPV, it is time to evaluate health law regarding IPV screening (i.e., California) and assess its potential harms and benefits. More importantly, the potential for harm appears even greater in regard to mandatory reporting. Mandating health providers to report IPV victims to law enforcement was enacted without evidence for its helpfulness. Without such evidence it is difficult to continue to justify the violation of patient confidentiality that compliance with the law requires of healthcare providers.
- *Link people to needed health services.* Many IPV victims consider their health provider to be a preferred resource for IPV care, so providing financial incentives to hospitals and other health systems willing to add on-site services for patients may be helpful. A source for these funds might be from increased marriage license fees, as allowed in recent legislation in several states.
- *Enforce laws and regulations that protect health and safety.* Interventions for batterers have been mostly disappointing in reducing recidivism of convicted offenders (22–25). Criminal justice efforts should focus on perpetrator assessment in an attempt to match intervention to offender characteristics. IPV gun violence must be addressed. One suggestion is to act quickly and aggressively to remove firearms from homes where IPV has occurred and to increase barriers to access to firearms.

The CDC is the lead agency in regards to injury and violence prevention, with an overall goal of reducing injuries, disabilities, and deaths due to unintentional injuries and violence. Of 45 objectives that addressed injury prevention in the Healthy People 2000 initiative, 19 were specific for violence prevention. Healthy People 2010 has as one targeted objective in regards to IPV, and that is to reduce physical assaults by an intimate partner from 4.4 (1998 baseline) to 3.3 physical assaults per 1,000 persons aged 12 years and older (26). As we move into developing goals for healthy people 2020, it is important to include objectives that also measure the impact of healthcare interventions on health status as well as reduction of number of assaults in IPV victims.

CAN SUCCESSFUL STRATEGIES IN REDUCING TOBACCO USE BE APPLIED TO VIOLENCE?

The issues of tobacco use and violence share certain characteristics: both are behavior-based health problems; a widespread desire exists to reduce the prevalence of violence and the use of tobacco; and both issues have generated complex advocacy, scientific, and social structures to address each problem.

However, according to Biglan and Taylor, although a generalized reduction in tobacco use has occurred, minimal progress has been made in reducing rates of violence crime (27).

Unlike the clear evidence for the benefits of tobacco use reduction programs, less agreement exists in the scientific community about the factors contributing to violence and the best strategies to use for prevention and intervention. Although opinion polls have consistently shown violent crime to be among the greatest concerns of Americans, the means of addressing violence are slow to change; historically, the major cultural practice for addressing violence has been punishment. The challenge now is to take the behavioral science–based literature regarding at-risk populations for violence, protective factors, and interventions to reduce risk of perpetration or victimization and translate these into program development and funding priorities.

Although numerous programs are funded by governmental and private monies to combat violent crime, many fewer are funded to address violence as a public health and healthcare problem. To see a real shift in prevention of IPV, on a scale approaching that of tobacco use prevention, health policy will need to promote (a) an investment in research on prevalence and healthcare responses to IPV and (b) strong collaborations among advocacy groups, professional health associations, and federal agencies to model clinical and community-based responses to IPV.

CONCLUSION

Intimate partner violence is a stigmatized health issue, much like alcoholism or drug addiction, and thus is hidden, underrecognized, and under-reported as a major public health issue. Intimate partner violence erodes the health of patients, consumes healthcare dollars, and compromises the present and future health and safety of children and communities. U.S. health policy has changed over time in regards to enacting new statutes and health policies that support women's health in general and IPV in particular. These policies have improved identification, documentation, surveillance; law enforcement responses; community prevention efforts; and funding of services for victims of violence. However, policy to advance a public health and healthcare approach to IPV is rare. No single

health policy change will dramatically decrease the incidence of IPV or improve the health system's ability to respond to victims. A public health approach and a national health policy, similar to those applied to tobacco smoking or motor vehicle accidents, can be expected to have an effect in reducing domestic violence (28).

IMPLICATIONS FOR POLICY, PRACTICE, AND RESEARCH

Policy

- To try to meet national health objectives such as Healthy People 2010 in regards to reducing physical assaults by intimate partners, a call to action at the NIH, CDC, national and state public health department levels will be required to gain the commitment of the public health workforce and to mobilize the range of public health activities that will be necessary (29).
- The WHO recommends a national strategy and action plan to reduce interpersonal violence with goals to:
  - Increase the capacity for collecting data on violence
  - Expand research on violence, its causes, consequences, and prevention
  - Promote the primary prevention of violence
  - Promote gender and social equality and equity to prevent violence
  - Strengthen care and support services for victims

Practice

- The most pressing need is for the development of health policy and practices that support health professionals and their efforts to address the health and safety needs of patients exposed to violence and abuse (30).
- Health professionals should obtain education and training to acquire skill proficiency in the identification, intervention, and prevention of violence.
- Health professionals should accurately diagnose and document violence-related illness and injury to aid public health surveillance that in turn influences health policy and resource allocation.

- Health professionals should advocate for policy change that addresses the health and safety needs of patients exposed to violence and abuse.

Research

- Encourage outcome evaluations of health policy and practice efforts to reduce interpersonal violence through funding and oversight.
- Provide the resources necessary to answer the question of whether health professional reporting mandates contribute or compromise patient safety.
- Foster international conferences and communication to compare and learn from the varying national strategies used to reduce interpersonal violence implemented around the world.
- The approach to IPV interventions has been relatively inflexible, particularly in regard to the response within the criminal justice system. A small body of literature has emerged, however, and this research should be expanded to examine more flexible, victim-centered interventions (31).

References

1. World Health Organization. *World report on violence and health.* Geneva: Author, 2002.
2. Tjaden P, Thoennes N. *Full report of the prevalence, incidence, and consequences of violence against women: Findings from the National Violence Against Women Survey.* Washington DC: National Institute of Justice Centers for Disease Control and Prevention (NIJCDC), 2000.
3. Centers for Disease Control and Prevention. Adverse health conditions and health risk behaviors associated with intimate partner violence. *MMWR.* February 8, 2008;57(05):113–117.
4. Ptacek J. *Battered women in the courtroom: The power of judicial responses.* Boston: Northeastern University Press, 1999.
5. Koop C. Foreword. In: Rosenberg M, ed. *Violence in America: A public health approach.* New York: Oxford University Press, 1991.
6. Freire P. *Education for critical consciousness.* New York: Seabury Press, 1973.
7. Zimmerman M, Israel B, Checkoway B. Further explorations in empowerment theory: An empirical analysis of psychological empowerment. *Am J Comm Psychol.* 1992;20(6):707–727.
8. Rapport J. Terms of empowerment/exemplars of prevention: Toward a theory for community psychology. *Am J Comm Psychol.* 1987;15:121–148.
9. Kar S. Empowerment of women in health promotion: a meta-analysis. *Soc Sci Med.* 1999;49(11):1431–1460.
10. Peter D. Hart Research Associates on behalf of the Family Violence Prevention Fund and Verizon Wireless. Father's day poll on fathers and family dialogs about healthy non-violent relationships, 2007.
11. Cohn F, Salmon ME, Stobo JD, eds. *Institute of Medicine report. Confronting chronic neglect: The education and training of health professionals on family violence.* Washington DC: National Academy Press, 2002.
12. Mitchell C. *Guidelines for the health care of intimate partner violence: For California health professionals.* Sacramento: California Office of Emergency Services, 2004.
13. Campbell JC, Coben JH, McLoughlin E, et al. An evaluation of a system-change training model to improve emergency department response to battered women. *Acad Emerg Med.* 2001;8(2):131–138.
14. World Health Organization. *Preventing violence: A guide to implementing the recommendations of the World Report on Violence and Health.* Geneva: Author, 2004.
15. Roper W, Baker E, Dyal W, Nicola R. Strengthening the public health system. *Pub Health Rep.* 1993;107(6):609–615.
16. Health Security Act, Title III—Public Health Initiatives. HR3600, 1993.
17. Chalk RKP. *Violence in families: Assessing prevention and treatment programs,* 1st ed. Washington DC: National Academy Press, 1998.
18. Sullivan CM, Bybee DI. Reducing violence using community-based advocacy for women with abusive partners. *J Consult Clin Psychol.* 1999;67(1):43–53.
19. McFarlane J, Malecha A, Gist J, et al. Increasing the safety-promoting behaviors of abused women. *Am J Nurs.* 2004;104(3):40–50; quiz 50–41.
20. Turnock B. *Public health: What it is and how it works,* 3rd ed. Sudbury, MA: Jones & Bartlett, 2004.
21. United States Preventive Services Task Force. Screening for family and intimae partner violence. *Ann Intern Med.* 2004;140(5):382–386.
22. Babcock J, La Taillade J. Evaluating interventions for men who batter. In: Vincent J, Jouriles E, eds. *Domestic violence: Guidelines for research-informed practice.* London: Jessica Kingsley Publishers, 2000:37–77.
23. Gondolf EW. A comparison of four batterer intervention systems: Do court referral, program length, and services matter? *J Interpers Violence.* January 1999;14(1):41–61.
24. Jackson S, Feder L, Forde DR, et al. *Batterer intervention programs: Where do we go from here?* Washington, DC: US Department of Justice, Office of Justice Programs; June 2003. NCJ195079.

25. Arias I, Dankwort J, Douglas U, et al. Violence against women: The state of batterer prevention programs. *J Law Med Ethics*. 2002;30(3 Suppl): 157–165.

26. Healthy People 2010. htp://www.healthypeople.gov. Accessed 1/15/08.

27. Biglan A, Taylor TK. Why have we been more successful in reducing tobacco use than violent crime? *Am J Comm Psychol*. 2000;28(3):269.

28. Saltzman L, Green YT, Marks JS, Thacker SB. Violence against women as a public health issue: Comments from the CDC. *Am J Prevent Med*. 2000;19(4):325–329.

29. Mitchell C. Shaping California's health policy for victims of intimate partner violence. *Harvard Public Policy Review*. October 2001.

30. Plichta S. Interactions between victims of intimate partner violence against women and the health care system: Policy and practice implications. *Trauma Violence Abuse*. 2007;8(2):226–239.

31. Goodman LA, Epstein D. Refocusing on women: A new direction for policy and research on intimate partner violence. *J Interpers Violence*. 2005;20(4): 479–487.

Chapter 2

Defining Intimate Partner Violence: Controversies and Implications

Christina Nicolaidis and Anuradha Paranjape

KEY CONCEPTS

- There are many different conceptualizations—and thus definitions—of intimate partner violence (IPV).
- These various conceptualizations are at times contradictory and may generate controversy.
- Controversial aspects of the definition of IPV include:
  - Who is considered to be an "intimate partner";
  - What types of actions constitute physical or sexual violence;
  - Whether or not emotional abuse or threats of violence constitute IPV;
  - The importance of power and control; and
  - The necessity of understanding the patterns, antecedents, and consequences of violent acts.
- Differences in the conceptualization of IPV may result from differences in which populations are sampled, how data are collected, and what aspects of violence are measured. All these factors play into important ongoing debates such as the existence of gender-symmetry in IPV.
- Simplistic conceptualizations may not be adequate to understand the complex phenomenon of IPV.

TERMINOLOGY

Before addressing the important controversies in the definition of intimate partner violence (IPV), it is worthwhile to comment on the terminology used. The feminist movement of the 1970s brought a new awareness of violence against women, and terms such as "wife battering" and "spouse abuse" were adopted to label a phenomenon that had previously been largely ignored by science, the criminal justice system, and the public health system. As it became evident that violence against women was not limited to married couples, these terms were replaced by the more generic

19

"domestic violence"; a term that is still in wide use today, especially by the lay public and advocacy communities. In 1999, over two decades after the issue was put on the map, the Centers for Disease Control and Prevention (CDC) suggested the use of the term "intimate partner violence"(1), in an attempt to describe the problem more accurately and to differentiate it from other forms of family violence that can occur in a domestic setting (e.g., child maltreatment and elder abuse). In keeping with this recommendation, this textbook primarily uses the term *intimate partner violence* (IPV), although may still at times refer to *domestic violence* (DV) especially when discussing DV services or the DV advocacy community.

This chapter first describes the different perspectives that influence the definition of IPV. The controversies in defining IPV are then addressed, followed by a discussion of ways in which to reconcile these differences. The chapter ends with a brief outline of the practical implications of the different definitions of IPV.

PERSPECTIVES INFLUENCING INTIMATE PARTNER VIOLENCE DEFINITIONS

How one defines IPV determines how one measures it, which in turn affects what conclusions can be drawn about the prevalence, patterns, gender differences, and health consequences of IPV. These findings can affect clinical decisions regarding how to counsel IPV victims and perpetrators, as well as policy decisions regarding legislation and funding. It may be naïve, however, to think that one starts by creating a definition of IPV de novo. Instead, the definition of IPV is largely driven by one's own conceptualization of the problem, which, in turn, is dependent on one's background, training, experience, research methodology, and political agenda. Multiple conceptualizations of IPV exist, and there are just as many ways that one can define IPV. A brief overview of the various perspectives is presented here (Table 2.1).

Advocates and researchers learning from the experiences of women in domestic violence shelters have

Table 2.1 Perspectives Influencing Intimate Partner Violence (IPV) Definitions

	Population Most Commonly Studied	Common Conceptualizations of IPV	Common Data Collection Instruments/Approaches
"Family violence" researchers	Male and female college students (and some general populations)	Violence as a response to intermittent conflict	Conflict tactics scale
Grassroots domestic violence movement and "feminist" researchers	Women seeking domestic violence services; men in batterer intervention programs	Violence is part of a pattern of coercive behaviors meant to establish power and control	Qualitative interviews; Index of Spouse Abuse, Women's Experience of Battering, Psychological Maltreatment of Women Inventory, Severity of Violence Against Women Survey
Legal system	Crime victims and perpetrators	Violence as a criminal act	National Incident Based Reporting System, Uniform Crime Reporting Program
Public health system	General populations	Violence victimization as a risk factor for morbidity and mortality	Public health surveillance systems
Healthcare delivery system	Patients seeking health care	Need to "screen" for IPV and refer for services; IPV as a cause for presenting symptoms or as barrier to care; trauma as pathologic condition	Abuse Assessment Screen, 3–4 item assessment instruments (HITS, WAST, PVS, STaT), clinical interviews

come to understand and define IPV as an ongoing pattern of behaviors in which a batterer uses violence as only one of many means to exert power and control over an intimate partner (2–5). Although these advocates and researchers recognize the existence of violence in same-sex relationships (as well as male victims and female batterers), and appreciate the great variation in women's individual experiences, the archetypal picture of IPV that emerges from this perspective is that of a controlling, jealous man progressively taking away his female partner's self-esteem, independence, resources, social support network, sense of safety, and health (6,7). Given this conceptualization and their desire to help abused women recognize what is happening before the violence escalates to even more dangerous levels, many advocates have argued for a broad definition of IPV that includes both severe and mild instances of physical or sexual assaults, as well as subtle forms of emotional abuse that add to the batterer's ability to control his partner (8). However, because the emphasis is placed on the power dynamics in the relationship, the intent of the violence, and the consequences to the victim, minor forms of violence perpetrated in isolation (the classic example being a woman slapping a man in response to a rude comment) would not be considered to constitute IPV. Of note, much of the work coming from this perspective has been attributed to "feminist researchers." Although many of these researchers welcome the label, it may give the impression that this perspective is based on politics whereas other approaches are based on law or science. We use this label acknowledging that all perspectives, not just the feminist one, are influenced by political agendas.

The second commonly used framework—that of "family conflict researchers"—stems from the work of Murray Straus and colleagues. Using the Conflict Tactics Scale (9–11) to survey college students or general populations, they have come to see a very different picture of IPV, in which violence is a response to intermittent conflicts and is perpetrated by both men and women at similar rates (12). Here, the focus is on specific behaviors perpetrated by either partner. Unlike the feminist perspective, relationship dynamics, antecedents to violence, intent, and consequences are purposely not included in this definition of IPV. Similarly nonviolent tactics used to gain power and control are not measured. In contrast, the "harmless slap" is included in their definition of IPV, the argument being that such acts are morally reprehensible and not really harmless at all (13).

Many other professionals have developed their own conceptualizations of IPV, and then have defined, measured, or treated it based on which aspects of IPV are most relevant to their work. To a prosecutor or criminologist, the most important aspect of IPV might be whether an assault, either simple or aggravated, as defined by the local penal code, was committed in the process (14). As noncriminal abusive behavior may be less important to the prosecution, and as such behaviors are also often more difficult to prove in an objective manner, information about emotional abuse or controlling behaviors are not consistently elicited in police reports, crime reporting systems, or national crime surveys, and these behaviors play less of a role in the legal system's conceptualization and definition of IPV. Local penal codes vary by state and, although there may be some elements of the legal definition of IPV that are common to all states, a heterogeneity exists in what is considered criminal behavior and therefore measurable as IPV (14).

Public health researchers approach IPV using a surveillance framework, in which the goal is to quantify, monitor, and reduce risk factors that negatively affect the health of populations (1,15). They may ask about noncriminal behaviors, such as emotional abuse, if there is reason to believe that such behaviors affect the risk or health consequences of IPV. However, public health surveys (and therefore, IPV definitions) may focus more on victimization and its health consequences, and less on the complexities that exist within individual intimate relationships. From a public health perspective, surveillance has a positive and scientific connotation. To an IPV survivor or advocate, however, the term "surveillance" may have negative connotations related to a batterer's behavior. Although much is to be gained from applying a public health model to IPV research, treatment, and prevention, bridging such perspectives may not come naturally (16).

Although a large literature about IPV in the healthcare setting exists, there is no consensus as to how to conceptualize, define, and measure IPV in health care. On the one hand, most training programs for healthcare providers conceptualize IPV in a manner similar to that of so-called "feminist researchers," in which IPV is seen as a pattern of coercive behaviors meant to gain power and control over an intimate (8,17,18). On the other hand, most screening instruments used in healthcare settings ask only a small number of simple items about the types of violence a woman has experienced, with little to no emphasis on whether a pattern of coercive behaviors exists (19–22). Such instruments may be useful in terms of assessing the prevalence of IPV in health-seeking populations or referring women for more in-depth assessments. However, in clinical practice, healthcare professionals still need to make a diagnosis of whether a patient is experiencing IPV and how that experience may be affecting the patient's health. It is still unclear what the clinical diagnostic criteria should be for IPV. Does a patient who has experienced a single episode of physical violence from a partner meet such criteria if there has been no pattern of controlling behavior or emotional abuse? How about a patient who is experiencing severe emotional abuse, threats, and control, with resultant symptoms of a stress response, but no physical or sexual abuse? Further work is needed to establish the diagnostic criteria and assessment instruments that help make a diagnosis. Even less is known about IPV perpetration in health-seeking populations or issues of gender symmetry.

Within health care, different specialties may approach IPV with different conceptualizations. For example, to a mental health professional, the details of the abusive relationship may be of less interest than knowing whether the patient has experienced a trauma on the list of qualifying traumas for a DSM-IV diagnosis of posttraumatic stress disorder (PTSD). Over time, the mental health professional may form a picture of IPV that is based on cumulative patients' histories of mental illness, childhood abuse, personality disorders, substance use, and their symptoms of depression, anxiety, or PTSD. That picture may be very different from the picture that a emergency medicine provider or a primary care provider develops over time—the former potentially focusing more on acute injuries, and the latter potentially focusing more on somatic complaints or the difficulties in adequately managing chronic illness.

violence is divided into interpersonal violence, collective violence (e.g., war, terrorism, or mob violence), or self-harm (e.g., suicide). Interpersonal violence is divided into family violence, community violence (e.g., stranger rape, muggings), and institutional violence (e.g., abuse of inmates). Family violence can then be separated into child abuse, IPV, and elder abuse. Intimate partner violence is defined as violence between intimates, but considerable variation exists in what constitutes "intimate partners." Some researchers define intimates as spouses or ex-spouses alone; others include nonmarried cohabiting partners, while still others include partners in any romantic relationship. Given data about the prevalence, severity, and impact of violence in dating relationships (23), a broader definition of intimates seems to be warranted that includes more than just married or cohabiting couples; however, in doing so, one will run into difficulties while trying to decide what constitutes an intimate relationship. For example, if a woman is raped on a first date, should that be considered IPV or acquaintance rape? If she has no emotional or financial attachment to her perpetrator, her experience and counseling needs may be quite different from those of a woman who has been abused by her husband for many years. What if the rape happened on the tenth date? What would one call it if it happened in the midst of a 5-year tumultuous relationship with two children in common? The latter example clearly appears to fall into the category of IPV, but may be excluded in studies or surveillance systems that only inquire about cohabiting couples. What if she is a teenager dating an older man, or an elderly woman being beaten by her caretaker-husband; should she be considered a victim of IPV, child abuse, or elder abuse? As these examples demonstrate, there many possible ways to define intimate partners, and therefore one must carefully consider what choices were made in defining "intimate partners" whenever interpreting or generalizing results of IPV studies.

CONTROVERSIAL COMPONENTS OF THE DEFINITION OF INTIMATE PARTNER VIOLENCE

Defining an Intimate Partner

Figure 2.1 shows a system that classifies all forms of violence based on the relationship between the perpetrator and the victim. In such a classification system,

Defining Abusive Behaviors

The different definitions of IPV, influenced by different perspectives of IPV, also differ on which types of behaviors they include. *Physical assaults* are included in almost all definitions of IPV, but the importance placed on minor physical assaults varies from perspective to perspective. For example, advocates or researchers working with battered women regularly

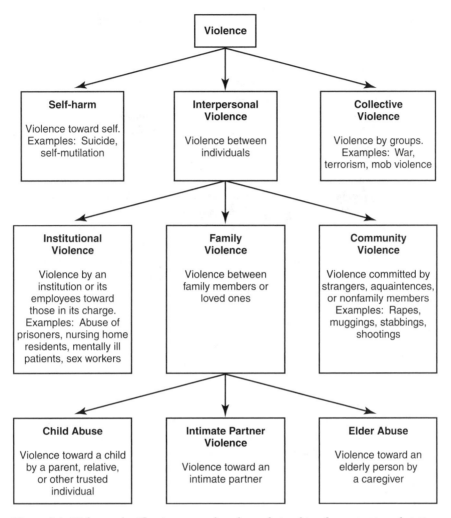

Figure 2.1 Violence classification system based on relationship of perpetrator and victim.

hear of the importance of pushes and shoves in allowing a batterer to maintain power and control over his
or her partner or in paving the way for more severe
abuse (3,7). Moreover, McCauley and colleagues
have found that even minor physical assaults, such
as pushes or shoves, are associated with worse physical and health outcomes in women recruited from
primary care clinics (24). Less is known, however,
about the effect of low-level violence on men or about
the significance of one-time minor physical assaults.
Should a woman be considered an IPV survivor if her
husband pushed her once during an argument, but
the violence never recurred and it was not accompanied by other forms of emotional abuse, threats, or
control? How about the man who was slapped by his

wife after he made a rude joke? As mentioned earlier,
feminists focusing on patterns of behavior or crimi-
nologists focusing on criminal acts would likely not
include either of these examples in their definition of
IPV, whereas family conflict tactics researchers focusing on specific physical actions would likely include
them. Sometimes researchers create hybrid definitions that include any severe assault, but only include
minor assaults if they are repetitive or accompanied by
emotional abuse (25,26).

Significant variation also exists in how to further
classify physical assaults. In the criminal justice system, physical assaults are often divided into *aggravated assaults*, which include serious injury or use of a
weapon, versus *simple assaults*, which involve neither.

One large national crime reporting system, the National Incident Based Reporting System (NIBR), includes both simple and aggravated physical assaults, whereas the older Uniform Crime Reporting (UCR) Program of the Federal Bureau of Investigation (FBI) only includes aggravated assaults (27) in reporting IPV. Non–crime based surveys tend to assess for a variety of physical assaults, but there is little consensus as to how to categorize or analyze the resulting data. The original and revised Conflict Tactics Scales (CTS and the CTS2) (9,11) divide physical aggression into a minor subscale that includes behaviors such as pushing, shoving, or slapping, and a major subscale that includes behaviors such as choking, kicking, punching, or using a weapon. The Abuse Assessment Screen scores physical assaults by fitting them into six ordered categories of increasing severity (28). The Index of Spouse Abuse, which has a subscale for physical violence, assigns different weights to each item (29). Individual studies using these instruments vary as to whether they include in their definition of IPV any physical assault or limit it to those experiencing severe assaults.

Sexual assault is increasingly being included in most definitions of IPV, although it is inconsistently measured. Most definitions of sexual assault include any forced sexual act, including rape and attempted rape. Coerced sexual acts, on the other hand, are not uniformly included in definitions of sexual assault across disciplines. Although DV advocates and feminist researchers operating from the perspective of patriarchal terrorism have always recognized coerced sexual acts as abusive, the crime reporting systems have not always measured sexual intimidation or coercion, especially when there is no perceived harm from the same. Global public health experts recognize denial of the right to use contraception and forced abortion as forms of sexual IPV, but the definition of assault recommended by the CDC for the purposes of surveillance is limited to an intentional sexual act against the person's will or in someone unable to provide consent. The original CTS did not measure sexual assault or coercion. The Revised CTS (CTS2) does have a scale on sexual aggression, which is divided into a major subscale (including acts such as rape) and a minor subscale (which includes insisting on sexual acts) (30).

Threat of violence, be it sexual assault or physical, has been included in most definitions of IPV. The point at which the experts begin to disagree is what constitutes a threat. Domestic violence advocacy and survivor groups consider any intent of harm expressed by a partner against themselves, their intimate partner, their family members, friends, or possessions as a threat of violence if it used as a means of control. The CTS, on the other hand, has only two items—threats of physical assault or threats made with a weapon—in its IPV scale. Unlike the advances made in understanding the impact of low-level physical violence on the health of the survivor, little is known at present regarding the long-term effect of repeated threats of violence on the health and well-being of those affected. It is conceivable to think that such threats can have long-term health effects, particularly mental health effects; however, one again is faced with the question of what threats are bad enough to cause harm. Does the gender or personality of the perpetrator matter? Is the effect of the threat linked to the ability of the perpetrator to carry out the threat, and if so, are threats a part of physical violence (as in legal definitions) or part of coercive control (as in feminist definitions)?

Emotional abuse is only included in some definitions of IPV. Qualitative studies focusing on battered women's experiences often highlight the great impact of emotional abuse (31). Similarly, quantitative studies have found an association between emotional abuse and worse health outcomes (32). Subtle psychological abuse has even been found to be more highly correlated with women's emotional state than overt acts of physical or sexual violence (33). Still, emotional abuse is hard to quantify. The CDC definition of IPV only includes physical or sexual assaults (1). Thus, most surveillance studies and many studies of the health consequences of IPV limit the abuse to physical or sexual assaults. Emotional abuse is also rarely included in the penal code or criminology studies. The CTS2 includes a psychological aggression scale that captures some forms of emotional abuse. Numerous scales have been developed from a feminist perspective that attempt to measure emotional abuse, including the Psychological Maltreatment of Women (34) and the Severity of Violence Against Women Scale (35). Most of these scales focus on emotionally abusive actions (for example name-calling or put-downs). The Woman's Experience of Battering (WEB) scale (36) focuses not on actions, but on how a woman experiences her situation (e.g., feeling unsafe or feeling ashamed).

Power and control are central in the feminist definition of IPV and are occasionally included in public health definitions of violence against women (3,8,37,38). They are generally not included in legal definitions or in family conflict studies. Numerous qualitative studies focus on the importance of controlling behaviors (7,31,39). Quantitative studies find that having a highly controlling partner is associated with higher risk of injury or homicide (40–42). How to best measure power and control, however, is less clear. The Danger Assessment (43) has a single item on a highly controlling partner. The Psychological Maltreatment of Women Inventory (34) includes a control subscale. Although the original psychometric testing of the Index of Spouse Abuse (ISA) only yielded two subscales (physical and nonphysical) (29), two subsequent re-analyses have supported the existence of a third subscale that relates to controlling behaviors (44,45). More recently, several researchers have developed more detailed instruments to specifically measure controlling behaviors (46) or coercive control (47). No consensus exists, however, as to how much control is "normal" in a relationship and what is abusive, or as to the significance of controlling behavior that is unaccompanied by physical, sexual, or emotional abuse. Studies that focus on the experiences of battered women often highlight additional abusive behaviors.

Stalking is increasingly seen as a crime, although there is still considerable variation in whether states have stalking laws or if stalking is considered to be a part of the definition of IPV. The HARASS scale (48) specifically measures stalking behaviors. Stalking is rarely included in family conflict studies, surveillance programs, or studies of health consequences. Other behaviors such as *pet abuse* may potentially be very significant to IPV survivors, but are not often included in definitions or measures of IPV(49).

ATTEMPTS TO RECONCILE DIFFERING DEFINITIONS AND FINDINGS

Differences in how one conceptualizes, defines, and measures IPV have engendered decades of heated debate, especially around the issue of gender symmetry (12,13,50–54). Feminists have argued that by ignoring the antecedents, intent, and consequences of violence, studies using the CTS or CTS2 falsely equate behaviors that are inherently different and gendered (51). Family conflict researchers have argued that by not

routinely measuring violence by women against male partners, or by making culturally based assumptions about gender roles, society is ignoring male IPV victims, much as it had ignored female IPV victims a few decades ago (13).

Several researchers have attempted to reconcile, or at least explain, how different camps may come to diametrically opposed conclusions. Many have pointed out that limiting violence to severe forms tends to highlight gender differences, whereas including more minor forms tends to increase gender symmetry (12). This finding is not only true for IPV but for most forms of crime. For example, if limiting juvenile delinquency to severe violence, most perpetrators are male. If including more minor forms such as school truancy, then greater gender symmetry is seen. A similar pattern is seen on the continuum of armed robbery to shoplifting (55). Straus himself points out that general population studies such as his own and others find much higher rates of IPV and much more gender symmetry than crime-based studies. He feels that this difference is a consequence of the population sampled (those recruited from the general population versus from within the legal system), the severity of the violence, and the context of the interview (e.g., whether the participant feels he or she is participating in a survey about normal relationship conflicts or criminal acts) (13).

Johnson has proposed a framework to reconcile the feminist and family conflict perspectives. He hypotheses that several distinct types of IPV exist (56–58). He defines "intimate terrorism" by "the attempt to dominate one's partner and to exert general control over the relationship, domination that is manifested in the use of a wide range of power and control tactics, including violence." This type of violence fits the classic picture of IPV and is the form of violence seen by people working with women seeking domestic violence services and by the legal system. The assumption is that this form is largely perpetrated by men against women and that this is the type of violence that tends to progressively escalate over time. A second type, which he calls "situational couples violence," is defined as "violence that is not embedded in a general pattern of controlling behaviors." Here, specific arguments may escalate into violence, but there is no relationship-wide evidence of one partner trying to exert control over the other, and no progressive escalation in the frequency and severity of violence. This second type, he hypothesizes, is the form most likely seen when surveying general populations, in which frequent examples of occasional violence among intimates may occur, but with a low prevalence of violence severe enough to necessitate domestic violence services or legal action. He also hypothesizes that men and women are equally likely to perpetrate this form of violence. In more recent work, he has described two additional types of IPV. "Violent resistance" occurs when the victim of an intimate terrorist responds with violence, but there is still clearly a power differential between the two partners. Again, he hypothesizes that men are more likely to be the intimate terrorists and women the violent resistors. Finally, he recognized the possibility of "mutual violent control," in which two intimate terrorists vie for control of the relationship, but he hypothesizes that this form is relatively rare.

Johnson's framework is theoretically appealing to many working in the field of IPV, as it has allowed for a more productive discussion around issues that were previously at an impasse. Relatively scant empiric evidence exists, however, to prove his hypotheses. One study compared results of the CTS and controlling behavior scale in four distinct populations—women in domestic violence shelters, men in batterers treatment programs, male and female college students, and men incarcerated for nonviolent crimes—and found at least partial support for Johnson's model (46). Johnson has used data from the Violence Against Women Survey to show that female victims of intimate terrorism are attacked more frequently, experience violence that is less likely to stop, suffer more injuries, exhibit more symptoms of posttraumatic pain disorder, use more pain killers, and miss more work than are female victims of situational couples violence (59). Many other aspects of the model, however, have not yet been tested, or have not been supported by empiric studies. Graham-Kevan and colleagues' study found gender symmetry to exist even within the couples with intimate terrorism (60). The study, however, used a general population sample and had overall much lower rates of controlling behaviors than were seen in their prior work with a domestic violence sample (46), leading to the possibility of misclassification. Moreover, it is unclear what the consequences are of situational couple violence. Qualitative work with women who have survived a homicide attempt by an intimate partner—presumably the most severe outcome of IPV—found that there was a wide spectrum of severity of controlling behaviors (39). There is a risk that, using

Johnson's framework, many of the women would have been classified as experiencing situational couple violence, and thus could potentially receive less counseling about safety issues than in a traditional model in which all domestic violence is expected to escalate. Similarly, concern exists that relationships that have reciprocal or bidirectional violence may be more dangerous than relationships in which the violence is perpetrated by only one partner. An analysis of a large national survey (N = 11,370) found that half of the violent relationships included violence by both partners and that bidirectional violence was associated with greater injury than was unidirectional violence, regardless of the gender of the perpetrator (61). More work is needed to operationalize and test Johnson's model, or to create other models that can bridge multiple perspectives about IPV.

Finally, McHugh has proposed using a postmodern perspective to understand the inconsistencies and contradictions in IPV research (62). She recognizes that every approach represents an ideological position, and that what we measure determines what we find. She argues against binary thinking and essentialism, concluding that interpersonal violence always involves gender, that men and women are violent in similar and different ways, and that research is needed to study the gendered patterns of violence in couples within the larger cultural context.

IMPLICATIONS FOR POLICY, PRACTICE, AND RESEARCH

Policy

- Narrowing the definition of IPV will result in lower IPV prevalence and incidence rates. Since policy makers and grant funders pay more attention to bigger problems, underestimation of IPV prevalence may result in reduction of funds for programs for IPV survivors and perpetrators.
- Broadening the definition of IPV may give the appearance that IPV is gender symmetric. Such data has at times been used to argue against gender-specific legislation, such as the Violence Against Women Act. Any discussion of the complexities of IPV must not ignore the inherently gendered nature of IPV, the differential consequences of IPV, and the need for gender-specific services.

Practice

- Narrowing the definition of IPV may trivialize a survivor's experience of IPV.
- Similarly, by limiting which behaviors are considered to be abusive, narrow IPV definitions may limit a survivor's ability to recognize a pattern of behavior as abusive or seek help for herself and her children, and may eventually hinder attempts to extricate herself from abusive relationships.
- Broader definitions, if applied to general populations, may potentially label common behaviors as IPV. It is unclear what the best counseling practices are for male and female victims of such violence, what the prognostic value is of these behaviors on an intimate relationship, or what the health consequences are for either partner.
- IPV survivors or perpetrators who do not fit a classic picture of IPV may find it difficult to identify with and respond to counseling that assumes the existence of unidirectional violence, traditional gender roles, or underlying issues of power and control.

Research

- Researchers and consumers of research need to be aware of the role that measurement instruments, sampling strategy, IPV definitions, personal perspective, and political agenda may have on their research findings.
- Further research is needed:
  - To clarify the impact of threats of violence on a survivor's health and well-being;
  - To clarify the impact of IPV on the health and well-being of the perpetrator;
  - To understand the antecedents, intent, and consequences of IPV in nonclassic situations, including violence perpetrated by women against men, violence in same-sex relationships, bidirectional violence, sporadic violence, and violence not embedded in a framework of power and control;
  - To operationalize and empirically test theoretical frameworks, such as that of Michael Johnson, to see if they accurately describe the experience of IPV survivors and perpetrators from different populations and to see if they help predict or explain social and health consequences; and
  - To develop appropriate counseling practices for IPV survivors and perpetrators that may not fit a classic model of IVP.

References

1. Saltzman LE, Fanslow J, McMahon P, Shelley G. *Intimate partner violence surveillance: Uniform definitions and recommended data elements.* Atlanta: National Center for Injury Prevention and Control, Center for Disease Control and Prevention, 1999; NCJ 181867.
2. Alpert EJ, Cohen S, Sege RD. Family violence: An overview. *Acad Med.* 1997;72(1 Suppl):S3–6.
3. Dutton MA, Goodman LA. Coercion in intimate partner violence: Toward a new conceptualization. *Sex Roles.* 2005;52(11–12):743–756.
4. *Power and Control Wheel.* Duluth, Minnesota: Domestic Abuse Intervention Project; 1983.
5. Gordon M. Definitional issues in violence against women: Surveillance and research from a violence research perspective. *Violence Against Women.* 2000;6(7):747–783.
6. Pence E. The Duluth domestic abuse intervention project. In Aldarondo E, Mederos F, eds. *Programs for men who batter: Intervention and prevention strategies in a diverse society.* NJ: Civic Research Institute, 2002: 6.1–6.46.
7. Nicolaidis C. The Voices of Survivors documentary: Using patient narrative to educate physicians about domestic violence. *J Gen Intern Med.* 2002; 17(2):117–124.
8. Family Violence Prevention Fund. *The national consensus guidelines on identifying and responding to domestic violence victimization in health care settings.* San Francisco: Author; September, 2002.
9. Straus MA. Measuring intrafamily conflict and violence: The Conflict Tactics Scales. *J Marriage Fam.* 1979;41:75–88.
10. Straus MA. The conflict tactics scale and its critics: An evaluation and new data on validity and reliability. In: Staus MA, Gelles RJ, eds. *Physical violence in American families: Risk factors and adaptation to violence in 8,145 families.* New Brunswick, NJ: Transaction; 1990:49–73.
11. Straus MA, Hamby SI, Boney-McCoy S, Sugarman D. The revised Conflict Tactics Scale (CTS2). *J Fam Issues.* 1996;17:283–316.
12. Archer J. Sex differences in aggression between heterosexual partners: A meta-analytic review. *Psychol Bull.* 2000;126(5):651–680.
13. Straus MA. The controversy over domestic violence by women: A methodological, theoretical, and sociology of science analysis. In: Arriaga XBEO, Stuart E, eds. *Violence in intimate relationships.* Thousand Oaks, CA: Sage; 1999:17–44.
14. Kilpatrick DG. What is violence against women? Defining and measuring the problem. *J Interpers Violence.* 2004;19(11):1209–1234.
15. Saltzman LE. Issues related to defining and measuring violence against women: Response to Kilpatrick. *J Interpers Violence.* 2004;19(11): 1235–1243.

16. Campbell JC. Promise and perils of surveillance in addressing violence against women. *Violence Against Women.* 2000;6(7):705–727.

17. *The Voices Of Survivors: Domestic Violence Survivors Educate Physicians.* [Educational Documentary]. Philadelphia: American College of Physicians-American Society of Internal Medicine, 2000.

18. Alpert EJ, Tonkin AE, Seeherman AM, Holtz HA. Family violence curricula in US medical schools. *Am J Prev Med.* 1998;14(4):273–282.

19. Feldhaus KM, Koziol-McLain J, Amsbury HL, et al. Accuracy of 3 brief screening questions for detecting partner violence in the emergency department. *JAMA.* 1997;277(17):1357–1361.

20. Sherin KM, Sinacore JM, Li XQ, et al. HITS: A short domestic violence screening tool for use in a family practice setting. *Fam Med.* 1998;30(7):508–512.

21. Brown JB, Lent B, Brett PJ, et al. Development of the Woman Abuse Screening Tool for use in family practice. *Fam Med.* 1996;28(6):422–428.

22. Brown J, Lent B, Schmidt G, Sas G. Application of the Woman Abuse Screening Tool (WAST) and the WAST-Short in the family practice setting. *J Fam Pract.* 2000;49(10):896–903.

23. Slashinski MJ, Coker AL, Davis KE. Physical aggression, forced sex, and stalking victimization by a dating partner: An analysis of the National Violence Against Women Survey. *Violence Vict.* 2003; 18(6):595–617.

24. McCauley J, Kern DE, Kolodner K, et al. Relation of low-severity violence to women's health. *J Gen Intern Med.* 1998;13(10):687–691.

25. Paranjape A, Liebschutz J. STaT: A three-question screen for intimate partner violence. *J Womens Health.* 2003;12(3):233–239.

26. Nicolaidis C, Curry M, McFarland B, Gerrity M. Violence, mental health, and physical symptoms in an academic internal medicine practice. *J Gen Intern Med.* 2004;19(8):819–827.

27. Rantala R. *Effects of NIBRS on crime statistics.* Washington, DC: US Department of Justice, 2000. NCJ 78890.

28. Soeken S, McFarlane J, Parker B, Lominack M. The Abuse Assessment Screen. In: Campbell J, ed. *Empowering survivors of abuse: Health care for battered women and children.* Thousand Oaks, CA: Sage; 1998:195–203.

29. Hudson WW, McIntosh SR. The assessment of spouse abuse: Two quantifiable dimensions. *J Marriage Fam.* 1981;43:873–885.

30. Straus MA, Hamby SL, Boney-McCoy S, Sugarman DB. *The revised conflict tactics scales (CTS2).* Durham, NH: Family Research Laboratory, 1995.

31. Sleutel MR. Women's experiences of abuse: A review of qualitative research. *Issues Ment Health Nurs.* 1998;19(6):525–539.

32. Coker AL, Smith PH, Bethea L, et al. Physical health consequences of physical and psychological intimate partner violence. *Arch Fam Med.* 2000;9(5): 451–457.

33. Marshall LL. Effects of men's subtle and overt psychological abuse on low-income women. *Violence Vict.* 1999;14(1):69–88.

34. Tolman RM. The validation of the Psychological Maltreatment of Women Inventory. *Violence Vict.* 1999;14(1):25–37.

35. Marshall LL. Development of the Severity of Violence Against Women Scale. *J Fam Violence.* 1992;7:103–121.

36. Smith PH, Earp JA, DeVellis R. Measuring battering: Development of the Women's Experience with Battering (WEB) Scale. *Womens Health.* 1995;1(4):273–288.

37. Dobash RE, Dobash RP. *Rethinking violence against women.* Thousand Oaks, CA: Sage, 1998.

38. Dobash R, Dobash RP. How theoretical definitions and perspectives affect research and policy. In: Douglas JB, ed. *Family violence: Research and public policy issues.* Washington, DC: AEI Press; 1990: 108–129.

39. Nicolaidis C, Curry MA, Ulrich Y, et al. Could we have known? A qualitative analysis of data from women who survived an attempted homicide by an intimate partner. *J Gen Intern Med.* 2003;18(10): 788–794.

40. Follingstad DR, Bradley RG, Laughlin JE, Burke L. Risk factors and correlates of dating violence: The relevance of examining frequency and severity levels in a college sample. *Violence Vict.* 1999;14(4): 365–380.

41. Campbell JC. 'If I can't have you, no one can': Power and control in homicide of female partners. In: Radford J, Russel DEH, eds. *Femicide: The politics of woman killing.* Boston, MA: Twayn, 1992.

42. Campbell JC, Webster D, Koziol-McLain J, et al. Risk factors for femicide in abusive relationships: Results from a multi-site case control study. *Am J Public Health.* 2003;93:1089–1097.

43. Campbell JC. *Assessing dangerousness: Violence by sexual offenders, batterers, and child abusers.* Thousand Oaks, CA: Sage, 1995.

44. Campbell DW, Campbell JC, King C, et al. The reliability and factor structure of the index of spouse abuse with African-American battered women. *Violence Vict.* 1994;9:259–274.

45. Cook SL, Conrad L, Bender M, Kaslow NJ. The internal validity of the index of spouse abuse in African American women. *Violence Vict.* 2003; 18(6):641–657.

46. Graham-Kevan N, Archer J. Physical aggression and control in heterosexual relationships: The effect of sampling. *Violence Vict.* 2003;18(2):181–196.

47. Cook SL, Goodman LA. Beyond frequency and severity: Development and validation of the brief coercion and conflict scales [see comment]. *Violence Against Women.* 2006;12(11):1050–1072.

48. Williams-Evans SA, Sheridan DJ. Exploring barriers to leaving violent intimate partner relationships. *ABNF Journal.* 2004;15(2):38–40.

49. Ascione FR, Weber CV, Thompson TM, et al. Battered pets and domestic violence: Animal abuse reported by women experiencing intimate violence and by nonabused women. *Violence Against Women.* 2007;13(4):354–373.

50. Archer J. Sex differences in physical aggression to partners: A reply to Frieze (2000), O'Leary (2000), and White, Smith, Koss, and Figueredo (2000) [comment]. *Psychol Bull.* 2000;126(5):697–702.

51. Dobash RP, Dobash RE, Wilson M, Daly M. The myth of sexual symmetry in marital violence. *Soc Probl.* 1992;39(1):71–91.

52. Dutton DG. Patriarchy and wife assault: The ecological fallacy. *Violence Vict.* 1994;9(2):167–182.

53. Frieze IH. Violence in close relationships: Development of a research area: Comment on Archer (2000) [comment] [see comments]. *Psychol Bull.* 2000;126(5):681–684.

54. White JW, Smith PH, Koss MP, Figueredo AJ. Intimate partner aggression: What have we learned? Comment on Archer (2000). *Psychol Bull.* 2000;126(5):690–696.

55. Hamby S. Measuring gender differences in partner violence: Implications from research on other forms of violent and socially undesirable behavior. *Sex Roles.* June, 2005.

56. Johnson MP, Ferraro KJ. Research on domestic violence in the 1990s: Making distinctions. *J Marriage Fam.* 2000;62(4):948–963.

57. Johnson MP. Patriarchal terrorism and common couple violence: Two forms of violence against women. *J Marriage Fam.* 1995;57:283–294.

58. Johnson MP. Conflict and control: Gender symmetry and asymmetry in domestic violence. *Violence Against Women.* 2006;12(11)1003–1018.

59. Johnson MP, Leone JM. The differential effects of intimate terrorism and situational couple violence: Findings from the National Violence Against Women Survey. *J Fam Issues.* 2005;26(3):322–349.

60. Graham-Kevan N, Archer J. Using Johnson's Typology to classify men and women in a non-selected sample. Paper presented at 9th International Family Violence Research Conference, Portsmouth, NH, 2005.

61. Whitaker DJ, Haileyesus T, Swahn M, Saltzman LS. Differences in frequency of violence and reported injury between relationships with reciprocal and nonreciprocal intimate partner violence. *Am J Public Health.* 2007;97(5):941–947.

62. McHugh MC, Livingston NA, Ford A. A postmodern approach to women's use of violence: Developing multiple and complex conceptualizations. *Psychol Women Q.* 2005;29(3):323–336.

Chapter 3

Prevalence of Nonfatal and Fatal Intimate Partner Violence in the United States

Linda E. Saltzman and Debra Houry

KEY CONCEPTS

- Many data sources exist on intimate partner violence (IPV)-specific events and prevalence both within health and justice data resources.
- Intimate partner violence rates vary greatly by data source.
- Intimate partner violence rates vary by incidence, 1-year prevalence, and lifetime prevalence.
- Many reported IPV rates are not inclusive and do not take into account all forms of IPV (physical, emotional, or sexual).
- *Intimate partner violence* is a term coined by the Centers for Disease Control and Prevention (CDC); *domestic violence* is a criminal justice term; "adult maltreatment" is the nomenclature used in the International Classification of Diseases for IPV, further complicating surveillance efforts.

MEASURING RATES OF INTIMATE PARTNER VIOLENCE PREVALENCE AND INCIDENCE

Intimate partner violence (IPV) is a worldwide problem, and 25% of women in the United States have reported victimization during their lifetime (1). Forms of IPV include physical, emotional, and sexual abuse. In addition, when we refer to IPV, it can be ongoing, intermittent, or based on a previous experience. Thus, reported prevalence and incidence rates of IPV vary greatly.

In epidemiology, *prevalence* refers to the proportion of a specific population with a particular disease or health condition at a given time (2,3). This is sometimes also called *point prevalence* (3). The numerator is the number of people with the condition; the denominator is the number of people in the population at risk of having it. Sometimes we refer to *annual prevalence* or *past year prevalence*. In such cases, we are referring to the proportion of the population having the disease or condition during the specified calendar year or 12-month period. We use the information about prevalence to estimate the number of people affected and to calculate associated costs for the healthcare system or to society. That information is also critical for prevention purposes. To plan interventions targeting those at risk, we must know the size of the group being targeted.

When we calculate prevalence for diseases, people who have previously had the disease but who have recovered from it are not counted in the numerator. For some chronic diseases or health conditions (e.g., epilepsy or hemophilia), once a person is identified as having it, they stay in the numerator for the remainder of their lifetime. For IPV, however, determining prevalence is less straight-forward. Knowing whether people in the population "have" IPV (i.e., what is a "case"?) depends both on the question being asked about its prevalence and on how IPV is defined. Whereas for many diseases the focus is on the proportion of people sick or infected, for IPV our focus can be on several possible groups: people who are victimized, people who perpetrate IPV, or on people with involvement of any kind, whether that be victimization, perpetration, or even witnessing it. Intervention can be focused at each of those groups. For example, the research agenda at the CDC focused on IPV highlights strategies targeting perpetration (4).

The measurement of IPV prevalence will obviously differ depending upon which of these groups we refer to. For illustration purposes, let's assume that we want to know the proportion of the population victimized. We would then need to know whether we are referring to people victimized by any form of IPV (e.g., physical, sexual, or emotional victimization) or whether we are referring only to a particular subset measurable by specified outcomes, such as physical injury. The prevalence again differs depending upon the answer. For example, let's assume that we want to include people victimized by any form of IPV. We would then need to specify what constitutes victimization. If someone has suffered violence at the hands of an intimate partner, but is now free from victimization, should that person be counted as a victim for prevalence purposes? In other words, is someone who has been physically assaulted by her husband in the past, but who is no longer being victimized by him, counted as having been victimized? Similar to the person with a recurring chronic disease, we would be

saying that once someone has been an IPV victim, they remain a victim and continue to be counted in the numerator for prevalence purposes. For annual prevalence, that would translate to counting anyone who had been victimized during the year, regardless of whether the violence terminated or continued unabated. Alternatively, we could count IPV victimization prevalence similarly to the way we treat people who have influenza. Even if they have had influenza in a prior year, if the person has not suffered IPV victimization during the year in question, they would not be counted in the numerator for prevalence purposes. To do that, however, necessitates establishing a period of time after which we will consider the absence of violence to be an indication of it having ceased. Because IPV is often episodic, typically with periods of time between episodes, it is important to differentiate a person whose victimization has stopped from a person who is between episodes of victimization. To address this, IPV prevalence is frequently cited as either a 1-year prevalence rate or a lifetime prevalence rate. Once we decide the time period to be used to measure prevalence, we still need to address the question regarding the types of IPV counted for prevalence purposes. That is, if physical violence has not occurred for more than a year, but emotional abuse is ongoing, does that situation warrant inclusion in the numerator for annual prevalence?

Whereas prevalence focuses on disease status at a given time, *incidence* refers to the rate of development of a health problem over a period of time (3). To calculate an incidence rate, we divide the number of disease onsets in a given period by the sum of the lengths of time the members of the population are at risk of getting that disease. Usually the denominator is calculated by multiplying the average size of the study population by the length of the period of time being studied. If we are talking about a year, the incidence rate would reflect the number of people in the population who get the disease during the year. For IPV, this measure is affected by the same issues that we identified for prevalence. To measure how many people "get" IPV in a year still depends on how we define it and how we determine whether it has ceased. If IPV victimization is considered to have ceased, then the prior victim is once again eligible to contribute to the numerator when a new event occurs.

Underlying these measurement issues is the question of *case definition*. That is, does a "case" of IPV refer to the person involved (i.e., is this a new victim or a new perpetrator?) or to the events that involve that person (i.e., a hit, slap, or punch). We may want to know the number of people who are punched by an intimate partner, or we may be interested in the number of times someone is punched by an intimate partner. Both are legitimate questions to ask, but the answers will obviously differ. For example, the National Violence Against Women Survey (1) refers to victims and victimizations to reflect both number of people affected and number of events occurring to them.

Because IPV prevalence and incidence can be defined and measured in a variety of ways, comparing data sources is complicated unless the operational definition of IPV prevalence or incidence is provided. Unfortunately, the prevalence of IPV is often discussed without provision of explicit information regarding what is being included in the numerator. When information about IPV prevalence from different sources varies, it is important to determine whether the variation simply reflects different underlying definitions of the numerator.

We will now focus on specific fatal and nonfatal data sources. We will review the focus, what was measured, IPV studies conducted with these databases, and strengths and limitations of these national datasets. Table 3.1 lists these databases, their sources, and their websites.

Table 3.1 Data Sources for Incidence and Prevalence Estimates of Intimate Partner Violence			
Database	Website	Source	Info Obtained From
Fatal			
UCR-SHR	http://www.fbi.gov/hq/cjisd/ucr.htm	FBI	Crime reports
NVSS	http://www.cdc.gov/nchs/nvss.htm	CDC-NCHS	Death certificates
NVDRS	http://www.aast.org/nvdrs.html	CDC	Crime reports, death certificates, coroner
Nonfatal			
NIBRS	http://www.fbi.gov/hq/cjisd/ucr.htm	FBI	Crime reports
NVAWS	http://www.ojp.usdoj.gov/nij/pubs-sum/172837.htm	NIJ/CDC	Random-digit-dial telephone survey
NCVS	http://www.ojp.usdoj.gov/bjs/cvict.htm	BJS	National household survey
NHAMCS	http://www.cdc.gov/nchs/about/major/ahcd/ahcd1.htm	CDC-NCHS	Emergency department records
NEISS	http://www.cdc.gov/ncipc/wisqars/		
	CPSC/CDC-NCIPC	Emergency department records	
BRFSS	http://www.cdc.gov/brfss/		
	CDC-NCCDPHP	Random-digit-dial telephone survey	

BJS, Bureau of Justice Statistics; BRFSS, Behavioral Risk Factor Surveillance System; CDC, Centers for Disease Control and Prevention; CPSC, Consumer Product Safety Commission; FBI, Federal Bureau of Investigation; NCCDPHP, National Center for Chronic Disease Prevention and Health Promotion; NCHS, National Center for Health Statistics; NCIPC, National Center for Injury Prevention and Control; NCVS, National Crime Victimization Survey, NEISS, National Electronic Injury Surveillance System; NHAMCS, National Hospital Ambulatory Medical Care Survey; NIBRS, National Incidence-Based Reporting System; NIJ, National Institue of Justice; NVAWS, National Violence Against Women Survey; NVDRS, National Violence Death Reporting System; NVSS, National Vital Statistics System; UCR-SHR, Uniform Crime Reports–Supplemental Homicide Reports.

FATAL INTIMATE PARTNER VIOLENCE

Since 1961, the Federal Bureau of Investigation (FBI)'s *Uniform Crime Reports – Supplemental Homicide Reports (UCR-SHR)* has collected incident-level homicide data from law enforcement agencies. Although reporting is voluntary, the SHR obtains information on over 90% of homicides in the United States. In general, criminal justice statistics focus on perpetrators, because law enforcement agencies routinely obtain perpetrator information as part of the arrest, and information on the victim may not be as rigorously collected. UCR-SHR does include information about the relationship of the perpetrator to the victim of the homicide. However, this dataset reports only on homicide, so IPV assaults are not captured by this database. Because these are homicides, only incidence rates can be reported.

Several studies have looked specifically at IPV homicides using the UCR-SHR database. Puzone and colleagues found that, although most homicide victims are men (78%), most adult victims of IPV homicide are women (60%) (5). Using SHR data from 1976–1995, Puzone and colleagues (5) also found that 34% of women were killed by an intimate partner (husband, ex-husband, boyfriend, or same-sex partner) compared to only 6% of men. Kellermann and colleagues (6) reported that in 60% of homicides by women, the victim was a spouse, intimate acquaintance, or a family member. By contrast, men killed nonintimate acquaintances or strangers in 80% of cases.

The strength of UCR-SHR data is that they are population-based and national in scope. Unlike vital records, they also include some information about the homicide perpetrators. However, a major limitation to using SHR data is that information on perpetrators and their relationship to the victims is often unknown or incomplete. Other limitations include underreporting of cases to police, as many victims do not report crimes committed against themselves; voluntary participation by police agencies; and errors in the way that relationships are recorded in police reports (thus affecting identification as IPV). Deaths included in SHR data are classified by place of occurrence rather than place of death (7).

National Incidence Based Reporting System (NIBRS) data are reported for 46 types of crime incidents and arrests, including homicide. Information collected includes data on victim and offender demographics, offender–victim relationship, substance use, weapon type, location of offense, and criminal activity. Both state and local law enforcement agencies participate in reporting to NIBRS; however, participation is voluntary, so only a proportion of the population is represented. The majority of information abstracted from these reports is on the perpetrator, so that only events or incidence rates can be reported. Most of the offenses included in NIBRS are nonfatal, so this dataset is discussed in more detail in the Nonfatal section.

The National Vital Statistics System (NVSS) collects and disseminates the nation's official vital statistics. Each state jurisdiction responsible for vital registration statistics submits information on births, deaths, marriages, divorces, and fetal deaths. Only demographic information regarding the victim of a fatal incident is recorded. The only study relevant to violently inflicted injuries we found stated that the 2002 death rate for firearm injuries was 10.4 deaths per 100,000 U.S. standard population. Men had a firearm injury rate that was 6.6 times higher than that of women; African Americans had a rate 2.1 times that of Caucasians (8). The NVSS does not provide information on relationships of victims and perpetrators for intentional injuries, thus specific information regarding IPV is not available.

In 2002, Congress approved funding for the *National Violence Death Reporting System (NVDRS)* (9). Currently, 17 states are funded, with plans to eventually expand to all 50 states and Washington D.C. Each state obtains information from death certificates, medical examiner files, law enforcement records, and crime laboratories. The NVDRS supplements current databases by providing much more detailed information regarding both victim and offender characteristics and circumstances surrounding the death. Two recent studies have looked at fatalities associated with IPV. Among participating NVDRS states, 20% of homicides were directly associated with intimate partner conflict (10). In addition, among cases of homicide followed by a suicide, it was found that most victims (58%) were a current or former intimate partner of the perpetrator (11). Limitations of this database include compliance with reporting of deaths and reconciling information from diverse databases.

NONFATAL INTIMATE PARTNER VIOLENCE

Police data are a systematic, ongoing collection of information about crime and a valuable resource in examining the epidemiological patterns and causes of violence among intimates. In keeping with the *Uniform Crime Report's* (UCR) crime hierarchy, assaults that occur during incidents of homicide, rape, and robbery are classified in those "higher-order" crime categories, and not as assaults. Similarly, several "lower-order" categories include incidents among intimate partners and family members that involve physical contact, use of weapons, or verbal or weapon threats. Some researchers have suggested that IPV research should take into account incidents classified in nonassault crime categories (12). Although the majority of assaultive incidents were classified as assaults, the number of IPV incidents classified as nonassault crimes was not negligible. However, this database is based on crimes reported to the police, and the police must report this information to UCR. Additionally, information is not collected on perpetrator–victim relationship for any nonfatal crimes. However, this dataset is national, ongoing, and, despite being voluntary, covers most of the country.

National Incidence-Based Reporting System (NIBRS) data are reported for 46 types of crime incidents and arrests (Group A offenses) within 22 categories. For 11 additional offenses (Group B), only arrest data are reported. Information collected includes data on victim and offender demographics, offender–victim relationship, substance use, weapon type, location of offense, and criminal activity. There is no specific category for IPV, but this information can be obtained by looking at the offender–victim relationship for both assaultive and nonassaultive crimes. As with all crime datasets, the majority of information reported is on the perpetrator. In addition, both state and local law enforcement agencies participate in reporting to NIBRS; but, participation is voluntary, so only a proportion of the population is represented. For example, a study conducted using Massachusetts information found that the data represented 34% of the state's population and only 20% of the state's reported crime (13). Using data from one state to look at IPV, investigators reported that 10% of women victimized by an intimate partner actually experienced more than one crime during the incident (13). Another study found that the majority of IPV incidents reported to police involved heterosexual couples (99%) and that incidents with both same-sex couples and heterosexual couples were equally likely to result in an arrest (14).

Using NIBRS, crime offense data can be broken down and combined into specific information. In addition, NIBRS collects data on all crimes associated with each incident, allowing for more detailed information about the nature of the incident. Obvious limitations to NIBRS include voluntary participation by agencies, abstraction of data from police reports, and missing crimes not reported to law enforcement.

Each year since 1973, the *National Crime Victimization Survey* (NCVS) is conducted to obtain information on criminal victimization from a nationally representative sample of 42,000 households comprising nearly 76,000 people. In this survey, households are surveyed over a 3-year period, and current household members respond to the survey (if someone leaves the household they are not contacted). This survey does collect demographic information and information on relationships between perpetrator and victim, although the focus, because of the self-reporting, is on victimization. Intimate partner violence is defined as any violent crime of rape, robbery, or assault that was perpetrated by an intimate partner. Current reports from the NCVS show that IPV comprised 20% of violent crime against women and that 85% of victimizations by intimate partners were against women (15). Another study used the NCVS to look at recurring violence-related injury and found that those who did not receive medical treatment, who did not report the incident to the police, and who have been victimized by someone known to them are at greatest risk for recurring injuries (16). Thompson and colleagues also reported that women assaulted by an intimate partner or ex-partner were more at risk of sustaining an injury than were those assaulted by any other type of male offender (17). Despite these findings, the NCVS is limited in that it relies on self-report in a crime context, which may result in underreporting as victims may choose not to report that a crime occurred. Finally, the NCVS does not include victims of fatal violence.

The *National Hospital Ambulatory Medical Care Survey* (NHAMCS) collects data on the utilization and provision of ambulatory care services from approximately 400 hospital emergency and outpatient departments during randomly assigned 4-week reporting periods. Data collected includes reason for visit, patient demographics, and medications given. The focus is on injuries the victim sustained and needs medical treatment for. However, documentation in medical records may not be complete and coders may not list IPV as the cause of injury or as a medical problem. Adult abuse or IPV can be listed as an ICD Code (International Classification of Diseases) diagnosis on medical records, although compliance with this is usually mediocre. To further complicate the issue, ICD uses the term "adult maltreatment" to include IPV and other forms of violence; however, there is a code specific for the relationship of the perpetrator. E-codes can further clarify the mechanism of injury and V-codes can be used to indicate a prior history of IPV, but no active problem currently. Alternatively, IPV can be abstracted from intentional assault cases in which the victim–perpetrator relationship is recorded. As reported in one study, only 93 diagnoses of child or adult abuse were coded for 351,359 patient visits during a 4-year period (18), whereas some studies have reported that 3% of women are treated in emergency departments for an injury from IPV (19). This suggests that NHAMCS is not picking up the majority of IPV cases. Strengths of this dataset include that it is updated nationally on an annual basis and provides a snapshot of injury patterns. However, documentation rates of IPV are low, and the majority of cases are not recorded.

The *National Electronic Injury Surveillance System* (NEISS) reviews emergency department medical records from emergency departments selected to represent various geographic areas and hospital sizes. The NEISS codes for intentional injuries and records relationship of perpetrator and victim. This information can be helpful in identifying incidence rates of those who seek medical care in the emergency department. For example, 40% of injured victims of violence were assaulted by someone known to them (20). However, prevalence rates for IPV cannot be determined by NEISS, and only those who seek medical care in the emergency department *and* report that their injury was due to IPV will be included in the NEISS database.

The CDC established the *Behavioral Risk Factor Surveillance System* (BRFSS) in 1984 and developed standard core questions for states to use to provide data that could be compared across states. Since 1994, all states participate in the BRFSS; however, there were no standard violence questions. Currently, 18 states and territories collect this information. The IPV questions in the module define IPV as lifetime physical or sexual violence. Overall, 26.4% of women and 15.9% of men reported experiencing some combination of physical violence (threatened, attempted, or completed) and/or unwanted sex in their lifetime. Interestingly,

compared to white non-Hispanic women, multiracial women were significantly more likely to have experienced lifetime IPV, whereas Asian women and Hispanic women were significantly less likely to report ever having experienced IPV (21). Women who reported lifetime IPV on the BRFSS were also more likely to have high cholesterol, heart disease, and arthritis as well as risk behaviors including smoking and binge drinking (22). Thus, the BRFSS is useful in obtaining state prevalence rates, but national estimates cannot be determined. In addition, the BRFSS is limited by self-report and recall bias.

The *National Violence Against Women Survey* (NVAWS) was a random-digit-dial telephone survey conducted with 8,000 men and 8,000 women. Validated tools, including the Conflict Tactics Scale and Health Survey Short Form (SF)-36, were used to assess IPV incidence, and past-year and lifetime prevalence. The focus of this survey was on victimization, and was based on self-report. However, unlike most of the other datasets discussed, this survey also included emotional and sexual IPV in their rates. The report found that 22% of women and 7% of men surveyed had been physically assaulted by a partner at some point in their lifetime (1). They also reported that 1.3% of women and 0.9% of men were assaulted by a partner within the past year. Slashinski and colleagues (23) stated that 4.3% of women and 1.2% of men had experienced physical aggression by a dating partner. Other studies using this database have added that physical IPV was associated with an increased risk of poor health, depressive symptoms, and substance use (24). The NVAWS report adds to current knowledge because it is one of the few population-based surveys, and it includes emotional and sexual violence. As with all surveys, this database is limited by recall bias as well as the inability to validate whether or not claims of abuse are true. Finally, this survey was administered once, so changes in rates and in the severity of violence cannot be measured.

Other surveys have been conducted, such as the *National Family Violence Surveys*; however, these surveys are usually conducted at a single point in time and do not allow temporal comparisons. In addition, other hospital databases, such as the *National Hospital Discharge Survey* and the *National Health Interview Survey*, collect information based on ICD and e-coding; therefore they miss the majority of IPV cases and do not collect specific information regarding IPV.

In summary, many datasets are available for estimates of IPV prevalence and incidence rates. However, given the complexities around type of IPV, ongoing IPV, and annual versus lifetime prevalence, a true rate cannot be stated. The CDC recently established guidelines for uniform definitions for IPV surveillance that should help investigators develop standard definitions of IPV (25). Using these definitions in combination with official records for morality (death certificates), records for morbidity (hospital records), and surveys, a more accurate assessment of IPV rates can be conducted.

IMPLICATIONS FOR POLICY, PRACTICE, AND RESEARCH

Policy

- Since the true incidence and prevalence of IPV are still not clear, resources should be directed appropriately to further elucidate the scope of this major health problem.
- Surveillance data should be collected according to national guidelines within every state.
- Hospital discharge data from emergency departments could provide information regarding incidence rates of IPV in this population.

Practice

- Document and record IPV where identified.
- Use standardized terminology and codes such as ICD 10 coding for "adult maltreatment."

Research

- Establish common terminology for reporting incidence and prevalence data for IPV.
- Continue to address the central question: What is the true incidence and prevalence of IPV in the United States?

References

1. Tjaden P, Thoennes N. Full Report of the Prevalence, Incidence, and Consequences of Violence Against Women. Findings from the National Violence Against Women Survey: Research report (NCJ 183781). Washington, DC: National Institute of Justice, 2000.

2. Ahlbom A, Norell S. *Introduction to modern epidemiology*. Chestnut Hill, MA: Epidemiology Resources Inc., 1984.

3. Rothman KJ. *Modern epidemiology*. Boston: Little, Brown and Company, 1986.

4. National Center for Injury Prevention and Control. *CDC injury research agenda*. Atlanta, GA: Centers for Disease Control and Prevention, 2002.

5. Puzone CA, Saltzman LE, Kresnow M, et al. National trends in intimate partner homicide, United States, 1976–1995. *Violence Against Women*. 2000;6: 409–426. Erratum: *Violence Against Women* 2000;6:1179–1184.

6. Kellermann AL, Mercy JA. Men, women, and murder: Gender-specific differences in rates of fatal violence and victimization. *J Trauma*. 1992;82(7): 1018–1020.

7. Paulozzi LJ, Saltzman LE, Thompson MP, et al. Surveillance for homicide among intimate partners: United States, 1981–1988. *MMWR CDC Surveill Summ*. 2001;50(3):1–15.

8. Kochanek KD, Murphy SL, Anderson RN, et al. Deaths: Final data for 2002. *Natl Health Stat Report*. 2004;53(5):1–116.

9. Paulozzi LJ, Mercy J, Frazier Jr., L, et al. CDC's national violence death reporting system: Background and methodology. *Inj Prev*. 2004;10:47–52.

10. Patel N, Webb K, White D, et al. Homicides and suicides: National Violent Death Reporting System, United States, 2003–2004. *MMWR Morb Mortal Wkly Rep*. 2006;55(26):721–724.

11. Bossarte RM, Simon TR, Barker L. Characteristics of homicide followed by suicide incidents in multiple states, 2003–2004. *Inj Prev*. 2006;12(Suppl 2): ii33–ii38.

12. Saltzman LE, Mercy JA, Rhodes PH. Identification of nonfatal family and intimate assault incidents in police data. *Am J Pub Health*. 1992;82(6):1018–1020.

13. Thompson MP, Saltzman LE, Bibel D. Applying NIBRS data to the study of intimate partner violence: Massachusetts as a case study. *J Quant Crim*. 1999;15(2):163–180.

14. Pattavina A, Hirschel D, Buzawa E, et al. A comparison of the police response to heterosexual versus same-sex intimate partner violence. *Violence Against Women*. 2007;13(4):374–394.

15. Rennison CM. Intimate partner violence, 1993–2001. Washington, DC: Bureau of Justice Statistics;2003:NCJ 197838.

16. Gallagher CA. Injury recurrence among untreated and medically treated victims of violence in the USA. *Soc Sci Med*. 2005;60(3):627–635.

17. Thompson MP, Simon TR, Saltzman LE, Mercy JA. Epidemiology of injuries among women after physical assaults: The role of self-protective behaviors. *Am J Epidemiol*. 1999;150(3)235–244.

18. Rovi S, Johnson MS. Physician use of diagnostic codes for child and adult abuse. *J Am Med Womens Assoc*. 1999;54(4):211–214.

19. Abbott J, Johnson R, Koziol-McLain J, Lowenstein SR. Domestic violence against women. Incidence and prevalence in an emergency department population. *JAMA*. 1995;273(22):1763–1767.
20. Rand MR, Strom K. Violence-related injuries treated in hospital emergency departments. Washington, DC: Bureau of Justice Statistics;1997:NCJ 156921.
21. Breiding MJ, Black MC, Ryan GW. Prevalence and risk factors of intimate partner violence in eighteen US states/territories, 2005. *Am J Prev Med*. 2008;34(2):112–118.
22. Black MC, Breiding MJ. Adverse health conditions and health risk behaviors associated with intimate partner violence: United States, 2005. *MMWR Morb Mortal Wkly Rep*. 2008;57(5):113–117.
23. Slashinski MJ, Coker AL, Davis KE. Physical aggression, forced sex, and stalking victimization by a dating partner: An analysis of the National Violence Against Women Survey. *Violence Vict*. 2003;18(6):595–617.
24. Coker AL, Davis KE, Arias I, et al. Physical and mental health effects of intimate partner violence for men and women. *Am J Prev Med*. 2002;23(4): 260–268.
25. Saltzman LE, Fanslow JL, McMahon PM, Shelley GA. *Intimate partner violence surveillance: Uniform definitions and recommended data elements*, Version 1.0. Atlanta: National Center for Injury Prevention and Control, Centers for Disease Prevention and Control, 1999.

Chapter 4

Explanatory Frameworks of Intimate Partner Violence

Connie Mitchell and Magdalena Vanya

KEY CONCEPTS

- Although the family is often imagined as a "haven in a heartless world," women and children are more likely to be hurt or killed by someone they live with than by a stranger on the street.
- The cultural pressure to perpetuate the loving family ideal in "front stage" contributes to the fact that intimate partner violence (IPV) frequently remains concealed from the public audience in the family's "back stage" for a long time.
- According to Goffman's *typology of stigmas*, living in a violent relationship would fall into the category of "blemishes of individual character," and therefore victims of spouse abuse are often seen as having a personal flaw or a deviant trait.
- Five explanatory frameworks exist: the psychological, the biobehavioral, the sociological, feminist theory, and an integrative

multidimensional approach. It is unlikely that IPV can be explained by any single theory and therefore theory-based interventions will also be diverse.
- Ongoing interpersonal dynamics have been described as cyclical in nature, as motivated by the need to control, as domestic terrorism, or as couple conflict, thus demonstrating that the interactions in abusive relationships can take many forms.

From the rise of industrialization, when people started to migrate to big cities for work in the factories, the family has been imagined as a "haven in a heartless world," a safe and protective shelter from the dangers of the public world (1). Intimate partner violence (IPV) challenges this long-held notion by highlighting the family home as a possibly more dangerous place than the street. Family violence accounts for about 1 in 10 violent victimizations (2). Nearly 25% of women and 7.6% of men were raped and/or physically assaulted by an intimate at some point in their lifetime (3). A survey of public attitudes conducted in the mid-1990s found that domestic violence preceded street crime, child poverty, and teenage pregnancy as the most pressing societal issue in the United States, which reveals the magnitude of change in public perceptions of the issue since the 1960s (4).

Nevertheless, despite widespread scholarly and media attention, intimate partner violence remains a delicate subject for discussion. The continuing social and cultural taboo surrounding intimate partner abuse complicates not only public forums, but also the introduction of effective professional approaches. In this chapter, we review the general theoretical explanations for the stigmatized nature, sources, causes, and expression of IPV in the contemporary United States, to provide the health professional with a framework for understanding this complex issue.

Gelles and Straus (5), the first to conduct a nationally representative survey on the extent and nature of spouse abuse in the United States, list seven myths commonly associated with IPV: (1) IPV is rare or it is epidemic (thus indicating our difficulties with measurement and surveillance); (2) abusers are aliens, victims are innocents (dichotomies seem easier to grasp and comprehend); (3) abuse is confined to poor, minority families (attributing it to "others" as a way of avoiding a complex issue or a way to avoid anxiety of proximity); (4) alcohol and drugs are the real problem (a variation of #3); (5) children who are abused grow up to be abusers (we tend to focus on risks and not learn enough about resiliency); (6) battered women like being hit (thank you, Dr. Freud); and (7) violence and love are incompatible (this is what makes IPV so insidious; the fact that the abused and the abuser are so tightly connected). Great progress has been made over the last two decades to debunk these myths by marshalling evidence from a range of disciplines, most of which is reviewed extensively in other chapters of this book.

REALITY AND ILLUSION REGARDING FAMILY DYNAMICS

When compared to other types of violence, the main distinctive characteristic of IPV is the private nature of its occurrence, defined by the intimate relationship between the victim and perpetrator and the location of violent behavior. The cultural pressure to perpetuate the loving family ideal in the "front stage" contributes to the fact that IPV frequently remains concealed from the public audience in the "back stage" of the family for a long time. The front stage of social life often serves as the setting "where illusions and impressions are fabricated" just to meet the cultural standard of caring and adoring spouses (6). Conversely, the back stage can be viewed as the repository of the "secrets of a show" that insiders strive to keep concealed from the audience of outsiders (6). The rigid boundary between the front and back stage is maintained by both insiders (the victim and the perpetrator or other family members) and outsiders (non–family members). Victims and perpetrators of spouse abuse work hard to avoid publicly contradicting the cultural expectations of the family as a peaceful retreat, while outsiders' shock, disbelief, or discomfort, after learning about partner abuse, fortifies the stigma attached to private violence.

THE ROLE OF STIGMA IN INTIMATE PARTNER VIOLENCE

Goffman's (7) definition of stigma as "[a]n attribute that is deeply discrediting within a particular social interaction" helps us understand many victims' efforts to keep their "dirty secret" within the bounds of their family's or relationship's back stage. Since U.S. culture remains rather resistant to viewing the family as a possible place of conflict and tension, victim-blaming attitudes (a form of the devaluing and discrediting reactions that Goffman associated with stigma in general) are still common regarding IPV. In Goffman's *typology of stigmas*, living in a violent relationship falls into the category of "blemishes of individual character" (7), as victims of spouse abuse are often seen as having a personal flaw or a deviant trait. Just like a person with a disease, victims of IPV are sometimes seen by the public as responsible for the violence inflicted upon them. Such victim-blaming attitudes are generally combined with the public's lack of understanding of the complex dynamics of violence in relationships.

EXPLANATORY FRAMEWORK: PSYCHOLOGICAL

Early Victim-blaming Theories

Until the 1960s, psychoanalytical theories individualized and pathologized violent incidents between married couples as the outcome of maladjusted individual personalities, and usually they directly or indirectly blamed women for the violence of their husbands (8). These accounts invested women clients with deviant, typically masochistic, personality traits (9).

Frustration-Aggression Theory

Frustration-aggression Theory was first described in 1939 by Dollard, who proposed frustration as a precursor to aggression. Frustration can provoke a variety of responses, but in some individuals, the response is anger/aggression. However, his hypothesis was attacked for failing to differentiate justified versus nonjustified frustration. Berkowitz later reformulated the theory to define aggression as the link between unpleasant stimuli and negative affect that triggers a "fight or flight" response. Berkowitz's theory has been criticized as being oversimplistic, and aggression has been redefined as a reaction calculated to manipulate a specific benefit. Relative to IPV, marital/dating frustrations can trigger anger (justified frustration) or aggression (unjustified frustration). Since the frustration is unjustified, it is postulated that the aggression is intended to manipulate a desired outcome (10,11).

Social Learning Theory

Learning theory advocates totally reject the aggression-as-instinct theory and instead ask "if aggression is innate, why aren't all societies and all individuals aggressive?" Albert Bandura instead proposed that "Human aggression is a learned conduct that, like other forms of social behavior, is under stimulus, reinforcement, and cognitive control" (12). The general appeal of the Social Learning Theory is that if aggression is learned, then nonaggressive responses to behavior can also be learned. What is not clear is whether aggression can be "unlearned."

Cognitive-Behavioral Theories

In this framework, aggressive behavior is a product of aggressive thoughts that are in turn "scripted" or learned in early development (13). The scripts are encoded at a young age and later retrieved in response to triggering events (14,15). In this model, five cognitive steps operate sequentially: (1) encoding, (2) interpretation, (3) response search, (4) response decision, and (5) enactment (16). Aggressive persons recruit fewer environmental cues to help interpret an event, and so the event is interpreted as hostile; because the response search is also narrowed, aggression is selected (13). Interventions, then, would be directed to widening the information processing process and expanding the choices for response.

EXPLANATORY FRAMEWORK: BIOBEHAVIORAL INFLUENCES

Genetic

Genes don't code directly for violence perpetration but do code for personality traits and cognitive styles that are associated with violence. Some evidence from twin studies supports the heritability of antisocial behavior, but evidence for a genetic basis of violent offending is weaker (17). Two major streams of research using twin and adoption studies examine for aggression and predictors of juvenile delinquency. The conclusions are: (a) a trend points toward a genetic effect on adult and adolescent antisocial behavior; (b) evidence for a genetic effect in offenses related to aggression is weak; (c) evidence exists for a genetic association between antisocial behavior and alcohol abuse; and (d) in adoption studies, an urban environment predicted adoptee criminal behavior independent of genetic background.

Neurochemical Mechanisms

The reader is referred to the extensive review of the National Research Council on biobehavioral influences on violence and violent behavior (17); a few key summary statements follow. Androgens can influence aggressive behavior but the strength of the association appears to decrease in more complex social animals. However, external factors can also alter hormonal levels (e.g., stress decreases testosterone and achievement/winning increases testosterone levels). Although medications to control violence act principally at dopamine receptors, there does not appear to be a marker for dopamine activity that is specific to violent or aggressive behavior. Although norepinephrine levels are correlated with arousal and either positive or negative affect, as well as adrenergic "flight or fight" readiness, increased levels are not associated with a specific behavior, such as a violent act. Drugs that target serotonin receptors seem to specifically target several types of aggressive behaviors. Violent acts have been linked to certain hallucinogens that act at distinct serotonin receptors. γ-aminobutyric acid (GABA) is present in 30% of all brain synapses but has been found to have inhibitory as well as excitatory influences on behavior.

EXPLANATORY FRAMEWORK: FEMINIST THEORY

Feminist theories explain IPV as a result of a "historically created gender hierarchy and sexual division of labor in the home, by which men dominate and control women" (18). Accordingly, IPV is seen as a mechanism of domination and control used by men over women.

The feminist perspective aims at raising public awareness of the seriousness of the problem of violence against women, including IPV directed against women, while deconstructing the idyllic image of the traditional, peaceful family. The attribute "feminist" implies a fundamental objective to challenge existing social conditions and change them by naming the unspoken. The feminist approach is related to the sociological one, to the extent that it considers social factors in addition to the personal histories of the involved people, but with the objective of achieving social change (9,19).

The feminist perspective emphasizes culturally constructed gender categories and the unequal power struggles these categories engender. Central to this approach is a reexamination of the institution of family and its contestation. Another imperative of a feminist approach is to create a wider arena for the expression of women's experiences, thus challenging the "male-constructed understandings of women, abuse, and intimate relationships" (20). Finally, feminist perspectives on wife abuse go beyond the description and explanation of violence; their main purpose is to change women's actual situations and eliminate violence against women (19).

Feminist research on domestic violence distinguishes itself by conducting social action research aimed at social change (20,21). Although many feminist researchers challenged the quantitative findings of Straus and Gelles for ignoring the difference between violence in an attack versus violence in self-defense, feminists embraced the overall conclusions of Straus and Gelles that accentuated the significance of social structure in understanding domestic violence and repudiating individualistic, pathologizing explana-

tions of spousal abuse (22).[1] Some of the most important sociological claims endorsed by feminist scholars of domestic violence link family violence to the ubiquity of street and media violence in the United States, the endurance of capital punishment, and the common occurrence of economic stress or professional failure, as well as men's dominance (23,24).

Both sociological and feminist accounts approach the institution of the family similarly, as a site of conflict in which often opposing emotions prevail. Consequently, both sociological and explicitly feminist studies of domestic violence view the family as a more dangerous place than the public streets—the prototypical domain of crime in U.S. popular discourse. However, the feminist perspective underscores culturally constructed gender roles intertwined with complex ramifications of power, and it advocates for social research that challenges and transforms existing patriarchal social conditions.

Living Without Fear of Violence as a Human Right

The recently developed human rights approach, motivated by the feminist vision, attempts to raise awareness of domestic violence as a human rights issue. Thomas and Beasley (25) claim that domestic violence cases are often ignored by state authorities and their prosecution is often suspended, thus providing for the inadequate protection of female victims abused behind the closed doors of private domain while perpetrators are not convicted. The human rights approach to domestic violence argues for prioritizing the right to a safe and healthy life through state protection from violence over the right to privacy, which is often used by authorities across the world as an argument against state intervention in domestic "disputes."

EXPLANATORY FRAMEWORK: SOCIOLOGICAL APPROACHES

The sociological approach focuses on macro-social factors, such as norms and cultural expectations, as well

---

[1] Straus and Gelles, in their repeated study in 1985, decided to include some dimension of purpose through additional questions on the motivation and aftermath of the violent incident. The sample this time consisted of 6,002 couples (Gelles, 1993).

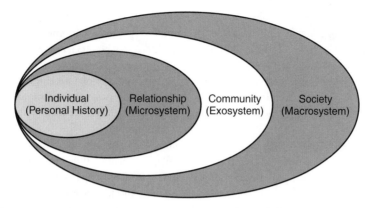

Figure 4.1 The social ecology model. Heise LL. *Violence against women: An integrated, ecological framework.* Violence Against Women. Adapted and reproduced with permission of Sage Publications.1998;4(3): 262–290.

as power structures within and outside the family (21). The institution of family is not treated as harmonic, but instead as a site of contestation where often controversial emotions can prevail. In addition, sociological theories transcend the individualizing approach of early psychological theories by emphasizing the effect of social, cultural, and economic context on violence in the family (26–28).

The first sociological approach to violence in the family was Goode's resource theory. According to Goode, violence between couples is used as the final instrument to take control of one's life and others' actions after all other potential resources, such as prestige or economic resources, have been exhausted or removed (28).

As a result of the growing public visibility of the issue, more sociologists became interested in assessing the extent and nature of domestic violence as well. In 1975, Straus (29) and Gelles (27) conducted the first representative study on family violence in the United States, including the dimension of wife abuse.[2] They correlated domestic violence with households below the poverty line, racial minority households, and heads of households being 18–30 years of age. These characteristics produce high levels of social stress, a common triggering mechanism of domestic violence. Additionally, sociologists report domestic violence in white middle- or upper-class families to be much more socially sheltered and less reported than in lower-class families (27). Middle- and upper-class victims of domestic violence can take advantage of their financial and social resources before contacting the police or calling a crisis line for shelter referrals.

EXPLANATORY FRAMEWORK: AN INTEGRATIVE MULTIDIMENSIONAL APPROACH

No single theoretical construct may sufficiently explain IPV, and contributory factors may operate on multiple levels, some to a greater degree than others, but multidimensionally nonetheless (29). A multidimensional approach was proposed by Bronfenbrenner (30) and Belskey (31) and then later applied by theorists to IPV (32,33).

Belsky's explanatory framework consists of four nested layers that emphasize the interaction and dynamic interplay between factors operating on multiple levels (Figure 4.1):

- *Individual*: The personal biological, experiential, or ontogenic profile that the individual brings to relationships
- *Family or primary relationships*: A microsystem of communication, interaction, and close contact
- *Community*: The exosystem that encompasses institutions, services, and proximal social structures (neighborhood, peer group) surrounding the relationship
- *Society*: The macrosystem that establishes policy, laws, cultural norms, attitudes, and biases

---

[2] The sample consisted of 2,143 married and cohabiting couples.

In 1998, Heise used the social ecology model as a framework for synthesizing available knowledge on the etiology of and risk factors for IPV (34). This model is further strengthened in that both factors associated with perpetration and/or victimization can be incorporated. A few examples of etiologic factors are described for each layer of the model in Table 4.1.

The Social Ecology Model for IPV is a valuable explanatory framework. By providing a model for identifying all possible variables for perpetration of IPV, matched sets of perpetrators can be analyzed to see which variables account for the most variance. The framework can operate on a case-by-case basis to determine the factors contributing to the violence and possible points of intervention. The model helps to explain the complexity of the issue, that different factors can play a different role in each case, and that risk factors can exist without IPV occurring until a tipping point is reached—that one last event that implodes the individual and the relationship.

Since it is likely that no single factor is the sole cause of one person's violent or aggressive behavior to another, then it follows that no single intervention or prevention tactic is likely to be successful. Bronfenbrenner contended that any successful interventions must not only be positive in and of themselves but must create "supportive linkages" between them (78). Multidisciplinary community organizations can examine the tactics and services available to address each level of the model and furthermore define the tactic as primary, secondary, or tertiary prevention (Table 4.2). Communities can use the model to identify strengths or gaps in services and move from shorter-term impact of tertiary prevention approaches to longer-term impact of primary prevention.

Table 4.1 Using the Social Ecology Model to Sort Factors Associated with IPV

Individual

- Genetic liability (35)
- Impaired neuropsychological mechanisms (36)
- Witnessing marital violence as a child (37–41)
- Experiencing physical or sexual abuse as a child (37,42)
- Absence of a consistent and available father as a risk for violent behavior in adults (43,44)
- Alcohol as a disinhibitor (45–48)
- Stimulant use (49–51)
- Individual psychopathology, personality deviance, attachment style (52,53)

Family or primary relationships (microsystem)

- Male dominance in economic issues and decision making (54–56)
- Wife is economically dependent on husband (57)
- Husband exhibits high interpersonal dependency on wife (58)

Community (exosystem)

- Lower socioeconomic status and unemployment (57)
- Social isolation of victim and/or family (59)
- Delinquent peer associations that encourage violence (60–62)
- Availability and ease of access to alcohol (63–65)
- Availability and ease of access to firearms (66)

Society (macrosystem)

- Socioeconomic factors (67–69)
- Cultural constructs of masculinity and femininity (54,70–72)
- Laws that describe wives as property (73,74)
- Laws or cultural practices that approve of physical chastisement of women (73)
- Male aggression as a cultural norm (75–77)

Social Ecology Model	Primary Prevention: (so that it never occurs)	Secondary Prevention: (so that it doesn't occur again)	Tertiary Prevention: (so that this episode doesn't get worse and function is restored)
Individual	Programs to promote maternal child bonding Healthy stress and coping strategies Education and job training Promotion of resiliency, "salutogenesis" Impulse control models in classrooms	Education/training for economic dependence of victims Routine assessment for prior to exposure in health care Relocation assistance Counseling for children exposed to IPV Foster placement	Safe houses for victims Mandatory reporting Mandatory arrest Mild traumatic brain injury intervention protocols Posttraumatic stress disorder (PTSD) prevention protocols
Family/ relationship	Promotion of empathy, cooperative learning, and group problem-solving in schools Home nurse visitation with monitoring and skills training Conflict resolution education Parenting skills training Mentoring programs for young boys	Batterer's intervention Supervised visitation of IPV perpetrators with children	Emergency protective orders Mandatory detention/separation post arrest
Community	Public education campaigns on risks of violence and constructs of healthy relationships	Danger assessments and safety planning Peer support groups Fatality review teams Substance abuse services Mental health services Access to providers in rural areas Neighborhood watch groups trained to address IPV	Multidisciplinary crises intervention teams
Society	Egalitarian policies in government Faith-based efforts to promote egalitarianism Decreasing poverty and desperation Media messages that unlink masculinity from dominance and aggression	Destigmatize with public awareness campaigns Laws that prevent insurance or employment discrimination against victims	Removing guns in IPV home Increased barriers to firearm access by IPV perpetrators

Table 4.2 Social Ecology Model for Intimate Partner Violence Applied to Prevention Strategies

INTERPERSONAL DYNAMICS

Although not an explanatory framework for the etiology of IPV, an understanding of ongoing interpersonal dynamics is helpful, as relationships are fluid and potentially explosive.

Abuse of Power to Control

Based on case histories, IPV perpetrators use coercion, threats, or intimidation that focuses on their victim's particular vulnerabilities, such as their own personal welfare or that of their children or other loved ones. Control can be imposed through physical, social, or economic isolation that deprives the victim of social support, alternate viewpoints, or independence. Through psychological tactics, the IPV perpetrator will denigrate, humiliate, or deny the victim's perceptions, such that the victim loses all confidence in her or his ability to think, process, or problem-solve. Physical or sexual violence or threats of violence to the victim, loved ones, or cherished objects achieves control through the use of fear, physical dominance, pain, or torture.

According to power motivation theory, and first conceptualized by McClelland, all of these behaviors are used to assert or maintain power within a relationship, particularly the power to be victorious in confrontation (79). In 1987, Dutton and Strachan (80) hypothesized that men who view intimacy with women as threatening will resort to violence as a means of controlling their partners and thus reduce their own anxiety and anger. Prince and Arias (81) further suggested that assaultive men may have high self-esteem but have a poor sense of control over their lives; these men use violence as a way of gaining control. According to Browning and Dutton (82), the men they studied perceived an impending loss of control as their partners attempted either greater autonomy or, in the reverse, greater intimacy, and they became physically aggressive to restore the balance of power and control.

Cycle of Violence

Lenore Walker (83) described a pattern of interaction based on three phases: (a) tension-building leading to (b) an abusive event that was followed by (c) remorse and renewed hope. The periods of relative calm could be long or short, but gradually tensions within the relationship escalate, culminating in another act of violence or abuse. The underlying theory for Walker's work is traumatic bonding and intermittent reinforcement. *Traumatic bonding* is defined as the formation of strong emotional ties between two individuals, one of whom intermittently harasses, beats, threatens, abuses, or intimidates the other (84). The intermittent nature of the violence is critical to traumatic bonding.

Walker's classic work *The Battered Woman* (85) represented a turning point in domestic violence literature. The abundant use of qualitative data in the form of interviews and life stories in the book allowed Walker to dispel the myth of provocative, self-indulgent wives perpetuated by many psychologists in the 1950s (21). Although her approach and findings contested earlier psychopathological explanations of domestic violence, Walker never transcends the realm of individual psychology, and her analysis elides discussions of socio-cultural factors, central to subsequent feminist and sociological perspectives on domestic violence.

Many feminist scholars critique Walker's conceptualization of the cycle of violence for its exclusively individualistic approach, which preempts a systemic analysis of domestic violence, thus reinforcing dominant gender relations. Similarly, Heberle (86) finds the concept of the cycle of violence inadequate in addressing the different experiences of battered women with diverse social locations, particularly after they start dealing with the police, the justice system, and/or the social service system. She suggests using the *web of effects* instead of the cycle of violence in order to dislodge the various individualizing, pathologizing, as well as paternalizing effects of these systems not addressed by the cycle of violence. Heberle argues that, by using the web of effects framework, we can imbue victims of domestic violence with more agency because we redirect the attention from helpless victim to active survivor, who must then negotiate the "effects" of multiple systems. Moreover, Heberle claims that the web of effects can reveal the racializing and classing effects of these systems because it examines how domestic violence victims experience the court or welfare system differently based on their class and/or racial background. Walker's cycle of violence, concludes Heberle, has limited explanatory power because it homogenizes battered women's experiences into a singular psychological profile.

Nevertheless, by the 1980s, the language of *learned helplessness* and the cycle of violence have quickly diffused from battered women's shelters to the more formal organizations of law enforcement and social services. The success of Walker's psychological theory among justice and mental health professionals was due to the persistent endeavors of feminist activists to access and train various professional groups about the psychology of battered women and thereby challenge the stereotypical, victim-blaming images of them.

Are There Two Sides to the Coin?

Some scholars distinguish two types of IPV: patriarchal terrorism and common couple violence. *Patriarchal terrorism* refers to systematic, severe bouts of physical aggression used by male batterers as a means of controlling their female victims. In contrast, common couple violence is used to indicate occasional, minor, violent incidents instigated by either the husband or the wife (87). Johnson believes that during verbal arguments, some partners can attack one another in ways that diminish self-esteem, create feelings of vulnerability, and promote fears of rejection and abandonment. In his model, either partner may escalate the attacks until one partner feels so overwhelmed and vulnerable that he or she reacts violently. He refers to this as *common couple violence* and, as the name implies, it is more widespread in U.S. families than patriarchal terrorism. He further defines couple violence as a response to the occasional conflicts of everyday life motivated by the need to control a specific situation. In contrast, patriarchal terrorism refers to a more general need to control the relationship by any means necessary. Patriarchal terrorism escalates whereas couple violence may not.

Johnson later expanded his model to four typologies based on the level of dyadic control (88):

1. *Intimate terrorism*: The abuser is violent and very controlling
2. *Violent resistance*: The abuser is violent and controlling, but the other partner is also violent but not controlling
3. *Situational couple violence*: One partner is violent while the other is not
4. *Mutual violent control*: Both persons are violent and very controlling

Considerable controversy has surrounded the question of whether husbands and wives inflict IPV in equal measure. According to the First National Family Violence Survey conducted in 1976, wives and husbands engage in almost equal proportions of physical aggression. Women actually reported higher rates of IPV than men (89). The debate around the possible gender symmetry of IPV became especially heated when a sociologist—relying on data from the first representative family violence survey—coined the term *battered husband syndrome* (90). From his analysis of prevalence and survey data, Johnson concludes that situational couple violence dominates in general survey responses, whereas intimate terrorism and violent resistance dominate in population data that is shelter- or agency-based. He contends that his model accounts for gender symmetry in IPV in some studies. Johnson cautions that all forms of IPV can be dangerous and impact the short- and long-term health and safety of women. These differences are most important when designing interventions. Klostermann and Fals-Stewart argue (91) that effective intervention is often hampered by professionals' and community organizations' failure to distinguish between these types while treating IPV.

Stockholm Syndrome

When considering domestic terrorism, one can conceptualize the IPV victim as hostage. Graham (92) wanted to know why some hostage victims appear so defensive and even attached to their captors. He identified a composite of behaviors that he named after a bank robbery with hostages that occurred in Stockholm, Sweden, in which the hostages seemed to be remarkably aligned with their captors. A hostage experiencing Stockholm syndrome will be hypervigilant to their captor's needs, find it difficult to leave or attempt escape from the captor, and fear the captor will come back and find the hostage even if escape does occur. Hostages are more likely to manifest the syndrome in scenarios in which the hostages believe their survival is threatened, they have been shown some small kindness by their captor, they are isolated from any views other than those of their captor, and they believe they have no escape. In 1995, Graham expanded Stockholm syndrome to some cases of IPV as a means of describing the attachment of victims to their abusers despite continued physical abuse (93). An IPV victim may appear suspicious of anyone trying to help, remain allied with the abuser, appear grateful for any acts of kindness, and may even attribute these acts of kindness to the underlying goodness and benevolence of the abusive captor partner.

Process of Change

The Transtheoretical Model describes five major stages in the process of change (94–96) and has been successfully applied to health problems of substance abuse, tobacco addiction, and obesity (97). The cycle might be repeated various times with slight variations before the change is manifested and maintained over time. The model does not translate well when applied to IPV, because IPV does not have a single variable outcome, such as stopping smoking, and the problem involves at least two people. So, the process of a victim trying to change to feel more safe and secure will be heavily influenced by the actions or inactions of the abusive partner (98,99). If IPV is thought of more from the perspective of a chronic disease with occasional flare up, however, the Transtheoretical Model provides a structure for creating an intervention plan for each step over time and for measuring outcomes of care (100).

Although some believe the model may prove useful in facilitating and measuring change in IPV victims, the model may also help explain interpersonal dynamics in IPV relationships. During the *pre-contemplation stage*, the victim may be able to identify the problem but doesn't see the potential or need for change. The victim may be ashamed, isolated, depressed, or numb, and there are neither questions asked of nor behavioral challenges made to the partner. During the *contemplation stage*, as the victim seeks clarification of the issue and understanding of possible alternatives, there may be more anger, confusion, and questioning, possibly provoking turmoil and increasing tension in the relationship and anxiety in the abuser. In the *preparation stage*, the victim has greater clarity, attempts practical problem-solving, and often prepares and practices new behaviors or strategies. The partner may observe the new behaviors or verbalized insight and perceive them as threatening; and then augments activities to suppress or control. In the *action stage*, the victim risks a concrete step toward change, whether it is confrontation, calling police, seeking a protective order, counseling, or packing a bag to leave. The perpetrator, if aware of these actions, could take action too by seeking help, retaliating, withdrawing, or increasing efforts to control. In the fifth, but often not final, phase of *maintenance*, some victims may experience elation at success while others express relief, sadness, or self-doubt that may expose vulnerabilities and lead to another phase of pre-contemplation as opposed to permanent healing.

CONCLUSION

Just as we attempt to unravel the mystery of the abusive relationship so must we endeavor to comprehend and elucidate the tenants of healthy relationships. For every hour spent on recognition and risk reduction of IPV, more time should be devoted to promoting behaviors associated with nurturing interactions such as shared decision-making, mutual trust, mutual regard for autonomy, and effective negotiation and communication skills. Emotional intimacy requires a certain vulnerability that is treasured and protected in healthy relationships and exposed and violated in unhealthy ones.

But IPV does not simply occur as a relationship unravels. Its roots are usually far more insidious and complex, with forces operating at the individual, familial, community, and societal levels. Both physiologic and psychological influences may be present; then, the complexity is squared because IPV involves at least two people. Layered onto the complexity is both stigma and taboo, which impedes our efforts to gain clarity. The Social Ecology Model appears to be a helpful construct for sorting through the complexity, and it can be adapted to a variety of power dynamics. The model provides direction without being excessively reductionistic.

Intimate partner violence is unacceptable, because it erodes the health of individuals, families, and communities, but it can be understood. The explanations for the human potential for violence are vast and a review of the research has filled volumes (13,17,58). The framework presented here provides a structure upon which further research and understanding about the etiology and dynamics of IPV can be built.

IMPLICATIONS FOR POLICY, PRACTICE, AND RESEARCH

Policy

- A need exists to expand beyond a one-size-fits-all approach to IPV interventions, and more attention should be devoted to the assessment of the victim, perpetrator, and family dynamics to ascertain how best to proceed. However, the first priority for any assessment and intervention is to provide for the immediate health and safety needs of the family.
- Despite its complexity, some intervention research suggests that widespread programs could be introduced to children to facilitate cognitive processing of events that lead to non-aggressive reaction choices. In addition, efforts to identify aggressive children and provide ameliorative intervention to children, parents, and families may also prove to be helpful.

Practice

- The reality that IPV is complex in its etiology means that its intervention will be equally complex. Some practitioners may feel equipped to address the short and long-term needs of families. However, most practitioners welcome specialty consultation services and on-site clinic or hospital programs, partnering with community agencies to assess and manage the care needs of the IPV victim.

- Clinicians must be alert to signs of aggression in children and provide early assessment and intervention.

Research

- Additional research on the typologies of IPV may better inform intervention strategies.
- The Transtheoretical Model may provide a structure for IPV intervention and measurement of outcomes but will need to be tested in a variety of settings. However, the model may be limited in that change in an abusive relationship, by definition, includes change in more than one person.
- It must be determined if the typologies of IPV are accurate and helpful in defining appropriate responses and in designing intervention studies.
- Studies must be undertaken to determine if intervention programs that target aggressive children impact the rates of IPV.

References

1. McClelland D. *The inner experience.* New York: Irvington Publishers; 1975.
2. Durose MR, Harlow CW, Langan PA, Motivans M, Tantala RR, Smith EL. *Family violence statistics: Including statistics on strangers and acquaintances:* US Department of Justice Statistics; 2005.
3. Tjaden P, Thoennes N. *Extent, nature, and consequences of intimate partner violence.* Washington, D.C.: U.S. Department of Justice; 2000.
4. Klein E. *Ending domestic violence: Changing public perceptions, halting the epidemic.* Thousand Oaks: Sage Publications; 1997.
5. Gelles RJ, Straus MA. *Intimate violence.* New York: Simon and Schuster; 1988.
6. Goffman E. *The presentation of self in everyday life.* New York: Doubleday; 1959.
7. Goffman E. *Stigma: Notes on the management of spoiled identity.* Englewood Cliffs, New Jersey: Prentice-Hall; 1963.
8. Kirkwood C. *Leaving abusive partners: From the scars of survival to the wisdom for change.* London: Sage Publications; 1993.
9. Hyden M. *Woman battering as marital act: The construction of a violent marriage.* Oslo: Scandinavian University Press; 1994.
10. Dollard J, Doob LW, Miller NE, Mowrer O, Sears RR. *Frustration and aggression.* New Haven: Yale University Press; 1939.
11. Berkowitz L. The Frustration-Aggression Hypothesis. In: Falk R, Kim S, eds. *The war system: An interdisciplinary approach.* Boulder, CO: Westview Press; 1980.
12. Bandura A. The Social Learning Theory of Aggression. In: Falk R, Kim S, eds. *The war system: An interdisciplinary approach.* Boulder, CO: Westview Press; 1980.
13. Reiss AJ RJ. *Understanding and preventing violence.* Vol 1. Washington D.C.: National Academy Press; 1993.
14. Huesmann L, Enron L. Cognitive processes and the persistence of aggressive behavior. *Aggressive Behav.* 1984;10:243–251.
15. Huesmann L, Eron L. Individual differences and the trait of aggression. *Eur J Personal.* 1989;3:95–106.
16. Dodge K. A social information processing model of social competence in children. In: Perlmutter M, ed. *Minnesota symposium in child psychology.* Vol 18. Hillsdale, NJ: Erlbaum; 1986:77–125.
17. Reiss AJ MK, Roth JA. *Biobehavioral influences.* Vol 2. Washington DC: National Academy Press; 1994.
18. Messerschmidt JW. *Capitalism, patriarchy, and crime: Toward a socialist feminist criminology.* Totowa, J.J.: Rowman and Littlefield; 1986.
19. Bograd M. Family systems approaches to wife battering: a feminist critique. *Am J Orthopsychiatry.* 1984;54(4):558–568.
20. Bograd ML. Feminist Perspectives on Wife Abuse. In: Bograd ML, Yllo K, eds. *Feminist perspectives on wife abuse.* Newbury Park.: Sage Publications; 1988:11–26.
21. Hydén M. *Woman battering as marital act: The construction of a violent marriage.* Oslo: Scandinavian University Press 1994.
22. Kurz D. Social science perspectives on wife abuse: Current debates and future directions. *Gender and Society.* December 1989;3(4).
23. Hughes HM. Research concerning children of battered women: Clinical implications. In: Gefffner K SS, Lundberg-Love PK, ed. *Violence and sexual abuse at home: Current issues in spousal battering and child maltreatment.* Haworth Press, Inc.; 1997:2225–2244.
24. Gelles RJ, Loseke DR. *Current controversies on family violence.* London: Sage Publications; 1993.
25. Thomas DQ, Beasley ME. Domestic violence as a human rights issue. *Human Rights Quarterly.* 1993;15:36–61.
26. Denzin N. Toward a phenomenology of domestic, family violence. *Am J Sociol.* November 1984;90:482–511.
27. Strauss M, Gelles R. Societal change and change in family violence from 1975 to 1985 as revealed by two national surveys. *J Marriage Fam.* 1986;48:465–479.
28. Goode WJ. Force and Violence in the Family. *J Marriage Fam.* 1971(33):624–636.
29. Crowell NA BA. *Understanding violence against women.* Washington DV: National Academy Press; 1996.
30. Bronfenbrenner U. *The ecology of human development: Experiments by nature and design.* Cambridge, MA: Harvard University Press; 1979.
31. Belsky J. Child maltreatment: An ecological integration. *Am Psychol.* 1980;35(4):320–335.

32. Edleson JL, Toman RM. Intervention for men who batter: An ecological approach; Thousand Oaks CA: Sage, 1992.

33. Dutton D. An ecologically nested theory of male violence toward intimates. *Internatl J Womens Studies.* 1985;8(4):404–413.

34. Heise LL. Violence Against women: An integrated, ecological framework. *Violence Against Women.* June 1998;4(3):262–290.

35. Hines DA, Saudino KJ. Intergenerational Transmission of Intimate Partner Violence: A Behavioral Genetic Perspective. *Trauma Violence Abuse.* July 1, 2002 2002;3(3):210–225.

36. Cohen R, Rosenbaum A, Kane R. Neuropsychological correlates of domestic violence. *Violence and Victims.* 1999;14:397–411.

37. Hotaling GT, Sugarman DB. A Risk Marker Analysis of Assaulted Wives. *Journal of Family Violence.* 1990;5(1):1–13.

38. Caesar PL. Exposure to violence in the families-of-origin among wife-abusers and maritally nonviolent men. *Violence Vict.* Spring 1988;3(1):49–63.

39. Ehrensaft MK, Cohen P, Brown J, Smailes E, Chen H, Johnson JG. Intergenerational transmission of partner violence: a 20-year prospective study. *J Consult Clin Psychol.* Aug 2003;71(4):741–753.

40. Coker A, Smith P, McKeown R, King M. Frequency and correlates of intimate partner violence by type: Physical, sexual and psychological battering. *American Journal of Public Health.* 2000;90(4):553–559.

41. Whitfield C, Anda R, Dube S, Felitti V. Violent childhood experiences and the risk of intimate partner violence in adults: Assessment in a lare health maintenance organization. *Journal of Interpersonal Violence.* 2003;18(2):166–185.

42. Hotaling GT, Sugarman DB. An Analysis of Risk Markers in Husband to Wife Violence: The Current State of Knowledge. *Violence and Victims.* 1986;1(2):1986.

43. Aldridge ML, Browne KD. Perpetrators of spousal homicide: a review. *Trauma Violence Abuse.* Jul 2003;4(3):265–276.

44. Mauricio AM, Gormley B. Male Perpetration of Physical Violence Against Female Partners: The Interaction of Dominance Needs and Attachment Insecurity. *Journal of Interpersonal Violence.* 2001;16(10):1066–1081.

45. Caetano R, Schafer J, Fals-Stewart W, O'Farrell T, Miller B. Intimate partner violence and drinking: new research on methodological issues, stability and change, and treatment. *Alcohol Clin Exp Res.* Feb 2003;27(2):292–300.

46. Caetano R, Schafer J, Field C, Nelson SM. Agreement on Reports of Intimate Partner Violence Among White, Black, and Hispanic Couples in the United States. *J Interpers Violence.* December 1, 2002 2002;17(12):1308–1322.

47. Cunradi CB, Caetano R, Schafer J. Alcohol-related problems, drug use, and male intimate partner violence severity among US couples. *Alcohol Clin Exp Res.* Apr 2002;26(4):493–500.

48. Murphy C, Winters J, O'Farrell T. Alcohol consumption and intimate partner violence by alcoholic men: Comparing violent and nonviolent conflicts. *Psychology of Addictive Behavior.* 2005;19(1):35–42.

49. El-Bassel N, Gilbert L, Wu E. Relationship between durg abuse and intimate partner violence: A longitudinal study among women receiving methadone. *American Journal of Public Health.* 2005;95(3):465–470.

50. Grisso JA, Schwarz DF, Hirschinger n, et al. Violent Injuries amoung Women in an Urban Area. *New England Journal of Medicine.* December 16 1999;341(25).

51. Miller B. Partner violence experiences and women's drug use: Exploring the connections. In: Wetherington C, Roman A, eds. *Drug Addiction Research and the Health of Women.* Rockville, MD: National Institutes of Health; 1998:407–416.

52. Ehrensaft M, Moffit T, Caspi A. Clinically abusive relationships in an unselected birth cohort: Men's and women's participation and developmental antecedents. *Journal of Abnormal Psychology.* 2004;113:258–270.

53. Dutton D, Saunders K, Starzomski A. Intimacy, anger and insecure attachments as precursors of abuse in intimate relationships. *Journal of Applied Social Psychology.* K Martholomew;24:1367–1386.

54. Coleman DH, Straus MA. Marital power, conflict, and violence in a nationally representative sample of American couples. *Violence and Victims.* 1986;1(2): 141–157.

55. Fitzpatrick M, Salgado D, Suvak M. Associations of gender and gender-role ideology with behavioral and attitudinal features of intimate partner aggression. *Psychology of Men and Masculinity.* 2004;5:91–102.

56. Smith M. Patriarchal ideology and wife beating: A test of a feminist hypothesis. *Violence and Victims.* 1990;5:257–273.

57. Farmer A, Tiefenthaler J. An economic analysis of domestic violence. *Review of Social Economics.* 1997;55(3):337–358.

58. Murphy C, Meyer S, O'Leary K. Dependency charactristics of partner assaultive men. *Journal of Abnormal Psychology.* 1994;103:729–735.

59. Michalski JH. Making Sociological Sense Out of Trends in Intimate Partner Violence: The Social Structure of Violence Against Women. *Violence Against Women.* June 1, 2004 2004;10(6):652–675.

60. DeKeseredy WS, Kelly K. Women Abuse in University and College Dating Relationships: The Contribution of the Ideology of Familial Patriarchy. *Journal of Human Justice.* Spring 1993;4(2):25–52.

61. Arriaga XB, Foshee VA. Adolescent dating violence: do adolescents follow in their friends', or their parents', footsteps? *J Interpers Violence.* Feb 2004;19(2): 162–184.

62. Gwartney-Gibbs PA SJBS. Learning courtship aggression: the influence of parents, peers, and personal experiences. *Family Relations.* 1987;36:276–282.

63. McKinney C, Caetano R, Harris T, Ebama M. Alcohol availability and intimate partner violence among US couples. *Alcohol Clin Exp Res.* 2009;33(1):169–176.

64. Livingston M. A longitudinal analysis of alcohol outlet density and assault. *Alcohol Clin Exp Res.* 2008;32(6): 1074–1079.   ⁻

65. Reid R, Hughey J, Peterson N. Generalizing the alcohol outlet-assaultive violence link: evidence from a US midwestern city. *Substance Use and Misuse.* 2003;38(14):1971–1982.

66. The Impact of Guns on Women's Lives. *Amnesty International International Action Network on Small Arms and Oxfam International.* Oxford, UK; 2005.

67. Kyriacou DN, Anglin D, Taliaferro E, et al. Risk Factors for Injury to Women from Domestic Violence. *New England Journal of Medicine* December 16 1999;341:1892–1898.

68. Honeycutt T, Marshall L, weston R. Toward ethnically specific models of employment, public assistance and victimization. *Violence Against Women.* 2001;7(126–140).

69. Raj A, Silverman J, Wingood G, DiClemente R. Prevalence and correlates of relationship abuse among a community-based sample of low-income African American women. *Violence Against Women.* 1999;5(3):272–291.

70. Woods S. Normative beliefs regarding the maintenance of intimate relationships among abused and nonabused women. *Journal of Interpersonal Violence.* 1999;14(5):479–491.

71. Moore T, Stuart S. Effects of masculine gender role stress on men's cognition, affective, physiologial and aggressive responses to intimate conflict situations. *Psychology of Men and Masculinity.* 2004;5: 132–142.

72. Jakupeak M, Lisak D, Roemer L. The role of masculine ideology and masculine gender role stress in men's perpetration of relationship violence. *Psychology of Men and Masculinity.* 2002;3:97–106.

73. Smith A. Domestic Violence Laws: The Voices of Battered Women. *Violence and Victims.* 2001;16(1): 91–111.

74. Dobash RE, Dobash R. *Violence Against Wives: A Case Against the Patriarchy.* New York, NY: The Free Press; 1979.

75. Levinson D, ed. *Violence in Cross-Cultural Perspective.* Newbury Park, CA: Sage; 1989.

76. Posner E. Symbols, signals and social norms in politics and law. *Journal of Legal Studies.* 1998;27: 765–798.

77. Cohen D. Culture, social organizations and patterns of violence. *Journal of Personality and Social Psychology.* 1998;75:408–419.

78. Bronfenbrenner U. Ecology of the family as a context for human development: Research perspectives. *Dev Psychol.* 1986;22:723–742.

79. McClelland D. *Power: The inner experience.* New York: Irvington Publishers; 1975.

80. Dutton DG, Strachan CE. Motivational needs for power and spouse-specific assertiveness in assaultive and nonassaultive men. *Violence and Victims.* 1987;2(3):145–146.

81. Prince JE, Arias I. The role of perceived control and the desirability of control among abusive and nonabusive husbands. *Am J Fam Ther.* 1994;22(2):126–134.

82. Browning J, Dutton D. Assessment of wife assault with the conflict tactics scale: Using couple data to quantify the differential reporting effect. *J Marriage Fam.* 1986;46:375–379.

83. Walker LE. *The battered woman.* 1st ed. New York: Harper & Row; 1979.

84. Dutton D, Painter S. Emotional attachments in abusive relationships: A test of traumatic bonding theory. *Violence and Victims.* 1993;8(2):105–120.

85. Walker LE. *The battered woman.* 1st ed. New York: Harper & Row; 1979.

86. Heberle R. Keeping victims safe and holding offenders accountable: The privatizing effects of criminalizing domestic violence. 2001:25.

87. Johnson MP. Patriarchal terrorism and common couple violence: Two forms of violence against women. *J Marriage Fam.* 1995;57(2):283–294.

88. Johnson M. Conflict and control: gender symmetry and asymmetry in domestic violence. *Violence Against Women.* 2006;12(11):1019–1025.

89. Straus MA, Gelles R, Steinmetz S. *Behind closed doors—Violence in the American family.* New York: Doubleday; 1980.

90. Steinmetz S. The battered husband syndrome. *Victimology.* 1978(2):499–509.

91. Klostermann KC, Fals-Stewart W. Intimate partner violence and alcohol use: Exploring the role of drinking in partner violence and its implications for intervention. *Aggression and Violent Behavior.* 2006;11(6):587–597.

92. Graham DLR, Rawlings E, Rimini N. Survivors of terror: Battered women, hostages, and the Stockholm Syndrome. In: Yllo K, Bograd M, eds. *Feminist perspective on wife abuse.* Newbury Park, CA: Sage Publications; 1988:217–223.

93. Graham DLR, Rawlings EI, Ihms K, et al. A scale for identifying "Stockholm Syndrome" reactions in young dating women: Factor structure, reliability, and validity. *Violence and Victims.* 1995; 10(1):3–22.

94. Prochaska JO, DiClemente CC. Integration of stages and processes of change. *The transtheoretical approach: Crossing traditional boundaries of therapy.* Malabar, FL: Krieger Publishing Company; 1994:45–56.

95. Prochaska JO, DiClemente CC. The Stages of Change. *The transtheoretical approach: Crossing traditional boundaries of therapy.* Malabar, Florida: Krieger Publishing Company; 1994:21–32.

96. Prochaska JO, DiClemente CC. The Transtheoretical Approach: Crossing Traditional Boundaries of Therapy. Malabar, Florida: Krieger Publishing Company; 1994:21–32 & 41–56.

97. Prochaska JO, DiClemente CC, Norcross JC. In Search of How People Change: Applications to Addictive Behaviors. *Am Psychol.* September 1992; 47(9):1102–1114.

98. Cluss PA, Chang JC, Hawker L, et al. The Process of Change for Victims of Intimate Partner Violence: Support for a Psychosocial Readiness Model. *Women's Health Issues.* 2006;16:262–274.

99. Burke JG, Denison JA, Gielen AC, McDonnell KA, O'Campo P. Ending intimate partner violence: an application of the transtheoretical model. *Am J Health Behav.* Mar-Apr 2004;28(2):122–133.

100. Zink TM, Lloyd K, Isham G, Mathews D, Crowson T. Applying the planned care model to intimate partner violence. *Managed Care.* 2007; 16(3):54–61.

101. Reiss AJ RJ. *Social influences.* Vol 3. Washington DC: National Academy Press; 1994.

Chapter 5

Economic Analysis and the Prevention of Intimate Partner Violence

Phaedra S. Corso

KEY CONCEPTS

- Economic analysis, as applied to preventing intimate partner violence (IPV), may include cost of illness analyses, programmatic cost analyses, and such economic evaluation techniques as cost-effectiveness analysis (CEA) and benefit–cost analysis (BCA).
- A monetary assessment of the economic burden of IPV is typically referred to as a cost-of-illness (COI) analysis, which estimates the costs of health outcomes associated with disease or injury by quantifying the (direct) medical expenditures resulting from a condition and the resulting (indirect) value of lost productivity.
- By comparing average intervention costs across sites and populations, programmatic cost analyses are useful as tools to determine the efficient allocation of resources within a particular intervention to prevent IPV. Cost analyses are also essential components of future analyses of economic evaluation and should, therefore, be collected during the program start-up and development phase.
- Economic evaluation is characterized by experimental and quasi-experimental methods and is used to produce information that compares intervention outcomes to costs. The main analytic tools used to conduct economic evaluations include CEA and BCA.
- In a CEA, the health benefit is measured in units of health, such as cost per injury prevented or cost per life year saved. In a BCA, health outcomes are valued in monetary terms.

The public health approach to preventing the adverse physical and mental health outcomes associated with intimate partner violence (IPV) relies on a range of disciplines to: (a) describe the public health burden associated with IPV, (b) identify risk and protective factors associated with IPV, (c) evaluate the interventions and policies designed to prevent IPV, and (d) implement and disseminate interventions and policies proven efficacious and effective. These disciplines include epidemiology, social and behavioral science, health, communication, and criminal justice. Incorporating the principles of economic analysis is a natural extension of the public health approach to preventing IPV, in which the scarcity of public health resources requires policy makers to contemplate the economic burden of IPV and the economic efficiency of interventions designed to prevent IPV. In this chapter, the public health approach for preventing IPV is expanded to include some applications from the field of economic analysis, specifically focusing on the economic impact of IPV and the economic evaluation of interventions designed to prevent IPV. This chapter is motivated by the desire to provide a framework that can help to more closely integrate public health with economic analysis in terms of informing public health researchers and policy makers about the practical value of applying the tools of economic impact analyses and economic evaluation to the traditional public health approach for preventing IPV.

THE PUBLIC HEALTH APPROACH TO PREVENTING INTIMATE PARTNER VIOLENCE

The public health approach described in Figure 5.1 provides a multidisciplinary, scientific approach that is explicitly directed toward identifying effective approaches to preventing IPV (1–3). The public health approach to prevention begins with defining the burden and characteristics of IPV in the populations at risk. This data collection phase seeks to answer the questions who, what, where, when, and how by gathering information on incidence, prevalence, morbidity, and mortality. Public health concerns can be identified through traditional surveillance techniques; that is, the ongoing, systematic collection of data, registries, or surveys, or, through descriptive and observational studies. The next step in the model involves identifying risk and protective factors or answering the question about why IPV occurs. This step can also be used to define populations at high risk and to suggest specific interventions. Risk and protective factors can be identified through a variety of research techniques including rate calculations, cohort studies, and case control studies.

The next public health objective is to develop interventions or policies based, in part, on the information provided in the previous steps. These policies and interventions subsequently need to be evaluated. Evaluation is the systematic investigation of the merit, worth, or significance of an object, for example, interventions that prevent or ameliorate violence. Interventions are typically evaluated first within a controlled research setting (efficacy) and then at the community or population level (effectiveness). Evaluations at this stage are outcomes-focused, designed to test for internal

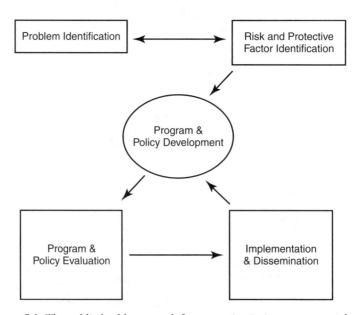

Figure 5.1 The public health approach for preventing intimate partner violence.

and external validity, and typically include study designs with randomized or nonrandomized controlled settings. For example, Foshee and colleagues' (4) examination of the effectiveness of the Safe Dates program to prevent dating and intimate partner violence was conducted in a randomized controlled setting and showed sustained decreases in IPV over a 4-year period in the intervention group compared to controls.

The final stage of the public health approach for preventing disease and injury is to ensure widespread adoption of interventions that have proven efficacious and effectiveness. Implementation implies translating research into practice by identifying the essential elements of the intervention, identifying acceptable alternatives when necessary, providing guidance, developing field-oriented materials, and pilot-testing. The successful dissemination of an intervention requires development of a public health infrastructure that allows adaptation with adherence to fidelity, feasibility, acceptability, and sustainability. Evaluation and monitoring play a role when assessing whether the intervention still works out in the field and whether it looks promising for alternative implementation settings and populations. Evaluation at this stage may emphasize process more than outcomes, and may include case studies or pre-, post-, or controlled study designs. One example includes evaluating the

statewide dissemination of evidence- and/or theory-based domestic violence prevention interventions through a pre-/post-study design.

Although the model proceeds sequentially, in reality many of these steps occur simultaneously. An opportunity also exists to gather feedback, in that, for example, lessons learned about potential risk factors for IPV can be applied to improve systems developed for surveillance and identification.

INCORPORATING ECONOMIC ANALYSIS INTO THE PUBLIC HEALTH APPROACH TO PREVENTING INTIMATE PARTNER VIOLENCE

The public health model for preventing disease and injury can be enhanced by incorporating the tools and techniques of economic analysis along its continuum (Figure 5.2).

Problem Identification

Economic analysis contributes to defining the public health problem by first defining *burden* in monetary terms or in quality of life. A monetary assessment of the economic burden is typically

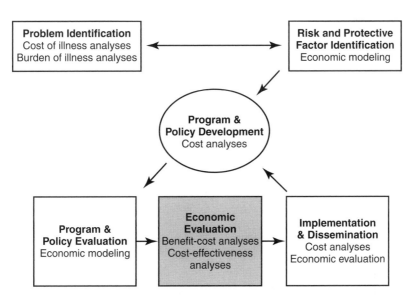

Figure 5.2 The expanded public health approach for preventing intimate partner violence, incorporating economic analysis.

referred to as a cost-of-illness (COI) analysis, which estimates the costs of health outcomes associated with disease or injury.

Cost-of-illness analyses, which are the most common type of economic analysis used in this field, summarize the economic burden of an outcome of interest, such as IPV, by quantifying the (direct) medical and nonmedical expenditures resulting from a condition and the resulting (indirect) value of lost productivity (5–8). Information on COI, and economic burden in general, is valued because it provides answers to such normative questions as: Why is this problem important? And, How does the impact of this problem on medical and mental health costs, educational costs, criminal justice system costs, and losses in productivity, etc., compare to other problems of interest?

Cost-of-illness analyses can be prevalence- or incidence-based. Prevalence-based estimates are cross-sectional estimates of costs that occur during a specified period (typically a year) and are not dependent on when the violent event occurred. For example, a prevalence-based estimate of IPV occurring in 2005 would include the costs occurring in 2005 for new cases of IPV occurring in that year, but also the costs occurring in 2005 for follow-up care of IPV occurring prior to the year 2005. In contrast, incidence-based analyses quantify the lifetime costs for all new violence events that occur during a particular time frame. For example, an incidence-based estimate of IPV costs from the base year of 2005 would include all lifetime expenditures associated with all new cases of IPV occurring in that year. Incidence-based, or lifetime COI estimates, can also be used to define cost per case prevented for use in full economic evaluations.

Most COI estimates of IPV are prevalence-based; that is, reflective of annual costs. For example, it has been estimated by the Centers for Disease Control and Prevention (CDC) that IPV costs U.S. society $5.9 billion annually in health-related costs (in 1995 $US), including $4.1 billion in direct medical and mental health care services and $1.8 billion in productivity losses associated with lost wages (9). Using data from the same survey—the National Violence Against Women Survey—Max and co-workers estimated the annual economic toll of IPV in the United States to be $8.3 billion when updated to 2003 U.S. dollars (10). Intimate partner violence impacts other countries as well. For more information on the impact

of IPV internationally, see the work by Waters and colleagues (11) from the World Health Organization for an international literature review of the annual costs associated with interpersonal violence and Yodanis and colleagues (12) for an earlier review. Not surprisingly, these reviews found that IPV disproportionately affects poorer countries, although the evidence of the economic impact in these countries is scarce. At the U.S. state level, the annual economic impact of IPV has also been quantified. For example, Oregon estimated that IPV costs $35 million every year for medical and mental healthcare services for victims of intimate partner rape and physical assault, in addition to $9 million in lost productivity (13).

Although these economic burden of disease estimates represent a measure of the health-related toll that IPV has on society and can be used by public health advocates to appeal for more investment in interventions that will prevent future acts of IPV (14), they represent only the tip of the iceberg. Other costs that are not included in these analyses include lifetime costs associated with IPV, costs associated with fatal IPV, and criminal justice system costs. For example, Miller and colleagues (15) estimated that each sex-offense homicide costs as much as $3 million (1996 $US). One could consider costs from the business sector perspective as well, such as the cost to replace those victimized workers who never return to the workplace and need to be replaced, and losses in on-the-job productivity (or "presenteeism") that are often not captured in these studies. Rothman and Corso (16) have recently conducted pilot work to assess on-the-job productivity losses associated with potential IPV batterers, which has shown some interesting results. They found that men who scored higher on a batterer index were more likely than their nonbattering peers to have more days missed from work, make more errors at work, and to take more breaks. The next step in this research is to assess the impact that IPV has on the productivity of victims, particularly how productivity measures may be biased against women, as recently suggested by Jones and Frick (17).

Another limitation in the previous COI estimates is that medical costs included in the analyses were for those that were specifically violence-related. If it is true that violence, particularly egregious and repeated violence, has impacts on other health outcomes, then the annual costs are underinflated. For example, Wisner and colleagues (18) found an annual difference of $1,775 (1994 $US) in overall healthcare costs, or 92% more for victims of IPV compared to a general female population of enrollees in a large health plan in Minnesota. Ulrich and co-workers (19) found that women with medical-record–documented domestic violence had 1.6-fold higher utilization and costs of health care compared to women with no documented violence. Coker and colleagues (20) explored the healthcare utilization and Medicaid cost data for self-identified survivors of IPV. The authors found that expenditures were different for women experiencing different levels of IPV, although utilization of health-care services was not significantly different. However, Snow and associates (21) found that average medical costs for women enrolled in a health maintenance organization (HMO) reporting abuse was on average $1,700 (2005 $US) higher over a 3-year period compared to women enrolled in the same HMO who did not report abuse. And Rivara and colleagues (22) found that even 5 years after abuse, healthcare costs were 19% higher (or $439 annually in 2004 $US) for abused compared to nonabused women. The costs of IPV likely extends to children of the victims as well. In a longitudinal cohort study, Rivara and associates (23) found that children whose mothers experienced IPV had higher healthcare utilization and costs, even if the abuse stopped before they were born.

In addition to COI analyses, economic analyses included as part of the problem identification stage of the public health model may also include quality of life assessments. Measures of disease and injury burden that incorporate quality of life are called burden-of-illness (BOI) analyses; these analyses rely on the use of health indices that combine the effects of a disease, illness, or injury on mortality (length of life) and morbidity (quality of life). Quality-adjusted life years (QALYs) and disability-adjusted life years (DALYs) are two commonly used indices of general health (24,25). These measures allow for a comparison of interventions that affect disparate health outcomes and populations.

Only a few studies have measured the impact of IPV on quality of life in a way that can be useful for economic evaluations. Wittenberg and colleagues (26) found, in a convenient sample of abused and nonabused women, that quality of life, as measured using the Health Survey Short Form (SF)-12, was lower in abused women compared with their nonabused counterparts. Further, they found that this decrement in quality of life was correlated with severity of abuse. And in a study of Norwegian women, Alsaker and co-workers (27) found a two-fold lower self-rating of quality of life, as measured by the SF-36, among battered women compared with their nonbattered peers. Despite these advances in research, much more work is needed in assessing acute losses in quality of life for victims of abuse and in long-term losses in quality of life as well.

Risk and Protective Factor Identification

One major contribution of economic analysis to public health is in exploring the ways in which behavior, such as violence, is influenced by economic considerations. Economic theories designed to explain rational economic behavior are important in identifying risk and protective factors for adverse outcomes. To test those theories, the field of *econometrics* develops and applies mathematical and statistical methods for use with empirical evidence. Econometrics includes many advanced quantitative techniques, such as structural equation modeling and instrumental variable analysis, which are often used in other social science disciplines. Empirical data are typically obtained from official records, population surveys, and other data sources, and can be used to test cause-and-effect relationships suggested by economic theory.

Econometrics, for example, has been used to examine risk factors for IPV. In an analysis of domestic violence, Farmer and Tiefenthaler (28) present an economic model predicting that a woman's income and other financial support received from outside the marriage will decrease the level of violence within the family because they increase the woman's *threat point* (the level of happiness/satisfaction achieved in the marriage that is at least as great as that which could be achieved outside the marriage). Using empirical evidence from longitudinal victim interview data, the results support the hypothesis that improved economic opportunities for women serve as a protective risk factor for the level of violence they experience in abusive relationships.

Program and Policy Development

Statistical analysis can similarly be used to determine which resources required to develop a program will most strongly influence total program costs. For example, in developing a school-based program to reduce the incidence of dating violence, is it personnel costs (as in type of provider) or space requirements (as in location of intervention) that are likely to drive total program costs? More specifically, cost analyses conducted prospectively during the program and policy development phase can assist policy makers in understanding how the structure, setting, or scope of an intervention ultimately influences implementation costs. Thus, cost analyses are useful as tools to determine the efficient allocation of resources within a particular intervention program by comparing average intervention costs across sites and populations. Cost analyses are also essential components of future analyses of economic evaluation and should, therefore, be collected during the program start-up and development phase.

The cost of most public health programs is an issue of interest to public health advocates, implementers, and program funders. For example, Jones (29) conducted a cost analysis of an intervention designed to stop assaults on and threats to participants' female partners—a batterer program. She found that the cost per batterer session across four different sites varied only slightly, from $22 to $32 (in 1995 $US), despite differences in program structure and level of service provision. When the total costs to complete all sessions were estimated, program costs were more varied, ranging from $264 to $864, and reflecting the costs to the men who complete the program (participant costs) and the opportunity cost to develop a policy that would increase the likelihood of men completing each program.

Program and Policy Evaluation

Given sound and well-tested theoretical models developed in the second phase of the public health approach—risk and protective factor identification—economic models can be used to predict the impact of legislation and public policy initiatives or of any other change affecting the public health outcome of interest. In this sense, economic models are developed prospectively to inform decision making. Applications of prospective economic models are often useful when considering legislative changes to prevent violence, such as the passage of the 1994 Brady Handgun Violence Prevention Act. In practice, however, economic models are most often used to evaluate legislation ex post passage. For example, Ludwig and Cook (30) conducted a pre-/post-study time series analysis comparing a control group that included 18 states already meeting the Brady Act requirements to a treatment group that included states required to implement the

new, more stringent procedures associated with the Act. They found that the change in rates of homicide and suicide for treatment and control states were not significantly different, except for firearm suicides among persons aged 55 years or older.

Economic Evaluation

Sometimes referred to as the nontraditional application of health economics, economic evaluation is characterized by experimental and quasi-experimental methods and is used to produce information that compares intervention outcomes to costs (24,25). The main analytic tools used to conduct economic evaluations include cost-effectiveness analysis (CEA) and benefit–cost analysis (BCA). Primers on how to use these methods specifically for public health interventions have been described in detail elsewhere (25). In a CEA, the health benefit is measured in units of health, such as cost per injury prevented or cost per life year saved. If length of life and quality of life are of interest in the economic evaluation, the health outcome measure in the CEA can use BOI measures discussed previously—that is, QALYs or DALYs—such that the summary measure is cost per QALY saved. In a BCA, health outcomes are valued in monetary terms, such that the summary measure is presented as net benefits (total benefits minus total costs) or as a benefit-to-cost ratio (total benefits divided by total costs). The COI analysis discussed previously is one approach for monetizing benefits in a BCA. *Contingent valuation* is another technique for monetizing benefits in a BCA; it includes an approach that measures society's willingness to pay for reductions in morbidity or mortality risks. For example, when people in a national survey were asked to state their willingness to pay for a 30% reduction in gun violence, their answers suggest that the benefits of reducing gun violence are worth approximately $24.5 billion in 1998 $US (31).

Very few published economic evaluations of IPV interventions exist (14). This is due, in part, to limited data on program effectiveness of IPV interventions (32). An example of a BCA of an intervention associated with IPV is a study of domestic violence shelter services by Chanley and colleagues (33). In this study, the authors quantified only the short-term costs and benefits of the shelters (including operating expenses and public assistance for the women and their children) as the costs, and quantified assaults averted and improved mental health as the benefits. The authors found that, even in the short-term, the social benefits of the shelters far outweighed the social costs of the shelters, nearly 7 to 1 on the low side, to 18 to 1 on the high side. Another example is a BCA of the Violence Against Women Act (VAWA) of 1994, conducted by Clark and colleagues (34). In this study, the authors included costs to implement the VAWA ($1.6 billion over 5 years) and calculated benefits as averted costs associated with direct property losses, medical and mental health care, police response, victim services, lost productivity, reduced quality of life, and death. The results of the analysis showed that VAWA saved $14.8 billion in net averted social costs, suggesting that the VAWA is an affordable and beneficial social program.

Implementation and Dissemination

Finally, the tools of economic analysis can be applied at multiple levels of program and policy implementation and dissemination. First, cost analyses can assist policy makers considering a specific intervention proven efficacious and effective. The objective is to minimize costs (a cost-minimization analysis) for a given output. And second, economic evaluations become useful when choosing between interventions for which both costs and effectiveness levels differ. For example, CEAs can answer questions regarding technical or production efficiency, such as: Given a fixed health budget and interest in preventing a specific outcome such as IPV, what are the costs associated with the various alternative means for reaching that objective?

CONCLUSION

From assessing burden of illness in the problem identification phase of the public health model, to cost analysis and economic evaluation in the implementation and dissemination phase, this chapter has outlined the possibilities for expanding the public health model for preventing IPV to include applications from the field of economic analysis. In this era of scarce public health resources, now more than ever will policy makers need to contemplate the economic burden of IPV and the economic efficiency of interventions designed to prevent IPV.

IMPLICATIONS FOR POLICY, PRACTICE, AND RESEARCH

Policy

- Economic burden of disease estimates represent a measure of the health-related toll that IPV has on society and can be used by public health advocates, researchers, and policy makers to appeal for more investment in interventions that will prevent future acts of IPV.
- Specifically, programmatic cost analyses can assist policy makers considering a specific intervention already proven efficacious and effective.
- Economic evaluations become useful for making policy decisions when choosing between interventions in which both costs and effectiveness levels differ.

Practice

- The field of economic analysis fits very well within the public health model for preventing IPV, thus complementing epidemiologic interest in etiology, efficacy, effectiveness, implementation, and dissemination.
- Unfortunately, a paucity of data regarding the application of economic analysis to public health outcomes, particularly in violence prevention, still exists.

Research

- Future research needed for incorporating economic analysis into the public health model for preventing IPV includes (a) longitudinal studies to assess the outcomes associated with IPV and their costs, particularly mental health implications, impact on educational attainment, and future productivity; (b) assessment of long-term economic impacts of IPV on children; and (c) studies to assess both the short- and long-term impacts that IPV has on quality of life for use in future economic evaluations. More investment in research dollars should be directed to these areas to justify the expenditure of scarce public health dollars toward prevention.

References

1. Foege WH, Rosenberg ML, Mercy JA. Public health and violence prevention. *Curr Issues Public Health.* 1995;1:2–9.

2. Mercy JA, Rosenberg ML, Powell KE, et al. Public health policy for preventing violence. *Health Aff.* 1993;12(4):7–29.
3. Potter LB, Mercy JA. Public health perspective on interpersonal violence among youths in the United States. In: Stoff DM, Breiling J, Maser JD, eds. *Handbook of antisocial behavior.* New York: John Wiley and Sons, 1997.
4. Foshee VA, Bauman KE, Ennett ST, et al. Assessing the long-term effects of the Safe Dates program and a booster in preventing and reducing adolescent dating violence victimization and perpetration. *Am J Public Health.* 2004;94:619–624.
5. Hodgson TA. The state of the art of cost-of-illness estimates. *Adv Health Econ Health Serv Res.* 1983;4:129–164.
6. Hodgson TA, Meiners MR. Cost-of-illness methodology: A guide to current practices and procedures. *Milbank Memorial Fund Q Health Sociol.* 1982;60:429–462.
7. Rice DP. Estimating the cost of illness. *Am J Public Health Nations Health.* 1967;57:424–440.
8. Rice DP. Cost of illness studies: What is good about them? *Inj Prev.* 2000;6:177–179.
9. Centers for Disease Control and Prevention. *Costs of intimate partner violence against women in the United States.* Atlanta: National Center for Injury Prevention and Control, 2003.
10. Max W, Rice DP, Finkelstein E, et al. The economic toll of intimate partner violence against women in the United States. *Violence Vict.* 2004;19(3):259–272.
11. Waters HR HA, Rajkotia Y, Basu A, Butchart A. The costs of interpersonal violence: An international review. *Health Policy.* 2005;73:303–315.
12. Yodanis CL, Godenzi A, Stanko EA. The benefits of studying costs: A review and agenda for studies on the economic costs of violence against women. *Policy Studies.* 2000;21(3):263–276.
13. Drach L. *Costs of intimate partner violence against Oregon women.* Portland: Oregon Department of Human Services, Office of Disease Prevention and Epidemiology, 2005.
14. Laurence L, Spalter-Roth RM. *Measuring the costs of domestic violence against women and the cost-effectiveness of interventions: An initial assessment and a proposal for future research.* Washington: Institute for Women's Policy Research, 1996.
15. Miller TR, Cohen MA, Wiersema B, eds. *Victim costs and consequences: A new look.* Washington, DC: US Department of Justice, Office of Justice Programs, National Institute of Justice, 1996.
16. Rothman E, Corso PS. Propensity for intimate partner abuse and workplace productivity: Why employers should care about changing the behavior of men who batter. *Violence and Women.* 2008;14(9):1054–1065.
17. Jones AS, Frick K. Gender bias in economic evaluation methods: Time costs and productivity losses. *Womens Health Issues.* 2008;18:1–3.
18. Wisner CL, Gilmer TP, Saltzman LE, Zink TM. Intimate partner violence against women: Do victims cost health plans more? *J Fam Pract.* 1999;48(6):439–443.
19. Ulrich YC, Kain KC, Sugg NK, et al. Medical care utilization patterns in women with diagnosed domestic violence. *Am J Prev Med.* 2003;24:9–15.
20. Coker AL, Reeder CE, Fadden MK, Smith PH. Physical partner violence and Medicaid utilization and expenditures. *Public Health Rep.* 2004;119:557–567.
21. Jones AS Dienemann J, Schollenberger J, Kub J et al. Long-term costs of intimate partner violence in a sample of female HMO enrollees. *Women's Health Issues.* 2006;16:252–261.
22. Rivara FP Anderson M, Fishman P, et al. Health-care utilization and costs for women with a history of intimate partner violence. *Am J Prev Med.* 2007;32(3):89–96.
23. Rivara FP AM, Fishman P, Bonomi AE, et al. Intimate partner violence and health care costs and utilization for children living in the home. *Pediatrics.* 2007;120:1270–1277.
24. Gold MR, Siegel JE, Russell LB, Weinstein MC, eds. *Cost-effectiveness in health and medicine.* New York: Oxford University Press, 1996.
25. Haddix A, Teutsch S, Corso PS, eds. *Prevention effectiveness: A guide to decision analysis and economic evaluation.* New York: Oxford University Press, 2003.
26. Wittenberg E, Lichter EL, Ganz ML, McCloskey LA. Community preferences for health states associated with intimate partner violence. *Med Care.* 2006;44(8):738–744.
27. Alsaker K, Moen BE, Nortvedt MW, Baste V. Low health-related quality of life among abused women. *Qual Life Res.* 2006;15:959–965.
28. Farmer A, Tiefenthaler J. An economic analysis of domestic violence. *Rev Soc Econ.* 1997;55(3):337–358.
29. Jones AS. The cost of batterer programs. *J Interpers Violence.* 2000;15(6):566–586.
30. Ludwig J, Cook PJ. Homicide and suicide rates associated with implementation of the Brady Handgun Violence Prevention Act. *JAMA.* 2000;284:585–591.
31. Ludwig J, Cook PJ. The benefits of reducing gun violence: Evidence from contingent valuation survey data. *J Risk Uncertain.* 2001;22(3):207–226.
32. Wathen CN, MacMillan HL. Interventions for violence against women: Scientific review. *JAMA.* 2003;289(5):589–600.
33. Chanley SA Chanley JJ, Campbell HE. Providing refuge: The value of domestic violence shelter services. *Am Rev Pub Administr.* 2001;31(4):393–413.
34. Clark KA, Biddle AK, Martin SL. A cost-benefit analysis of the violence against women act of 1994. *Violence Against Women.* 2002;8(4):417–428.

Chapter 6

International Perspectives on Intimate Partner Violence

Gregory Luke Larkin and Stephen C. Morris

KEY CONCEPTS

- Intimate partner violence (IPV) is a global problem, and the reported prevalence and incidence varies widely.
- Micro-, meso-, and macro-level forces combine to put individuals at risk of partner violence within specific environments and cultural contexts.
- Cultural forces represent both risk and protective IPV factors.
- Culturally appropriate strategies are particularly important for developing nations.
- Global public health and medical institutions are leading the way toward violence prevention and a more shared understanding of IPV around the world.

Despite being shrouded in shame and secrecy, intimate partner violence (IPV) is a widespread problem of global proportions (1). Although no society is immune from IPV, its varying prevalence across time and space suggests the importance of cultural influences on violence perpetration and prevention. Indeed, the understanding and recognition of domestic abuse varies widely from country to country. Although IPV involves dynamics of power and control between individuals, it is also affected by the interplay between gender, socio-political structure, religious beliefs, attitudes toward violence in general, criminal justice systems, migration, civil unrest, resource allocation, the environment, and other contextual factors. Understanding the global landscape of IPV is difficult due to its extreme heterogeneity, but reviewing IPV in different cultural settings permits insight into IPV's shared or root causes. Understanding these root causes leads, in turn, to a mosaic of IPV prevention efforts that may be transferable to new societies and settings.

SEEKING A CROSS-CULTURAL MODEL FOR INTIMATE PARTNER VIOLENCE

Although Heise (2) has proposed an ecological framework for interpersonal violence based on four concentric circles of individual, relationship, social structures, and socio-economic environments, other less tidy models may better locate IPV in a modern world undergoing tumultuous change. A modified model acknowledging the influence and intersection of multiple macro-, meso-, and micro-level forces would be more responsive to our current notions of relationships within dynamically changing environments.

This model might adapt another theory regarding "family" or "domestic" violence that has been proposed to give structure to the unique elements of violence that occur within the family group or home environment. This concept includes multiple forms of violence, such as child abuse and elder abuse, and ignores many of the nonfamilial aspects of IPV, such as those occurring in nonformalized relationships. In addition, because the concept of "family" is poorly defined within and across cultural and societal landscapes, it is difficult to translate to international IPV.

Because the perpetrator is usually male and the victim female, the terms *violence against women* and *gender-based violence* (which are often used interchangeably) are inclusive of most IPV. These terms help frame and define IPV because they underscore the exploited status of women worldwide. Other systemic types of violence against women that are not associated with IPV include human trafficking and female genital mutilation (3).

Although no model can completely represent the complex interplay between factors that influence and allow IPV, an understanding of the forces involved is critical to an analysis of the problem. Internationally, the prevalence of IPV is influenced by a society's views of IPV, public problem-solving discourse, the role and status of women, the role of religious and political leadership, economic conditions, general levels of safety, and social stability.

A molecular analogy may present a helpful model of an IPV event. An individual is at the center, the nucleus; their partner or partners are at the center of their own nuclei, each bringing with them a cluster of personal traits, values, experiences, genetics, expectations, and resources that make up their atomic mass. All partners bring to the relationship a certain sphere of influence that includes family structure, competing relationships, religious or organizational memberships, community resources, friendships, and occupational affiliations that further influence how any two individual elements combine in a compound relationship structure. Relationships are further situated in a dynamic milieu of other influences that can either help the two cohere or split them apart. These influences may enter at the individual, relationship, or environmental level, but include community structures, legal and ethical mores, religiosity, economic stresses, cultural forces, media influences, peer and nonpeer relationships, physical and mental health, children, family, acquaintances, social networks, and other relationship and environmental forces. These dynamic clouds of influence must also contend with larger, macro-level forces to a greater or lesser degree, depending on the particular relationship and context.

GLOBAL PREVALENCE

The exact prevalence of IPV across the globe is not known with any precision for at least three reasons. First, the problem of partner violence is not clearly defined within and between populations. Although most definitions discuss a pattern of abusive physical, sexual, or psychological maltreatment, the less nuanced definitions of the adjectives "domestic" or "family" can sometimes cloud the scope or nature of the problem, thus complicating measurement (2). Even the labels "violence" and "abuse" are sometimes misapplied, as there are few internationally accepted operational definitions for these constructs. In Japan, for example, "family violence" more traditionally connotes children's violence against their parents (4). Second, most IPV data are derived from surveys and other self-report measures, which are seldom objective or reliable. Injured or threatened individuals must feel safe in order to report reliably, which is rare. Third, gathering and comparing data across cultures is complicated by linguistic, ethnic, and sociological differences.

In this chapter, instead of attempting to catalogue all possibilities of IPV in every continent, country, and context, we will seek a nuanced view of just a few cultures to allow a more subtle comparison. We will strive to describe factors reported in the public health and peer-review literature that illuminate both the commonalities and differences in prevalence and management of domestic violence in non-Western societies.

BUILDING PUBLIC HEALTH RESEARCH AT THE GLOBAL LEVEL

Until recently, violence-related research and intervention was largely outside of the domain of the medical sciences. In the last 20 years, a change in the perception of IPV as a health concern has arisen, encouraging healthcare workers and researchers to explore the subject and its consequences from a health perspective (5). Because groups affected by IPV have differing perspectives, research about IPV may be approached in completely different ways. Criminal justice, social science, survivors' advocates, and humanitarian groups all see IPV through different lenses. The previous lack of health-related IPV research has resulted in a dearth of reliable information from a health perspective, so the true impact of IPV on health is incompletely understood. Comprehension will grow, as the strict scientific methodology and interdisciplinary approach common to the medical sciences has much to offer in studying this complex problem.

Efforts by health-focused groups in the developing world have resulted in improved understanding of the impacts of IPV within these resource-poor settings. However, as with other influences, it remains unclear how many of these findings are translatable to other countries. Rigorous health services and public health research approaches to studying the IPV problem and solution have been encouraging. Efforts by the global healthcare community, as evidenced by work of the World Health Organization (WHO) and other United Nations (UN) health-related agencies, nongovernmental organizations (NGO) foundations, and international health advocacy groups, have all embraced the concept of IPV as a global public health concern. Understanding IPV from a global health perspective will supplement work in other related fields to yield more holistic improvements in IPV intervention and prevention. Indeed, targeting individuals in the healthcare field taps perhaps the most trusted professionals to intervene in public education and awareness programs, targeted prevention activities, public safety, and community-based interventions.

Work by the WHO's Departments of Violence and Injury Prevention and Disability (VIP) and the Department of Gender, Women, and Health (GWH) highlights the role that the health field can play in IPV research, education, advocacy, intervention, and prevention (Table 6.1). The publication of the *World Report on Violence and Health* by the WHO in 2002

Table 6.1. Key Public Health Documents Concerning Global Intimate Partner Violence

WHO *multi-country study on women's health and domestic violence against women*. World Health Organization, Geneva, Switzerland (6)

World report on violence and health. 2002 World Health Organization, Geneva, Switzerland (7)

Guidelines for medico-legal care for victims of sexual violence. 2003 World Health Organization, Geneva, Switzerland (8)

Intervening with perpetrators of intimate partner violence: A global perspective. 2003 Department of Injuries and Violence Prevention, World Health Organization, Geneva, Switzerland (9)

Handbook for the documentation of interpersonal violence prevention programmes. 2004 World Health Organization, Geneva, Switzerland (10)

Guide to United Nations resources and activities for the prevention of interpersonal violence. 2002 Department of Injuries and Violence Prevention, World Health Organization, Geneva, Switzerland (11)

The economic dimensions of interpersonal violence. 2004 Department of Injuries and Violence Prevention, World Health Organization (12)

helped establish violence as a serious public health concern (7). The report is aimed at those involved in healthcare delivery and social work and at workers in the field of violence prevention and intervention; it attempts to describe the epidemiology and impact of violence on a global scale, address the risk factors and roots of violence, document current interventions and policy responses and, finally, makes recommendations for policy makers and workers in the field.

Other documents and campaigns by the WHO that have directly addressed IPV include the following:

- *Guidelines for medico-legal care for victims of sexual violence* is a guide to healthcare providers on the complexities of the provision of care to sexual assault victims (8). The book addresses the need for a compassionate and but comprehensive approach to working with victims of sexual assault and provides guidelines for standards and program establishment.
- *Intervening with perpetrators of intimate partner violence: A global perspective* is a report of research into the efficacy of programs aimed at resolving the problem of IPV, emphasizing programs aimed at the perpetrators of IPV (9).

- *Handbook for the documentation of interpersonal violence prevention programmes* is a framework document for the classification, comparison, and analysis of interpersonal violence prevention programs (10).
- *Guide to United Nations resources and activities for the prevention of interpersonal violence* documents the work of 15 UN agencies in relation to prevention and intervention (11).
- *The economic dimensions of interpersonal violence* documents what is known about the costs associated with interpersonal violence. Although the studies in developing countries are limited, the results indicate a higher level of economic consequences from IPV in resource-poor settings (12).

Following the publication of the *World Report on Violence and Health*, the Global Campaign for Violence Prevention was begun. This initiative is mandated to implement the recommendations of the report, and in particular to "raise awareness about the problem of violence, highlight the crucial role that public health can play in addressing its causes and consequences, and encourage action at every level of society" (13). Another organization, the Violence Prevention Alliance (VPA), was formed. The VPA is made up of WHO Member State Governments, nongovernmental and community-based organizations, and private, international and intergovernmental agencies working to prevent violence. The VPA provides policy guidelines as well as coordinating and organizing efforts and building the capacity of member organizations that work on violence research and prevention from a scientifically based, public health perspective.

INTERNATIONAL INTIMATE PARTNER VIOLENCE RESEARCH

International IPV research is fundamentally problematic: Difficulties arise from the conflict between researchers' definitions of IPV and their subjects' beliefs; inconsistent and incompatible methodology and design makes interstudy comparison and cross-country meta-analysis difficult. Inherent challenges also exist in conducting research across cultural and dynamically changing geopolitical lines. Threats to science are common in many countries. In addition, external validity is also at issue when attempting to generalize study results. It is challenging to find coherence and consistency within communities, let alone consistency between disparate settings. Population-based data and demographics, essential for understanding the context of social and health-related research, are absent or incomplete in much of the world. Most studies of IPV focus on physical violence and ignore other aspects of IPV, such as deprivation and psychological abuse. Research has been tacitly stifled or deliberately blocked in closed societies for fear of misogynistic exposure. Many other factors have contributed to poor research quality and gaps in international IPV research, such as financing issues, religious influences, and geographical, political, and cultural heterogeneity.

Monitoring the significant ethical and safety concerns for both researchers and study participants is another critical component of international IPV research (14). Studies have demonstrated an escalation in violent behavior during times of victim help-seeking and, therefore, similar concerns arise when a victim is being contacted by researchers. Researchers may also become victims of violence if they are viewed as a threat to the violent offender or to the community. This situation presents a possible ethical conflict, however unintended, when hopes of safety and intervention are raised where none exist.

As the international health community has become more involved in IPV, the lack of critical data has become more apparent. A concerted effort to amend this situation has been made by many within the field and is exemplified by the three efforts documented in the following list. It is likely that our understanding of IPV, from a public health perspective, will increase as quality data slowly accumulates.

- *World Studies of Abuse in Family Environments* (WorldSAFE), from the WorldSAFE International Clinical Epidemiology Network (INCLEN). A group of physicians and researchers are conducting parallel studies of domestic violence and child abuse in 33 countries. Addressing factors such as social beliefs, community beliefs, family dynamics and stresses, and societal and economic characteristics, it is hoped that this information will be used to guide future planning and interventions. In addition, cross-cultural comparison may offer insight to the common roots of IPV and thereby inform prevention efforts.

- *Researching Violence Against Women: A Practical Guide for Researchers and Advocates* (15).

This work by the WHO and a nongovernmental organization, PATH, attempts to provide a comprehensive tool for those engaged in researching violence against women. By providing background on health and developmental concerns, this text addresses critical theoretical topics and practical issues such as ethical concerns and working in the field. The book provides a model for guiding efficient and thoughtful research in the field.

– *The WHO Multi-country Study on Women's Health and Domestic Violence Against Women* (6). A survey of 24,000 women in 10 countries (Bangladesh, Brazil, Ethiopia, Japan, Peru, Namibia, Samoa, Serbia and Montenegro, Thailand, and the United Republic of Tanzania) was conducted in collaboration with the London School of Hygiene and Tropical Medicine (LSHTM), PATH, U.S. research institutions, and local women's organizations. The report documents the prevalence and nature of IPV, highlighting its negative association with physical, mental, sexual, and reproductive health.

Preliminary results from the study demonstrate disturbing but enlightening trends about the global problem of IPV. Significant variation is the norm, with differences in prevalence seen both between and within countries. The conservative definitions employed were more likely to underestimate rather than overestimate the IPV problem. Results include data on attitudes condoning or justifying physical abuse. For example, although over 80% of women in urban Brazil did not accept any of six reasons for justifying physical IPV, almost 80% of women in rural Ethiopia accepted disobeying their husband as a justification to be hit. Women who were victims of IPV were more likely than nonvictims to accept justification of violence. This study also unmasked significant discordance (up to 16% in urban Namibia,) among women who reported sexual abuse in a face-to-face versus anonymous settings. The terrible scope of the problem was highlighted by the sheer numbers of women who reported being victims of various types of IPV (examples are given in the country sections below). Significant overlap between physical and sexual abuse was common, with up to 56% of victims reporting both types of IPV. Effects on the mental health of victims included up to 47% victims in urban Brazil reporting that they had experienced suicidal thoughts. Protective factors against IPV included higher education, empowerment, and being married. Factors that

were identified as placing women at risk for IPV included youth, being in a separated or cohabiting relationship, and partner's use of alcohol. Although the full results of the study are not yet available or analyzed, it is clear that this landmark study has done much to shed light on the vast global problem of IPV.

The WHO Multi-country Study on Women's Health and Domestic Violence Against Women makes 15 recommendations to help countries tackle the problem of IPV (6). The report's recommendations fall into thematic categories:

- Strengthening national commitment and action
- Promoting primary prevention
- Involving the education sector
- Strengthening the health sector response
- Supporting women living with violence
- Sensitizing criminal justice systems
- Supporting research and collaboration

The recommendations are:

1. Promote gender equality and women's human rights and compliance with international agreements.
2. Establish, implement, and monitor multisectoral action plans to address violence against women.
3. Enlist social, political, religious, and other leaders in speaking out against violence against women.
4. Enhance capacity for data collection to monitor violence against women and the attitudes and beliefs that perpetuate it.
5. Develop, implement, and evaluate programs aimed at primary prevention of IPV and sexual violence.
6. Prioritize the prevention of child sexual abuse.
7. Integrate responses to violence against women into existing programs, such as those for the prevention of HIV/AIDS and for the promotion of adolescent health.
8. Make physical environments safer for women.
9. Make schools safe for girls.
10. Develop a comprehensive health sector response to the various impacts of violence against women.
11. Use the potential of reproductive health services as an entry point for identifying women in abusive relationships and for delivering referral and support services.
12. Strengthen formal and informal support systems for women living with violence.

13. Sensitize legal and justice systems to the particular needs of women victims of violence.
14. Support research on the causes, consequences, and costs of violence against women and on effective prevention measures.
15. Increase support to programs to reduce and respond to violence against women.

An egregious failure to enroll men into IPV research or the IPV conversation is one limitation in this study and in much of the WHO's other work on IPV. Research with adolescent female perpetrators, same-sex male and female couples, and large household surveys suggest other stakeholders be included if nations are to meaningfully address violence at its root cause. Men are as much a part of the solution as they are the problem and yet they have been systematically excluded from most of the WHO research agenda. Until researchers, policy makers, and women see men as their partners in solving the IPV problem, research will continue to be about screening and risk factors rather than the eradication/elimination and prevention of interpersonal violence.

FIVE INFLUENCES ON GLOBAL INTIMATE PARTNER VIOLENCE

Poverty

The influence of poverty on human interaction is well-known; it is less well known how deprivation contributes to violence, including IPV. The uncertainty, degradation, and environmental deprivation associated with material poverty are significant social stressors. Changing economic fortunes can complicate relationships. Although numerous studies demonstrate that IPV exists at all socioeconomic levels, those living in poverty suffer disproportionately higher levels of IPV. Tension within a partnered relationship may include disputes over limited resources, absence of privacy when living in close quarters or high-density areas, and limited educational and professional options. Poverty may force changes in traditional gender roles—if, for example, financial circumstances demand that a women work outside the home, it may foster jealousy and anger. The unemployed victim in an abusive relationship may hesitate to report family violence and risk the loss of the primary breadwinner. Similarly, the victim may be reluctant to leave the relationship without the means to financially support herself and her children.

Poverty also affects violence on a more global, societal level. Impoverished nations with infrastructure problems may be too unstable and unwilling to create unpopular legislation to curtail violence within the home. Even if strong policies are designed, they cannot easily be implemented or enforced without adequate funding for mental health, program staff, police, and legal enforcement. Although not all protection of the vulnerable depends on funding, a lack of resources for protective services or interventions is a significant obstacle in many nations. Most macro-level measures of health are improved with poverty reduction, and IPV is no exception.

Family Dynamics and the Role of Women

The role of women within their society and culture and within family structures is related to risk of IPV (16). Most of the world's women lack control over their domestic situations. The resultant vulnerability establishes fertile ground for discordant power sharing and, ultimately, IPV. The status of women within their cultural and social context has been linked to the prevalence of IPV (17). Societies in which men have sole economic decision-making power and in which women do not have easy access to legal divorce are havens for high rates of IPV (18).

Religion

The relationship between religion and IPV is quite complex, given the cultural and behavioral cofactors associated with religion. Studies of religious permission or condemnation of IPV are inconclusive, but reveal the complexity of religious attitudes in regards to the domestic sphere (19). Although much can be inferred from understanding orthodox religious influences on other areas of life, it would be erroneous to subscribe overt changes in IPV prevalence to religion alone. Most religious authorities influence social structure (from private spiritual beliefs to secularly dominated social structures). Although the influence of personal beliefs is not always coherent with religious teachings, religious justification for violent actions is the most clear-cut example of influence. In particular, religious decrees or cultural traditions that subordinate the role of women within the family structure or within society are most troubling. Although the Bible, Torah, and Koran do not actively encourage either IPV or the subjugation of women, some scriptural interpretations have traditionally subjugated women (20,21). Ultra conservative interpretation of Islamic law by the Taliban, for example, is one example of a misplaced religiously influenced belief system that likely promotes tolerance of IPV. However, religious leaders' condemnation of IPV and supportive intervention offers a wonderful opportunity in societies lacking a strong criminal justice system to harness established networks of religious support—in developing and developed countries alike. Moreover, religious practices and exercises have repeatedly been shown to offer protection against the emotional sequelae and psychological burden of violence exposure.

Social Disruption

Natural and manmade disasters are often associated with social change, an escalation of family violence, and changing political boundaries and governmental systems that may result in regime shifts that are more or less tolerant of violence and the repression of women. For example, the 2nd Intifada in both Gaza and the West Bank led to significant increases in family violence that paralleled Palestinian unemployment in the region. Other geopolitical forces such as wars, drought, famine, floods, disease, and a host of supervening influences can stress individuals and, by extension, relationships in any society, but especially those most contingent and fragile.

Mobile Populations

Displaced populations and those in turmoil are known to suffer from higher levels of IPV, and justifiably deserve special attention. Research on populations in crisis is lacking due to the inherent difficulty of working in these environments and the necessity of critical resource allocation to urgent interventions. However, existing evidence suggests that high levels of IPV are normative in times of social stress migration and political turmoil (22–24). In addition, immigrants demonstrate a higher tolerance for and susceptibility to IPV than surrounding host populations (25–28).

Global-level Prevention and Intervention Strategies

Published in 2004, *Preventing Violence: A Guide to Implementing the Recommendations of the World* *Report on Violence and Health* (29) provides conceptual and practical suggestions on how to implement IPV prevention policies, focusing on the following principles:

- Increasing the capacity for collecting data on violence.
- Researching violence, its causes, consequences, and prevention.
- Promoting the primary prevention of violence.
- Promoting gender and social equality and equity to prevent violence.
- Strengthening care and support services for victims.
- Bringing it all together to develop a national action plan of action.

Social Institutions and Intimate Partner Violence Prevention

Globally, social institutions exert significant influence on IPV. Women's groups in the developed and developing world provide support for many activities, such as economic development. These groups in particular are strong advocates of IPV education, prevention, and intervention. Additionally, many of these groups have provided some forms of intervention (normally part of governmental structures) such as safe houses, medical services, and research programs on IPV.

Nongovernmental agencies focusing on gender issues, human rights, health care, and justice have long been involved in addressing IPV around the world. In some developing and disrupted societies, these organizations may be the only organized service provider available. For example, in past conflict societies, international NGOs may provide nutrition, healthcare education, and even security. These organizations are variably adept at addressing issues of IPV, but efforts by international and governmental agencies are often in flux.

CASE STUDIES: ASIA

By highlighting well-documented examples of IPV research and literature from a variety of countries and continents, it is hoped that a mosaic of IPV as a global phenomenon can be better appreciated. Although not representative, each country's example reveals regional trends. We begin with Asia, where we find housed nearly one-third of all the planet's inhabitants. We will focus on India, Bangladesh, China, Japan, and Russia due to their sheer epidemiologic import, population density, and relatively high prevalence of IPV compared to other societies.

Bangladesh

Despite its relative poverty, Bangladesh is one country that has bravely attempted to accurately report the prevalence of IPV within its own borders. Large, well-designed, population-based studies estimate lifetime prevalence of physical IPV against women in rural areas from 47% to 67% and report annual incidence rates of 19%–35% (30,31). Other large population-based studies of physical violence in partnered women in rural Bangladesh estimate current IPV to be as shockingly high as 32%–42%. (32,33). Over two-thirds (68%) of these current Bengali victims report never having told anyone about the physical abuse and mistreatment (32).

Other studies have shown that increased education, higher socioeconomic status, non-Muslim religion, and extended family residence to be protective. In culturally conservative areas, short-term membership in savings and credit groups was associated with elevated risks of violence; this was not true in less culturally conservative areas (17). Other studies in rural Bangladesh confirm the protective effects of education, but also suggest that women with more than nominal personal earnings had an increased risk of IPV. Dowry costs were also associated with IPV (30). Pressures to marry women early to keep dowry costs down were also pervasive. Thus, in rural women, economic circumstances influence risk in complex and often contradictory ways (34).

The relationship of religion to all aspects of life in this region of the world is profound, and its influence of the problem of IPV is likely substantial. Islam is the religion of the majority in Pakistan and Bangladesh; neighboring countries such as India, Sri Lanka, Bhutan, and Nepal are more likely to follow Hinduism, Buddhism, and Sikhism, but some follow Christianity as well as Islam. When the Prophet Muhammad started Islam in Mecca 1,400 years ago, women were accorded new rights to choose a marriage partner, a right to divorce, and a right to an inheritance, among others (35). The Prophet himself married both divorced and widowed women to encourage other men to follow his example.

Over time, however, the religious patriarchy has largely suppressed women's rights to obtain a divorce freely, and in many settings (including Egypt and Iran) only men may initiate religious divorce (*Talaq*) proceedings. Although men may enter into four separate religious marriages (called *Nikah* agreements) through the Imam, a woman may marry only one man at a time. Even in the wake of a civil divorce, she may not remarry unless a religious divorce is first granted. Muslim men, however, may sometimes get a civil divorce from their wives but never initiate the *Talaq*, in order to keep the estranged wife from remarrying.

Although Islam condemns violence against women, a verse in the Quran (verse 4:34) refers to a man's right to beat his wife if he fears willfulness from her. The literal or symbolic meaning of this admonition is widely debated and seems inconsistent with other passages in the Quran calling for kindness and justice toward women. The Islamic religious community has been criticized on the issue of spouse abuse and is seen as generally condemning those women who seek outside assistance for marital IPV as bringing dishonor and shame upon their household. One criticized concept is that a woman should remain obsequious, patient, loyal, self-sacrificing, and accepting of their kismet (fate) so that after death she may more readily reap the rewards of being a tolerant and devoted wife. Conservative clothing, such as the Hijab head scarf, can hide a woman's beauty from the outside world, and may also carry the dual use of hiding bruises. The religious patriarchy of Islam recommends "chador and char diwar" (the veil and the four walls of the house) as a woman's best protection; but one must sometimes ask, "Protection for whom?"

India

As in Bangladesh, India also has a very high reported prevalence of IPV—in fact, some of the highest rates ever recorded anywhere in the world. In Tamil Nadu and Uttar Pradesh, incidence rates in current relationships vary from 37% to 45%, respectively (36). A study of nearly 7,000 males in five districts of Uttar Pradesh validate these high numbers, revealing that 30% of men admit to using violence against their spouse (37).

Further evidence of the severity of the problem in India was provided more recently by the WorldSAFE consortium. From 1997 to 2003, the consortium ambitiously conducted a series of population-based, cross-sectional household surveys in selected communities in four countries: Temuco, Chile; Ismailia, Egypt; Lucknow, Trivandrum, and Vellore non-slum areas of India; and in Manila, the Philippines. The percentages of lifetime and current physical IPV against women were 24.9 and 3.6 (Santa Rosa, Chile), 11.1 and 10.5 (El-Sheik Zayed, Egypt), 34.6 and 25.3 (Lucknow, India), 43.1 and 19.6 (Trivandrum, India), 31.0 and 16.2 (Vellore, India), and 21.2 and 6.2 (Paco, the Philippines). This study also showed that repeated severe physical IPV was more common in the three communities within India (9.0%, 5.9%, and 8.0% in Trivandrum, Lucknow, and Vellore) than within the other three communities (Santa Rosa 2.1%, El-Sheik Zayed 2.9%, and Paco 1.9%) (38).

Similar to Western societies, Indian marriage and motherhood provide women with their primary role identities. As in Islamic cultures, Hindi households judge the woman as a failure if she cannot maintain her marriage and provide her children with a father, regardless of his behavior. Divorce and single motherhood are largely anathema in Indian society. Marital-based IPV is often interpreted as wife's predestined fate or karma, a result of past acts in a prior life. Such religious and cultural norms can provoke a kind of learned helplessness and fatalism in many women who are resigned to accepting IPV as an inevitable part of relationships with Indian men.

As dramatically publicized in international satellite broadcasts, dowry transactions have become increasingly expensive and commercialized on the Indian subcontinent. When dowry demands are not met after a marriage, new wives are sometimes driven or forced into "suicide" (often from pesticide overdoses or immolation), so that the husband may start over and pursue another wife and dowry (39). If the woman tries to return to her natal home, her own family will often shun her for fear of having to pay yet another dowry downstream. Unfortunately, the Indian census, based in Chennai, has not always been successful in unmasking legitimate suicides from dowry-related murders, thus accurate population data on the incidence of IPV-related suicides and dowry murders is lacking. However, observational data of the author (GLL) and colleagues in New Delhi, Chennai, and Mumbai indicate that IPV is a common denominator in most of these deaths, suicides or not.

A promising development in both India and Bangladesh is the practice of implementing local systems of justice, referred to as the *salishe*, whereby an appointed person or persons come into the village and consult with the individuals and families involved. This collective bargaining or mediation strategy can enlist the involvement of the community to arrive at a fair and just solution, which is then put in writing and monitored by a local committee made up of both men and women (40). These new developments in justice notwithstanding, both countries have a long way to go before they will lose the distinctions of having some of the highest reported rates of IPV on the planet.

China

The largest of the world's countries in population terms remains one of the most mysterious in terms of IPV epidemiology. The Chinese Central Government has not routinely welcomed investigators from abroad to study embarrassing or politically damaging subjects such as IPV. Indeed, good population-based data on the nature and prevalence of IPV in China are sorely lacking. Within Chinese family systems, as in many other societies, males dominate and maintain a strict gender-based hierarchy that discourages discussion or full disclosure of domestic problems outside of the home. One study in China revealed that the lifetime and 12-month prevalence of IPV was 43% and 26%, respectively. This study involved surveys of only 600 women attending an urban gynecologic clinic in Fuzhou (41). The strongest predictors of IPV in this cross-sectional cohort were partner refusals to share money, partners having affairs, and frequent quarreling. Other patriarchal values and traditional gender roles are linked to IPV in Chinese society. These included having refused a job because of a partner, believing a wife is obliged to have intercourse with her husband, and holding traditional beliefs about wife beating such as "it is important for a man to show his wife who is boss." Protective factors included having a partner who worked as a manager or supervisor and, quite unexpectedly, agreeing that family problems should be discussed only within the family. Those women who grew up in rural areas had higher odds of reporting abuse (2.0–2.1, depending on the setting). Age and female-gendered children were not associated with IPV, in contrast to expectations (41,42).

Another community-based face-to-face survey of women who had a child aged 6–18 months in 32 communities of Tianjin, Liaoning, Henan, and Shaanxi provinces revealed that the prevalence of domestic abuse (emotional, sexual, or physical) occurring in any period (before, during, or after pregnancy) was

12.6% (43). The prevalence of abuse during pregnancy (4.3%) was relatively lower than the prevalence of abuse during the 12 months before pregnancy (9.1%) and after delivery (8.3%). Factors associated with abuse during pregnancy included women previously witnessing domestic violence, a poor relationship with the partner, socioeconomic level, alcohol consumption, and smoking.

Partner violence exposure is a major risk factor for suicide, and China has consistently had one of the highest suicide completion rates for women of any country in the world; it is the only country to have near parity in completion rates between the sexes (44). Disproportionate numbers of the suicides occur in rural areas, where the suicide rates of married women exceed the suicide completion rates of married men (42 versus 31 per 100,000). In rural areas, the roles of married women are often subordinate to their husbands, as well as to their mothers-in-law. The wives are expected to do hard labor, endure arranged marriages, produce male offspring, and tend to the needs of their spouse and his mother without complaint. It is unsurprising then that rural China is a hotbed of domestic violence as well; women here frequently ingest organophosphate pesticides with fatal results. (In Western societies, women exposed to IPV also overdose at a high rate, but the sedative and analgesic types of drugs used are seldom lethal.) Unfortunately, given the context of a woefully under-resourced emergency medical care system in rural China, the lethality of the gesture is often assured, regardless of intent. Few rural Chinese physicians have had training in toxicology or emergency medicine, and the availability of needed antidote (atropine and 2-pralidoxime) is severely limited. Although preventive strategies are easily imaginable, the Central Government has supported neither lock boxes nor the development of Western-style emergency medicine in rural China, where IPV is rampant and terra cotta wives[1] come remarkably cheap.

---

[1] "Terra cotta wives" is a reference to the 3,000 wives and concubines of the First Emperor of China, Qin Shi Huang, who amassed the warriors of the Terra Cotta Army. The term is used here to signify the generally low regard for females, and cavalier attitude to the ready availability, acquisition, and expendability of wives implied by the Emperor's quantity of wives.

Japan

As in China, Japan has had relatively few large population-based studies of IPV. In one study, using a sample of both men and women, the prevalence of IPV was reported as high as 46.4% and the prevalence of perpetration of IPV was nearly as high at 43.1% (45). Women reported experiencing more sexual IPV than males, and males admitted to more perpetration. Both victimization and perpetration were strongly associated with being a childhood witness of IPV or with exposure to child abuse.

The awareness of domestic violence in Japan is increasing (46), although in rural areas the term still largely refers to the physical and emotional violence of children against their parents (4). The Japanese penchant tendency for copying Western approaches to modernization has meant many more opportunities for women than elsewhere in Asia. It has also meant a faster recognition of women's rights and is perhaps related to a lower prevalence of IPV than in other less industrialized societies in the region.

Russia and the Former Soviet Union

Because of its immense size, large population, and distinctive and changing social institutions, Russia offers a unique perspective on the global problem of IPV. Studies of IPV in Russia however, like studies in much of the world, have yet to shed comprehensive insight into magnitude of the IPV problem. Indeed, underreporting by government-related agencies is widely accepted as the norm. The Russian Federation's 1994 National Report 1993 concluded that 14,500 women were killed and 56,400 injured by their male partners (47). A 2000 U.S. Centers for Disease Control and Prevention (CDC) study of Russian women age 15–44, in three different provinces, demonstrated physical assault by a partner at rates of 7% and 22% for the last 12 months and ever, respectively (48). A population-based cross-sectional study from the Ukraine of 3,587 ever-married women aged 17–44 demonstrated that 7.2% had experienced physical abuse in the previous year and that these women were more likely to have had more than one sexual partner and less likely to have used condoms in the past year, thus putting them at additional risk for sexually transmitted disease (49). This is a particularly concerning element of IPV, given the rapidly expanding HIV/AIDS epidemic in Russia and the former Soviet Union (50).

Cultural issues specific to the region may have a strong influence on IPV prevalence. Historically, the low social status of women and cultural acceptance of IPV was common. Intimate partner violence has been considered a private family matter, and low levels of public discourse on the subject was the norm until the past two decades. Structural protection of women during the Soviet era was assured on paper but was not prioritized. In addition, legal avenues to protect victims of IPV have been limited at best. Finally, social disruption, such as loss of previously strict policing and community structure and economic equity since the fall of the Soviet Union has resulted in increased vulnerability for women (47). Anecdotal evidence of an increase in IPV since the breakup of the Soviet Union concurs with what is understood about violence during times of social stress (7).

Opportunities for help in the region are hampered by limited services and the continued dysfunctional legal system. One result of this is that many victims are accustomed to resorting to family and friends and not institutions for assistance. Interestingly, many of the patterns of abuse and response to abuse have been demonstrated in Russian-speaking women who have emigrated to other countries as well (51). Many advocacy groups currently work in the region to raise awareness about, prevent, and protect victims of IPV. In particular, major public awareness campaigns have been undertaken, and some have advocated the introduction of international techniques to combat the problem (52). An example of such advocacy groups is the Association of Crisis Centres' Stop Violence program, which represents a web of 45 NGOs with 435 employees across Russia. In addition, research and public policy groups have become more active in addressing an understanding of the issues influencing IPV and its prevention.

CASE STUDIES: AFRICA

Nigeria

The most populous country in Africa, the Federal Republic of Nigeria has over 250 distinct cultural groups speaking 500 languages and living within unique social structures. The country is also experiencing significant social stresses, such as some of the world highest fertility rates, absolute poverty, cultural and religious tension, and political instability. High rates of IPV have been demonstrated in many studies.

Perhaps more concerning, levels of acceptance of IPV are also high. In the 2003 Nigeria Demographic and Health Survey (NDHS), 66.4% of ever-married and 50.4% of unmarried women agreed that a man is justified in beating or hitting his wife (53).

A study of 600 men in two tertiary healthcare centers in South Eastern Nigeria found high levels of violence within the home, with 92% of the victims being women. Factors associated with violence included lower social class, alcohol consumption, increasing age disparity between couples, and unemployment. Although only 8% of the victims informed someone of the abuse, the family doctor was the recipient of disclosure in 88% of those cases.

In this same study, 21% of the abuse occurred while the partner was pregnant (54). The study also indicated that of the 6% of men who were victims of IPV by a female partner, influencing factors were financial disparity in favor of the female, influential in-laws, and educated women mimicking the gender inequality seen in more common IPV situations.

Intimate partner violence occurring during pregnancy has many associated social and health outcomes. A study of 400 pregnant women at National Hospital, Abuja, Nigeria showed that 35.4% of them had experienced IPV during pregnancy and, of those who where victims of physical or sexual abuse, 21.2% required medical attention of injuries resulting from the IPV. In this study, 85.2% of those surveyed had a tertiary education and all knew of the potential for pregnancy complications that could result from domestic violence, such as abortion, premature labor, and depression (55). In another study of 418 pregnant women in Lagos, Nigeria, 49.2% reported abuse by a family member during the current pregnancy, and 11.7% reported that they first experienced abuse during pregnancy. Importantly, 99% of the abused women were not prepared to report the abuse to the police (56).

A study of 308 communities of Imo State, Nigeria demonstrated very high rates of IPV, including rates of physical abuse of 84.6% and 73.5% in urban and rural areas, respectively. Abuse is often culturally condoned, reflected by the low status of women within the culture and the high rates of female genital mutilation (52%–73%) (57).

Nigeria has been slow to react to international efforts to reduce IPV. Legal protection for victims and criminal prosecution of perpetrators is only slowly becoming a reality. Even with laws in place, it seems that the culture of acceptance of IPV will prevent widespread justice in the foreseeable future. Resources and sanctuary are largely absent for the majority of the population. Women's groups and international organizations are making some headway in raising awareness, but changing perceptions are occurring at a glacial rate.

Tanzania

With a population of over 38 million and more than half of them living on less than $2 a day, Tanzania is one of the world's poorest countries. In addition, with an estimated 1.4 million people living with HIV/AIDS, Tanzania has some of the world's highest demonstrated rates of IPV (58). With poor infrastructure and limited resources, Tanzania faces many barriers to fully understanding and acting to prevent IPV.

As one of the ten sites from the WHO Multi-country Study of Women's Health and Domestic Violence Against Women, Tanzania has more data available on the subject than most other countries in the region. Two sites were selected for the WHO study: one urban (Dar es Salaam; 2002 population estimate 2,500,000) and one rural (Mbeya District; 2002 population estimate 521,000). A total of 2,698 women who had ever been in a partnered relationship completed interviews at the two sites. Significant differences in outcomes between sites were demonstrated. Prevalence of IPV in the urban setting were physical 32.9% (ever) and 14.8% (in last year) and sexual abuse 23.0% (ever) and 12.8% (in last year). This contrasts with significantly elevated rates in the rural setting, where the prevalence of IPV was physical 46.7% (ever) and 18.7% (in last year) and sexual abuse 30.7% (ever) and 18.3% (in last year). In addition, overall lifetime rates of having been a victim of either physical or sexual IPV or both were 41.3% and 55.9% in urban and rural settings, respectively. Controlling behavior was also commonly endorsed, with almost 90% of urban women reporting controlling behavior such as being prevented from seeing family and friends, enduring suspicion of being unfaithful, and having access to health care controlled (6,59). The scope and magnitude of these results have serious implications for Tanzania.

Understanding the causes of high levels of IPV in Tanzania and neighboring countries will be critical to improving the problem. Studies in the region have demonstrated that low education levels, multiparity,

and a history of childhood sexual abuse are associated with increased risk. In addition, men who participate in violence outside of the home, are heavy alcohol consumers, or have multiple partners have been shown to have an increased likelihood of IPV perpetration (60). A 2002 study of 1,444 urban women in Moshi, Tanzania showed that being unable to bear children or having more than five children, having less than a primary level of education, and having a partner who either did not contribute financially to the relationship or who had other partners were all associated with an increased likelihood of IPV (61). The strict patriarchal family structure and gender inequity, as represented by economic and sexual decision making power by men, are likely contributions to the high prevalence. In addition, very low levels of education, youth, and passivity among females is narrative and contributes greatly to gender inequity.

A link between the risk of risk of HIV exposure and IPV has been established and may represent an opportunity to heighten awareness about IPV and improve resources for victims (62,63). Assistance for IPV is relatively nonexistent for the majority of the Tanzanian population. International organizations and sponsorship may provide the best hope for combating the problem in the short-term, but the Ministry of Health must prioritize the health/IPV relationship and address gender inequity and miseducation at the earliest possible ages.

CASE STUDIES: SOUTH AMERICA

Peru

With a population of almost 30 million, Peru is home to 100 distinct cultural groups living in diverse ecological environments including tropical and temperate forests, desert, mountains, and coastal regions. Although the central government provides nationalized health care, much of the population lives in isolation from the infrastructure and support of the modern world.

Two sites were chosen in Peru as part of the WHO Multi-country Study of Women's Health and Domestic Violence Against Women: Lima (2000 population estimate 7.5 million) and the Department of Cusco, a rural mountainous area in the south of the country. Of the 2,620 partnered women who completed the study, 51.2% in the urban setting and 69.0% in the rural setting reported lifetime IPV. In addition, 16.4% of responders in the urban setting and 37.7% in the urban setting reported ever having being forced to have sexual intercourse (rape) by their intimate partner (6,59).

Factors influencing high levels of IPV in Peru have been speculated to include the high levels of non-IPV, the strict roles of women, and male aggression as evidenced by the concept of *machismo* (64). Investigation as to the causes of such high levels of IPV in Peru have included an analysis of the 2000 Peru Demographic and Health Survey. Using a logistical regression model of a sample of almost 16,000 women, Flake and colleagues were able to demonstrate risk factors at the individual, family, and community level. At the individual level, low education achievement, a history of prior family violence, and early marriage were associated with increased IPV risk. Large extended families living together, male partner's alcohol use, and women's unemployment were also associated with IPV. Community-level indicators of increased IPV risk were living in a noncoastal or urban area. The increase in urban IPV contradicts the WHO study, but may be accounted for by differences in study definitions and methods. In a study of 2,167 women who had just delivered babies in Lima, 40% had been victims of either physical or sexual IPV, and 65% reported unintended pregnancies. In fact, IPV exposure was an independent predictor of having an unintended pregnancy (65), increasing the risk by 3.3-fold.

As a response to the IPV epidemic, the Peruvian government has strengthened laws, established specially trained policing units, and encouraged the development of women's advocacy groups.

CASE STUDIES: OCEANIA

Australia

As with most developed nations, Australia and New Zealand have well-developed IPV research and response programs. However, aspects such as historical and cultural identities, immigrant and indigenous populations, geographical isolation, and heavy alcohol consumption continue to elevate IPV risk in the Antipodes.

Two large studies by the Australian government directly addressed issues of IPV: the Women's Safety Study of 1996 and the Personal Safety Study of 2005 both found rates of physical and sexual IPV of less than 7.1% (66).

In *The Cost of Domestic Violence to the Australian Economy*, the annual cost of IPV in Australia was reported to be AU$8.1 billion with AU$388 million being spent in direct healthcare costs. Additionally, Australia estimates that the lifetime cost per victim of IPV is AU$224,000 (67).

An analysis of 9,683 women surveyed as part of the 1996 Australian national health insurance database demonstrated that early intercourse was associated with increased risk for IPV; specifically, intercourse before age 14 is associated with 7 to 14 times more risk of IPV than those experiencing first intercourse after the age of 17 (68). In a subanalysis of 14,776 women in the Australian Longitudinal Study on Women's Health, young women aged 18–23 years who terminated pregnancies were three times more likely to have been victims of IPV compared with those who didn't have an elective abortion (69).

POLICY CONSIDERATIONS: ECONOMICS, BARRIERS TO INTERVENTION, AND SERVICE GAPS

Economic Consequences of Violence Against Women

In all countries and cultures studied to date, victims of abuse incur more medical costs, surgeries, prescription drug use, office visits, hospital stays, and mental health visits than those not afflicted by abuse. However, in addition to the increased costs of medical and mental health care, IPV undermines the economic development of nations at the macro level by lowering productivity and reducing women's collective participation in the workforce. One example of combating the controlling behavior of IPV is through the use of micro-credit schemes that advance small loans to women textile workers in Southeast Asia and Latin America. Although this type of program empowers women, it can backfire; in order to maintain control, males have sometimes undermined this process, despite the shared economic benefits of allowing a woman to work in the home making clothes, furniture, or other housewares. In many poor countries, women are not empowered to work outside the home, and those who travel beyond their neighborhoods or villages often risk rape and other unsafe or abusive situations. In much of the Arab world, for example, women are not permitted to take taxis alone to work, and women caught driving cars without their heads covered have been killed. Although employment may be seen to lessen dependence on the abuser in the long term, it is often threatening to males and poses a risk factor for escalating jealousy, fears of abandonment, and abuse in the near term.

Cultural Barriers to Addressing Intimate Partner Violence Within Countries

Regardless of the culture, most women who are victims of violence are often ashamed to report the experience. In cultures in which the role of women is often constrained to domestic life, this shame is magnified. Isolation further exacerbates this phenomenon, as communications and mobility out of a rural village, for example, may be severely limited. In encounters with family, physicians, police, or others, many women are afraid to mention their experiences with violent partners for fear of reprisal or being blamed for the abuse itself. In addition to limited options for travel or communication, women also have limited options for health care. Many women are unable to obtain needed health care without their partner's permission and presence to pay for the care, making confidentiality and privacy all but impossible. Access to mental health care is also severely limited, even in highly industrialized societies.

Other cultural practices can also threaten the health of women. For example, requiring the husband to pay his in-laws for a bride (bridewealth) has perpetuated the idea that husbands "own" their wives in many parts of Africa and Asia. If a woman from such a commoditized union subsequently leaves her husband, the parents must then repay the bridewealth, resulting in economic hardship and a familial reticence to take their daughter back, even in the throes of abuse.

In some Middle Eastern cultures, patriarchal terrorism and the demands for sexual purity are so great that women are often subjected to hostile sexism and virginity exams before marriage. To preserve their purity, many are subjected to female genital mutilation that ostensibly destroys clitoral function and lessens sexual pleasure. Furthermore, in both Arab and Latin American cultures, those who are raped or have sex outside of marriage are often killed in order to restore family honor. In a study from Alexandria, Egypt, nearly half (47%) of all femicides occurred at the hand of a relative after the victim had been raped (70).

Professional Barriers to Addressing Intimate Partner Violence

Healthcare workers, police, social service agents, and others who should be seen as allies by victims of violent crime may also be obstacles to meaningful solutions. Like all citizens within a given culture, clinicians and police may carry negative biases or disparaging stereotypes about women who are hit by their partners, thinking that such physical abuse is justified as a form of domestic discipline. In addition, many societies do not recognize forced sex within the bounds of marriage as an actual rape. Unpublished data from the West Bank demonstrates that many physicians and most police reported that the hitting of wives by husbands was often justified and necessary discipline, supported both by cultural norms and the Koran. Further work in this population has shown patriarchal professions and paternalistic physicians, untrained in psychosocial matters and empathetic communication, frequently frighten female patients from honestly disclosing IPV.

Service Gaps

Many countries lack a well-developed infrastructure of social services, thus leading to large disconnects between the criminal justice and healthcare systems. This lack of service coordination for victims makes an IPV patient disposition exceedingly difficult. Often, victims are hampered from pursuing justice by unsympathetic or inefficient bureaucracies. Many countries in Sub-Saharan Africa, Latin America, and even India require victims of rape to submit to visits with government agents or physicians under government contract, adding days to an already challenging evaluation. Typical 3- to 5-day bureaucratic delays often result in the destruction of any forensic evidence, making the pursuit of justice all the more unlikely. The obstacles to getting help for abused women may be significant even in well-developed countries. In regions where women are denied education or economic participation, it is risky to engage in public pursuits. For many, leaving the village on foot to pursue an uncertain future is unthinkable. Many women are trapped physically, geographically, socio-culturally, politically, and economically. For these, suicide may present an attractive option.

CONCLUSION

Hope for the Future

The UN General Assembly passed the Declaration on the Elimination of Violence Against Women in 1993 (23). Momentum was further generated in 1999, when the UN Population Fund declared violence against women "a public health priority." Although many countries and cultures have yet to legitimize domestic violence as a serious public health concern, these outdated notions are slowly giving way to a wider acceptance of the gravity of this problem, even in less-developed countries. Despite decades of denial, many emerging nations are attempting to use creative strategies to mitigate this serious health concern, even in the context of familial, religious, and cultural expectations that the role of women as wife, daughter, and mother be consistently proscribed.

Changing the landscape of IPV around the globe will require sustained local action on many fronts, political, legislative, and cultural. An increasing number of countries have passed laws against sexual harassment, domestic violence, and marital rape. Some countries have resorted to the public shaming of men who abuse their wives, and others have increased the consequences of abuse within the legal framework. Although increasing penalties to abusers may have a mild deterrent effect, targeted punitive solutions that create an "us versus them" gender war are ultimately doomed to fail; in addition, such short-term solutions can have complex social consequences, such as loss of financial support and housing and repercussive violence by family members. Indeed, both sexes must share in the burdens and responsibilities of such penalties, and must work as a bipartisan cooperative team to develop shared solutions.

Education, life skills training, communication, employment, and decreasing cultural norms that produce gender inequity are essential. Skills training on conflict resolution and zero tolerance for physical violence in the home or in the context of interpersonal relationships should be the norm. Men and women must both learn not to resort to violence in the rearing of their children. Providing havens for physical safety, emotional support, legal aid, and economic empowerment are ideal, but for many developing countries, the use of women's support groups may be the most cost-effective first step. Women's shelters are used in Western capitalist societies but are far too expensive for general use; they also have the added disadvantage of translocating women to an area away from their only known community, with the inherent connections to schools, churches, friends, and family. Another candidate strategy for improving communications for help is through the use of mobile phones. Although U.S. citizens view cellular telephones as an expensive appliance, towers and satellites are widespread across most of the planet and using them is orders of magnitude less expensive outside of the U.S. The potential of this adjunctive communication solution for women in developing countries who need access to health care, criminal justice, or other forms of protection awaits further study.

Men still constitute many of the leaders, policemen, healthcare workers, and politicians throughout the world, and they represent a disproportionate share of the perpetrators. Thus, they are especially vital to this transformative process and must not be made to feel left out of any solution. Like women, they too need parallel training in life skills, healthy relationships, conflict resolution, and personal safety. It is critically important that young men be proactively enrolled in the notion that fairness, kindness, and treating women with dignity and respect is both masculine and honorable. Male role models, peer mentoring, support groups, and drug and alcohol treatment can all play an important part.

Finally, getting helpful, reinforcing, and culturally sensitive messages across to both perpetrators and potential perpetrators of violence is a cornerstone of any modern societal solution. As global access to radio and televised media increases, the potential to bend cultural norms and generate targeted and powerful messages of nonviolence to men and women around the world is unprecedented. Enrolling local celebrities, opinion leaders, and religious and political leaders as agents of change is central to this mission. International cooperation and the cross-pollination of successful strategies can reconnect us to each other in ways that promote peace and health inside our homes, our communities, our countries, and perhaps someday, our entire world.

IMPLICATIONS FOR POLICY, PRACTICE, AND RESEARCH

Policy

- Culturally sensitive solutions must be sought, so that societies can maintain their dignity, their religious practices, and their traditions in the light of new roles for both women and men.
- The media, criminal justice system, and religious leaders need to work together to create more consistent messages and cross-cutting solutions to IPV that teach both men and women the life skills needed for healthy relationships and nonviolent conflict resolution.
- Key stakeholders, opinion leaders, and other key contacts within villages, communities, faith organizations, cities, societies, governments, and nations must be mobilized to acknowledge the economic and human costs of this issue and seek shared solutions that involve both men and women.

Practice

- Economically viable candidate strategies for improving surveillance, identification, communications, and follow-up include sustainable, nonperishable technologies, such as the use of mobile phones. The potential of this and other promising adjunctive communication solutions for women in developing countries who need access to health care, criminal justice, or other forms of protection awaits further study.
- International aspects of knowledge uptake and knowledge translation are vital concerns for the local implementation of the latest evidence into practice; this is especially important when evidence and/or practice guidelines are being generated from homogeneous or well-resourced settings and are then being considered or applied to culturally diverse and economically disparate settings. Although policies can be set globally and regionally, best practices will be determined locally, in response to the culture, setting, demographics, politics, and resources of particular settings.
- The establishment of support groups for survivors of IPV is a cost-effective approach to providing emotional support, as well as a resource for legal aid and economic empowerment.
- The media may be used to bend cultural norms and target victims, perpetrators, and potential perpetrators with messages of nonviolence.

Research

- Academic experts and researchers in Western countries must partner with academicians and workers in other nations to further the accurate documentation of trends in IPV prevalence, as well as the risk factors, protective factors, costs, and outcomes for IPV-exposed persons across different contexts and cultures.
- International IPV research must go beyond the mere counting of victims and enumeration of risk factors. It must move toward intervention studies that create an evidence base for optimal and generalizable healthcare responses to IPV, as well as research that prevents violence at its very genesis.

References

1. Garcia-Moreno C. Violence against women: International perspectives. *Am J Prev Med.* 2000;19(4):330–333.
2. Heise L, Ellsberg M, Gottmoeller M. A global overview of gender-based violence. *Int J Gynaecol Obstet.* 2002;78(Suppl 1):S5–S14.
3. Rutherford A, Zwi AB, Grove NJ, Butchart A. Violence: A glossary. *J Epidemiol Community Health.* 2007;61(8):676–680.
4. Kozu J. Domestic violence in Japan. *Am Psychol.* 1999;54(1):50–54.
5. Campbell JC. Health consequences of intimate partner violence. *Lancet.* 2002;359(9314):1331–1336.
6. Garcia-Moreno C. *WHO multi-country study on women's health and domestic violence.* Geneva: World Health Organization, 2005.
7. Krug, EG. *World report on violence and health.* Geneva: World Health Organization, 2002.
8. Wells DT. *Guidelines for medico-legal care for victims of sexual violence.* Geneva: Department of Injuries and Violence Prevention, World Health Organization, 2003.
9. Rothman EF, Butchart A, Cerdá M. *Intervening with perpetrators of intimate partner violence: A global perspective.* Geneva: Department of Injuries and Violence Prevention, World Health Organization, 2003.

10. Sethi D. Marais S, Seedat M, et al. *A handbook for the documentation of interpersonal violence prevention programmes.* Geneva: Department of Injuries and Violence Prevention, World Health Organization, 2004.

11. World Health Organization. *Guide to United Nations resources and activities for the prevention of interpersonal violence.* Geneva: Department of Injuries and Violence Prevention, World Health Organization, 2002.

12. Waters HH, Rajkotia Y, Basu S, et al. A. *The economic dimensions of interpersonal violence.* Geneva: Department of Injuries and Violence Prevention, World Health Organization, 2004.

13. World Health Organization. Global campaign for violence prevention. http://www.who.int/violence_injury_prevention/violence/global_campaign/en/ (accessed November 12, 2008).

14. Ellsberg M, Heise L. Bearing witness: Ethics in domestic violence research. *Lancet.* 2002; 359(9317):1599–1604.

15. Ellsberg M Heise L, Shrader E. *Researching violence against women: A practical guide for researchersand advocates.* Geneva: World Health Organization, Program for Appropriate Technology in Health, Center for Health and Gender Equity 2005.

16. Fernandez M. Cultural beliefs and domestic violence. *Ann NY Acad Sci.* 2006;1087(1):250–260.

17. Koenig MA, Ahmed S, Hossain MB, et al. Women's status and domestic violence in rural Bangladesh: Individual- and community-level effects. *Demography.* 2003;40(2):269–288.

18. Levinson D. *Family violence in cross-cultural perspectives.* Thousand Oaks CA: Sage, 1989.

19. Ellison CG, Trinitapoli JA, Anderson KL, Johnson BR. Race/ethnicity, religious involvement, and domestic violence. *Violence Against Women.* 2007; 13(11):1094–1112.

20. Ammar NH. Wife battery in Islam: A comprehensive understanding of interpretations. *Violence Against Women.* 2007;13(5):516–526.

21. Levitt HM, Ware K. "Anything with two heads is a monster": Religious leaders' perspectives on marital equality and domestic violence. *Violence Against Women.* 2006;12(12):1169–1190.

22. Khawaja M, Barazi R. Prevalence of wife beating in Jordanian refugee camps: Reports by men and women. *J Epidemiol Community Health.* 2005; 59(10):840–841.

23. Hynes M, Cardozo BL. Sexual violence against refugee women. *J Womens Health Gend Based Med.* 2000;9(8):819–823.

24. Hynes M, Ward J, Robertson K, Crouse C. A determination of the prevalence of gender-based violence among conflict-affected populations in East Timor. *Disasters.* 2004;28(3):294–321.

25. Midlarsky E, Venkataramani-Kothari A, Plante M. Domestic violence in the Chinese and South Asian immigrant communities. *Ann NY Acad Sci.* 2006;1087:279–300.

26. Morash M, Bui H, Zhang Y, Holtfreter K. Risk factors for abusive relationships: A study of Vietnamese American immigrant women. *Violence Against Women.* 2007;13(7):653–675.

27. Shiu-Thornton S, Senturia K, Sullivan M. "Like a Bird in a Cage": Vietnamese women survivors talk about domestic violence. *J Interpers Violence.* 2005;20(8):959–976.

28. Bhuyan R, Senturia K. Understanding domestic violence resource utilization and survivor solutions among immigrant and refugee women: Introduction to the special issue. *J Interpers Violence.* 2005;20(8):895–901.

29. Butchart AP, Phinney A, Check P, Villaveces A. *Preventing violence: A guide to implementing the recommendations of the World Report on Violence and Health.* Geneva: Department of Injuries and Violence Prevention, World Health Organization, 2004.

30. Bates LM, Schuler SR, Islam F, Islam K. Socioeconomic factors and processes associated with domestic violence in rural Bangladesh. *Int Fam Plan Perspect.* 2004;30(4):190–199.

31. Schuler SR, Hashemi SM, Riley AP, Akhter S. Credit programs, patriarchy and men's violence against women in rural Bangladesh. *Soc Sci Med.* 1996;43(12):1729–1742.

32. Koenig M, Hossain MB, Ahmed S, Haaga J. *Individual and community-level determinants of domestic violence in rural Bangladesh.* Baltimore, Johns Hopkins School of Public Health. Department of Population and Family Health Sciences. (Hopkins Population Center Paper on Population No. WP-99–04);1999:32.

33. Steele F, Amin S, Naved RT. The impact on an integrated micro-credit program on women's empowerment and fertility behavior in rural Bangladesh. *Policy Research Division Working Papers: New York, Population Control.* New York Population Council;1998:39.

34. Ahmed SM. Intimate partner violence against women: Experiences from a woman-focused development programme in Matlab, Bangladesh. *J Health Popul Nutr.* 2005;23(1):95–101.

35. Ayyub R. Homeless DV in South Asian Muslim immigrants. *J Soc Distress.* 2000;9(3):237–248.

36. Jejeebhoy SJ. Wife-beating in rural India: A husband's right? *Econ Political Weekly (India).* 1998;23: 588–862.

37. Martin SL, Tsui AO, Maitra K, Marinshaw R. Domestic violence in northern India. *Am J Epidemiol.* 1999;150(4):417–426.

38. Hassan F, Sadowski LS, Bangdiwala SI, et al. Physical intimate partner violence in Chile, Egypt, India and the Philippines. *Inj Control Saf Promot.* 2004;11(2):111–116.

39. Rao V. Wife-beating in rural south India: A qualitative and econometric analysis. *Soc Sci Med.* 1997;44(8):1169–1180.

40. Datta B, Motihar R. *Breaking down the walls: Violence against women as a health and human rights issue*. New Delhi Ford Foundation, 1999.

41. Xu X, Zhu F, O'Campo P, et al. Prevalence of and risk factors for intimate partner violence in China. [see comment]. *Am J Public Health*. 2005; 95(1):78–85.

42. Hollander D. Traditional gender roles and intimate partner violence linked in China. *Int Fam Plan Perspect*. 2005;31(1):46–47.

43. Guo SF, Wu JL, Qu CY, Yan RY. Domestic abuse on women in China before, during, and after pregnancy. *Chin Med J*. 2004;117(3):331–336.

44. Phillips MR, Yang G, Zhang Y, et al. Risk factors for suicide in China: A national case-control psychological autopsy study. *Lancet*. 2002;360(9347): 1728–1736.

45. Hasegawa M, Bessho Y, Hosoya T, Deguchi Y. [Prevalence of intimate partner violence and related factors in a local city in Japan]. *Nippon Koshu Eisei Zasshi*. 2005;52(5):411–421.

46. Yoshihama M, Sorenson SB. Physical, sexual, and emotional abuse by male intimates: Experiences of women in Japan. *Violence Vict*. 1994;9(1):63–77.

47. Horne S. Domestic violence in Russia. *Am Psychol*. 1999;54(1):55–61.

48. Centers for Disease Control and Prevention. *Russia Women's Reproductive Health Survey: Follow-up study of three sites: Final report*. Russian Center for Public Opinion and Market Research, Centers for Disease Control and Prevention, 2000.

49. Dude A. Intimate partner violence and increased lifetime risk of sexually transmitted infection among women in Ukraine. *Stud Fam Plann*. 2007;38(2): 89–100.

50. Kalichman SC, Kelly JA, Shaboltas A, Granskaya J. Violence against women and the impending AIDS crisis in Russia. *Am Psychol*. 2000;55(2): 279–280.

51. Crandall M, Senturia K, Sullivan M, Shiu-Thornton S. "No Way Out": Russian-speaking women's experiences with domestic violence. *J Interpers Violence*. 2005;20(8):941–958.

52. Johnson JE. Domestic violence politics in post-Soviet states. *Soc Pol*. 2007:jxm015.

53. Oyediran KA, Isiugo-Abanihe U. Perceptions of Nigerian women on domestic violence: Evidence from 2003 Nigeria Demographic and Health Survey. *Afr J Reprod Health*. 2005;9(2):38–53.

54. Obi SN, Ozumba BC. Factors associated with domestic violence in south-east Nigeria. *J Obstet Gynaecol*. 2007;27(1):75–78.

55. Efetie ER, Salami HA. Domestic violence on pregnant women in Abuja, Nigeria. *J Obstet Gynaecol*. 2007;27(4):379–382.

56. Ezechi OC, Kalu BK, Ezechi LO, et al. Prevalence and pattern of domestic violence against pregnant Nigerian women. *J Obstet Gynaecol*. 2004;24(6): 652–656.

57. Okemgbo CN, Omideyi AK, Odimegwu CO. Prevalence, patterns and correlates of domestic violence in selected Igbo communities of Imo State, Nigeria. *Afr J Reprod Health*. 2002;6(2):101–114.

58. World Health Organization. WHO multi-country study on women?s health and domestic violence against women. 2005. http://www.who.int/gender/violence/who_multicountry_study/en/index.html (accessed March 18, 2008).

59. Garcia-Moreno C, Jansen HAFM, Ellsberg M, et al. Prevalence of intimate partner violence: Findings from the WHO multi-country study on women's health and domestic violence.[see comment]. *Lancet*. 2006;368(9543):1260–1269.

60. Jewkes R, Levin J, Penn-Kekana L. Risk factors for domestic violence: Findings from a South African cross-sectional study. *Soc Sci Med*. 2002;55(9): 1603–1617.

61. McCloskey LA, Williams C, Larsen U. Gender inequality and intimate partner violence among women in Moshi, Tanzania. *Int Fam Plan Perspect*. 2005;31(3):124–130.

62. Maman S, Mbwambo JK, Hogan NM, et al. HIV-positive women report more lifetime partner violence: Findings from a voluntary counseling and testing clinic in Dar es Salaam, Tanzania. *Am J Public Health*. 2002;92(8):1331–1337.

63. Sa Z., Larsen U. Gender inequality increases a woman's risk for HIV in Moshi, Tanzania. *J Biosoc Sci*. 2008;40(4):505–525.

64. Rondon MB. From Marianism to terrorism: The many faces of violence against women in Latin America. *Arch Womens Ment Health*. 2003;6(3): 157–163.

65. Cripe SM, Sanchez SE, Perales MT, et al. Association of intimate partner physical and sexual violence with unintended pregnancy among pregnant women in Peru. *Int J Gynecol Obstet*. 2008;100(2):104–108.

66. Carrington K. *Domestic violence in Australia: An overview of the issues*. Parliament of Australia, Parliamentary Library, 2006.

67. *The Cost of Domestic Violence to the Australian Economy*. Partnerships Against Domestic Violence: An Australian Government Initiative, 2004.

68. Watson LF, Taft AJ, Lee C. Associations of self-reported violence with age at menarche, first intercourse, and first birth among a national population sample of young Australian women. *Womens Health Issues*. 2007;17(5):281–289.

69. Taft AJ, Watson LF. Termination of pregnancy: Associations with partner violence and other factors in a national cohort of young Australian women. *Aust N Z J Public Health*. 2007;31(2):135–142.

70. Graitcer R, Yousseff Z. *An analysis of: Injuries as a health problem*. Washington DC and Cairo U.S. Agency for International Development and Ministry of Health; 1993.

Chapter 7

Culture and Cultural Competency in Addressing Intimate Partner Violence

Sujata Warrier

KEY CONCEPTS

- The essentialist picture represents cultures as being distinct and separate, thus obscuring the reality that all boundaries between cultures are human constructs and that time and space bind the labels used to demarcate these boundaries.
- Assigning traditions, values, beliefs, and practices to any culture as stable elements obscures the ways in which historical and political processes shape how a particular tradition or practice comes to occupy a central position.
- One of the lessons learned in the early feminist movement is that a serious danger exists of imposing sameness on different groups of women, yet numerous problems arise when too much focus is placed on difference.
- To accommodate rapid changes in a complex world, culture must be critically redefined to also account for power, its structures, and its manifestations.
- Many terms are misused to describe diversity, such as multiculturalism; cultural sensitivity is quite different from cultural competency.
- A critical understanding of culture should include the intersections and interconnections existing between various aspects of identity and oppression, in order to move away from essentialist and one-dimensional notions of identity and oppression.
- Understanding the specificity of the cultural contexts that shape intimate partner violence (IPV) is essential, so that both similarities and differences in the lives of survivors can be examined in more nuanced ways using the "world traveling" methods of cultural competency.
- Cultural competency is not a set of behaviors to use simply to understand victims/survivors, but is a lifelong practice that combines critical thinking, dialog, self-reflection, and interrogation.

As the population of the United States has grown more diverse and healthcare professionals have had to work with people different from them, culture and cultural competency have emerged as areas of concern. Various agencies and written materials[1] provide many ways with which individual practitioners and healthcare agencies can learn to deal with diverse populations. Much of the material centers on individual actions that professionals can undertake in order to become culturally competent. Some additionally contain information on institutional concerns about diversity. These materials and training are useful, as professionals continue to integrate diversity.

That there is a concern on how to deal with diversity is truly remarkable and admirable; the problem lies with what is contained in the materials and what type of training is provided to assist healthcare providers (HCPs) in learning to be culturally competent. The majority of these materials contain a litany describing the characteristics of different groups and presenting solutions on how to work with those individuals who represent a particular racial or ethnic group. And although this approach may work for some professionals some of the time, serious gaps are evident. The complexity of cultural sensitivity is enhanced when the issue of dealing with and routinely screening for domestic violence or intimate partner violence (IPV) is added to the concerns of HCPs.

This chapter critiques the thinking on culture and cultural competency in the healthcare arena, especially in the context of IPV and women's health in an attempt to develop a critical framework for the issue and provide concrete ways in which to implement training. The goal is to persuade providers to use a more nuanced understanding of culture as they grapple with how to work with a diverse patient population.

[1]   To name a few, agencies such as the Multicultural Institute in Washington DC and the Cross-Cultural Health Care Program in Seattle provide training and technical assistance on the issue. Similarly, authors include Betancourt, J R., Green AR, Carrillo JE. *Cultural competence in health care: Emerging frameworks and practical approaches.* New York: The Commonwealth Fund, 2002; and The California Endowment. *Principles and recommended standards for the cultural competence education for health care professionals.* Woodland Hills, CA: The California Endowment, 2003.

"PACKAGED PICTURES OF CULTURE(S)"

Much of the material on culture and cultural competency contains behavioral characteristics of various groups of people, usually based on race or ethnicity, along with instructions on how to deal with individuals from these various groups. Many providers also attend seminars in which representatives from these groups also provide additional information on characteristic behaviors. In the context of IPV, this has meant that providers are taught how to work with victims from different communities, how to present the issue, how to screen, and how to determine feasible solutions for these victims, within the constraints of the culture. The same logic then applies to perpetrators as well. The fundamental flaw in this approach is that such a view of culture and cultural groups is fundamentally essentialist and based upon a binary or dichotomous view of the population—"whatever we are, they are not, and vice versa."

An essentialist and binary view gives rise to neat pictures of culture(s), or as Narayan (1) states, the "packaged picture of culture." The essentialist picture of cultures represents cultures as being distinct and separate, thus obscuring the reality that all boundaries between cultures are human constructs and that time and space bind all labels used to demarcate the boundaries (1). For example, a construct such as "the West" is bound by the time period in which it was constructed. Although today the idea of "the West" contains elements contributed from ancient Greece all the way to the modern United States, historically this has not been the case. Similar arguments can be made for all possible cultural groups. In the same vein, individuals are also assigned to specific cultures in obvious and uncontroversial ways. As a result, we then think that we know as a simple matter what culture or group we belong to. So, when we are assigned to a cultural group such as "American," do we really know what we have in common with the millions of other Americans? Critical reflection suggests that such assignment is less than simple and is affected by numerous methods of classification (1).

Assigning traditions, values, beliefs, and practices to any culture as stable elements of that culture obscures the ways in which historical and political processes shape how a particular tradition or practice comes to occupy a central position. Those holding the power in a community can take up any practice and discard others at will, at the same time disregarding those that might be important to other subgroups. This is especially true when it comes to women's issues and violence against women.[2] Many studies[3] in various parts of the world reveal ways in which dominant groups undercut the struggles for progress in women's rights, violence against women, and domestic violence by labeling changes in practices that affect women as *cultural loss* or *cultural betrayal*. The packaged pictures of cultures can pose serious problems for women's issues and, by extension, for domestic violence issues.

There is, therefore, a serious reason for moving away from static descriptions of culture that provide homogenous descriptions of people to one that reveals the sharp differences in values among people of the same group. Yet, we need to recognize that strong affinities exist among people of different groups; this allows us more hope for developing a cross-cultural agenda on IPV that meets the need of women in different groups. For example, in thinking about IPV, it is not enough to theorize male violence as occurring similarly across the globe. The very term "intimate partner violence" suggests that the phenomenon occurs in the same way in all cultures. Uncontested and uncritically accepted terminology imposes particular modalities of thinking and understanding. Many women from different parts of the world do not experience violence only at the hands of their intimate partners, but also from members of their extended families, both natal and affinal. How can the term IPV capture these nuances without missing out on an entire configuration of violence? Therefore, the understanding of IPV must be forged within those particular historical and cultural contexts within which male violence occurs, and it must be

interpreted within the context of specific communities. Only when we can describe, understand, and challenge how context shapes the experience of violence, can we draw universal inferences. The normal practice to date has been to use alleged "universals" to determine in what ways communities are different or aberrant from a "universal" model.

One of the lessons learned from the early feminist movement is that a serious danger exists of imposing sameness on different groups of women, yet numerous problems arise when too much focus is placed on difference. Although there is a need to account for differences arising from differing contexts, there is an equal risk of replacing woman essentialist analysis with culturally essentialist analysis. Both sets of essentialisms can be problematic when it comes to understanding and developing helpful interventions for battered women and their health needs.

DEFINITION OF CULTURE AND CULTURAL COMPETENCY

Armed with this understanding, an attempt was made to develop a more complex understanding and definition of culture that would encompass the idea of cultural context and outline a set of principles on how to develop competency in the area of domestic violence. The traditional definition of culture—one that portrays it as a stable pattern of values, traditions, beliefs handed down from one generation to another so that the second generation could successfully adapt to the first—is unacceptable. This static view of culture leads to the production of a "packaged picture of culture," wherein group characteristics are exclusively focused on the dimensions of race or ethnicity. Thus, using this static view, behaviors, norms, and traditions could be traced, unchanging, over the course of generations, without taking into account class or gender differences. Such packaged pictures also lead to the continued production of cultural misinformation or stereotypes about groups of people.

A more critical definition of culture arises out of our current state of knowledge, which refers to the shared experiences or commonalties that groups and individuals within groups have developed in relation to changing political and social contexts (2). Thus, culture must also include the human constructs of race, ethnicity, gender, class, age, sexual orientation, immigration, disability, and all other axes of identification understood within the

---

[2] A number of scholarly works deal with the use of culture in the discussion of women's issues and violence against women. To cite two: Bhavnani KK et al. *Feminist futures: Re-imagining women, culture and development.* London: Zed Books; 2003; and Mohanty CT. *Feminism without borders: Decolonizing theory, practicing solidarity.* Durham, NC: Duke University Press, 2003.

[3] See above and also Okin S, ed. *Is multiculturalism bad for women?* Princeton (NJ): Princeton University Press 1999; and Nussbaum M, Glover J. *Women, culture and development: A study of human capabilities.* Oxford: Clarendon Press, 1995.

historical context of oppression. These categories however, cannot be understood as isolated and discrete from each other, but rather as intersecting and interconnecting to produce differences within and between groups. The intersections and interconnections change as the social and political landscape changes.

Thus, we must first move away from understanding culture only in terms of race and ethnicity and second, we must be sensitive to the fact that all of the categories that make up a culture intersect in complex and nuanced ways for both individuals and groups. How a poor Asian American woman experiences IPV in New York City might have certain elements in common with how a lesbian Italian American experiences IPV in Iowa, but not have much in common with how another Asian American woman might experience violence in California. Similarly, a fourth-generation African American man growing up in Louisiana may share something in common with a young African American lesbian living in Los Angeles and a young Iberian mother who just immigrated to New York. As a group, these three may also share something in common with a Chinese American gymnast who is an atheist living in Des Moines with a young Chinese adopted by Jewish parents, and with a disabled 10-year-old Chinese American girl growing up in Minneapolis (3). The examples illustrate that culture and cultural identities are complex, multifaceted, and changing. There is much that we know and much that we do not know or will ever know.

In the complex interplay around culture and cultural identity, we cannot overlook the long history of oppression in the United States and how each group has experienced and may continue to experience varied forms of oppression. Although it may appear that oppression is a linking factor for marginalized groups, nevertheless oppression should always be contextualized because intersectional analysis compels us to.

Ethnicity, class, and sexual orientation all share something in common; how individuals and groups might experience each separately or in conjunction varies by location and historical context. Space and time therefore bind cultures. In attempting to teach, screen, or intervene it is critically important that the HCP understand the context in which differential experiences are produced. Intersectional analysis[4]

shifts us away from the dichotomous, binary way of thinking about structures, power, organization, and privilege. *Intersectionality* focuses attention on specific contexts, distinct experiences, and the qualitative aspects of equality and discrimination. It allows us to understand complexity, including the structural and dynamic dimensions of the interplay of different policies and institutions, so that interventions for victims of IPV can meet their needs. Without a complex understanding of the social and cultural factors, interventions and programs cannot achieve their full potential. These issues and concerns cannot be overlooked in any teaching, practice, research, or policy development that focuses on culture and cultural competency.

An analysis of intersectionality also forces us to move away from the current practices surrounding training, research, intervention, and policy, which consist of providing practitioners with a list of characteristics that will enable them to intervene with survivors who are obviously different from them. This information often is provided by "cultural experts," or the pattern is developed by the provider himself, after working with particular groups of people over an extended period. Looking for and establishing a pattern is how we make sense of complexity. When dealing with people, however, using established patterns can lead us down the path of misinterpretation, causing us to overlook critical cues and indicators. Generalized information, and not one or two attributes that describe a whole group of people, is the starting point. It gives us an important starting point to begin eliciting information that might be helpful in determining possible best practices and interventions that will lead the individual victim to a path of safety and empowerment. Providers must understand how a patient interprets her "culture," because the cues for intervention lie in this interpretation. For example, if the provider has heard that Asian women do not like to be screened and that they will never take action against their partners because of the

---

[4] Intersectionality theory seeks to examine the ways in which various socially and culturally constructed categories interact on multiple levels to manifest themselves as inequality in society. Intersectionality holds that the classical models of oppression within society, such as those based on race, ethnicity, gender, religion, and the like do not act independently of one another; instead, these forms of oppression interrelate to create a system of oppression that reflects the "intersection" of multiple forms of discrimination. See Crenshaw KW. Mapping the margins: Intersectionality, identity politics and violence against women of color. *Stanford Law Review*. 1991;43(6):1241–1299.

cultural notion of shame, it does not mean that all Asian women accept that interpretation. First, Asia constitutes half the world and is extraordinarily diverse. Whereas some may accept the notion of shame, others may accept some variation of it and others might totally reject it. However, the idea that some Asian women may be experiencing shame might nudge the provider to ask questions about what the term "shame" means to the woman, her family, and her community. The answers will provide the cues necessary to give referrals and develop appropriate interventions. Similar examples of how and in what ways culture needs to be considered for the appropriate screening of African American and Latina survivors can be found in the literatures cited (4–6).

Any work on cultural competency has to move away from presenting a packaged picture of cultures to an interrogation of power in the analysis and include material on entangling complex issues without losing the nuances. It means that the work of cultural competency is a lifelong process—attending a certain number of trainings, presentations, and certificates does not make for a culturally competent person. Such thinking also means that cultural work should be the purview of all, including those from oppressed or marginalized groups who think that they do not need it since they understand oppression. The intersections and interconnections between oppressions means that being oppressed or lacking privilege in one area does not guarantee that one does not have privilege in another. One can be oppressed from the standpoint of gender and ethnic identity but may be in the position of oppressing someone from a lower class, region, or sexual orientation. It must be recognized that oppressions interconnect, and cultural competency work is for all, encompassing a more nuanced understanding of privilege and access.

As stated earlier, IPV occurs in specific cultural contexts. It is not enough to state that male violence occurs universally in the same manner across cultures. The understanding of IPV has to be forged within concrete historical and political contexts and interpreted within specific communities and societies. So, it would be critical to consider "intersectionality" and how these experiences manifest themselves in the patient population in the area of IPV; how the experiences of the HCP can either exacerbate or alleviate the symptoms for the patient; and how the context within a particular healthcare facility can structure both the experience of the patient as well as the provider.

CULTURAL WORK IN INSTITUTIONS

Developing cultural competency work is not just about training. Training is the first component. Standardized 1- or 2-hour presentations do not work—competency training has to include real-life case scenarios that are helpful in critically redefining the work on culture and cultural competency in the area of domestic violence. Practicing screening and intervening is an integral part of the training. Because the nature of the problem is complicated itself, and the topic of culture is equally complicated, and any training that deals with both has to ensure that the participants are able to deconstruct each topic. Part of the training must explore the culture of the professional and the system, since cultural competency is not just about the culture of the patient. Historically, in almost all cultural competency training, the focus is on the culture of the patient—the idea that guides the work is that if there is an understanding of the patient's culture then appropriate interventions can be designed. However, in shaping of any outcome, the issue at hand is not just the culture of the patient. The equation includes the culture of the provider and the culture of the institution, as well as the culture of the patient. The first two components are commonly excluded since they are often harder to change and work on. But these two components are also part of the ongoing process of bringing cultural change in providers and health care institutions, so that they can then truly address the needs of the patient. Therefore, continuous self-assessments have to be incorporated into the process, and this must recur frequently, so that accountability for change work occurs and providers are truly able to relate to a diverse group of people and design effective interventions.

Given the current state of knowledge on health disparities in marginalized communities (7), an examination of the role of institutions in promoting and treating all patients equitably should be part of all cultural competency work. An examination of both personal and institutional bias is key to changing the treatment of survivors from diverse cultural groups. Some work has been done on how institutions create systematic barriers by standardizing worker actions through their mission, administrative practices, rules and regulations, theories and concepts, and training (8). Standardization is important because it brings consistency to everyday practice. In the context of IPV, it provides consistency to screening, assessment, and intervention. The problem with standardized or generalized practices is that they often fail to recognize and account for the multiple social positions occupied by patients—some of which might place them in marginalized areas. For the majority of patients, it may be important to vary the general practices, so that the provider can understand the context that is producing the particular set of experiences, and with which the possible assessment and intervention will have to contend. The understanding that providers occupy different places in an intersectional web should be translated to the experiences of patients. Often, the confluence of the cultures of the provider, institution, and patient collide in ways that are unhelpful for the patient experiencing partner violence.

In conclusion, it is not just the mere recognition of difference that makes for cultural competency, but a critical interrogation of, and grounding in cross-cultural work in an analysis of how power shapes institutional, personal, and social cultures. Paying attention to the specificity of diversity and difference does not mean generalizations cannot exist; rather, cross-cultural work or "world traveling" requires us to be attentive to the micropolitics of context and to the macropolitics of global economic and political systems, leading us to recognize that we can work on and through "common differences" (9,10). The concept of "world traveling" as put forth by Gunning forces us to abandon arrogant perceptions of practices that we might be unaware of and/or are offended by or do not understand. The central thesis of Gunning's work is that the preservation of, respect for, and equality of others and their cultures helps us to find areas of shared concerns. This forces us to understand not only our own historical context, which has shaped our cultures and thinking, but to grant the same respect for the "Other." We have to then attempt to understand how the "other" perceives us. *Mirroring* as a practice enables us to be more humble about ourselves in order to analyze different cultures and attempt to understand the particular configurations that created particular practices. So, at a daily practice level, this means that we get rid of the word *compliance*[5] and focus on developing a *colloquy*

---

[5] The above and following are taken from Arthur Kleinman (Harvard Medical School) and quoted in Fadiman A. *The sprit catches you and you fall down.* New York: Farrar, Straus and Giroux, 1997. See also Gunning I. Female genital surgeries. *Columbia Human Rights Law Review.* 1992;23(2):189–248.

with the patient, one that recognizes the importance of culture in our lives as well as theirs and the interconnectedness among all.

IMPLICATIONS FOR POLICY, PRACTICE, AND RESEARCH

Policy

- Policies should require continuous assessment of the workplace, focusing on the development of culturally competent practices, diversity of the workforce, and conflict resolution between different cultural positions to promote greater shared areas of concern.

- In attempting to develop policy, there should be considerable internal as well as external debate on the meaning and significance of the policy to various members of diverse communities.

- In the area of violence against intimate partners, it is crucial to remember that cultural relativism has no place. Rather cultural competency requires interrogation of practices in a respectful manner that will lead to a negotiated understanding. Only in this way is the policy of the utmost benefit to many.

- Policies are needed to encourage standardization of practices; however, standardization cannot come at the hands of flexibility as practitioners come across more challenging cultural practices and learn to negotiate changes in patient behavior.

- A sustainable model policy must be capable of valuing differences while assuring that differences will be seen as contributive and nonlimiting, working against pigeonholing and negative views of difference.

- Institutional practice should set up a norm of expecting differences, assuming that these are not essential, and accepting that it is acceptable to notice differences.

- In interpreting any policy or legislation in the context of cultural competency, it is critical to expose all debate and disagreement. For example, in developing the International Convention of the Rights of the Child, many debates centered around certain fundamental questions. Similar questions and debate can be developed using a diversity of opinions, people, and communities.

Practice

- Remove the word "compliance" from health-care terminology. Patients, especially survivors from marginalized or different communities, cannot simply comply with recommendations from the provider, especially if it appears that these recommendations are being imposed from a viewpoint of privilege.
- In the area of IPV, cultural relativism—that one's beliefs and values can only be interpreted through one's own culture—is unacceptable. Neither is cultural imposition—the idea that everybody should conform to the majority (because we know best). The focus should be on developing a colloquy with the victim/survivor and negotiating the acceptance of new ideas or values.
- Be aware that just because someone looks like you, talks like you, or dresses like you it does not mean that they automatically think like you.
- Be aware of one's own blinding preferences and how they shape the ways in which we view the other person. Although we know that the clear and explicit expression of prejudice and bias is wrong, implicit bias (or where one's preference for one's own group lies outside awareness and often clashes with overtly expressed views or unconscious attitudes) can also have harmful results. "We do not see things as they are but as we are."[6]
- Attempt to understand the person's own interpretation of their culture rather than imposing your version on it.
- Recognize professional power and avoid the imposition of values.
- Negotiate the acceptance of a different set of values: It takes time for people to change—be patient.

Research

- All research should be cognizant of blinding preferences, acknowledge their existence, and determine how they may or may not impact the work.
- Research should attempt to historicize and describe the social nature of the issues uncovered.
- Researchers should be more nuanced in their understanding of culture, and expose how the intersection of different aspects of identity impact violence.
- Analyzing complexities requires making multidimensional conceptualizations that expose how socially constructed categories interact and lead to specific experiences of IPV. Without such research generalizations, replicability and scaling-up are nearly impossible or of limited value. This means that more detailed cross-tabulations and context analysis uncovers details.
- Researchers should actively involve the community and attempt to understand the idiosyncrasies, internal dissensions, conflicts, and gender roles within a particular community and their impact on individuals.
- Be careful with terminology, such as IPV, in specific communities. It may not resonate or mean the same as it does to researchers. Search for what research subjects understand by terms and points of agreements and disagreements within the conceptualization of terms.

References

1. Narayan U. Undoing the package picture of culture. *Signs.* 2000;25(4):1083–1086.
2. Warrier S, Brainin-Rodriguez J. *From sensitivity to competency: Clinical and departmental guidelines to achieving cultural competency.* San Francisco (CA): Family Violence Prevention Fund, 1998.
3. Minnow M. *Not only for myself: Identity, politics and the law.* New York (NY): The New Press, 1996.
4. Bent-Goodley T. Perceptions of domestic violence: A dialogue with African American women. *Health Soc Work.* 2004;29(4):307–316.
5. Campbell DW, Sharps PW, Gary FA, et al. Intimate partner violence in African American women. *Online J Issues Nurs.* 2002;7(1):5.
6. Adames SB, Campbell R. Immigrant Latinas conceptualizations of IPV. *Violence Against Women.* 2005;11(10):1341–1364.
7. Gunning I. Female genital surgeries. *Columbia Human Rights Law Rev.* 1992;2(2)189–248.
8. Mohanty CT. *Feminism without borders: Decolonizing theory, practicing solidarity.* Durham, NC: Duke University Press;2003:223.
9. Smith D. *Institutional ethnography: A sociology for the people.* Lanham, MD: AltaMira Press, 2005.
10. Pence E, Sheppard M. *Coordinating community responses to domestic violence.* Duluth, MN: The National Training Project, 1999.

---

[6] Anais Nin.

Chapter 8

Diagnosis Through Disclosure and Pattern Recognition

Deirdre Anglin

KEY CONCEPTS

- Intimate partner violence (IPV) is identified in the clinical setting by one of two means: patient disclosure that may be either spontaneous or prompted, or clinically suspected by means of pattern recognition in the history or physical examination.
- Fostering disclosure of IPV involves practitioner behaviors that promote privacy and safety, as well as addressing institutional, professional, and victim barriers to disclosure.
- During discussions with patients about stigmatized health issues such as IPV, healthcare providers (HCPs) must convey compassion, interest, and respect, and maintain a nonjudgmental perspective at all times.
- *Screening* is a public health term used to describe the application of a test to diagnose asymptomatic disease. *Assessment*, including routine inquiry, for IPV is a process for identifying asymptomatic (screening) as well as symptomatic (case finding) individuals with past or current partner violence that may be affecting their physical and mental health.
- Assessment or routine inquiry about IPV in the clinical setting may be conducted using written or verbal questionnaires or computer-based health assessments. Assessment for IPV should be flexible, and the specific questions will vary depending on the discussion between the patient and provider regarding current or past abuse.
- Most female patients believe that it is important for HCPs to ask patients about IPV.
- It is necessary to differentiate the act of diagnosing IPV from the diagnosis "adult maltreatment" for diagnostic or surveillance reasons, or the mandated reporting of IPV to legal or public health authorities.
- In the absence of outcome studies demonstrating the efficacy of IPV interventions to which

...or many years, intimate partner violence (IPV) has been viewed as a complex social issue that interfaces with the criminal justice and social justice systems. More recently, IPV has also been recognized as an important healthcare issue. Based on numerous studies, the prevalence of current IPV of any type among women in the primary care setting ranges from 8%–29%. Further, 21%–39% of women presenting to primary care providers have experienced IPV at some point in their lives (1). In a review of 13 studies on IPV during pregnancy, Gazmararian found that the prevalence ranged from 1%–20% (2). Summarizing a number of emergency department–based studies, between 1% and 7% of all adult and adolescent females present to the emergency department on account of acute physical abuse (3–6). In addition, 14%–22% of women presenting for any reason have a history of IPV in the past year (5,7), and 37%–54% of female patients have a lifetime history of IPV (5,8).

Increasingly, the adverse health sequelae of IPV are being acknowledged. Women who have experienced IPV suffer many physical health problems including trauma (9,10); cardiorespiratory problems, such as palpitations, chest pain, shortness of breath, hyperventilation, and asthma exacerbations; gastrointestinal disorders, such as functional bowel disease (11); gynecologic disorders, such as frequent urinary tract infections, sexually transmitted infections (STIs), HIV, and chronic pelvic pain; neurologic problems, such as headaches; and generalized constitutional symptoms such as fatigue, chronic pain, weakness, and weight loss or gain (12–14). In addition, these women have higher rates of mental health problems, including anxiety, depression, posttraumatic stress disorder (PTSD), suicidality (8), and alcohol and substance abuse (13). In addition, McCloskey identified that among women presenting to the healthcare setting who reported IPV in the previous year, 17% reported that their partners interfered with their health care, as compared to 2% of those women without past-year IPV (odds ratio [OR] 7.5, 95% confidence interval [CI] 4.7–11.9) (15). The women reporting partner interference disclosed poorer health than those without partner interference. Partner interference may result in limited access to care or noncompliance with scheduled appointments or medications.

Research has shown that women who are victims of IPV have increased utilization of healthcare services. Ulrich and colleagues compared the healthcare utilization of women who had medical record–confirmed IPV to those who had no evidence of IPV in their medical records, and who presented for an injury, chronic pelvic pain, depression, or a physical examination. They found that, with adjusting for comorbidity, women with IPV were 1.6 times more likely to use healthcare services than those without documented IPV. Further, when compared with a second population-based group, the women experiencing IPV were 2.6 times more likely to use healthcare services. Ulrich also noted that the IPV victims had greater annual healthcare costs (16). Wisner also found that victims of IPV had increased healthcare costs. In her study, she compared the annual costs of IPV patients in a large health plan to a random sample of women with no IPV history. She found that IPV patients cost the health plan $1,775 or 92% more annually (17).

The healthcare system offers numerous opportunities for women experiencing IPV to interact with healthcare providers (HCPs). Yet, numerous studies have documented the missed opportunities within the healthcare system for identifying patients experiencing IPV. Kothari reviewed hospital records for emergency department visits by IPV victims listed in a county prosecutor's IPV database in southwest Michigan. Within 1 year of the index assault, 63.9% IPV victims had sought care in at least one emergency department, and within 3 years of the index assault, 81.7% had one or more emergency department visits, with four being the mean number of visits. In 30.3% of the visits, assessment for IPV was documented, with only 5.8% being positive (18). In a study of 34 IPV homicides in Kansas City, Wadman found that 15 (44%) had presented to an emergency department within the previous 2 years, making a total of 48 visits. In two cases, IPV was identified, however, no interventions were documented (19). In Campbell's study of femicide victims, 22% of physically abused women saw an HCP within the year prior to the femicide, and

12% of the abused/stalked women saw a mental health provider prior to the femicide. Half of the women with injuries from IPV had been seen in the emergency department for their injuries. In addition, 20% of the femicide perpetrators had seen HCPs for physical or mental health care in the year prior to committing the femicide (20).

Given the varied presentations of women to HCPs, adverse effects of IPV on women's health, the high rates of physical and mental health problems of IPV victims, and the frequency with which IPV victims interact with the HCPs, advocates and experts recommend that HCPs identify IPV victims in order to improve their care and provide them with options to address their health and safety needs. However, the best way to undertake the identification of IPV patients in the healthcare setting is uncertain and has been the topic of substantial controversy recently. This chapter discusses the various ways that disclosure of IPV in the healthcare setting may occur, how to foster disclosure, and the barriers to disclosure. In addition, this chapter discusses the definition of the public health term *screening*, and will examine the evidence for and controversy surrounding IPV screening.

DISCLOSURE OF INTIMATE PARTNER VIOLENCE

The word *disclosure* means the act of revealing or uncovering (21). In the case of IPV in the healthcare setting, we use the term disclosure to refer to the act of a patient informing a practitioner about current or past abuse. Disclosure of IPV may be either spontaneous or prompted.

Spontaneous Disclosure

A patient may spontaneously disclose IPV as part of the chief complaint, or as part of the history of the presenting illness. For example, when a triage nurse asks a woman why she came to the emergency department, the response "My boyfriend punched me in the eye," would constitute a spontaneous disclosure. Likewise, when in the course of obtaining a more detailed medical history a practitioner asks a patient when she began having back pain, her response "Ever since my husband pushed me down a flight of stairs," is a spontaneous disclosure of IPV. Past abuse may also be spontaneously disclosed.

Prompted Disclosure

Prompted disclosure refers to the situation in which a patient discloses current or past IPV in response to routine inquiry or assessment for IPV by the HCP. It may also occur in response to the clinician asking additional questions in the course of the history or physical examination in order to ascertain the diagnosis via pattern recognition. *Pattern recognition* is the cognitive process by which clinicians sort historical clues, findings on the physical examination, and patient presentations into a particular diagnosis, based on known clinical findings of that particular health problem. As reviewed briefly earlier, certain clinical conditions are suggestive of the underlying diagnosis of IPV. When faced with a clinical presentation suggestive of IPV, an HCP may specifically inquire about current or past abuse, and such an inquiry may prompt disclosure.

FOSTERING DISCLOSURE OF INTIMATE PARTNER VIOLENCE

Two major concerns surrounding prompted disclosure of IPV are privacy and safety. Breaches of privacy and safety have been cited by numerous authors as potential harms due to routine inquiry about IPV, and whereas privacy and safety is a priority for every patient, for IPV patients, a lapse in precautions could lead to further harm.

Behaviors for Promoting Privacy

To create an environment that fosters disclosure, it is important to provide the most private situation possible. While it is preferable to have a patient-only interview policy, patients will frequently request that friends or family members be present during an encounter with an HCP. Victims of IPV may feel shame or embarrassment about their abusive relationship and would likely choose not to disclose current or past abuse in front of friends, family members, or their children, even though these individuals may already be aware of the ongoing IPV. One survey of 140 women entering a domestic violence shelter found that women preferred to talk with HCPs alone, and felt uncomfortable with children, friends, or family members in the room (22). Healthcare providers must also be aware that a visitor of the same sex as the patient may be their intimate partner. Allowing some time for private interviews with each patient should be a matter of policy, whether it be in a clinic, office, or emergency department setting.

If interpretive services are required for communication with a patient about any personal issues, including IPV, only hospital, clinic, or office employees or a nationally based telephone translator service should be used. In smaller communities, if the interpreter is a hospital or clinic employee, the patient should always be asked if they know or are related to the interpreter, so as not to jeopardize their privacy or put them at additional risk. In that case, a nationally based telephone translator service should be used. In the event that no translator other than the partner can be found, the HCP should avoid asking questions about IPV and arrange for a follow-up visit when an interpreter can be obtained.

If a written or computerized health questionnaire is being used to gather pertinent medical and social information, including about sensitive topics such as IPV, patients must be provided with a private environment in which to complete the questionnaire. When promoting privacy in fostering disclosure, it is also important to make patients aware of the limits of confidentiality. In the past several years, some states have enacted laws regarding the mandatory reporting of injuries from IPV. Healthcare practitioners must be aware of the laws in the state(s) in which they practice regarding the reporting of abusive behaviors such as IPV. In some states, HCPs are only mandated to report firearm injuries; in others they are mandated to report all injuries from knives or stabbing instruments; and in some, all injuries suspected to be from assaultive or abusive behavior must be reported to law enforcement. Additionally, HCPs may be required to report sexual abuse and elder abuse. Some states may have requirements to report children who witness IPV. It is suggested that, prior to asking about IPV, HCPs inform their patients about the circumstances under which they would be required to report violence-related problems or other public health and safety risks. Further, if a patient expresses homicidal ideation in relation to a specific individual, the HCP has the duty to warn that other individual under the *Tarasoff vs. University of California Regents* decision (23,24).

Behaviors for Promoting Safety

Patient safety in the healthcare setting is of paramount importance. In the case of IPV, patient safety may be compromised in several ways: an abusive partner may be in the waiting room nearby or arrive unexpectedly at the healthcare facility, or he may be a patient himself at the same facility, perhaps even of the same HCP. To help a patient feel safe in an examination room, all doors should have locking mechanisms and the facility should have alternate routes of egress. In addition, the medical facility should have a protocol to deal with the eruption of violence by a batterer.

Provider Characteristics and Behaviors

Several studies describe HCP characteristics that foster disclosure of IPV by patients. The majority of these are qualitative studies involving focus groups or surveys of women who have experienced IPV. Chang found that when posters and other information about IPV were available in the healthcare setting, it made IPV patients feel that the HCP was a safe person to talk to about the abuse (25). Healthcare practitioner characteristics and behaviors that created a more comfortable environment for women to disclose IPV included listening attentively; demonstrating compassion and concern; acting in a caring, nonjudgmental manner; and being trustworthy (26–28). In addition, women expressed that an HCP's respect for a woman's desire to have control over decision-making in her life fostered disclosure (29). Some studies found that women experiencing IPV preferred to talk with female HCPs about their abusive situations (22,26,30,31). However, in other studies, there was no clear gender preference (27). Feder conducted a meta-analysis of qualitative studies of women's experiences when they encounter HCPs and found that the evidence for gender preference is conflicting (32).

POTENTIAL BARRIERS TO DISCLOSURE OF INTIMATE PARTNER VIOLENCE

Numerous barriers to the identification and disclosure of IPV in the clinical setting have been cited in the literature. The majority of studies regarding barriers to disclosure have utilized focus groups or surveys. These barriers may be categorized into institutional barriers, personal barriers of the IPV patient, and professional and personal barriers of the HCP.

Institutional Barriers

Both IPV patients and HCPs have expressed that HCP time constraints in today's clinical practice are a major institutional barrier to disclosure of IPV by patients (26,33–36). To avoid giving patients the perception of trivializing their experiences, adequacy of time is particularly important when addressing complex social problems such as IPV. In studies by Mezey and Minsky, HCPs stated that a lack of time to be alone with a patient, safety issues, and staff shortages were barriers to disclosure (34,35). Bacchus found that a lack of privacy and a lack of continuity of care in their primary care settings were also barriers to disclosure for IPV patients, who felt they lacked rapport with a specific HCP (26). Additional institutional barriers include the lack of a protocol and the lack of availability of translators and social services or peer counselors. Institutions that regularly assess for compliance with measures of quality for IPV care will gradually identify and address multiple barriers to providing IPV patient care.

Personal Barriers for the Intimate Partner Violence Patient

Women who had experienced IPV expressed numerous barriers to disclosure of IPV to HCPs. Shame, embarrassment, and denial were frequent reasons why they did not disclose IPV (26,27,37). In addition, batterers' threats of violence (29) and women's fear of retaliation by their partners (33,38) if they found out the woman had revealed IPV prevented many women from disclosing. Some IPV patients talked about being concerned about law enforcement being contacted (29), whereas others said that they were reluctant to initiate a conversation about their abusive situations (26,28). Several IPV patients spoke about their fears that they might lose control of being able to make decisions that impacted them if they were to disclose IPV to their HCP (37). Many IPV patients voiced that HCP behaviors deterred them from disclosing abuse. Behaviors such as appearing disinterested, unsympathetic, untrustworthy, too busy, and judgmental were barriers to patient disclosure (26,33,38). In addition, HCPs who did not provide validation of a woman's experience, or who seemed to have a lack of understanding of the complexity of IPV dissuaded IPV patients from discussing their situation further (33,38).

Professional and Personal Barriers for the Healthcare Provider

The most frequent barriers to asking about IPV that HCPs cite are time constraints (34), a lack of education about IPV and IPV interventions (35,36), and a lack of

effective interventions to which to refer patients (36). In addition, issues related to reimbursement for potentially time-consuming interactions with IPV patients dissuade HCPs from inquiring about IPV. Other barriers include a fear of offending patients, frustration that patients do not disclose and do not take the HCP's advice, mandatory reporting to authorities (35,36), and the fear of having to make court appearances. In addition, an HCP's own experiences with IPV may prevent her or him from inquiring of a patient about IPV (34). Further, misconceptions about batterers and victims, personal biases, and the belief that IPV is a private not healthcare problem may affect the ability of HCPs to identify IPV among their patients.

Overcoming Barriers to Disclosure of Intimate Partner Violence

Although substantial research has been conducted on barriers to disclosure, even greater effort must be made into how to break down the barriers and assist HCPs to routinely inquire about IPV. Numerous studies have shown that educating HCPs about IPV increases rates of inquiry; however, the educational efforts have not all been effective and have not demonstrated long-lasting effects. Studies that have combined educational programs with additional interventions such as chart prompts (4) or advocacy programs (39) have resulted in improved rates of identification of IPV. Further, healthcare settings in which a comprehensive system-wide approach to support HCPs and IPV patients has been instituted (40) has been shown to be effective in increasing rates of identification and referral by clinicians.

DISCUSSING STIGMATIZED HEALTH ISSUES

In the course of routine clinical assessment HCPs frequently ask patients questions about health risks that are related to stigmatized health conditions. For example, HIV infection, STIs, alcohol and substance abuse, and mental health problems are all stigmatized health issues. Likewise, IPV is a stigmatized health condition, and patients who have experienced IPV are vulnerable to being revictimized. First, HCPs need to address their own barriers and biases related to IPV, so that they are able to respond to their patients in a nonjudgmental, compassionate, respectful way.

The use of *framing questions* is one way to convey a nonjudgmental attitude and make patients feel that they are not being singled out based on preconceived biases (25). For example, prior to directly asking about IPV, an HCP could state, "I ask all my female patients these questions" or "Because violence is such a common problem among women, I have begun asking about it routinely in my practice." Further, HCPs need to reflect on their own feelings related to interacting with IPV patients and be aware of any emotional responses that IPV patients may trigger, such as frustration, impatience, or a desire to tell the patient what is best for her.

Some patients may provide HCPs with cues, hoping that the HCP will ask further questions and thus enable them to provide an *invitational disclosure*. An invitational disclosure occurs when a patient hints or alludes to an HCP about a problem, such as a stigmatized health condition, hoping that the provider will pick up on the cues and ask more about it, thus inviting the patient to disclose the nature of the issue (27,41).

SCREENING FOR INTIMATE PARTNER VIOLENCE

With the increased recognition of IPV as a healthcare and public health problem, several professional medical organizations and regulatory bodies have endorsed routine "screening" for the identification of IPV in the clinical setting. These organizations include the American Medical Association (42), American College of Obstetricians and Gynecologists (43), American College of Emergency Physicians (44), and the American Academy of Family Practice (45). Further, the Joint Commission on Accreditation of Healthcare Organizations has requirements for the identification of victims of violence among patients. The Family Violence Prevention Fund in their *National Consensus Guidelines on Identifying and Responding to Domestic Violence Victimization in Health Care Settings* also recommends routine screening by those working in the healthcare setting (46). However, the optimal way for this "screening" to be conducted remains unclear.

What Is Screening?

Screening is a public health term that refers to the identification of an unrecognized disease or condition in asymptomatic individuals through the use of a spe-

cific test, examination, or procedure (47). The goal of screening is to recognize a disease process early in its course in healthy individuals, thereby decreasing morbidity and mortality on account of the early referral to effective interventions. The population being screened may be selected based on certain criteria, such as age, gender, or other risk factors. The tests and procedures that are used for screening are validated to ensure that they are effective in identifying truly positive cases while minimizing the number of false-negative results. The diagnosis is then confirmed using a "gold standard" test (for example, a biopsy).

Does the term "screening" apply to the identification of IPV in the clinical setting? Are IPV patients asymptomatic? It has been recommended that women should be routinely "screened" for IPV due to the high prevalence and varied presentations of IPV among female patients. However, in doing so, not only are asymptomatic patients being questioned, but also patients who fall all along the spectrum of IPV. This includes patients who have never experienced IPV and are not at risk for IPV, those who are at risk for IPV but have not yet experienced it, those who have experienced IPV but do not yet have adverse physical and mental health sequelae, and those who have experienced IPV and are very symptomatic—suffering from severe adverse physical and mental health sequelae, including near fatalities—and fully recognize that they are experiencing IPV, even if the HCPs do not.

Is there a validated test to use for screening, and is there a gold standard for confirming the diagnosis? Several questionnaires or instruments have been developed to identify IPV and will be discussed later in this chapter. Almost all have been developed for use in questioning women; many have been validated in selected populations or in specific clinical situations. However, rather than a standardized instrument, HCPs often use a variety of other questions in the course of obtaining a history to identify IPV among patients. Not all forms of IPV (physical, sexual, psychological) are identified by all questionnaires. In addition, IPV may only be identified by a clinician if the IPV-exposed patient chooses to disclose at that particular encounter. Further, no gold standard test exists with which to confirm the diagnosis of IPV. There is also a lack of research on the effectiveness of interventions to which IPV patients can be referred. In summary, the traditional public health term "screening" does not apply to the currently advocated questioning of patients about IPV by HCPs.

ASSESSMENT FOR INTIMATE PARTNER VIOLENCE

The overall process by which HCPs identify current or past IPV is probably best referred to as *assessment*. Assessment applies to all patients who present for care, including those within the full spectrum of exposure to IPV. Patients may have nonexposure, exposure/asymptomatic (screen), or exposure/symptomatic (case finding). But given that IPV is not readily disclosed due to both fear and stigmas, routine assessment may lead to identification of patients anywhere along the spectrum (Figure 8.1). Intimate partner violence, in and of itself, is not a disease but describes an unhealthy relationship. However, due to the health impact of the relationship, it may have a course similiar to that of a chronic disease.

Whether the routine inquiry is verbal or is initiated by means of patients completing a paper or computerized health questionnaire prior to being seen by the HCP, ultimately the assessment will result in a conversation between the patient and HCP. The exact way that the conversation is carried out must be individualized, so that it is sensitive to the patient's presenting problems, race and ethnicity, language barriers, cultural beliefs, and sexual orientation.

Gerbert (48) conducted a qualitative study of how physicians with expertise in managing IPV approach the identification of IPV patients in their practices. Participants included 45 emergency physicians, obstetricians/gynecologists, and primary care physicians who regularly identify IPV patients and refer them to resources. The physicians described several behaviors they use in assessing patients for IPV. First, they try to make the patients feel more comfortable by normalizing the inquiry about IPV through framing questions. They also ask about IPV during the social history, along

with other questions about safety issues such as wearing seat belts. These physicians also described that, during the evaluation of a patient, certain symptoms and clinical findings (pattern recognition) "switched on a light bulb" in their minds and prompted them to ask additional questions. In addition, these providers described approaching identification through indirect as well as direct inquiry. Many instruments that have been developed for inquiring about IPV use direct questions that ask about being hit, hurt, or threatened. These providers frequently found that indirect questions such as "Is there anything else on your mind that you would like to tell me?" or "Is there something going on at home that might be causing you to feel this way?" were more likely to facilitate disclosure. Finally, these physicians spoke about redefining success in prompting disclosure. Rather than the actual disclosure constituting a successful outcome of routine inquiry, they defined success as an assessment in which they convey compassion and caring to the patient, let the patient know that it is a safe environment in which to talk about abuse when they were ready, and provide the patient with information and resources. Chang (25) found that women who have experienced IPV want to be offered information and resources, whether or not they choose to disclose.

In a study by Rhodes, in which clinical encounters between patients and physicians in the emergency department were audiotaped, certain provider communication behaviors were associated with disclosure of IPV. These included providing patients with an open-ended opportunity to speak, asking one or more additional questions after the first question about IPV, and asking further questions when a patient mentioned any type of psychosocial problem. However, even with awkward provider–patient communications, patients still disclosed IPV (49). This confirms that, although

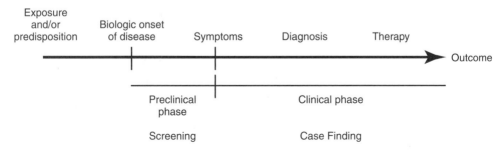

Figure 8.1 What is the natural history of a disease?

some provider behaviors will foster disclosure and the identification of IPV in the healthcare setting, no one single way exists for an assessment to be conducted. More importantly, as discussed by Gerbert and confirmed by Chang, there needs to be a response by providers to provide further information and referrals to healthcare- and community-based resources whether or not IPV was disclosed (25,50).

Routine inquiry in itself is an intervention, providing patients with validation that IPV is unacceptable, whether or not they have experienced abuse, and whether or not they choose to disclose at that particular time (51). Nondisclosure does not mean that the patient has not been helped.

INTIMATE PARTNER VIOLENCE DISCLOSURE: METHODS OF ROUTINE INQUIRY

Routine inquiry may be conducted via person-to-person interviews or through written or computer-based questionnaires. A couple of research studies have used audiotaping for disclosure, but because this method of inquiry has not been widely studied, it will not be discussed in this chapter (52). Patient preferences for the three techniques for routine inquiry need to be taken into account, as this will affect the rates of IPV disclosure. However, since disclosure depends on patients who are experiencing IPV to choose to disclose the abuse at that specific time, rates of disclosure alone should not be used to decide which method of inquiry is best. Advantages and disadvantages apply to each of the approaches.

Person-to-Person Interviews

In some studies, person-to-person interviews have been found to be preferred by patients (50,53). In-person interviews have the advantage that the HCP may be able to pick up on patient cues, such as body language or affect during the questioning. In addition, providers can ask additional questions as part of their assessment for IPV and provide support and validation at the time of the interview. Disadvantages of interviews include HCPs having to remember to ask about IPV, and individual variations between HCPs' styles of questioning and comfort with questioning, which may affect patients' likelihood of disclosing.

Written Questionnaires

Other studies have revealed patients' preferences for disclosing IPV as part of written questionnaires (54,55). One advantage of written questionnaires is that patients can complete them prior to meeting with the HCP, hence saving time. Questions related to IPV may be included in a more comprehensive health questionnaire. Also, patients may feel that they have greater privacy with written questionnaires. However, language barriers and patient literacy may make written questionnaires more difficult for some patients to complete. In addition, patients must be provided with a private, safe location (not the waiting room) in which to complete the questionnaires.

Computer-based Questionnaires

Recently, computer-based questionnaires have been used to assist in identifying patients experiencing IPV. Comprehensive health and safety assessments, including questions about IPV, can be completed prior to the provider–patient interaction, and a print-out of the patient's responses placed with the medical record. Several studies have shown a patient preference for this method of inquiry about IPV (56), although other studies have found computer-based questionnaires to have similar acceptance among patients as written questionnaires (57). Due to the technology, some patients may not feel comfortable using a computer, or may have limited literacy. Therefore, assistance must be readily available. In addition, computers are expensive and require available technical support. Despite these issues, computer-based questionnaires for identifying IPV show promise.

ASSESSMENT TOOLS FOR INQUIRY ABOUT INTIMATE PARTNER VIOLENCE IN THE HEALTHCARE SETTING

Numerous assessment tools have been developed for use by HCPs for the purposes of identifying IPV in the healthcare setting. In general, due to time constraints in the healthcare setting, when routine inquiry is in-person, brief tools are most useful. The tools described in Table 8.1 assess for one or more forms of IPV. Most of the tools have been validated against one of two lengthier questionnaires that are considered gold

Table 8.1 Assessment Tools for Use in Identification of Intimate Partner Violence (IPV) in Patients in Healthcare Settings

Assessment Tool/Author	Description of Tool	Psychometrics	Method of Administration	Target Population
Abuse Assessment Screen (AAS) (McFarlane, 1992)	5-item tool, asks about physical, sexual and psychological abuse, and the relationship of the perpetrator to the patient; Spanish version available	93% sensitive, 55% specific vs. ISA	Verbal	Multiethnic pregnant and nonpregnant women in healthcare settings
Composite Abuse Scale (CAS) (Hegarty, 1999)	30-item scale, 4 subscales measuring physical and psychological abuse and harrassment	Internal consistency for physical abuse: 0.94; psychological abuse: 0.93; harassment: 0.87	Verbal or written	Women with current or former partners for more than 1 month
Revised Conflict Tactics Scales (CTS2) (Strauss, 1996)	39-item victimization scales, measures use of reasoning, verbal aggression, physical violence in resolving family conflict, as well as familial interpersonal conflict. 7-point Likert scale	Internal consistency 0.79–0.95 construct and discriminant validity	Verbal or written	Women and men in relationships
HITS (Hurt-Insult-Threaten-Scream) (Sherin, 1998, Chen, 2005, Shakil, 2005)	4-item tool, asks about the frequency of IPV; Spanish version also available	Women: 86–96% sensitive, 91–99% specific vs. CTS or ISA Men: 88% sensitive, 97% specific vs. CTS Spanish: 100% sensitive, 86% specific vs. WAST	Verbal or written	Women in primary care settings, men in clinical settings
Index of Spouse Abuse (ISA) (Hudson, 1981)	30-item tool, asks about intensity of physical and nonphysical violence to women by their partners; Likert scale	Data based on approximately 500 women	Verbal or written	Women being evaluated and monitored for progress in treatment
Partner Violence Screen (PVS) (Feldhaus, 1997)	3-item tool, asks about past-year physical violence and safety	64.5% sensitive, 80.3% specific vs. ISA 71.4% sensitive, 84.4% specific vs. CTS	Verbal	Women patients in emergency departments
Woman Abuse Screening Tool (WAST) (Brown, 2000)	8-item tool, asks about physical, sexual, and emotional IPV; Spanish version available	Construct validity: correlation with Abuse Risk Inventory 0.69 Cronbach's α–0.75	Written	Women in healthcare settings and shelters
Women's Experience of Battering (WEB) (Smith, 1995)	10-item tool, asks about psychological IPV and battering	86% sensitive, 91% specific vs. ISA Cronbach's α–0.95	Written	African-American and White women in primary care settings

standards, either the Conflict Tactics Scale (CTS) (58) or the Index of Spouse Abuse (ISA) (59). These two instruments were developed for use in research or in evaluating the clinical progress of women experiencing IPV in the treatment setting, and were not developed or validated in the healthcare setting. A more comprehensive review of IPV assessment tools is provided in the two CDC publications, *Measuring Intimate Partner Violence Victimization and Perpetration: A Compendium of Assessment Tools* (60) and

Intimate Partner Violence and Sexual Violence Victimization Assessment Instruments for Use in Healthcare Settings (61). As stated previously, these tools may be used to facilitate routine inquiry and assessment for IPV by HCPs in the clinical setting. In research, their use provides a standardized method of identification of IPV patients.

SUPPORT OR NONSUPPORT FOR ROUTINE INQUIRY

Patients Experiencing Intimate Partner Violence

Several researchers have studied the issue as to whether patients, including those experiencing IPV, support routine inquiry about IPV in the healthcare setting. Some studies were qualitative, involving focus groups, whereas others used survey methodology. The participants in the studies involving focus groups were women who had been or still were in abusive intimate relationships.

Many of the women in these studies expressed that they favored routine inquiry about IPV by HCPs (28–30,38,62). Several women stated that they were reluctant to initiate a conversation about IPV and preferred that the HCP introduce the topic, as long as they did it in a sensitive manner (28). In most of the studies, women commented that HCPs should not force the issue if a woman was not ready to disclose.

In a survey of 171 women who either were in a shelter, attending support groups, or were primary care patients (abused and nonabused), McNutt found that approximately 75% of primary care patients favored routine inquiry compared to 88% of support group clients and shelter residents (37). Burge surveyed family practice patients about whether family physicians should ask about family conflict. She found that 67% thought physicians should ask sometimes and 29% thought they should ask always (63). Hurley surveyed a convenience sample of 514 emergency department patients; 86% favored routine inquiry, 10% did not, and 3% had no opinion (64). In Zeitler's survey of 645 young women about their opinions regarding routine inquiry, 90% responded that it was a "very good" or "good" idea (31). In a telephone interview of active-duty military women, 60% of those abused agreed with routine inquiry compared to 56% of nonabused women (65).

These studies demonstrate that, contrary to what was previously believed, substantial support exists from women for routine inquiry about IPV by HCPs.

Systematic Reviews and Preventive Care Task Forces

United States Preventive Services Task Force

In 2004, the third United States Preventive Services Task Force (USPSTF) published its updated recommendations on screening for family and intimate partner violence based on its assessment of the evidence related to these forms of violence (66). Their findings were that insufficient evidence existed to recommend *for* or *against* routine IPV screening. In addition, the USPSTF did not find any studies that examined the accuracy of screening tools for the identification of IPV, and it found little evidence that interventions decreased harm to women. Further, the USPSTF found no studies determining the harms of screening and interventions for IPV. Therefore, it could not make an assessment as to whether IPV screening was more beneficial or harmful. This recommendation has caused enormous controversy and resulted in concerns among advocacy groups and HCPs alike that the movement to improve the health care of IPV patients might suffer substantial setbacks. Chamberlain wrote a thorough review of the USPSTF recommendation, raising concerns about methodolo-gical issues in its evaluation of the evidence, identifying the gaps in the evidence, questioning its emphasis on the potential adverse effects to women from screening, and calling for IPV to be evaluated as a counseling service rather than a prevention service (67).

The Canadian Task Force on Preventive Health Care

The Canadian Task Force on Preventive Health Care evaluated the evidence for universal IPV screening in pregnant and nonpregnant women and men (68). They came to a similar conclusion as the USPSTF, stating that there is insufficient evidence *for* or *against* universal IPV screening, but that HCPs should be alert to the possibility of IPV and may want to consider inquiring about abuse if concerned. They also pointed out the lack of evidence regarding the potential harms of IPV screening among women. The Canadian Task Force did mention the potential harm of HCPs *not* addressing IPV in the healthcare setting.

Other Systematic Reviews of the Evidence for Screening for Intimate Partner Violence

In 2002, Ramsay and co-workers published a systematic review of the evidence for acceptability and effectiveness of IPV screening by HCPs (69). They found a paucity of research on the outcomes of interventions, no randomized controlled trials assessing intervention outcomes, and no studies measuring the potential harm to women due to screening. Their conclusion was that until evidence existed that demonstrated a benefit from interventions in the form of decreased violence and a lack of harm from screening, routine screening is not justified. They did not consider that a lack of evidence existed both for and against routine inquiry.

A systematic review by Anglin and Sachs reviewed the evidence for IPV screening in the emergency department setting (70). This review found that due to a lack of outcomes research in this field, there was insufficient evidence *for* or *against* routine screening in the emergency department. However, due to the adverse mental and physical sequelae, morbidity and mortality, societal cost, and effect on children, HCPs should strongly consider routinely inquiring about IPV when assessing adolescent and adult women.

When considering the findings and recommendations of the USPSTF, Canadian Task Force, and other systematic reviews, it is important to take into consideration the following points:

- Women and IPV patients are in favor of routine inquiry about IPV by HCPs.
- All reviews of the evidence demonstrated a lack of evidence *for* or *against* routine IPV screening. Therefore, no evidence suggests that HCPs should *not* screen.
- HCPs are not "screening" for IPV as defined in traditional public health terms. Rather, they are conducting an assessment for IPV among their patients. Therefore, there is no burden of proof placed on the predictive effectiveness of questions used to ask patients about IPV, nor to measure the outcomes of interventions in terms of only morbidity and mortality.
- The potential adverse effects of routine inquiry are also the effects of ongoing and escalating IPV. The likelihood that IPV patients will suffer continued physical, sexual, and psychological abuse is great, given the nature of IPV.

Therefore, the harms of not assessing patients for IPV in the clinical setting are significant and should not be ignored.

Practice-based Evidence

In this day and age of emphasis on evidence-based practice, it is important not to forget about practice-based evidence (48,71). Qualitative studies of IPV patients and women who have experienced IPV have revealed that they do not feel comfortable initiating a conversation about IPV with their HCPs (28,48). However, they have derived benefit from HCPs having caring, compassionate conversations with them about their abusive situations. Some of the feelings that women describe as a results of the HCPs asking them about IPV or talking with them about their situations are validation, relief that someone knows about the abuse, believing that there is someone they can talk to even if they choose not to disclose at that time, change in the way they view their situation, and help in realizing that they have choices (50). Even if patients choose not to disclose IPV, they may receive benefit from being provided with information and resources. From clinical experience, experts in the field also believe that assessment and routine inquiry for IPV remains the recommended approach, despite the lack of research evidence for or against it. Clinical judgment may outweigh lack of evidence. Patients perceive their HCP as an appropriate person to talk to about IPV; IPV is a health problem; and there is face validity in the idea that talking to patients about their health issues is a good first step. As stated so aptly by Lachs (71), conveying the following message to IPV patients through words and actions during a clinical encounter may be the best evidence that we have:

> You are my patient; I know you are suffering. I care about you. You may not have perceived me as a resource to help you solve this problem, but I am ready to help you to the best of my ability now or in the future (71).

ASSESSING FOR INTIMATE PARTNER VIOLENCE ACROSS THE LIFESPAN

Intimate partner violence adversely affects patients across the entire lifespan, including children who witness IPV at home, teens in violent dating relationships, pregnant and nonpregnant women, older women, and men. Therefore, it is important to assess patients at all stages of life for exposure to IPV. Since this book includes chapters on IPV at each of these specific stages of life, this section discusses issues about disclosure of IPV specific to each of these groups of individuals.

Identifying Children Who Witness Intimate Partner Violence

The American Academy of Pediatrics Committee on Child Abuse and Neglect has recommended routine inquiry for IPV among mothers in pediatric healthcare settings (72). Research has shown that in 33%–77% of homes where adult abuse occurs (72,73), children are also being abused, and 30%–59% of mothers of abused children have experienced IPV (74). Adverse childhood experiences have been demonstrated to be linked to poorer health outcomes in adulthood (75). Substantial research has been conducted on routine inquiry about IPV in the pediatric healthcare setting. In general, women are in favor of being asked about IPV in the pediatric setting (76). However, most women prefer that none but very small children be present during the assessment, which is often impractical in the clinical setting (77,78). Written, computerized, and audiotaped questionnaires have been found to be acceptable to women (79). When assessing women for IPV in the pediatric setting, it is important to be aware of the HCP reporting requirements for children who witness abuse and to inform the mothers of the limits of confidentiality prior to inquiring about IPV (80). Finally, children may spontaneously disclose ongoing IPV at home to an HCP. In these circumstances, the HCP should relate his concern to the child and speak with the nonoffending parent. Referrals to advocacy and counseling services should be made.

Disclosure of Teen Dating Violence

Due to the prevalence of dating violence, teens should also be routinely assessed for IPV. Assessment may be conducted in much the same way as with adults. Teens should be asked about relationship violence (bullying, dating violence, sexual coercion, harassment) at new visits, annual visits, and when they disclose a new dating relationship (81).

Disclosure of Intimate Partner Violence in Pregnant Women

Due to changing dynamics in a pregnant woman's relationship with her partner, she may be at increased risk of IPV. It is recommended that pregnant women be assessed for IPV during each trimester, and after delivery (46). McFarlane has conducted extensive research among pregnant abused women, using the Abuse Assessment Screen (82). HCPs should be sensitive to the reluctance of women to leave an abusive relationship during their pregnancy and the first 2 years of their baby's life due to their desire for a normal relationship and family, as well as their hopes for the future (83).

Disclosure of Intimate Partner Violence in Older Women

Older women may not be recognized as being IPV patients, due to the perception by many that IPV is a younger woman's problem. Like younger women, older women often have difficulty initiating conversations about IPV with their HCPs, partly because of the generational belief that IPV is a private, family matter. Zink conducted interviews with 38 abused women ranging from 55 to 90 years of age (84). The median length of their abusive relationships was 24 years. Approximately half of the women had ever disclosed IPV to an HCP. The older women experienced similar barriers to disclosure as younger women, both personal as well as on the part of their HCPs. However, older women had additional barriers to leaving their partners. After experiencing abuse for many years, before IPV was considered a healthcare problem, older women often felt their options were limited due to poor health, restricted financial resources, and a fear of being alone. Further, some older women are dependent on their abusive partners as caregivers. When assessing older women for IPV, HCPs must be sensitive to the fact that many are unwilling to leave their abusive situations.

Disclosure of Intimate Partner Violence in Men

When identifying male victims of IPV in the healthcare setting, the HCP needs to be aware that the context in which the violence occurred may have been perpetration rather than victimization. Muelleman found that when he compared male victims of IPV to male patients presenting to the emergency department for injuries from other reasons, 51% of the IPV male patients had previous arrests for IPV versus 22% for the non-IPV injured male patients (85). Several assessment tools that were developed for women have been used to identify IPV in male patients, however, few have been validated. The HITS tool has been validated for use in identifying IPV in men (see Table 8.1) (86), but does not determine the context of the violence. Clearly, further research of IPV assessment tools for men is necessary. In addition, although a few assessment tools are available to identify batterers, the majority are too lengthy for use in conducting a brief inquiry in the healthcare setting (87).

DIAGNOSING, DIAGNOSIS, REPORTING: THE NEED FOR CLARITY OF TERMS

When discussing the identification of IPV, it is important use common terminology. Certain terms are related to, but often confused with, identification of IPV: diagnosing, diagnosis, and reporting.

Diagnosing is a process used by clinicians to determine the underlying etiology of a patient's symptoms and signs. It combines the gathering of clinical data, scientific knowledge, and clinical interpretation. A *diagnosis* is the underlying cause of the presenting problem and generally follows the common nomenclature given to a disease or condition. The World Health Organization's *International Statistical Classification of Diseases and Related Health Problems* (ICD) has a name and code for each diagnosis. Diagnoses are used for communication about an individual's medical conditions, surveillance of diseases and conditions, reimbursement purposes, and research. The ICD general diagnosis for IPV is Adult Maltreatment. In ICD, Version 10 additional "T" modifiers are available for confirmed or suspicious abuse.

Reporting is an action that may be legally required of HCPs, depending on the condition of the patient and the state in which they practice. Reporting may be for surveillance purposes, such as the reporting of infectious diseases to public health departments. *Forensic reporting* involves reporting to the criminal justice system. In the case of IPV, some states mandate that HCPs submit a report to law enforcement regarding incidents in which a patient has sustained an injury due to IPV. In other states, the reporting is mandated only if the individual has sustained a penetrating injury (i.e., stab or gunshot wound). In addition, some states require HCPs to make a report to law enforcement if a child has been exposed to IPV in the home.

BENEFITS AND RISKS OF MAKING THE DIAGNOSIS

There are risks and benefits to diagnosing IPV and then documenting the diagnosis of adult maltreatment in the patient's medical record. Since IPV is a potentially stigmatizing health condition, it is important to realize that the way HCPs and healthcare systems treat patients with this diagnosis may result in the IPV patient being either empowered or revictimized. It is critical that the medical records of IPV patients be handled with utmost confidentiality, to prevent inappropriate disclosure of their health information that may result in safety as well as confidentiality issues. Not only may a batterer retaliate against a partner who has disclosed IPV, but so may others. For example, insurance companies, employers, the criminal justice system, and communities may discriminate against an individual with a diagnosis of adult maltreatment. It is particularly important for pediatric and adolescent HCPs to provide additional protections for the medical records of children if it has been documented that their mothers have disclosed IPV because the batterer may also have access to the child's medical record (46,81). Healthcare providers can block access to the medical record in the name of patient safety, although in the case of minors for whom both parents have custody, this would require a court order and thus defeat the original intent.

Making the diagnosis of IPV in a patient may also result in access to additional resources and support for the patient, including victims of crime funding. Further, documenting the diagnosis of adult maltreatment in the medical record may allow for improved epidemiological studies of IPV in the healthcare setting, as well as research into the health status of IPV patients and outcomes of health-based interventions. Improved health surveillance means improved health policy regarding IPV.

RISKS AND POTENTIAL HARMS RELATED TO INQUIRING

What Are the Risks and Potential Harms of Routine Inquiry?

As part of their recommendation, the USPSTF stated that it could not determine the risk-to-benefit ratio of screening, since no studies directly assessed the harms of IPV screening (66). So, what are the potential risks and harms of routine inquiry? In qualitative research using focus groups of women experiencing IPV, Gerbert found that women were afraid of retaliation if their partners discovered that they had disclosed abuse to their HCPs. In addition, the attitudes and behaviors of HCPs when the women disclosed caused them to feel ignored or trivialized (33). Other negative consequences of inquiry included a fear of being judged by HCPs, feeling anxious about the unknown consequences, feeling that the intervention was intrusive, and being disappointed in the manner with which the HCP responded to them (38,88,89). Gerbert also found that women were afraid that they might be more at risk for further abuse by their partner, that they might lose their health insurance, and that some women might be offended by being asked (89).

In a study of 548 women who had disclosed IPV in the emergency department, Houry assessed whether they had suffered negative consequences as a result. There were no problems related to safety identified during the emergency department visit. Of the 281 IPV patients interviewed or contacted by phone 1 week later, no women reported an increase in IPV or injuries. On reviewing police records of 911 calls, there was no increase in 911 calls in the 6 months following the women's emergency department visits. Finally, 35% of the women reported utilizing community resources within the subsequent 3 months (90). This is one of the first studies to directly assess whether the risks and harms of routine inquiry are potential or actual.

What Are the Risks and Potential Harms of Not Routinely Inquiring?

The risks and harms of not inquiring about IPV may be even more significant than the potential risks of inquiring. In focus groups, women have stated that they are unaware of many available resources. Women expressed that HCPs can offer compassion, validation and empowerment, a supportive environment, and referrals to community as well as social and legal resources (29). Increasing evidence suggests that referral to advocacy programs results in IPV patients feeling better and utilizing resources (39). McCloskey compared IPV patients who had left their partners and those who had not. She found that those who had left their partners were more likely to have spoken to their HCPs and to have used an intervention (OR = 3.9) (91). In addition, they reported better

physical health than those who were still with their partners. Given our knowledge about the escalation of violence in IPV relationships, sitting by and waiting for proof that asking patients about IPV is not harmful may be unethical.

IMPLICATIONS FOR POLICY, PRACTICE, AND RESEARCH

Policy

- There is neither evidence for nor evidence against routine screening for IPV. However, patient surveys indicate that IPV victims believe their HCP to be an appropriate person to talk to about the issue.
- Research indicates that rates of identification increase in the healthcare setting if referral mechanisms are in place and resources for care are readily available for the HCP and the patient.

Practice

- Healthcare providers should inform patients about confidentiality issues and mandatory reporting requirements prior to assessing them for IPV in adult and pediatric healthcare settings.
- Medical offices, clinics, and hospitals should evaluate specific performance measures (Delphi tool) related to the institution and staff that foster disclosure and provide patients with information about IPV resources.
- Patients should be provided with information about IPV resources and interventions, regardless of their readiness for disclosure.

Research

- Questions regarding the benefits and harms of routinely assessing for IPV should be included in other IPV studies.
- Outcomes research is needed to provide effective interventions to which to refer individuals exposed to IPV.
- Further research should be conducted on the best ways to identify men who present to the healthcare setting as a result of IPV and to differentiate perpetrators from victims.
- Research is needed to determine how to break down the barriers to routine assessment for IPV by HCPs.

References

1. Naumann P, Langford D, Torres S, et al. Women battering in primary care practice. *Fam Pract.* 1999; 16:343–352.

2. Gazmararian J, Lazorick S, Spitz A, et al. Prevalence of violence against pregnant women. *JAMA.* 1996;275:1915–1920.

3. Fanslow J, Norton R, Robinson E. Outcome evaluation of an emergency department protocol of care on partner abuse. *Aust N Z J Public Health.* 1998; 22:598–603.

4. Olson L, Anctil C, Fullerton L, et al. Increasing emergency physician recognition of domestic violence. *Ann Emerg Med.* 1996;27(6):741–746.

5. Dearwater SR, Coben JH, Campbell JC, et al. Prevalence of intimate partner abuse in women treated at community hospital emergency departments. *JAMA.* 1998;280(5):433–438.

6. Feldhaus KM, Koziol-McLain J, Amsbury HL, et al. Accuracy of 3 brief screening questions for detecting partner violence in the emergency department. *JAMA.* 1997;277(17):1357–1361.

7. McFarlane J, Greenberg L, Weltege A, Watson M. Identification of abuse in emergency departments: Effectiveness of a two-question screening tool. *J Emerg Nurs.* 1995;94(5):391–384.

8. Abbott J, Johnson R, Koziol-McLain J, Lowenstein SR. Domestic violence against women: Incidence and prevalence in an emergency department population. *JAMA.* 1995;273(22):1763–1767.

9. Kyriacou DN, Anglin D, Taliaferro E, et al. Risk factors for injury to women from domestic violence. *N Engl J Med.* 1999;341:1892–1898.

10. Muelleman R, Lenaghan P, Pakieser R. Battered women: Injury locations and types. *Ann Emerg Med.* 1996;28:486–492.

11. Drossman D, Leserman J, Nachman G, et al. Sexual and physical abuse in women with functional or organic gastrointestinal disorders. *Ann Intern Med.* 1990;113:828–833.

12. Campbell J, Jones AS, Dienemann J, et al. Intimate partner violence and physical health consequences. *Arch Intern Med.* 2002;162(10):1157–1163.

13. Coker A, Davis K, Arias I, et al. Physical and mental health effects of intimate partner violence for men and women. *Am J Prev Med.* 2002;23(4): 260–268.

14. Coker A, Smith PH, Bethea L, et al. Physical health consequences of physical and psychological intimate partner violence. *Arch Fam Med.* 2000;9(5): 451–457.

15. McCloskey LA, Williams CM, Lichter E, et al. Abused women disclose partner interference with health care: An unrecognized form of battering. *J Gen Intern Med.* 2007;22:1067–1072.

16. Ulrich YC, Cain KC, Sugg NK, et al. Medical care utilization patterns in women with diagnosed domestic violence. *Am J Prev Med.* 2003;24(1): 9–15.

17. Wisner CL, Gilmer TP, Saltzman LE, Zink TM. Intimate partner violence against women: Do victims cost health plans more? *J Fam Pract.* 1999;48(6): 439–443.

18. Kothari CL, Rhodes KV. Missed opportunities: Emergency department visits by police-identified victims of intimate partner violence. *Ann Emerg Med.* 2006;47(2):190–199.

19. Wadman MC, Muelleman RL. Domestic violence homicides: ED use before victimization. *Am J Emerg Med.* 1999;17(7):689–691.

20. Sharps PW, Koziol-McLain J, Campbell J, et al. Health care providers' missed opportunities for preventing femicide. *Prev Med.* 2001;33(5):373–380.

21. The American Heritage Dictionary of the English Language, 4th ed: Houghten Mifflin Company; 2004: http://dictionary.reference.com/browse/disclosure. Accessed 4/15/08.

22. Thackeray J, Stelzner S, Downs SM, Miller C. Screening for intimate partner violence: The impact of screener and screening environment on victim comfort. *J Interpers Violence.* 2007;22(6):659–670.

23. Oppenheimer K, Swanson G. Duty to warn: When should confidentiality be breached? *J Fam Pract.* 1990;30:179–184.

24. Bloom J, Rogers J. The duty to protect others from your patients: Tarasoff spreads to the northwest. *West J Med.* 1988;148(231–234).

25. Chang JC, Decker MR, Moracco KE, et al. Asking about intimate partner violence: Advice from female survivors to health care providers. *Patient Educ Couns.* 2005;59:141–147.

26. Bacchus L, Mezey G, Bewley S. Experiences of seeking help from health professionals in a sample of women who experienced domestic violence. *Health Soc Care Community.* 2003;11(1):10–18.

27. McCauley J, Yurk RA, Jenckes MW, Ford DE. Inside "Pandora's Box": Abused women's experiences with clinicians and health services. *J Gen Intern Med.* 1998;13:549–555.

28. Rodriguez MA, Bauer HM, Flores-Ortiz Y, Szkupinski-Quiroga S. Factors affecting patient-physician communication for abused Latina and Asian immigrant women. *J Fam Pract.* 1998;47(4):309–311.

29. Rodriguez MA, Szkupinski-Quiroga S, Bauer HM. Breaking the silence: Battered women's perspectives on medical care. *Arch Fam Med.* 1996;5: 153–158.

30. Lutz KF. Abuse experiences, perceptions, and associated decisions during the childbearing cycle. *Wes J Nurs Res.* 2005;27(7):802–824.

31. Zeitler MS, Paine AD, Breitbart V, et al. Attitudes about intimate partner violence screening among an ethnically diverse sample of young women. *J Adolesc Health* 2006;39(1):119.

32. Feder GS, Hutson M, Ramsay J, Taket AR. Women exposed to intimate partner violence. Expectations and experiences when they encounter health care professionals: A meta-analysis of qualitative studies. *Arch Intern Med.* 2006;166:22–37.

33. Gerbert B, K J, Caspers N, T B, Woods A, Rosenbaum A. Experiences of battered women in health care settings: A qualitative study. *Women Health.* 1996;24(3):1–17.

34. Mezey G, Bacchus L, Haworth A, Bewley S. Midwives' perceptions and experiences of routine enquiry for domestic violence. *Br J Obstet Gynaecol.* 2003;110:744–752.

35. Minsky-Kelly D, Hamburger LK, Pape DA, Wolff M. We've had training, now what? *J Interpers Violence.* 2005;20(10):1288–1309.

36. Waalen J, Goodwin MM, Spitz AM, Petersen R. Screening for intimate partner violence by health care providers: Barriers and interventions. *Am J Prev Med.* 2000;19(4):230–237.

37. McNutt L-A, Carlson BE, Gagen D, Winterbauer N. Domestic violence screening in primary care: Perspectives and experiences of patients and battered women. *J Am Med Womens Assoc.* 1999; 54(2):85–90.

38. Lutenbacher M, Cohen A, Mitzel J. Do we really help? Perspectives of abused women. *Public Health Nurs.* 2003;20(1):56–64.

39. Krasnoff M, Moscati R. Domestic violence screening and referral can be effective. *Ann Emerg Med.* 2002;40(5):485–492.

40. McCaw B, Berman W, Syme S, Hunkeler M. Beyond screening for domestic violence: A systems model approach in a managed care setting. *Am J Prev Med.* 2001;21:170–176.

41. Limandri B. Disclosure of stigmatizing conditions: The discloser's perspective. *Arch Psychiatr Nurs.* 1989;2:69–78.

42. American Medical Association. *Diagnostic and Treatment Guidelines on Domestic Violence.* Author, 1992.

43. American College of Obstetricians and Gynecologists: Domestic violence. ACOG technical bulletin no. 209. *Int J Gynaecol Obstet.* 1995;41:161–170.

44. American College of Emergency Physicians. Emergency medicine and domestic violence. *Ann Emerg Med.* 1995;25:442–443.

45. American Academy of Family Practice. Family violence. *Am Fam Physician.* 1994;50:1636–1646.

46. *National Consensus Guidelines on Identifying and Responding to Domestic Violence Victimization in Health Care Settings.* San Francisco, CA: Family Violence Prevention Fund, 2002.

47. Last JM, ed. *A dictionary of epidemiology,* 3rd ed. New York, NY: Oxford University Press, 1995.

48. Gerbert B, Caspers N, Bronstone A, et al. A qualitative analysis of how physicians with expertise in domestic violence approach the identification of victims. *Ann Intern Med.* 1999;131(8):578–584.

49. Rhodes KV, Frankel RM, Levinthal N, et al. "You're not a victim of domestic violence, are you?" Provider-patient communication about domestic violence. *Ann Intern Med.* 2007;147(9):620–627.

50. Gerbert B, Abercrombie P, Caspers N, et al. How health care providers help battered women: The survivor's perspective. *Women Health.* 1999; 29(3):115–135.

51. Warshaw C, Alpert E. Integrating routine inquiry about domestic violence into daily practice. *Ann Intern Med.* 1999;131(8):619–620.

52. Furbee P, Sikora R, Williams J, Derk S. Comparison of domestic violence screening methods: A pilot study. *Ann Emerg Med.* 1998;31:495–501.

53. McFarlane J, Christoffel K, Bateman L, et al. Assessing for abuse: Self-report versus nurse interview. *Public Health Nurs.* 1991;8:245–250.

54. Kataoka Y, Yaju Y, Eto H, et al. Screening of domestic violence in the perinatal setting: A systematic review. Kango Tenbo [*Jap J Nurs Sci*]. 2004;1:77–86.

55. MacMillan HL, Wathen NC, Jamieson E, et al. Approaches to screening for intimate partner violence in health care settings. *JAMA.* 2006;296(5): 530–536.

56. Rhodes KV, Lauderdale DS, He T, et al. "Between me and the computer": Increased detection of intimate partner violence using a computer questionnaire. *Ann Emerg Med.* 2002;40(5):476–484.

57. Hamby S, Sugarman DB, Boney-McCoy S. Does questionnaire format impact reported partner violence rates? An experimental study. *Violence Vict.* 2006;21(4):507–518.

58. Straus M, Hamby S, Boney-McCoy S, Sugarman DB. The Revised Conflict Tactics Scale (CTS2): Development and preliminary psychometric data. *J Fam Issues.* 1996;17(3): 283–316.

59. Hudson W, McIntosh S. The assessment of spouse abuse: Two quantifiable dimensions. *J Marriage Fam.* 1981:873–888.

60. Wax W, Rice DP, Finkelstein E, et al. The economic toll of intimate partner violence against women in the United States. *Violence Vict.* 2004;19(3): 259–272.

61. Basile K, Hertz M, Back S. *Intimate partner violence and sexual violence victimization assessment instruments for use in healthcare settings: Version 1.* Atlanta, GA: Centers for Disease Control and Prevention, National Center for Injury Prevention and Control, 2007.

62. Zink T, Elder N, Jacobson J, Klostermann B. Medical management of intimate partner violence considering the stages of change: Precontemplation and contemplation. *Ann Fam Med.* 2004;2(3): 231–239.

63. Burge SK, Schneider FD, Ivy L, Catala S. Patients' advice to physicians about intervening in family conflict. *Ann Fam Med.* 2005;3(3):248–254.

64. Hurley K, Brown-Maher T, Campbell S, et al. Emergency department patients' opinions of screening for intimate partner violence among women. *Emerg Med J.* 2005;22:97–98.

65. Gielen AC, Campbell J, Garza MA, et al. Domestic violence in the military: Women's policy preferences and beliefs concerning routine screening and mandatory reporting. *Mil Med.* 2006;171(8):729–735.

66. USPSTF. Screening for family and intimate partner violence: Recommendation statement. *Ann Intern Med.* 2004;140(5):382–386.
67. Chamberlain L. The USPSTF recommendations on intimate partner violence: What we can learn from it and what we can do about it. *Fam Violence Prevent Health Pract.* 2005;1(1):1–24.
68. Wathen NC, MacMillan HL. Prevention of violence against women: Recommendation statement from the Canadian Task Force on Preventive Care. *Can Med Assoc J.* 2003;169(6):582–584.
69. Ramsay J, Richardson J, Carter YH, et al. Should health professionals screen women for domestic violence? Systematic review. *Br Med J.* 2002;325:314–318.
70. Anglin D, Sachs C. Preventive care in the emergency department: Screening for domestic violence in the emergency department. *Acad Emerg Med.* 2003;10(10):1118–1127.
71. Lachs MS. Screening for family violence: What's an evidence-based doctor to do? *Ann Intern Med.* 2004;140(5):399–400.
72. The role of the pediatrician in recognizing and intervening on behalf of abused women. *Pediatrics.* 1998;101(6):1091–1092.
73. Ernst AA, Weiss SJ, Enright-Smith S. Child witnesses and victims in homes with adult intimate partner violence. *Acad Emerg Med.* 2006; 13:696–699.
74. Phelan MB. Screening for intimate partner violence in medical settings. *Trauma Violence Abuse.* 2007;8(2):199–213.
75. Felitti V, Anda R, Nordenberg D, et al. Relationship of childhood abuse and household dysfunction to many of the leading causes of death in adults. *Am J Prev Med.* 1998;14:245–258.
76. Newman JD, Sheehan KM, Powell EC. Screening for intimate partner violence in the pediatric emergency department. *Pediatr Emerg Care.* 2005;21(2):79–83.
77. Zink T. Should children be in the room when the mother is screened for partner violence. *J Fam Pract.* 2000;49(2):130–136.
78. Zink T, Levin L, Putnam F, Beckstrom A. Accuracy of five domestic violence screening questions with nongraphic language. *Clin Pediatr.* 2007;46(2):127–134.
79. Bair-Merritt MH, Feudtner C, Mollen CJ, et al. Screening for intimate partner violence using an audiotape questionnaire. *Arch Pediatr Adolesc Med.* 2006(311–316).
80. Zink T, Kamine D, Musk L, et al. What are providers' reporting requirements for children who witness domestic violence? *Clin Pediatr.* 2004;43:449–460.
81. *Identifying and responding to domestic violence: Consensus recommendations for child and adolescent health.* San Francisco, CA: Family Violence Prevention Fund, 2002.
82. McFarlane J, Parker B, Soeken K, Bullock L. Assessing for abuse during pregnancy, severity and frequency of injuries and associated entry into prenatal care. *JAMA.* 1992;267(23):3176–3178.
83. Lutz KF. Abused pregnant women's interactions with health care providers during the childbearing year. *JOGNN.* 2005;34:151–162.
84. Zink T, Jacobson J, Regan S, Pabst S. Hidden victims: The healthcare needs and experiences of older women in abusive relationships. *J Womens Health.* 2004;13(8):898–908.
85. Muelleman RL, Burgess P. Male victims of domestic violence and their history of perpetrating violence. *Acad Emerg Med.* 1998;5(9):866–870.
86. Shakil A, Donald S, Sinacore JM, Krepcho M. Validation of the HITS domestic violence screening tool with males. *Fam Med.* 2005;37(3):193–198.
87. Thompson M, Basile K, Hertz M, et al. *Measuring intimate partner violence victimization and perpetration: A compendium of assessment tools.* Atlanta, GA: Centers for Disease Control and Prevention, National Center for Injury Prevention and Control, 2006.
88. Chang JC, Decker M, Moracco KE, et al. What happens when health care providers ask about intimate partner violence? A description of consequences from the perspectives of female survivors. *J Am Med Womens Assoc.* 2003;58(2):76–81.
89. Gielen AC, O'Campo P, Campbell JC, et al. Women's opinions about domestic violence screening and mandatory reporting. *Am J Prev Med.* 2000;19(4):279–285.
90. Houry D, Kaslow NJ, Kemball RM, et al. Does screening in the emergency department hurt or help victims of intimate partner violence? *Ann Emerg Med.* 2008;51(4):433–442.
91. McCloskey LA, Lichter E, Williams CM, et al. Assessing intimate partner violence in health care settings leads to women's receipt of interventions and improved health. *Public Health Rep.* 2006;121:435–444.
92. Sherin KM, Sinacore JM, Li XQ, et al. HITS: A short domestic violence screening tool for use in a family practice setting. *Famy Med.* 1998;30:508–512.
93. Chen PH, Rovi S, Vega M, et al. Screening for domestic violence in predominantly Hispanic clinical settings. *Fam Pract.* 2005;22:617–623.
94. Brown JB, Lent B, Schmidt G, et al. Application of the woman abuse screening tool (WAST) and WAST-short in the family practice setting. *J Fam Pract.* 2000;49:896–903.
95. Smith PH, Tessaro I, Earp JA. Women's experiences with battering: A conceptualization from qualitative research. *Womens Health Issues.* 1995;5:173–182.
96. Hegarty K, Sheehan M, Schonfeld C. A multidimensional definition of partner abuse: Development and preliminary validation of the Composite Abuse Scale. *J Fam Violence.* 1999;14:399–415.

Chapter 9

Risk Factors for Victimization of Intimate Partner Violence

Sheryl L. Heron

KEY CONCEPTS

- Individual, dyadic (e.g., the relationship between a man and woman), institutional, and societal determinants increase the risk of intimate partner violence (IPV) toward women.
- Individual risk factors include primarily violence in the family of origin, such as witnessing parental violence, as well as a childhood history of physical and sexual abuse.
- Dyadic risk factors include stress between partners, as well as a woman's ability to meet the needs of her partner to maintain the relationship.
- Institutional risk factors such as schools that may reinforce socialization supporting violent behavior or religious institutions with conservative theological views, require more research and support programs to protect women against IPV.
- Societal risk factors for victimization include partner unemployment, low insurance status, neighborhood poverty, and low levels of partner education.
- Ongoing and systematic assessment of IPV victims is needed to determine the contextual risk factor, whether individual, dyadic, institutional, or societal.

For the past 20 years, intimate partner violence (IPV) has gained much attention within the literature, with increased research aimed at identifying the risk factors for this global public health problem. In related chapters of this text, we note that IPV is the most common cause of injury to women in the United States (1,2), and that more than one-third of all female homicide victims in the United States were killed by their husband or partner (3). The health consequences for IPV victims and healthcare professionals (HCPs) on

the front line caring for them has been well documented (4–8). Further, the criminal justice system,
policy makers, and legal strategists have been charged
with being a part of a coordinated response to IPV.
Salazar and colleagues note from their work that if
a legitimate authority, such as the criminal justice
system, does not condone, but rather condemns
domestic violence, then community norms may change
so as to be aligned with the views of the system (9).

In 1996, the National Research Council issued a
report, "Understanding Violence Against Women,"
that explored two lines of questioning: Why do people
batter? And, what factors place women at increased
risk for victimization? Analysis of risk factors for IPV
included individual, dyadic, institutional, and societal determinants for victimization (10). This chapter
examines these four areas of inquiry in an attempt to
analyze IPV, as well as explore the implications for
direct HCPs, public health and policy analysts, and
the patients and families who seek care in the healthcare environment. Without a comprehensive lens for
identifying these risks, appropriate and targeted interventions in the public health and clinical practice arenas would be impossible to implement.

INDIVIDUAL RISK FOR
VICTIMIZATION

All forms of family-of-origin violence were predictive
of all forms of relationship abuse (11). Violence in the
family of origin, such as witnessing parental violence
as a child, has been cited as one of the primary risk factors for IPV (10,12–16). This intergenerational transmission of violence is not an independent marker, but
rather is confounded by other social and/or psychological processes, such as marital conflict and socioeconomic status (17). In the Adverse Childhood Experiences study, a large study of patients within a health
maintenance organization, Whitfield and colleagues
studied three forms of violent childhood experiences.
They included childhood physical abuse, childhood
sexual abuse, and growing up with a battered mother.
This study examined whether persons who had all
three forms of violent childhood experiences would
be at risk of victimization or perpetration. They concluded that, among persons who had all three forms of
violent childhood experiences, the risk of victimization and perpetration was increased 3.5-fold for women
and 3.8-fold for men (16). One of the limitations of

studies that examined the intergenerational theory is
the lack of a longitudinal design examining the effect
of clinically relevant developmental risk factors for
partner violence programs. Ehrensaft and colleagues
conducted such an analysis by following a sample of
543 children over 20 years. They concluded that childhood behavior problems, such as conduct disorder,
were the most predictive of partner violence and that
exposure to violence between parents increased the
risk for using violent conflict resolution within intimate relationships (18). These findings suggest that it
would be appropriate to design target prevention programs for youth with these behavioral problems.

McCauley and colleagues note in their study of
characteristics of women that increase the risk for IPV,
that these women were more likely to be younger than
35 years of age; to be single, separated, or divorced; to
be receiving medical assistance or to have no insurance; to have had more physical symptoms; to have
had higher scores on instruments for depression, anxiety, somatization, and interpersonal sensitivity; were
more likely to have a partner abusing drugs or alcohol
(as previously stated); were more likely to be abusing drugs or alcohol; and were more likely to have
attempted suicide (19).

Despite the reference to younger women at
increased risk for IPV, IPV is also a problem in older
women. Reasons for nondisclosure were similar to
those of younger women, but were compounded
by the generational mores of privacy about domestic affairs and society's lack of understanding and
resources for IPV (20).

Alcohol abuse has been well documented as a
risk factor for perpetration of violence by men against
women, as well as by women against men (21–23).
Caetono noted in his study that 30%–40% of the men
and 27%–34% of the women who perpetrated violence against their partners were drinking at the time
of the event. Alcohol's role in partner violence may
be explained by people's expectations that alcohol will
have a disinhibitory effect on behavior or by alcohol's
direct physiological disinhibitory effect (21,22). Murphy and colleagues also note that alcohol consumption is a proximal risk factor for partner violence in
alcoholic men (24,25). Moreover, women in abusive
relationships were at increased risk of injury when
alcohol was used by their male partners (20,26,27)
or cocaine (2). The presence of alcohol in partner
relationships is a demonstrated risk factor for IPV,
thus supporting the need for targeted interventions.

For example, by routinely assessing substance use and abuse as part of batterer interventions programs, these programs could be improved by offering adjunct or integrated alcohol treatment (28).

Similarly, women's drinking, women's general violence, and partner drinking all contributed to some form of violence perpetration or victimization. These problems should be assessed routinely as part of violence intervention programs for women; intervention programs would thus be improved by offering adjunct or integrated alcohol treatment (29,30). One study further noted that after the women became pregnant, the links between women's experiences of IPV and their use of substances became stronger, with the women who experienced each type of partner violence being more likely to use both alcohol and illicit drugs (31). The success of future practice, policy, and research in this arena will depend on the identification of violence-related issues important to women with alcohol and other drug problems, and on the implementation of treatment strategies that address the role of violence within their lives (32).

Recently, literature has addressed the impact of culture and minority status in the United States on women's experience of IPV, considering family structure, immigration, acculturation, oppression, and community response (33). Although some data suggest that African Americans are at increased risk for partner violence (34,35), after controlling for both victim gender and annual household income, the victim's race is no longer significant (3). Further, with varying cultures within the Black community, researchers have noted a need for increasing research to include more diverse Black samples, considering how living at the intersection of multiple forms of oppression shapes Black women's experience of violence (36,37).

One of these least studied areas on IPV risk factors is among women with disabilities. In one of the most recent publications, Nosek and colleagues note that women with disabilities experience rates of emotional, physical, and sexual abuse that are comparable to, if not greater than women without disabilities (38). A review within her study noted five risk factors that increase vulnerability to abuse: (a) cultural devaluation of women, with the belief that women with disabilities have fewer opportunities to learn sexual likes and dislikes, often perceiving celibacy or violent sexual encounters as their only choices; (b) overprotection of caretakers, with abuse being the price the woman must pay; (c) denied sexuality, leading to the

woman's belief that violent sexual encounters may be the only choice; (d) cognitive impairment in some disabled women, limiting the ability to recognize abuse; and (e) lack of economic independence (38). As with nondisabled persons, collaborations between domestic violence and disability service providers are necessary for improving the service and care delivered to women with disabilities who experience domestic violence (39).

Finally, a woman's perceived sense of risk has emerged as a risk factor for the likelihood for repeat assault. Gondolf and Heckert noted in two studies that women's perceived likelihood of reassault increased with men who were divorced or separated, heavy drinkers, and severely abusive in the past. The strongest determinant for perceptions of safety was the perceived likelihood of reassault. The women's perceptions appear, therefore, to be grounded in practical circumstances and correspond to established predictors of reassault (40,41).

RISK IN DYADIC CONTEXT

In examining the relationship between men and women, it has been noted that stress between partners has been cited in the literature as an IPV risk factor (14). This dyadic context in which a man carries out violence against a woman includes features of the relationship, characteristics of the woman, and their communication styles (10). Men notably exhibit violence once their partners have made an emotional commitment to them. One study on interaction effects showed that men, more than women, rated the actions of the married perpetrator as more of a human rights violation than the same actions of the acquaintance perpetrator (20).

Within the societal context and how women communicate within the relationship dyad, Woods indicated that abused and nonabused women with low self-esteem tended to have higher levels of belief in societal norms and gender-specific socializations regarding how women should maintain their relationships (42). Specifically, they note that women who are battered disconnect from their feelings and thoughts to meet the partner's needs or to maintain the relationship. In addition, continued emotional attachment appears to play a significant role in past and future decisions for a woman to return to her batterer (43).

INSTITUTIONAL RISK FOR VICTIMIZATION

Families, schools, organized religion, and media exposure have been cited as institutional factors that contribute to IPV (10). Violence in the family has been previously discussed as an individual risk factor, but it also is specific to the institutional framework for risk exposure because family is the first "institution" within which we develop our individual ideas, values, and beliefs.

To the extent that schools reinforce sex role stereotypes and attitudes that condone the use of violence, they may contribute to socialization that supports violent behavior (10). Other institutions, such as organized religion, also have been implicated in contributing to the socialization process of violence against women. In particular, men who hold much more conservative theological views than their partners are especially likely to perpetrate domestic violence (44). Despite the few studies on religious involvement and IPV, Ellison and co-workers noted in a later study that regular attendance at religious services is inversely related to commission of domestic violence in both self-reported and partner-reported abuse (45), thus serving as a protective factor against IPV.

Within the media, studies have shown that violence exposure and lack of parental monitoring were the most influential contributors in explaining children's violent behaviors (2). Further, Robinson and colleagues found that an intervention to reduce television, videotape, and video game use decreased aggressive behavior in elementary school children, thereby supporting the causal influences of these media on aggression and the potential benefits of reducing children's media use (46).

Within the criminal justice system (CJS), increased risk for IPV can be attributed to the experiences a woman encounters while accessing the legal system. Compared to nonpartner assault victims, victims of assault by an intimate partner were consistently less likely to report satisfaction with the professionals involved in the CJS as well as with the CJS in general (47). In addition, women entering the court system face a challenging experience, in part because a courtroom can be an intimidating and difficult place for any person, and in part because women victimized by crimes in which the offender is known to them face distinct difficulties when they seek the court's remedies (48). Controversial in its response, Erez reviewed

the history of domestic violence as a criminal offense and the justice system response to woman battering incidents over time (49).

Law enforcement, likewise, has been reluctant to arrest batterers (20,49), despite mandatory arrest policies (50,51), and prosecutors have been unwilling (at times unable) to prosecute cases of IPV (52,53). Despite these institutional risk factors for ongoing IPV, Ames suggests probation as one alternative outcome of criminal prosecution that can offer justice for some victims and perhaps keep some victims safer (5).

SOCIETAL RISKS FOR VICTIMIZATION

Socioeconomic Factors

Individuals with low socioeconomic status, low insurance status, partner unemployment, and low levels of partner education have sociodemographic variables that put them at risk for IPV (12,13,15,26,54,55).

Further, Wenzel and colleagues, in one of the few prospective studies on impoverished women, demonstrated that physical or sexual abuse during childhood, having two or more sexual partners as opposed to just one, experiencing psychological distress/risk for mental health problems prior to baseline interview, and reporting poor social support at baseline predicted the physical victimization of women at follow-up (56). When including neighborhood poverty, particularly among Blackcouples, there is an increased risk of partner violence (22). Therefore, it is recommended that policies be aimed at reducing community poverty, which may contribute to effective partner violence prevention strategies.

With regards to homelessness as a risk factor for abuse, Bassuk and associates have noted in several studies that sheltered homeless mothers had fewer economic resources and social supports and higher cumulative rates of violent abuse and assault over their lifespan than their housed counterparts (57,58). The link between IPV and homelessness has been noted in other studies; the reality is that inadequate income, lack of affordable housing, and fleeing domestic violence are key factors in making women homeless (59).

Immigration Status

The immigrant community represents another vulnerable population that has had limited IPV research.

The common belief is that immigrants may be at increased risk for IPV. In a review by Menjivay, however, he notes that the incidence of domestic violence is no higher than it is in the native population, but rather that the experiences of immigrant women in domestic violence situations are often exacerbated by their specific position as immigrants, such as limited host language skills, isolation from and contact with family and community, lack of access to dignified jobs, uncertain legal status, and experiences with authorities in their origin countries (60). An entire chapter of this book is dedicated to the sociocultural considerations of women and IPV.

CONCLUSION

Intimate partner violence victimization has multilevel, multifactorial causes, including individual, dyadic, institutional, and societal determinants. The relevance of identifying these risk factors has far-reaching impact for both public health and clinical practice. Indeed, from a societal level, in 2003, the economic cost of IPV perpetrated against women in the United States—including expenditures for medical care and mental health services, and lost productivity from injury and premature death—totals over $8.3 billion (61). Moreover, the relevance of continued and increased engagement of healthcare and social science professionals is of obvious importance. It is well know that the health arena is an entry point for many victims of violence (4,6,44,62–65), and this fact should heighten our vigilance in determining those factors related to victimization as well as perpetration. As a result, professional organizations encourage clinicians to identify IPV victims and to refer them to community resources (66–68).

Although several reviews in scientific journals cite a lack of evidence on the effectiveness of identifying abused women in the healthcare setting (69–71), with many completed studies criticized for methodological weaknesses (72), this lack of evidence should not dampen our clinical alertness or our clinical judgment in determining those risk factors associated with victimization (20,73,74).

Risk factors from each of the four domains—individual, dyadic, institutional, and societal—will require persistent, consistent identification, intervention, and evaluation to monitor the effectiveness of the health and social science professional's response to IPV.

IMPLICATIONS FOR POLICY, PRACTICE, AND RESEARCH

Policy

- Ongoing and systematic assessment of IPV victims is needed to determine the contextual risk factor, whether individual, dyadic, institutional, or societal.
- Institutions such as healthcare systems, religious groups, and legal/law enforcement offices should create policies on IPV in their respective domains. These policies should be evaluated to ensure effectiveness in identifying women at risk for IPV.
- Policy makers should align with researchers in determining how to implement or augment existing policies on IPV.

Practice

- Translation of research and policy into practice will need to be collaboratively based to ensure that practice outcomes are in alignment with the research findings and policy recommendations.
- A primary prevention focus requires targeting those attitudes or behaviors that result in victimization of women (75).
- Focus groups have been noted to elicit strategies for protecting women from returning to violent relationships. The findings suggest a need for health communications messages and interventions to help women vulnerable to abuse (76).
- To the extent that shared risk factors that affect child abuse, youth violence, and IPV can become identifiable, prevention efforts and intervention strategies can be developed and adopted in community practice (77).

Research

- Much work is still to be done to develop a research agenda that will be useful to health and social science professionals (78).
- Given the methodological challenges of performing the gold standard randomized control trial, realistic expectations of what can be done in IPV research in the clinical setting are needed (72) to determine interventions for the known risk factors for victimization and perpetration, as well as whether these risk

factors change or remain the same during the lifespan.

- Ways to influence social norms about violence (e.g., attitudes about the acceptability of men's violence against women) should also be explored (75).
- The continued dialogue that has been set forth by Jordan and colleagues on reaching a national research agenda on violence against women includes what women need to know about the risk of victimization (79,80).
- Campbell highlights three categories of risk (factors that increase the risk of reassault or revicitimization, those that increase risk of lethality, and those that keep women who are battered safer or reduce their risk of being battered) and the relationship of these risk factors for IPV (81).
- There is also a shortage of primary research studies based in medical specialties, dental care, and the allied health fields, such as physical and occupational therapy. Determining the prevalence of IPV in these patient populations would enlarge the research body in determining those risk factors that affect the women these professionals encounter (77).
- Although considerable agreement exists in the United States and internationally about the importance of uniform terminology and measurement related to violence against women, a strategy is needed for choosing standardized definitions and measures (82) that would contribute specifically to studies that examine the prevalence, consequences, and risk and protective factors of violence by intimate partners in different cultural settings using standardized methodologies (83).

References

1. Grisso JA, Wishner AR, Schwarz DF, et al. A population-based study of injuries in inner-city women. *Am J Epidemiol.* 1991;134(1):59–68.
2. Grisso JA, Schwarz DF, Hirschinger N, et al. Violent injuries among women in an urban area. *N Engl J Med.* 1999;341(25):1899–1905.
3. Rennison CM. *Intimate partner violence, 1993–2001.* Washington, DC: Bureau of Justice Statistics, Crime Date Brief; February, 2003 2003. NCJ 197838.
4. Abbott J, Johnson R, J Koziol-M, et al. Domestic violence against women: Incidence and prevalence in an emergency department population. *JAMA.* 1995;273:1763–1767.

5. Alpert EJ, Milstein A, Marks JS, et al. "Challenges and Strategies" and "Evidence-Based Care": Excerpt from day 1 plenary sessions. *Violence Against Women.* 2002;8(6):639–660.
6. McGrath ME, Hogan JW, Peipert JF. A prevalence survey of abuse and screening for abuse in urgent care patients. *Obstet Gynecol.* 1998;91(4):511–514.
7. McKenzie KC, Burns RB, McCarthy EP, Freund KM. Prevalence of domestic violence in an inpatient female population. *J Gen Intern Med.* 1998; 13(4):277–279.
8. Plichta SB, Falik M. Prevalence of violence and its implications for women's health. *Womens Health Issues.* 2001;11(3):244–258.
9. Salazar L, Baker C, Price A, Carlin K. Moving beyond the individual: Examining the effects of domestic violence policies on social norms. *Am J Community Psychol.* 2003;32(3/4):253–259.
10. Council NR. *Understanding violence against women.* Washington, DC: Institute of Medicine, 1996.
11. Kwong MJ, Bartholomew K, Henderson AJ, Trinke SJ. The intergenerational transmission of relationship violence. *J Fam Psychol.* 2003;17(3): 288–301.
12. Coker AL, Smith PH, McKeown RE, King MJ. Frequency and correlates of intimate partner violence by type: Physical, sexual, and psychological battering. *Am J Public Health.* 2000;90(4):553–559.
13. Ernst AA, Nick TG, Weiss SJ, et al. Domestic violence in an inner-city ED. *Ann Emerg Med.* 1997; 30(2):190–197.
14. Huang C, Gunn T. An examination of domestic violence in an African American community in North Carolina: Causes and consequences. *J Black Stud.* 2001;31(6):790–811.
15. Wyatt G, Axelrod J, Chin D, et al. Examining patterns of vulnerability to domestic violence among African American women. *Violence Against Women.* 2000;6(5):491–514.
16. Whitfield CL, Anda RF, Dube SR, Felitti VJ. Violent childhood experiences and the risk of intimate partner violence in adults: Assessment in a large health maintenance organization. *J Interpers Violence.* 2003;18(2):166–185.
17. Hotaling G, Surgaman D. A risk marker analysis of assaulted wives. *J Fam Violence.* 1990;5(1):1–13.
18. Ehrensaft M, Cohen P, Brown J, et al. Intergenerational transmission of partner violence: A 20-year prospective study. *J Consult Clin Psychol.* 2003;71(4): 741–753.
19. McCauley J, Kern DE, Kolodner K, et al. The "battering syndrome": prevalence and clinical characteristics of domestic violence in primary care internal medicine practices. *Ann Intern Med.* 1995;123(10):737–746.
20. Campbell JC, Webster D, Koziol-McLain J, et al. Risk factors for femicide in abusive relationships: Results from a multisite case control study. *Am J Public Health.* 2003;93(7):1089–1097.

21. Caetano R, Schafer J, Cunradi CB. Alcohol-related intimate partner violence among white, black, and Hispanic couples in the United States. *Alcohol Res Health.* 2001;25(1):58–65.

22. Caetano R, Cunradi CB, Clark CL, Schafer J. Intimate partner violence and drinking patterns among white, black, and Hispanic couples in the US. *J Subst Abuse.* 2000;11(2):123–138.

23. Cunradi CB, Caetano R, Clark CL, Schafer J. Alcohol-related problems and intimate partner violence among white, black, and Hispanic couples in the US. *Alcohol Clin Exp Res.* 1999;23(9): 1492–1501.

24. Murphy CM, Winters J, O'Farrell TJ, et al. Alcohol consumption and intimate partner violence by alcoholic men: Comparing violent and nonviolent conflicts. *Psychol Addict Behav.* 2005;19(1):35–42.

25. Murphy CM, O'Farrell TJ, Fals-Stewart W, Feehan M. Correlates of intimate partner violence among male alcoholic patients. *J Consult Clin Psychol.* 2001;69(3):528–540.

26. Kyriacou DN, Anglin D, Taliaferro E, et al. Risk factors for injury to women from domestic violence against women. *N Engl J Med.* 1999;341(25): 1892–1898.

27. Kyriacou DN, McCabe F, Anglin D, et al. Emergency department-based study of risk factors for acute injury from domestic violence against women. *Ann Emerg Med.* 1998;31(4):502–506.

28. Holtzworth-Munroe A, Meehan JC, Herron K, et al. Do subtypes of maritally violent men continue to differ over time? *J Consult Clin Psychol.* 2003; 71(4):728–740.

29. Stuart GL. Improving violence intervention outcomes by integrating alcohol treatment. *J Interpers Violence.* 2005;20(4):388–393.

30. Stuart GL, Moore TM, Ramsey SE, Kahler CW. Hazardous drinking and relationship violence perpetration and victimization in women arrested for domestic violence. *J Stud Alcohol.* 2004; 65(1):46–53.

31. Martin S, Beaumont J, Kupper L. Substance use before and during pregnancy: Links to intimate partner violence. *Am J Drug Alcohol Abuse.* 2003; 29(3):599–617.

32. Miller BA, Wilsnack SC, Cunradi CB. Family violence and victimization: Treatment issues for women with alcohol problems. *Alcohol Clin Exp Res.* 2000;24(8):1287–1297.

33. Kasturirangan A, Krishnan S, Riger S. The impact of culture and minority status on women's experience of domestic violence. *Trauma Violence Abuse.* 2004; 5(4):318–332.

34. Rennison C, Welchans S. Intimate partner violence. In: U.S. Dept. of Justice, Office of Justice Programs, Bureau of Justice Statistics, *Intimate Partner Violence*, by Callie Marie Rennison & Sarah Welchans (2000, revised 2002). http://www.ojp.usdoj.gov/bjs/pub/pdf/ipv.pdf

35. Tjaden P, Thoennes N. *Extent, nature, and consequences of intimate partner violence: Findings from the National Violence Against Women Survey.* Washington DC: Government Printing Office, 2000.

36. Bent-Goodley TB. Culture and domestic violence: Transforming knowledge development. *J Interpers Violence.* 2005;20(2):195–203.

37. West CM. Black women and intimate partner violence: New directions for research. *J Interpers Violence.* 2004;19(12):1487–1493.

38. Nosek M, Foley C, Hughes R, Howland C. Vulnerabilities for abuse among women with disabilities. *Sex Disabil.* 2001;19(2):177–189.

39. Chang JC, Martin SL, Moracco KE, et al. Helping women with disabilities and domestic violence: Strategies, limitations, and challenges of domestic violence programs and services. *J Womens Health (Larchmt).* 2003;12(7):699–708.

40. Gondolf EW, Heckert DA. Determinants of women's perceptions of risk in battering relationships. *Violence Vict.* 2003;18(4):371–386.

41. Heckert DA, Gondolf EW. Battered women's perceptions of risk versus risk factors and instruments in predicting repeat reassault. *J Interpers Violence.* 2004;19(7):778–800.

42. Woods SJ. Normative beliefs regarding the maintenance of intimate relationships among abused and nonabused women. *J Interpers Violence.* 1999;14(5):479–491.

43. Griffing S, Ragin DF, Sage RE, et al. Domestic violence survivors' self-identified reasons for returning to abusive relationships. *J Interpers Violence.* 2002;17(3):306–319.

44. Ellison CG, Bartkowski JP, Anderson KL. Are there religious variations in domestic violence? *J Fam Issues.* 1999;20(1):87–113.

45. Ellison C, Kristin K. Religious involvement and domestic violence among US couples. *J Sci Study Relig.* 2001;40(2):269–286.

46. Robinson TN, Wilde ML, Navracruz LC, et al. Effects of reducing children's television and video game use on aggressive behavior: A randomized controlled trial. *Arch Pediatr Adolesc Med.* 2001; 155(1):17–23.

47. Byrne C, Kilpatrick D, Howley S, Beatty D. Female victims of partner versus nonpartner violence: Experiences with the criminal justice system. *Crim Justice Behav.* 1999;26(3):275–292.

48. Jordan CE. Intimate partner violence and the justice system: An examination of the interface. *J Interpers Violence.* 2004;19(12):1412–1434.

49. Erez E. Domestic violence and the criminal justice system: An overview. *Online J Nursing Issues.* 2002:1–30.

50. Haviland M, Frye V, Rajah V, et al. The Family Protection and Domestic Violence Intervention Act of 1995: Examining the Effects of Mandatory Arrest in New York City: A Report by the Family Violence Project of the Urban Justice Center. New York: Urban

Justice Center, 2001. http://www.connectnyc.org/cnyc_pdf/Mandatory_Arrest_Report.pdf

51. Schmidt JD, Sherman LW. Does arrest deter domestic violence? In: Buzawa E, Buzawa C, eds. *Do arrests and restraining orders work?* Thousand Oaks, CA: Sage Publications, Inc.,1996:43–53.

52. Davis RC, Smith B. Domstic violence reforms: Empty promises or fulfilled expectations. *Crime Delinq.* 1995;41:541–552.

53. Fagan J. The criminalization of domestic violence: Promises and limits (NCJ 157641). Washington, DC: Office of Justice Programs, 1996.

54. Honeycutt T, Marshall L, Weston R. Toward ethnically specific models of employment, public asssistance, and victimization. *Violence Against Women.* 2001;7:126–140.

55. Raj A, Silvermna J, Wingood G, DiClemente R. Prevalence and correlates of relationship abuse among a community-based sample of low-income African American women. *Violence Against Women.* 1999;5(3):272–291.

56. Wenzel SL, Tucker JS, Elliott MN, et al. Physical violence against impoverished women: A longitudinal analysis of risk and protective factors. *Womens Health Issues.* 2004;14(5):144.

57. Bassuk EL, Melnick S, Browne A. Responding to the needs of low-income and homeless women who are survivors of family violence. *J Am Med Womens Assoc.* 1998;53(2):57–64.

58. Bassuk EL, Weinreb LF, Buckner JC, et al. The characteristics and needs of sheltered homeless and low-income housed mothers. *JAMA.* 1996;276(8): 640–646.

59. Correia A, Rubin J. Housing and battered women. At http://www.vaw.umn.edu/documents/vawnet/arhousing/arhousing.html#rwarm1997. Accessed 4/10/2005.

60. Menjivar C, Salcido O. Immigrant women and domestic violence: Common experiences in different countries. *Gend Soc.* 2002;16(6):898–920.

61. Max W, Rice DP, Finkelstein E, et al. The economic toll of intimate partner violence against women in the United States. *Violence Vict.* 2004;19(3): 259–272.

62. Amaro H, Fried LE, Cabral H, Zuckerman B. Violence during pregnancy and substance use. *Am J Public Health.* 1990;80(5):575–579.

63. Dearwater S, Coben J, Nah G, et al. Prevalence of domestic violence in women treated at community hospital emergency department. *JAMA.* 1998;480:433–438.

64. Kyriacou DN, Anglin D, Taliaferro E, et al. Emergency department-based study of risk factors for actute injury from domestic violence against women. *Ann Emerg Med.* 1998;31(4):502–506.

65. Zink T, Jacobson CJ, Jr., Regan S, Pabst S. Hidden victims: The healthcare needs and experiences of older women in abusive relationships. *J Womens Health (Larchmt).* 2004;13(8):898–908.

66. American College of Emergency Physicians. Emergency Medicine and Domestic Violence. Policy #400163, Approved October 2002. At http://www.acep.org/webportal/PracticeResources/PolicyStatementsByCategory/ViolenceAbuse/EmergencyMedicineDomesticViolence.htm. Accessed 4/11/2005.

67. American College of Obstetricians and Gynecologists. Domestic violence: Educational bulletin. No. 257 ed. Washington, DC; 1999.

68. American Medical Association. American Medical Association diagnostic and treatment guidelines for domestic violence. *Arch Fam Med.* 1992; 1:39–47.

69. *Crawford v. Washington*, 541 US 36, 124 S.Ct. 1354 (2004).

70. Ramsay J, Richardson J, Carter YH, et al. Should health professionals screen women for domestic violence? Systematic review. *BMJ.* 2002; 325(7359):314.

71. Wathen CN, MacMillan HL. Interventions for violence against women: Scientific review. *JAMA.* 2003;289(5):589–600.

72. Zink T, Putnam F. Intimate partner violence research in the health care setting: What are appropriate and feasible methodological standards? *J Interpers Violence.* 2005;20(4):365–372.

73. Lachs MS. Screening for family violence: What's an evidence-based doctor to do? *Ann Intern Med.* 2004;140(5):399–400.

74. Nelson HD, Nygren P, McInerney Y, Klein J. Screening women and elderly adults for family and intimate partner violence: A review of the evidence for the US Preventive Services Task Force. *Ann Intern Med.* 2004;140(5):387–396.

75. Saltzman L, Green YT, Marks JS, Thacker SB. Violence against women as a public health issue: Comments from the CDC. *Am J Prev Med.* 2000;19(4).

76. Goodman LA, Dutton MA, Bennett L. Predicting repeat abuse among arrested batterers: Use of the danger assessment scale in the criminal justice system. *J Interpers Violence.* 2000;15(1):63–74.

77. Guterman, N. B. (2004). Advancing Prevention Research on Child Abuse, Youth Violence, and Domestic Violence: Emerging Strategies and Issues. *J Interpers Violence* 19(3): 299–321.

78. Plichta SB. Intimate partner violence and physical health consequences: Policy and practice implications. *J Interpers Violence.* 2004;19(11): 1296–1323.

79. Jordan CE. Toward a national research agenda on violence against women: Continuing the dialogue on research and practice. *J Interpers Violence.* 2004;19(11):1205–1208.

80. Jordan CE. Toward a national research agenda on violence against women: Continuing the dialogue on research and practice. *J Interpers Violence.* 2004;19(12):1365–1368.

81. Campbell JC. Helping women understand their risk in situations of intimate partner violence. *J Interpers Violence.* 2004;19(12):1464–1477.

82. Kilpatrick DG. What is violence against women: Defining and measuring the problem. *J Interpers Violence.* 2004;19(11):1209–1234.

83. Saltzman LE. Issues related to defining and measuring violence against women: Response to Kilpatrick. *J Interpers Violence.* 2004;19(11): 1235–1243.

Chapter 10

Risk Factors for Intimate Partner Violence Perpetration

Typologies and Characteristics of Batterers

L. Kevin Hamberger

KEY CONCEPTS

- Perpetrators of intimate partner violence (IPV) comprise a heterogeneous group based on personality style and violence profile.
- Understanding male batterers requires multidimensional assessment of psychological, demographic, cultural, and attitudinal variables.
- Male batterers will respond to questions about IPV.

HISTORICAL PERSPECTIVE

Intimate partner violence (IPV) has been a topic of great concern to social scientists, public health professionals, policy makers, clinicians, and community activists from the early days of the women's movement in the 1970s (1). Early conceptualizations of IPV focused on one of two sources believed to be etiologically linked to such violence. One analysis of the cause of IPV, particularly violence against women, focused exclusively on socio-political factors that supported male domination and oppression of women from a feminist perspective (2,3). Another analysis emerged from the psychotherapy and psychiatry fields and examined, variously, what it was about the *woman* that would cause her to be victimized (4) and what it was about the man's psychological make-up that would prompt him to batter his partner (5). Although theories that blamed the victim were dismissed fairly quickly, questions about men who battered their partners persisted, as researchers asked "Who are those guys?"(6). Early reports of batterer characteristics were based primarily on clinical observation of select patients who sought some form of psychotherapy (5). Another source of early research on male batterer characteristics was the battered woman (6,7). One reason why abusive men were not directly studied early on is that they were not readily available for study at that time. Few communities and states required the arrest of domestic violence perpetrators, and few clinical programs for treating abusive men existed until the late 1980s. Further, abusive men did not make themselves readily available for study or treatment (8). Hence, because battered women were available to study in shelters, they also constituted an early, convenient source of information about the men who harmed them.

With the advent of programs that specialize in the treatment of men who batter their female partners, men became increasingly available for study. Hamberger and Hastings (9) published the first typology study of male batterers based on systematically gathered psychological and demographic data. The advent and proliferation of mandatory arrest laws (10), which required police to arrest perpetrators for probable cause that domestic violence had occurred, resulted in even more men being arrested and mandated to specialized batterer treatment programs. Indeed, Hamberger and Arnold (11) reported that implementation of mandatory arrest resulted in a twofold increase in referrals of men for treatment in a single community—a trend that was noted in other settings as well (12). The increased availability of abusive men opened the door for in-depth study of their characteristics. As with early developments of conceptualizations of male IPV as rooted in socio-political dynamics or the internal psychodynamics of the abuser, subsequent research has attempted to address this debate.

The purpose of this chapter is to review relevant research on characteristics of men who abuse their intimate partners. Recent research with nationally representative samples, large community samples, and longitudinal cohorts of men and women have begun to elucidate factors related to the etiology and maintenance of IPV with nonclinical samples. However, in the present chapter, emphasis will be placed on samples that provide the most direct clinical implications for direct services to batterers, defined primarily as those who commit violence of sufficient severity as to warrant arrest, adjudication, and referral to a batterer intervention program. As such, these individuals are, by definition, labeled batterers, not merely aggressive individuals. Therefore, throughout the chapter, the term "batterer" will be used to denote perpetrators studied from clinical samples, and other terms (e.g., perpetrator, abusive person, etc.) will be used to denote individuals who use IPV but who have not yet been labeled as batterers.

MASCULINE POWER, IDEOLOGY, POWER, AND INTIMATE PARTNER VIOLENCE

The most influential views of male to female IPV may be characterized, broadly, as feminist or pro-feminist (13). These views assert that IPV occurs within a broader socio-political context of male oppression of women. Such oppression pervades all of society, including its institutions and individual, intimate relationships. Thus, it is appropriate to begin an exposition of risk factors for battering with consideration of research that has investigated the relationship of sexist beliefs, masculine ideology, and gender role orientation with perpetration of partner violence. Consistent with pro-feminist characterizations of male-initiated IPV, a number of studies have investigated its relationship with various manifestations of masculine power, sexism, gender role orientation, and masculine ideology. An early study reported by Coleman and Straus (14), using data from the First National Family Violence Survey (15), found that the lowest levels of conflict and violence were reported by couples characterized as "equalitarian" (p. 141). Male-dominated relationships reported the highest levels of conflict. Further, as conflict increases, Coleman and Straus observed largest violence increases in male-dominated relationships, and at high conflict, male-to-female violence increased even more dramatically within female-dominated relationships. Hence, asymmetrical power structures within intimate relationships may constitute a risk for violence in the face of escalating conflict, particularly when both partners do not agree with the power arrangement (14). Fitzpatrick and colleagues (16) also reported for college students that males with egalitarian gender role attitudes reported lower relationship aggression and lower threat when their partners engaged in aggressive behavior. Smith (17) reported that men, particularly those with low education and occupational status, and who hold patriarchal beliefs about men's and women's roles in relationships, are more likely to approve of violence against women and to physically assault their wives than men who do not. Dutton and Starzomski (18) compared abusive men and nonviolent men on a measure designed to assess dimensions of the Duluth Power and Control Wheel—a well-known graphic used to educate abusers and victims about different forms of abuse and control. Abusive men scored higher on tactics of emotional abuse, minimization and denial of abuse, and use of the children to control the partner. Although use of male privilege did not differentiate the two groups, it was highly correlated with the other factors for abusers, but not for non-violent men, thus suggesting an indirect relationship with aggression.

Another area of inquiry related to the role of patriarchal beliefs and IPV has been to investigate masculine gender role stress. *Masculine gender role stress* refers to the degree of stress experienced when a male deviates from stereotypical male norms and codes of conduct, such as possessing indices of success, physical adequacy, and perseverance, as well as the avoidance of femininity. Jakupcak, Lisak, and Roemer (19) found that men with high masculine ideology and high levels of masculine gender role stress exhibited higher levels of partner violence. On the other hand, men with low levels of gender role stress, even if they exhibited high levels of masculine ideology, exhibited low levels of partner aggression. Moore and Stuart (20) further reported that when men with high masculine gender role stress were exposed to hypothetical vignettes related to dating partner conflict, such men were more likely than those with low masculine gender role stress to experience anger, attribute negative intent to the woman's actions, and report more verbal aggression.

Taken together, these studies suggest two conclusions related to patriarchal attitudes, masculine gender role attitudes, masculine gender role stress, and IPV. First, attitudes and beliefs that support male dominance of women and the strict definition of men's and women's roles in relationships appear to be related to IPV. Related constructs, such as marital power and masculine gender role stress, are also related to attitudes and behaviors that lead to IPV. This conclusion is similar to that reached by Moore and Stuart (21) in a review of the literature on masculinity and partner violence. Second, these relationships do not appear to be straightforward. Rather, they appear to interact with numerous other variables to exert an effect. Thus, for example, men with high levels of masculine ideology but low levels of masculine gender role stress seem to have lower levels of partner violence (19). This suggests that men for whom a masculine ideology is well integrated into their identities may be less likely to be violent with their partners than men who espouse highly masculine beliefs but not in an integrated fashion. Indeed in an early study of sex role orientation, Rosenbaum (22) concluded that many batterers act

the way they *think* a man should behave, but without a genuine sense of masculinity.

Supportive of Rosenbaum's conclusion, a recent meta-analysis reported by Sugarman and Frankel (23) reported that assaultive husbands exhibit greater undifferentiated sex role orientation than nonabusive men. Similarly, Coleman and Straus (14) reported that conflict and violence were lower in male- and female-dominated relationships when both partners agreed with the power structure than if they did not. These findings are consistent with a path analysis reported by Stith and Farley (24) that showed egalitarianism was related to use of partner violence through its relationship with approval of marital violence. As approval of marital violence increased, egalitarianism decreased.

Although the findings are statistically significant and thus may lead to the conclusion that egalitarianism, sexism, and patriarchal attitudes are risk factors for IPV, the observed and reported effect sizes for many of the variables are not large. For example, Smith (17) reported that a combination of six variables, including patriarchal beliefs and approval of violence, accounted for 20% of the variance in partner violence. Jakupcak and colleagues (19) reported that masculine ideology and masculine gender role stress accounted for 12% of the variance in partner violence, and the path model reported by Stith and Farley (24) accounted for 19% of the variance in severe partner violence.

Due to the low amount of variance accounted for by gender-based, socio-political variables, Dutton (25,26) argues that it is inappropriate to confine analysis of IPV only to a socio-political level. Rather, Dutton argues that study of psychopathology and psychological processes in male batterers may yield data and increase our understanding of IPV at least as much as study of socio-political variables. Further, using a longitudinal birth cohort, Ehrensaft, Moffitt, and Caspi (27) found that males who used clinical levels of partner violence also showed evidence of psychopathology, stemming from childhood, as well as personality deviance. Such findings argue for the inclusion of study of psychological variables as risk factors for IPV. Hamberger and Lohr (28) have also argued that the study of psychological processes is a legitimate approach, as battering is a complex behavior governed by principles of learning and amenable to behavioral analysis. Further, study of psychopathology and psychological processes does not excuse the batterer for bad behavior. Rather, such study may increase our understanding of abuse and ways to prevent and end it. The following sections review research on psychological characteristics of abusive men, and how these may differ from nonviolent men.

PSYCHOLOGICAL CHARACTERISTICS OF MEN WHO BATTER THEIR PARTNERS

Study of the psychological characteristics of male partner violence perpetrators has proceeded along two primary paths. One approach has attempted to highlight the diversity and heterogeneity of abusive men by various means, such as cluster analysis and factor analysis, to determine different "types" or subgroups based on certain psychological and/or behavioral variables. One example is the early work of Hamberger and Hastings (9). These authors derived subgroups of batterers based on factor analysis of respondents' scores on a measure of personality and psychopathology, yielding three major subgroups. Hamberger and Hastings did not include a nonviolent cohort in their analysis, so their research describes characteristics of abusive men only. Further, Hamberger and Hastings did not include analysis of the relationship between psychological type and profile of violence.

A second approach to studying the characteristics of abusive men has been to compare cohorts of such men with comparison groups of nonviolent men who are either in distressed or nondistressed relationships. The latter case comparison approach helps answer the question of whether and how abusive men differ from nonviolent men, but typically does not highlight the heterogeneity of the violent men. Given these two approaches, a considerable amount has been learned about abusive men over the past several years that can provide guidance in determining risk factors for intimate partner abuse.

TYPOLOGIES OF ABUSIVE MEN

A number of typologies have been offered to describe the heterogeneity of abusive men. Most of these typologies are based on personality type (29), physiological reactivity (30), or type of violence (31,32). However, the physiological reactivity typology offered by Gottman and colleagues has not been successfully replicated, suggesting a need for more research before identifying batterers from measures of autonomic reactivity (33,34). In addition, although behaviorally based typologies show some promise for conceptualizing different types of IPV and the development of different types of psycho-social interventions, they are based on post-hoc assessment of violence that has already been committed. Thus, the information gleaned from such studies does not lend itself to the development of risk markers and will not be considered further in the present discussion. Because a primary goal of this chapter is to discuss risk factors for battering and IPV, the primary focus will be on identifying the most common characteristics of batterers (and, where appropriate, aggressive men) that can be identified and used by the practicing clinician. Further, the work of Holtzworth-Munroe and Stuart, as well as that of Hamberger and colleagues has been foundational in elucidating batterer types and is the most clinically descriptive. Thus, the latter typologies will constitute the centerpiece of the description of batterer types.

Holtzworth-Munroe and Stuart (35) conducted a comprehensive review of batterer typology research and determined, across study methodologies, three main subtypes of batterers, based on a combination of violence profile and personality psychopathology. The types identified by Holtzworth-Munroe and Stuart are family-only perpetrators, borderline/dysphoric, and antisocial/generally violent perpetrators. Hamberger, Lohr, Bonge, and Tolin (36) provided empirical support for the primary model hypothesized by Holtzworth-Munroe and Stuart (35), reporting three main types of batterers—nonpsychopathological, negativistic/dependent, and antisocial/narcissistic, consistent with the Holtzworth-Munroe and Stuart types, respectively. Relying primarily on data from Hamberger and Hastings (9) and Hamberger and colleagues (36), each of the primary perpetrator types will be described.

Borderline/Dysphoric Batterers

Hamberger and colleagues (36) identified a subtype of batterers they labeled *negativistic/dependent* who, psychologically, appears quite similar to Holtzworth-Munroe and Stuart's (35) dysphoric/borderline and Hamberger and Hastings' (9) schizoidal/borderline perpetrator. The different labels used may reflect specific personality scale elevations and profiles, and probably reflect the continuum of borderline personality organization more than a particular diagnostic category (37). Clinical experience suggests that such men have the capability of appearing pleasant (if brooding, at times), charming and effusive, insightful, and open about discussing their feelings. They can establish an intimate level of relating quickly and intensely. Partners of borderline/dysphoric men frequently comment on how, upon first meeting, the couple spent hours, long into the night, discussing their lives and experiences, including problems, leading the woman to believe that this was a man in touch with his feelings. Sometimes, such men also appear to be lost, and they enlist the aid of the woman in their search for identity. Hence, borderline/dysphoric batterers typically appear as very dependent on their intimate partner for a sense of identity, but experience tremendous conflict between their dependence and their fear of being "taken over" or engulfed by her. Thus, he may be viewed by others as unpredictably moody—clingy and fawning one moment, and angry and rejecting the next. Partners of such men frequently describe them as having a "Dr. Jeckyll-Mr. Hyde" personality, able to go from calm and controlled one moment to angry and oppressive the next, for no apparent reason. Borderline/dysphoric men are typically hypersensitive to subtle interpersonal slights that would not cause an impact on others. For example, a borderline/dysphoric man may interpret his partner's absence from the house when he returns from work as rejection of him or "proof" of her "screwing around" rather than related to her running errands for the family. The batterer's experience of rejection can result in a spectrum of emotions ranging from sadness and distress to anger and rage.

In addition to the basic personality features just described, borderline/dysphoric batterers also exhibit a number of other features related to psychopathology and violence profile. In particular, among the three primary batterer types, borderline/dysphoric batterers commit fairly high levels of violence toward their partners, especially compared to nonpathological, family-only batterers. Hamberger and colleagues (36) and Holtzworth-Munroe and associates (38) both reported borderline/dysphoric batterers to commit nonsignificantly lower levels of violence than antisocial/generally violent batterers, and significantly higher than nonpathological, family-only batterers. In addition, Hamberger and colleagues observed that female partners reported borderline/dysphoric batterers to exhibit the highest annual frequency of physical assault compared to antisocial/generally violent

and nonpathological/family-only batterers. However, antisocial/generally violent batterers were much more likely than borderline/dysphoric batterers to report violence toward a prior intimate partner.

Holtzworth-Munroe and associates (38) and Hamberger and colleagues (36) observed higher rates of alcohol and drug use among borderline/dysphoric batterers than among nonpathological/family only batterers. However, Hamberger and colleagues reported greater alcohol abuse among dysphoric/borderline batterers and higher drug abuse among antisocial/generally violent batterers, whereas Holtzworth-Munroe and associates reported highest levels of alcohol and drug abuse among the antisocial/generally violent batterers. Further, Hamberger and colleagues (36) observed that antisocial/generally violent batterers were more likely to report having sought alcohol or drug abuse treatment than the other two groups. Because Holtzworth-Munroe and associates (38) used multiple and independent measures of substance abuse, their findings are probably more reliable.

Borderline/dysphoric batterers show fairly high rates of annual police contact for a variety of violations of the law. Specifically, such batterers are intermediate between antisocial/generally violent and nonpathological/family-only batterers in number of annual arrests for violent offenses and acting-out offenses such as disorderly conduct, obstructing a police officer, or absconding from probation (36).

Borderline/dysphoric batterers appear to be the most depressed and suffer higher levels of anger proneness than the other two batterer types. Cognitively, these batterers also tend to express a high need for approval, have difficulty motivating themselves to take initiative, and are pessimistic about their ability to change negative behavior patterns (39). Borderline/dysphoric batterers also appear to have higher levels of fearful and dismissing attachment styles, relative to nonpathological/family-only and antisocial/generally violent batterers (38). Dutton, Saunders, Starzomski, and Bartholomew (40) further found that fearful attachment style was more highly correlated with borderline personality organization than was preoccupied attachment style. Hence, borderline/dysphoric batterers appear to enter intimate relationships with massive concerns about rejection and abandonment, feel highly anxious, and look to their intimate partners to provide them with a sense of self-worth, validation, and stability.

Dysphoric/borderline batterers reported witnessing significantly more parental violence than did nonpathological/family-only batterers. Further, compared to the other two types, dysphoric/borderline batterers reported the highest rates of experiencing abuse as a child (36), from both mother and father (38). Further, dysphoric/borderline batterers reported experiencing more rejection from their mothers than did nonpathological/family-only batterers.

Despite the large amount of work that has gone into studying the borderline/dysphoric batterer, recent research has called for caution in conceptualizing borderline/dysphoric batterers as a distinct clinical group. Two independent studies (41,42) were able to identify the three primary groups of batterers discussed in the present section. However, both groups of researchers were not able to report any meaningful differences between generally violent/antisocial batterers and borderline/dysphoric batterers. Hence, more work is needed to identify the clinical utility of typologies that distinguish between the latter two types of abusive men.

Antisocial/Generally Violent Batterers

The primary characteristics of the antisocial/generally violent batterer, sometimes also known as antisocial-narcissistic, are self-centeredness, self-absorption, and lack of empathy. Antisocial/generally violent batterers have little to no sense of the mutuality and reciprocation that characterizes many intimate relationships. Rather, others, including intimate partners, are viewed essentially as objects, possessions to be used for the gratification of the perpetrator's needs and ends. This lack of empathy is illustrated by the comment made by an antisocial/narcissistic batterer who related in treatment that his partner had finally left him. He commented, "I finally got rid of her. No big deal. I can just go out and get me another one."

Any appearance of reciprocity and mutuality exhibited by the antisocial/generally violent batterer is engaged in to his benefit rather than for the benefit of the relationship or another person. Hence, he may buy his potential partner expensive gifts to impress her with his generosity and status, not as a sign of his affection for her. Such individuals are typically seen as charming and interesting in superficial interactions. For example, reception staff at a medical clinic or mental health center may find such men to be fun to interact with during check-in or check-out. He may make pithy comments that result in much levity and laughter, or shower the staff with compliments. To a potential intimate partner, the antisocial/generally violent man appears confident and exciting, if competitive, unsentimental, and aloof. He may impress his potential partner as protective and caring, particularly if she is vulnerable. As the relationship progresses, the antisocial/generally violent batterer manipulates and imposes his values, perceptions, and brand of reality onto his partner and others with whom he has a relationship. He sets the rules, feels entitled to have them complied with, and claims the absolute right to determine and mete out punishment when they are violated in any way.

As noted earlier, antisocial/generally violent batterers commit violence toward their partners that is roughly equal to (36,38) or more severe than borderline/dysphoric batterers, and considerably more severe than the nonpathological/family-only batterers (43). Further, antisocial/generally violent batterers commit more severe sexual battery toward their partners than the other two subgroups, especially the nonpathological/family-only group (38), and more psychological abuse toward their partner than the nonpathological/family-only batterers (43).

In comparison with the other two subgroups, generally violent/antisocial batterers appear to exhibit more general violence outside the context of intimate relationships (36,43) and in previous intimate relationships (38). Further, antisocial/generally violent batterers experience significantly more arrests overall (38) and more violent crime than nonpathological/family-only batterers (36). Antisocial/generally violent men also report having more criminally deviant relationships than the other two batterer subtypes, especially the nonpathological/family-only batterers (38).

Antisocial/generally violent batterers tend to exhibit fairly low levels of depression, especially compared to borderline/dysphoric batterers. Although Hamberger and colleagues (36) found no differences in depression between antisocial/generally violent and nonpathological/family-only batterers, Saunders (43) did find generally violent batterers to score higher on depression than family-only batterers. However, Saunders did not assess for antisocial personality, and it is possible that his observed generally violent group also contained some batterers with borderline personality organization. On measures of irrational cognitions, antisocial/generally violent batterers appear to view their emotional problems and negative emotional reactions as the fault of and controlled by external sources, such as other people doing things they do not like. This batterer type also reports excessive worry about how things can go wrong for them, suggesting concerns about control of their environment. Hence, they tend to blame others for their problems while simultaneously working to control how others act toward them. Holtzworth-Munroe and associates (38) also found the antisocial/generally violent batterers to exhibit a dismissing attachment style, especially compared to nonpathological/family-only batterers, and lower levels of spouse-specific dependency than borderline/dysphoric batterers. Although Hamberger and colleagues (36) reported no significant differences between borderline/dysphoric and antisocial/generally violent men on a general measure of anger proneness, Saunders (43) observed that generally violent men exhibited significantly higher spouse-specific anger than did family-only batterers.

Family Only/Nonpathological Batterers

Across studies using different measures of psychopathology, a group of nonpathological batterers has been observed (35). Nonpathological batterers are typically labeled so not because their violence is somehow "normal" and not deviant, but because they rarely show evidence of psychopathology on any of the psychological measures they complete. A variation among nonpathological batterers is a group of men who show elevated scores on measures of passive dependency and compulsive personality features—personality styles that are not typically associated with the impulsivity noted in borderline/dysphoric batterers, or planned, instrumental violence and coercion noted in generally violent/antisocial batterers. Rather, family-only/nonpathological batterers appear, upon casual observation, as the stereotypic "man next door." They live highly conventional lives, have little or no contact with law enforcement for criminal violations, blend into their community fabric, and appear to all the world to be normal in every respect. Therefore, men with passive dependent or obsessive compulsive personality characteristics will be included in the discussion of family-only/nonpathological batterers.

Those batterers who show evidence of passive dependency or obsessive compulsive personality style typically have low self-esteem and engage in passive and ingratiating ways. The passive dependent batterer, in particular, may lack assertive skills for setting boundaries or negotiating conflict. Thus, he subordinates his rights in conflicts to "keep the peace," while building internal resentments that occasionally erupt in aggressive, rebellious outbursts of hostility and physical aggression. Such individuals may be seen as willing to go along to get along, and thus be viewed by others as cooperative, laid back or, on the negative side, as easily manipulated and intimidated to back down.

The batterer with a compulsive personality style also typically lacks confidence in self-assertion but has adapted by developing adherence to a set of rules that guides him. Compulsive batterers often view themselves as highly disciplined and reliable. They tend to be viewed by others as rigid, rule-bound, and unexpressive, although highly conventional, predictable, polite, and respectful. The struggle for the compulsive batterer is coping with the inherent differences in approach to solving life's problems that occur in any, including intimate, relationship. For example, the man might hold the belief that after work, everyone should stay home and engage in "family" activities. His partner may belong to organizations that meet in the evening. The compulsive batterer tends to view his partner's behavior as violations of the rules, resulting in his feeling anger and anxiety. Although he may comprehend intellectually, he cannot emotionally tolerate that his partner may view how time is used in the evening differently than he does. He may view her difference in this area as a betrayal of some earlier promise and understanding she made to him regarding how evening family time will be spent, and he will engage in behaviors designed to restore, what to him, is the proper order of things.

When compared to the other two primary batterer groups, family-only/nonpathological batterers appear to mainly confine their violence to their intimate relationships and families (36,38). Overall levels of partner violence are also lower than those observed among dysphoric/borderline and antisocial batterers, and they exhibit the lowest frequency of physical battering (36,43). Compared to the other two groups, family-only/nonpathological batterers engage in the lowest amounts of criminal behavior (36,38). Further, family-only/nonpathological batterers also show the lowest levels of depression, anger, jealousy, and alcohol and drug abuse compared to the other two batterer groups (36,38,43).

Given the diversity of psychological and violence types exhibited among men who batter their partners, one might ask about the clinical utility of dividing batterers up along the lines of violence severity and personality disturbance. Cavanaugh and Gelles (44) suggested that such typologies might be useful in determining the risk level of batterers. For example, family-only/nonpathological batterers show the lowest levels of violence and the least psychopathology, whereas the borderline/dysphoric batterer seems to exhibit moderate risk, and the generally violent/ antisocial batterer the highest risk. Although such a designation remains to be validated, dividing batterers by risk and personality type can lead to the development of treatment approaches matched to specific type and violence profile. Initial assessment to determine "type" may be somewhat expensive, given that personality testing, together with extensive history taking is required (45). Recent research has shown that psychologists with domestic violence training are able to accurately identify and classify batterers into the three main subtypes just described and discussed (46). Given that the vast majority of providers of batterer intervention services are not doctoral-level psychologists, more research needs to be done to determine the utility of typologies for nonpsychologist providers. Further, almost no research demonstrates the utility of batterer typologies in guiding treatment approach or predicting treatment outcomes. Despite such limitations, understanding common characteristics of men who batter their partners has value in helping clinicians to identify men at risk for IPV and lead to the development of appropriate screening approaches. However, another way to identify IPV risk factors is to examine studies that compare abusive men with those who are not abusive and note consistent differences. Examples of important case control studies will be reviewed next.

CASE-COMPARISON STUDIES OF ABUSIVE AND NONABUSIVE MEN

In addition to the rich descriptions of batterer characteristics provided by typology studies, another line of research has compared abusive men, as a group, with nonviolent men to elucidate characteristics that are unique, or at least more typical of abusive men that can function as risk markers and guide both theory building and treatment planning for abusive men. Generally, when case comparison studies have been conducted with clinical samples or large, community cohort

samples, they have been retrospective in nature. More recently, a number of studies have reported longitudinal, prospective cohort studies. As noted previously, because the primary interest of this chapter is to elucidate characteristics of clinical samples, retrospective case comparison studies will predominate the review. However, where prospective studies overlap with clinical studies, they will also be noted.

Case control studies have been conducted along a variety of dimensions. In an earlier section of this chapter, differences related to patriarchal, masculine ideology were reviewed. Other important variables include anger and hostility, alcohol and drug abuse, dependency and attachment style, marital satisfaction, and family of origin abuse experiences.

Anger and Hostility

Several early studies on batterer characteristics showed that men who batter their partners, as a group, struggle with anger and hostility, although not universally. For example, Hamberger and Hastings (9) revealed that while borderline/dysphoric batterers showed high levels of anger, nonpathological batterers and antisocial/ narcissistic batterers did not show as high of levels of anger proneness. Hershorn and Rosenbaum (47) showed that batterers experienced and expressed hostility in two different ways. Men with undercontrolled hostility were more frequently violent with their partners and more violent generally in their lives. Men with overcontrolled hostility showed less frequent episodes of violence, but the episodes were more severe. Further, men with overcontrolled hostility confined their violence to their intimate relationships.

Case comparison studies have also shown that abusive men show more hostility than nonviolent men. Abusive men show similar levels of hostility as those exhibited by generally violent men, but higher levels than nonviolent men (48). Further, batterers show different *types* of hostility compared to nonviolent men. For example, compared to criminally violent men who are not maritally violent, abusive men exhibit higher overall hostility but lower suspicion (49). Abusive men also score higher than nonabusive men on measures of *state anger* (i.e., anger at the moment) and *trait anger* (i.e., the tendency to become angry) (50,51). Further, compared to nonviolent men, abusers are more likely to exhibit hostility directed at themselves and toward others (50,52,53) and lower anger control (50,53).

Although not specifically related to anger and hostility, a number of studies have begun to investigate the types of attributions abusive men make, compared to nonviolent men, in situations related to relationship conflict. This research is important in that it provides insight into how an abusive man labels and interprets partner behavior that may lead to highly negative feelings, including anger, and subsequent abusive behavior. Holtzworth-Munroe and Hutchenson (54) reported that, compared to nonviolent men in satisfied or distressed relationships, abusive men attributed negative wife behaviors to the wife's negative intent rather than to other causes, especially in situations involving jealousy and rejection. Moreover, compared to nonabusive men, abusive men tend to attribute negative partner behavior as due to her selfishness and blameworthiness for the behavior (55). Other research has shown that abusive men tend to make such negative attributions of partner intent in situations that are moderately provocative. In highly provocative situations, nonabusive men also make such negative attributions. Hence, in situations where "anybody would be upset," both violent and nonviolent men make similar types of attributions. But, in less intense situations, abusive men continue to react as though their partner "did it on purpose," whereas nonviolent men do not (56).

Alcohol and Other Drug Abuse

A common question about partner violence is whether it is caused by alcohol or other drug abuse. Indeed, studies indicate that alcohol abuse is observed among abusive men at rates approaching 60%–70% (57). Using data from the second National Family Violence Survey (58), Kaufman-Kantor and Straus (59) demonstrated that, although alcohol did play a role in the violence of many relationships, it was neither a necessary nor sufficient factor. This finding is consistent with the idea that substance abuse is correlated with IPV but does not cause it. Heyman, O'Leary, and Jouriles (60) discovered from longitudinal research that the role of alcohol in predicting partner violence changes over the course of the relationship. From pre-marriage to 6 months after marriage, alcohol use was positively associated with serious partner violence. However, after 18 months of marriage, alcohol use interacted with aggressive personality style to predict level of marital violence. Further, Heyman and

colleagues (60) observed that alcohol abuse was not associated with the abused partners' marital satisfaction and plans for seeking divorce. Rather, it was the husband's premarital aggression that predicted the latter factors. Hence, as a correlate of IPV, alcohol appears to be rather weak. On the other hand, another longitudinal study suggested that on days when abusive men were drinking, the odds of them perpetrating partner violence were eight times higher than the chances of committing violence on days when they did not drink alcohol. The odds of severe marital violence on drinking days were even higher—11 times, than on days of no drinking (61). Further research suggests that it is the man's *expectations* of aggression following drinking that mediate the relationship between alcohol use and partner violence (62). Specifically, expectations that aggressive behavior will follow alcohol consumption increased the odds of partner violence by a factor of 3.2. Recent research by Snow and associates (63) further clarifies the indirect effect of alcohol on IPV. These researchers investigated the relationship between coping style and alcohol abuse on IPV in male batterers. Specifically, the authors found that greater use of avoidance coping styles (e.g., avoid the stressful situation or avoid thinking about it, denial, and minimization) was more characteristic of problem drinkers, whereas increased use of direct problem solving characterized men without problem drinking. Avoidance strategies, in turn, were directly related to the perpetration of physical and emotional abuse, and indirectly related through problem drinking. Hence, although the effects of alcohol on IPV may not be direct, alcohol abuse or problem drinking does appear to exert an indirect effect and should be considered a risk factor.

Dependency and Attachment Style

A common notion about batterers is that they are highly and abnormally dependent on their partners. Compared to maritally discordant and satisfied, nonviolent men, Murphy, Meyer, and O'Leary (64) found that abusive men exhibited both higher general interpersonal dependency and spouse-specific dependency. Such dependency appeared to be undergirded by high personal inadequacy while being highly invested in the intimate relationship. In contrast, happily married men felt both adequate and invested in their relationships. Hence, abusive men appear to feel incapable of effectively managing their intimate relationship, whereas happily married, nonviolent men do, even if they are highly invested in their relationships.

A number of studies have begun to examine attachment style and its relationship to abusiveness. *Attachment style* refers to the internal, mental template of relationships that one develops in childhood through early interactions with important caretakers. Attachment style is believed to provide information about how a person regulates emotion in the context of intimate relationships. *Secure attachment* refers to a relationship template that includes a positive image of self and other, resulting in confident, comfortable interactions with intimate others. *Preoccupied attachment* style is characterized by a negative view of self and positive image of others in relationship. *Fearful attachment* style consists of a negative internal model of both self and others with whom one has a relationship. Both preoccupied and fearful attachment styles are characterized by tension and anxiety, fear of rejection and abandonment, and high levels of negative affect, including anger, in intimate relationships. A *dismissing* style consists of a positive internal view of self and negative model of others, suggesting a disdainful style of relating to intimate others. Dutton and colleagues (40) compared abusive men referred for treatment and a demographically matched control group on measures of attachment and other variables found to be related to abusiveness—anger, jealousy, borderline personality organization, and trauma symptoms. Fearful attachment style correlated most strongly and positively with the other measures of abusiveness. Preoccupied attachment also correlated positively but not as strongly as fearful attachment style. Dismissing attachment style was not correlated with any of the other abusiveness measures. Other research also found abusive men compared to nonviolent, maritally distressed men to exhibit preoccupied and insecure attachment styles (65). In addition, insecure and preoccupied attachment was associated with the least amount of distancing during marital interactions. Further, for batterers with preoccupied attachment style, partner withdrawal during interaction significantly predicted violence. In contrast, dismissing attachment style was associated with the greatest amount of distancing and control. Such attachment difficulties among batterers, particularly those with preoccupied and fearful attachment styles, seems to stem from perceptions of deficits in maternal love and nurturing which, in turn, appear to be related to low self-esteem and the perception of less support from one's intimate partner (66).

Family-of-Origin Experiences

A common question about men who abuse and batter their partners is "Where did they learn this? Did they grow up in a violent home?" Many studies have included questions about family-of-origin exposure to abuse, generally focusing on direct abuse experiences and witnessing of parental violence. In general, compared to nonviolent men, abusive men report growing up in homes where they personally experienced violence and abuse against themselves (52,67,68). Abusive men also report having witnessed more parental violence than nonviolent men (67,68). However, other research has begun to show that the relationship between family-of-origin experiences and abusiveness is not always straightforward or strong. For example, in a meta-analytic review reported by Stith and co-workers (69), growing up in an abusive family was a weak to moderate predictor of adult involvement in IPV. Hamberger and Hastings (70) observed that witnessing and experiencing abuse as a child was significant only for batterers who reported alcoholic problems. Rosen, Parmley, Knudson, and Fancher (71) found that being abused as a child predicted partner violence for White, but not for Black perpetrators. For Black men, child abuse was related to depression, but not perpetration. Hanson and colleagues (68) reported that witnessing parental abuse was related to severe, but not moderate, violence perpetrators. Corvo and Carpenter (72) also found that abuse experiences and witnessing of abuse in the family of origin predicted violence; in addition, they reported that paternal substance abuse exerted a similar, independent effect on partner violence. Hence, the findings of Corvo and Carpenter, together with those of other researchers (40), reporting on other negative family-of-origin experiences (such as rejection and harsh punishment) suggest that broader family-of-origin experiences beyond being abused or exposed to parental violence may act to influence the development of personality and behavior patterns that increase vulnerability to perpetration of IPV.

Demographic Characteristics

Hastings and Hamberger (73) argue that demographic characteristics are neither specific nor sensitive enough to adequately predict violent offending. Nevertheless, almost every study of IPV collects such data in order to adequately describe populations and samples under study. Comprehensive reviews by Barnett, Miller-Perrin, and Perrin (74) and Hastings and Hamberger (73) suggest that younger age and lower socioeconomic status are typically characteristic of violent versus nonviolent men. Race has also been investigated as a predictor of partner violence, but when socioeconomic status is controlled for, race is usually washed out as a predictor (73,74).

Marital Satisfaction and Interaction

Studies routinely find that abusive relationships are also more distressed and unsatisfying than are non-violent relationships, even when these are distressed (7,68). However, marital dissatisfaction, by itself, does not predict partner violence (75). Rather, among newly married couples, it appears that acts of psycho-logical aggression are more important in predicting partner violence. *Psychological aggression* was defined as verbal aggression such as threats and nonverbal acts, such as doing the opposite of what one's partner asks. Murphy and O'Leary (75) found that marital dissatisfaction, however, was both correlated to physical aggression and a consequence of it. For men involved in abuse abatement treatment, Fals-Stewart, Lucente, and Birchler (76) found that number of days of face-to-face contact was significantly related to physical aggression but not verbal aggression. Specifically, men and their partners who reported more days away from each other in the previous year reported lower levels of physical violence. The authors reasoned that face-to-face contact is not needed for verbal aggres-sion, as this can be accomplished over the phone or via e-mail. Nevertheless, these studies suggest that relationship distress, coupled with reports of verbal aggression, a lot of day-to-day contact, and little time apart may function as risk markers for IPV that should be noted and monitored.

Head Injury, Brain Damage, and Neuropsychological Deficits

A small number of studies have investigated whether men who batter have different, and possibly deficient, neuropsychological functioning than men who do not abuse their partners. Warnken and associates (77) directly compared orthopedically injured and head-injured males, recruited from a hospital database, on measures of partner violence and a number of correlates of traumatic brain injury and psychological

characteristics. Although the two groups did not differ in rate of IPV, the researchers found that, compared to men with orthopedic injuries, head-injured men reported more problems with losing their tempers, controlling impulses, arguments with others, and decreased marital satisfaction. Further, head-injured men reported increased dependency, and decreased self-esteem and masculine self-image. Head-injured men also reported increased alcohol abuse and depression.

Cohen and associates (78) compared batterers referred for treatment with groups of maritally dis-tressed and satisfied, nonviolent men on a number of measures of neuropsychological functioning. Compared to the nonviolent men, batterers showed a number of deficits suggestive of compromised neu-ropsychological function, including cognitive flex-ibility, attention information processing efficiency, and executive control ability. Batterers also showed deficits in memory, learning, and verbal ability. Further, head injury alone did not account for the differences in neuropsychological function, nor is it known what amount of contribution to battering is accounted for by such processes in addition to other factors such as emotional state, substance abuse, psychopathology, and patriarchal values. Neverthe-less, the observed differences and effects of neuro-psychological functioning suggest their importance as risk markers for IPV.

RISK FACTOR PREDICTION OF INTIMATE PARTNER VIOLENCE BY MALES

Few studies have examined how the many variables elucidated here may combine to allow predictive statements about the risk of perpetrating IPV. Hanson and colleagues (68) found that abuse was associated with high levels of violence victimization during childhood, antisocial personality disorder, personal distress, marital distress, impulsivity, and positive attitudes toward violence against women. Further-more, Hanson and colleagues reported a linear rela-tionship between the latter variables and severity of violence. Thus, batterers who committed moderate levels of violence shared the same risk factors with those who perpetrated severe violence. However, as the level of risk factor increased, violence severity also increased.

In a study of over 15,000 members of the U.S. Army, Pan, Neidig, and O'Leary (79) observed that both moderate and severe IPV was predicted by lower income, alcohol problems, marital discord, and depression. Similar to the observations of Hanson and colleagues (68), severe IPV was predicted by the lowest income levels, the most marital discord, and the highest levels of depression. In addition, severe IPV was predicted by perpetrator drug abuse. Although the latter studies do not evaluate all possible risk markers for IPV, the available data do suggest that personal characteristics commonly observed in clinical practice sites can be useful for estimating IPV risk.

EXPANDING RESEARCH WITH CULTURAL MINORITIES

For most of the past two decades of research on characteristics of partner-abusive men, the focus has been on convenience samples of men who were typically arrested and referred through the criminal justice system for abuse abatement counseling. Although studies of such samples have typically been fairly ethnically diverse, by and large they have consisted primarily of Caucasian, heterosexual men. In recent years, researchers have begun to investigate characteristics of intimate aggressors among Mexican-American and African-American male batterers, gay and lesbian batterers, and heterosexual female batterers.

Ethnic/Racial Minority Batterers

A small but growing number of studies have begun examining correlates of IPV among Mexican Americans. In general, these studies are beginning to demonstrate that, compared to nonbatterers, Mexican-American batterers exhibit more alcohol and drug problems (80–82). Financial stress also predicts violence, particularly for married Mexican-American and Anglo couples (81). Conversely, higher income appears to reduce the odds of violence among Mexican-American, Anglo, and African-American couples (81). Other research has shown that immigration status may be related to abuse perpetration among Mexican Americans. In particular, Mexican Americans born in the United States showed significantly higher domestic violence rates than did Mexican Americans born in Mexico (83). Sorenson and Telles also found age and marital status related to abuse

among Mexican Americans. Older age and divorced or separated status were found to predict abuse perpetration. Further, psychopathology appears to predict IPV. Lifetime mental disorder/psychiatric diagnosis predicts IPV. In addition, Mexican-American batterers show more fear of rejection and closeness in intimate relationships, low self-esteem, and passive aggressive behavior patterns (82).

Research with Lesbian Batterers

Clinical work and burgeoning research with lesbian batterers has begun to elucidate characteristics that may differentiate them from nonviolent lesbians. Coleman (84) observed among her patient population that lesbian batterers show personality characteristics consistent with borderline personality organization and narcissistic/antisocial personality style. These clinical observations have been supported by empirical assessment of abusive and nonabusive lesbians that has shown batterers to score higher on measures of borderline personality and antisocial personality (85). Fortunata and Kohn also reported that lesbian batterers showed more alcohol and drug abuse, as well as childhood physical and sexual abuse victimization, than did nonviolent lesbians. McKenry, Serovich, Mason, and Mosack (86) found, in a small sample of gay male and lesbian participants, that individual factors differentiated perpetrators from nonabusive individuals to a greater extent than relationship factors or family-of-origin factors. In particular, compared to nonperpetrators, perpetrators showed greater masculine orientation and less secure attachment styles. Female perpetrators were more likely to report being abused as a child, but no more likely that nonperpetrators to report witnessing parental violence. However, perpetrators and nonperpetrators did not differ on measures of perceived relationship power differential, interpersonal dependency, or outing.

Heterosexual Female Batterers

Although a lot of research has been conducted on gender differences in perpetration of IPV (87,88), recent research has begun to investigate a small group of women who appear to be primary physical aggressors in their heterosexual intimate relationships. Conradi (89) reported that female batterers who had been arrested and ordered to participate in batterer intervention counseling showed a history of prior victimization, including physical abuse as a child, exposure to parental violence, and previous partner violence victimization. Further, female batterers report problems with substance abuse, a masculine sex role orientation, and a history of initiating violence in other situations not involving an intimate partner.

Clearly, the works just reviewed point to the importance of studying IPV risk among different groups. Although many of the risk factors identified in general research on IPV seem to also apply to specific, minority groups, these factors appear to do so in different ways that are unique to respective groups. More research is needed among different minority groups to further clarify culturally specific risk factors for IPV.

WILL MALE HEALTHCARE PATIENTS TALK ABOUT THEIR USE OF VIOLENCE?

Because men who batter have a tendency to deny and minimize the true extent of their violent and abusive behavior (90), the question naturally arises as to whether they will be willing to talk about their violent experiences when queried as part of routine, universal screening in healthcare settings. Little research guides the answer to this question, but that which does exist appears to offer some promising leads. Oriel and Fleming (91) assessed men in primary care settings and found that 13% reported committing minor acts of partner violence, and 4.2% reported using severe violence against their partners. Phelan and colleagues (92) studied prevalence of perpetration among men seeking emergency medical care and found that 25.6% reported being in a violent relationship. In both studies, participation rates were around 85%. Although the findings from the latter two studies were not corroborated with partner report or some other independent account and may thus represent an underestimate of the prevalence of partner assaulters in primary and emergency care, the prevalence rates do nevertheless suggest that men will discuss their use of violence when asked. Further, the high participation rates suggest that men are open to being asked and responding to questions about their use of IPV. Clearly, however, more work needs to be done in the area of asking men about IPV as part of their routine health care.

CHALLENGES TO HEALTHCARE PRACTITIONERS ASKING MALE PATIENTS ABOUT PERPETRATION

A fairly extensive literature has evolved that examines healthcare provider barriers to asking women about partner violence victimization and, although there is as yet no comparable literature regarding asking male patients about perpetration, some of the identified barriers for screening women patients seem applicable to screening men as well. In particular, despite training and development of appropriate, professional attitudes toward screening for partner violence, many providers continue to worry that they will offend their patients for doing so, and may even endanger themselves in the process (4). If these concerns inhibit asking women patients about partner violence victimization, it is difficult to imagine that many providers will feel comfortable asking men about their potential perpetration and related dynamics. Thus, prior to implementing policies for perpetration screening, it will be necessary to develop training programs that clearly and directly address these and related concerns, as well as ongoing staff support for coping with their uneasiness in this area (93). Hamberger and Phelan (94) also identify a number of other challenges that need to be addressed and resolved prior to developing screening protocols and programs to identify partner abusers. These include ensuring that appropriate community infrastructure is in place to provide services and support to identified perpetrators and their victims. This includes not only victim services, but specialized batterer intervention programming as well. In addition, healthcare providers and organizations will have to develop policies and procedures for dealing with problems related to having both perpetrator and victim dyads in the same practice. Not only is confidentiality important in such cases, but universal screening for victimization *and* perpetration will be necessary to reduce the likelihood that perpetrators will suspect that they are being asked because their partners disclosed first.

CONCLUSION

Over the past two decades, a considerable amount of work has been done to elucidate those characteristics that differentiate men who batter their partners from those who do not. Such research has focused on personality characteristics, psychopathology, alcohol and drug abuse, family-of-origin experiences, demographic characteristics, relationship problems, and violence profiles. Virtually all of these variables differentiate abusive from nonabusive men, with abusive men typically showing more problems, pathology, and poor premorbid functioning. Further, abusive men appear to be a heterogeneous group, as research has repeatedly demonstrated that no single "batterer profile" exists. In the absence of universal screening, healthcare professionals can rely on knowledge of these risk markers to cue inquiry about IPV perpetration. However, the research has not advanced sufficiently to offer appropriately sensitive and specific risk profiles. Therefore, inquiries targeting known risk markers only, as well as reliance only on self-report, will likely lead to underidentification of perpetrators. On the other hand, development of universal perpetration screening without developing and implementing appropriate community resources, clinic or health system policies and procedures, and provider training and support will not likely be successful and effective.

IMPLICATIONS FOR POLICY, PRACTICE, AND RESEARCH

Policy

- Research on men who batter their partners forms the basis for identifying families and children at risk and engaging in primary prevention efforts in the clinic, schools, and general community education.
- Research on male batterers in healthcare settings, including potential harms and benefits, has not sufficiently advanced to recommend routine screening or assessment of men for perpetration.
- Greater attention needs to be given to the development of interdisciplinary, community-collaborative practice to identify and help partner-abusive men.

Practice

- Healthcare providers must have a clear awareness that, like abuse victims, perpetrators of abuse are part of every medical practice.
- Clinician awareness of batterer dynamics leads to the establishment and enforcement of appropriate boundaries, particularly when both partners are patients within the same practice.

- Batterers will talk about violence in their lives, including their use of it. However, batterers also tend to underreport the severity and frequency of violence they commit. Both of these facts should be remembered and considered by practitioners.
- As a group, batterers are heterogeneous, necessitating a flexible clinical interpersonal style for interacting, asking, and intervening.

Research

- Longitudinal studies are needed to more keenly determine the developmental processes that increase risk and lead to onset of IPV.
- Research on men who batter has, to date, been primarily descriptive in nature. Theory-based research is needed to further enhance and advance understanding of the etiology and course of IPV.

References

1. Tjaden P. What is violence against women? Defining and measuring the problem. *J Interpers Violence.* 2004;19:1244–1251.
2. Schechter S. *Women and male violence: The visions and struggles of the battered women's movement.* Boston: South End, 1982.
3. Walker LE. *The battered woman.* New York: Harper and Row, 1979.
4. Martin D. The historical roots of domestic violence. In: Sonkin DJ, ed. *Domestic violence on trial: Psychological and legal dimensions of family violence.* New York: Springer;1987:3–20.
5. Elbow M. Theoretical considerations of violent marriages. *Social Casework.* 1977;58:515–526.
6. Gondolf EW. Who are these guys? Toward a behavioral typology of batterers. *Violence Vict.* 1988;3:187–203.
7. Rosenbaum A, O'Leary KD. Marital violence: Characteristics of abusive couples. *J Consult Clin Psychol.* 1981;49:63–76.
8. Hamberger LK, Hastings JE. Characteristics of spouse abusers: Predictors of treatment acceptance. *J Interpers Violence.* 1986;1:363–373.
9. Hamberger LK, Hastings JE. Personality correlates of men who abuse their partners: A cross-validation study. *J Fam Violence.* 1986;1:323–341.
10. Sherman LW, Berk R. The specific deterrent effects of arrest for domestic assault. *Am Sociol Rev.* 1984;57:680–690.

11. Hamberger LK, Arnold J. The impact of mandatory arrest on domestic violence perpetrator counseling services. *Family Violence Sexual Assault Bull.* 1990;6:11–12.

12. Jaffe PG, Wolfe DA, Telford A, Austin G. The impact of police charges in incidents of wife abuse. *J Fam Violence.* 1986;1:37–49.

13. Miller SL. Expanding the boundries: Toward a more inclusive and integrated study of intimate violence. In: Hamberger LK, Renzetti C, eds. *Domestic partner abuse.* New York: Springer;1996:191–212.

14. Coleman DH, Strauss MA. Marital power, conflict, and violence in a nationally representative sample of American couples. *Violence Vict.* 1986;1: 141–157.

15. Straus M, Gelles R, Steinmetz S. *Behind closed doors: Violence in the American family.* Garden City, NY: Doubleday, 1980.

16. Fitzpatrick MK, Salgado DM, Suvak MK, et al. Associations of gender and gender-role ideology with behavioral and attitudinal features of intimate partner aggression. *Psychol Men Masculinity.* 2004; 5:91–102.

17. Smith MD. Patriarchal ideology and wife beating: A test of a feminist hypothesis. *Violence Vict.* 1990;5:257–273.

18. Dutton DG, Starzomski A. Personality predictors of the Minnesota power and control wheel. *J Interpers Violence.* 1997;12:70–82.

19. Jakupcak M, Lisak D, Roemer L. The role of masculine ideology and masculine gender role stress in men's perpetration of relationship violence. *Psychol Men Masculinity.* 2002;3:97–106.

20. Moore TM, Stuart GL. Effects of masculine gender role stress on men's cognition, affective, physiological, and aggressive responses to intimate conflict situations. *Psychol Men Masculinity.* 2004;5:132–142.

21. Moore TM, Stuart GL. A review of the literature on masculinity and partner violence. *Psychology of Men and Masculinity.* 2005;6(1):46–61.

22. Rosenbaum A. Of men, macho, and marital violence. *J Fam Violence.* 1986;1:121–129.

23. Sugarman DB, Frankel SL. Patriarchal ideology and wife assault: A meta-analytic review. *J Fam Violence.* 1996;11:13–40.

24. Stith SM, Farley SC. A predictive model of male spousal violence. *J Fam Violence.* 1993;8:183–201.

25. Dutton DG. Patriarchy and wife assault: The ecological fallacy. In: Hamberger LK, Renzetti C, eds. *Domestic partner abuse.* New York: Springer;1996: 125–152.

26. Dutton DG, Nicholls T. The gender paradigm in domestic violence research and theory: The conflict of theory and data. *Aggression Violent Behav.* 2005;10:680–714.

27. Ehrensaft MK, Moffitt TE, Caspi A. Clinically abusive relationships in an unselected birth cohort: Men's and women's participation and developmental antecedents. *J Abnorm Psychol.* 2004;113:258–270.

28. Hamberger LK, Lohr JM. Proximal causes of spouse abuse: A theoretical analysis for cognitive-behavioral interventions. In: Caesar PL, Hamberger LK, eds. *Treating men who batter: Theory, practice, and programs.* New York: Springer;1989:53–76.

29. Tweed RG, Dutton DG. A comparison of impulsive and instrumental subgroups of batterers. *Violence Vict.* 1998;13:217–230.

30. Gottman JM, Jacobson NS, Rushe RH, et al. The relationship between heart rate, reactivity, emotionally aggressive behavior, and general violence in batterers. *J Fam Psychol.* 1995;9: 227–248.

31. Chase KA, O'Leary KD, Heyman RE. Categorizing partner-violent men within the reactive-proactive typology model. *J Consult Clin Psychol.* 2001; 69:567–572.

32. Johnson MP, Ferraro KJ. Research on domestic violence in the 1990s: Making distinctions. *J Marriage Fam.* 2000;62:948–963.

33. Babcock J, Green CE, Webb SA, Graham KH. A second failure to replicate the Gottman, et al. (1995) typology of men who abuse intimate partners... and the possible reasons why. *J Fam Psychol.* 2004;18:396–400.

34. Meehan JC, Holtzworth-Munroe A. Heart rate activity in male batterers. *J Fam Psychol.* 2001; 15:415–424.

35. Holtzworth-Munroe A, Stuart GL. Typologies of male batterers: Three subtypes and the differences among them. *Psychol Bull.* 1994;116:476–497.

36. Hamberger LK, Lohr JM, Bonge D, Tolin DF. A large sample empirical typology of male spouse abusers and its relationship to dimensions of abuse. *Violence Vict.* 1996;11:277–292.

37. Dutton DG, Starzomski A. Borderline personality in perpetrators of psychological and physical abuse. *Violence Vict.* 1993;8:327–337.

38. Holtzworth-Munroe A, Meehan JC, Herron K, et al. Testing the Holtzworth-Munroe and Stuart batterer typology. *J Consult Clin Psychol.* 2000;68: 1000–1019.

39. Lohr JM, Hamberger LK, Bonge D. The nature of irrational beliefs in different personality clusters of spouse abusers. *J Rational-Emotive Cognitive-Behavior Ther.* 1988;6:273–285.

40. Dutton DG, Saunders K, Starzomski A, Bartholomew K. Intimacy anger and insecure attachments as precursors of abuse in intimate relationships. *J Appl Soc Psychol.* 1994;24:1367–1386.

41. DelSol C, Margolin G, John RS. A typology of maritally violent men and correlates of violence in a community sample. *J Marriage Fam.* 2003;65: 635–651.

42. Waltz J, Babcock JC, Jacobson NS, Gottman JM. Testing a typology of batterers. *J Consult Clin Psychol.* 2000;68:658–669.

43. Saunders DG. A typlogy of men who batter: Three types derived from cluster analysis. *Am J Orthopsychiatry.* 1992;62:264–275.

44. Cavanaugh MM, Gelles RJ. The utility of male domestic violence offender typologies: New directions for research, policy, and practice. *J Interpers Violence.* 2005;20:155–166.

45. Hamberger LK. The Men's Group Program: A community-based, cognitive, behavioral, profeminist intervention program. In: Aldarondo E, Mederos F, eds. *Batterer intervention programs: A handbook for clinicians, practitioners, and advocates.* Kingston, NJ: Civic Research Institute, 2002.

46. Lohr JM, Bonge D, Witte TH, et al. Consistency and accuracy of batterer typology identification. *J Fam Violence.* 2005;20:253–258.

47. Hershorn M, Rosenbaum A. Over- vs. under-controlled hostility: Application of the construct to the classification of maritally violent men. *Violence Vict.* 1991;6:151–158.

48. Maiuro RD, Cahn TS, Vitaliano PP, et al. Anger, hostility, and depression in domestically violent versus generally assaultive and nonviolent control subjects. *J Consult Clin Psychol.* 1988; 56:17–23.

49. Barnett OW, Fagan RW, Booker JM. Hostility and stress as mediators of aggression in violent men. *J Fam Violence.* 1991;6:217–241.

50. Barbour KA, Eckhardt CI, Davison GC, Kassinove H. The experience and expression of anger in maritally violent and maritally discordant-nonviolentment. *Behavior Therapy.* 1998;29:173–191.

51. Beasley R, Stoltenberg CD. Personality characteristics of male spouse abusers. *Prof Psychol Res Pr.* 1992;23:310–317.

52. Else L, Wonderlich SA, Beatty WW, et al. Personality characteristics of men who physically abuse women. *Hosp Community Psychiatry.* 1993;44:54–58.

53. Dye ML, Eckhardt CI. Anger, irrational beliefs, and dysfunctional attitudes in vilent dating relationships. *Violence Vict.* 2000;15:337–350.

54. Holtzworth-Munroe A, Hutchenson G. Attributing negative intent to wife behavior: The attributions of maritally violent men versus nonviolent men. *J Abnorm Psychol.* 1993;102:206–211.

55. Tonizzo S, Howells K, Day A, et al. Attributions of negative partner behavior by men who physically abuse their partners. *J Fam Pract.* 2000; 15:155–167.

56. Moore TM, Eisler RM, Franchina JJ. Causal attributions and affective responses to provocative female partner behavior by abusive and nonabusive males. *J Fam Violence.* 2000 15:69–80.

57. Conner KR, Ackerley GD. Alcohol-related battering: Developing treatment strategies. *J Fam Violence.* 1994;9:143–155.

58. Straus MA, Gelles RJ. Societal change and change in family violence from 1975 to 1985 as revealed by two national surveys. *J Marriage Fam.* 1986;48: 465–479.

59. Kaufman-Kantor G, Straus MA. The "drunken bum" theory of wife beating. In: Straus MA, Gelles RJ, eds. *Physical violence in American families.* New Brunswick, NJ: Transaction Books;1990:203–224.

60. Heyman RE, O'Leary KD, Jouriles EN. Alcohol and aggressive personality styles: Potentiators of serious physical aggression against wives? *J Fam Psychol.* 1995;9:44–57.

61. Fals-Stewart W. The occurrence of partner physical aggression on days of alcohol consumption: A longitudinal study. *J Consult Clin Psychol.* 2003; 71:41–52.

62. Field CA, Caetano R, Nelson S. Alcohol and violence related cognitive risk factors associated with the perpetration of intimate partner violence. *J Fam Violence.* 2004;19:249–253.

63. Snow DL, Sullivan TP, Swan SC, et al. The role of coping and problem drinking in men's and women's abuse of female partners: Test of a path model. *Violence Vict.* 2006;21:267–285.

64. Murphy CM, Meyer SL, O'Leary KD. Dependency characteristics of partner assaultive men. *J Abnorm Psychol.* 1994;103:729–735.

65. Babcock JC, Jacobson NS, Gottman JM, Verington TP. Attachment, emotional regulation, and the function of marital violence: Differences between secure, preoccupied, and dismission violent and nonviolent husbands. *J Fam Violence.* 2000;15: 391–409.

66. Kesner JE, Julian T, McHenry PC. Application of attachment theory to male violence toward female intimates. *J Fam Violence.* 1997;12: 211–229.

67. Caesar PL. Exposure to violence in the families-of-origin among wife-abusers and maritally nonviolent men. *Violence Vict.* 1988;3:49–63.

68. Hanson RK, Cadsky O, Harris A, Lalonde C. Correlates of battering among 997 men: Family history, adjustment, and attitudinal differences. *Violence Vict.* 1997;12:191–208.

69. Stith SM, Rosen KH, Middleton KA, et al. Intergenerational transmission of spouse abuse: A meta-analysis. *J Marriage Fam.* 2000;62:640–654.

70. Hamberger LK, Hastings JE. Personality correlates of men who batter and nonviolent men: Some continuities and discontinuities. *J Fam Violence.* 1991;6:131–137.

71. Rosen LN, Parmley AM, Knudson KH, Fancher P. Intimate partner violence among married male US Army soldiers: Ethnicity as a factor in self-reported perpetration and victimization. *Violence Vict.* 2002;17:607–622.

72. Corvo K, Carpenter EH. Effects of parental substance abuse on current levels of domestic violence: A possible elaboration of intergenerational transmission processes. *J Fam Violence.* 2000;15: 123–135.

73. Hastings JE, Hamberger LK. Sociodemographic predictors of violence. *Psychiatr Clin North Am.* 1997;20:323–335.

74. Barnett OW, Miller-Perrin CL, Perrin RD. *Family violence across the lifespan: An introduction*. Thousand Oaks, CA: Sage, 1997.

75 Murphy CM, O'Leary KD. Psychological aggression predicts physical aggression in early marriage. *J Consult Clin Psychol*. 1989;57:570–582.

76 Fals-Stewart W, Lucente SW, Birchler GR. The relationship between the amount of face-to-face contact and partners' reports of domestic violence and frequency. *Assessment*. 2002;9:123–130.

77 Warnken WJ, Rosenbaum A, Fletcher KE, et al. Head-injured males: A population at risk for relationship aggression? In: Hamberger LK, Renzetti C, eds. *Domestic partner abuse*. New York: Springer;1996:103–124.

78. Cohen RA, Rosenbaum A, Kane RL, et al. Neuropsychological correlates of domestic violence. *Violence Vict*. 1999;14:397–411.

79. Pan HS, Neidig PH, O'Leary KD. Predicting mild and severe husband-to-wife physical aggression. *J Consult Clin Psychol*. 1994;62:975–981.

80. Van-Hightower NR, Gorton J, DeMoss CL. Predictive models of domestic violence and fear of intimate partners among migrant and seasonal farm worker women. *J Fam Violence*. 2000;15:137–154.

81. Neff JA, Holaman B, Schlter TD. Spousal violence among Anglos, Blacks, and Mexican American: The role of demographic variables, psychosocial predictors, and alcohol consumption. *J Fam Violence*. 1995;10:1–21.

82. Sugihara Y, Warner JA. Mexican-American male batterers on the MCMI-III. *Psychol Rep*. 1999; 85:163–169.

83. Sorenson SB, Telles CA. Self-reports of spousal violence in a Mexican-American and non-Hispanic white population. *Violence Vict*. 1991;6:3–15.

84. Coleman VE. Lesbian battering: The relationship between personality and perpetration of violence. In: Hamberger LK, Renzetti C, eds. *Domestic partner abuse*. New York: Springer;1996:77–102.

85. Fortunata B, Kohn CS. Demographic, psychosocial, and personality characteristics of lesbian batterers. *Violence Vict*. 2003;18:557–568.

86 McKenry PC, Serovich JM, Mason TL, Mosack K. Perpetration of gay and lesbian partner violence: A disempowerment perspective. *J Fam Violence*. 2006;21:233–243.

87. Archer J. Sex differences in aggression between heterosexual, a meta-analytic review. *Psychol Bull*. 2000;26:651–680.

88. Hamberger LK. Men's and women's use of intimate partner violence in clinical samples: Toward a gender sensitive analysis. *Violence Vict*. 2005;20:131–151.

89. Conradi L. An exploratory study of heterosexual females as dominant aggressors of physical violence in their intimate relationships. Psy.D Thesis, 2004.

90. Dutton DG, Hemphill KJ. Patterns of socially desirable responding among perpetrators and victims of wife assault. *Violence Vict*. 1992;7:29–39.

91. Oriel KA, Fleming MF. Screening men for partner violence in a primary care setting: A new strategy for detecting domestic violence. *J Fam Practice*. 1998;46:493–498.

92. Phelan MB, Hamberger LK, Guse C, et al. Domestic violence among male and female patients seeking emergency medical services. *Violence Vict*. 2005;20:187–206.

93. Minsky D, Hamberger LK, Pape D, Wolff M. We've had training, now what? Qualitative analysis of barriers to domestic violence screening and referral in a healthcare setting. *J Interpers Violence*. 2005;20:1288–1309.

94. Hamberger LK, Phelan MB. Screening men for intimate partner violence in health care settings: Some promises, challenges, and issues. *Wisconsin Coalition Against Domestic Violence*. 2003;22:13–15.

Chapter 11

Chronic Physical Symptoms in Survivors of Intimate Partner Violence

Christina Nicolaidis and Jane Liebschutz

KEY CONCEPTS

- Numerous studies confirm an association between intimate partner violence (IPV) and poorer general physical health, a wide range of physical symptoms, a greater number of symptoms, and more severe symptoms.
- Intimate partner violence may also be associated with somatic complaints or symptom syndromes such as irritable bowel disease or fibromyalgia, but it is unclear if functional conditions are any more common in IPV than in conditions with known organic causes.
- Little is known as to why and how IPV and physical complaints are related. Theories focus on factors that reinforce and sustain both posttraumatic stress disorder (PTSD) and pain, on physiologic changes that predispose sensitivity to trauma or occur as a result of trauma, and psychological mechanisms related to the experience of battering.
- Assessing for violence is important in understanding the patient's symptoms and can influence the provider–patient relationship.
- Qualitative data suggest that clinicians should incorporate certain specific approaches when treating a survivor of IPV, including emphasizing how a history of IPV impacts the experience of pain or other symptoms, focusing on the patient's survival skills, and explicitly addressing issues of power and control in the clinician–patient relationship.

Intimate partner violence (IPV) has many direct short- and long-term physical consequences, such as fractures, head trauma, internal organ damage, or even death. Survivors, however, may also present with physical symptoms that may not appear to have an obvious link to a particular physical assault. Sometimes no medical explanation can be found for such symptoms. In other cases, a pathologic diagnosis is made that is unrelated to trauma. An IPV survivor may experience more severe pain or more intense symptoms than a nontraumatized patient with a similar condition. In this chapter, we explore the relationship between IPV and physical symptoms that are not an immediate consequence of physical injury. We focus on studies linking IPV to general physical health, specific physical symptoms, an overall increased number or severity of symptoms, or a variety of symptom syndromes whose pathology has not yet been clearly defined. We then discuss how a history of IPV may influence the treatment needs of patients with chronic pain or other physical symptoms.

UNEXPLAINED PHYSICAL SYMPTOMS, SOMATIZATION, AND SYMPTOM SYNDROMES

Physical symptoms account for more than half of all outpatient visits (1). Often no medical explanation can be found for patients' symptoms. In one study of 1,000 patients followed over a 3-year period, two-thirds of symptoms prompted a medical evaluation, but an organic etiology was found in only 16% (2). Unexplained symptoms are associated with higher levels of depression, psychological distress, health-care utilization, and a history of prior physical and/or sexual abuse (2–5).

Some patients will present with patterns of symptoms that fit the descriptions of symptom-based syndromes such as fibromyalgia, chronic fatigue syndrome, multiple chemical sensitivity, temporomandibular disorder, tension headache, and myofascial pain disorder. These syndromes frequently overlap, and they share many important features such as fatigue or pain, disability out of proportion to physical findings, and an association with stress and psychosocial factors (6,7). Other patients present with multiple unexplained symptoms that do not fit any recognized pattern. Often clinicians label these patients as somatizers. A true *Diagnostic and Statistical Manual of Mental Disorders* (DSM-IV) diagnosis of somatization disorder is difficult to make, requiring two symptoms in the digestive tract, one symptom involving the sexual organs, one symptom related to the nervous system, and four symptoms of pain. The DSM-IV includes diagnoses of undifferentiated somatoform disorder or somatoform disorder not otherwise specified, but those conditions only need the presence of one unexplained symptom, and are thus too broad to be of practical use in a primary care population, where a majority of patients have at least some unexplained symptoms. Categorizations of abridged somatization (8) or multisomatoform disorder (9) may better describe the physical symptoms experienced by many abuse survivors, although such conditions are not yet included in the DSM-IV.

Despite a lack of firm evidence, somatization, somatoform disorder, or functional disorders imply a psychiatric etiology. There are many reasons why, in this chapter, we will frame these symptoms or syndromes as physical problems that are *comorbid with* mental illness and not necessarily *caused by* mental illness: (a) growing evidence suggests altered physiology in many of these conditions; (b) patients most commonly present to primary care providers or medical subspecialists, not psychiatrists, for these conditions; (c) regarding their symptoms as psychiatric often gives patients a marginalized status in the medical world; and (d) patients often refuse referrals to mental health services for these problems, interpreting such referrals as misguided or stigmatizing (1,10,11).

RELATIONSHIP BETWEEN INTIMATE PARTNER VIOLENCE AND PHYSICAL SYMPTOMS

Studies Assessing General Physical Health

Numerous large (N >1,000) cross-sectional studies show an association between IPV and poorer general health. These studies recruited women from the general population (12,13), female members of health-maintenance organizations (14,15), or women seeking health care in primary care settings (16). Most of these studies measured general physical health using a single self-report item taken from the Health Survey Short Form (SF)-36 (17). Sometimes additional single items address physical limitations (12) or compare current to prior health (13). Two recent large studies (N ≈ 3,000 in each) of obstetrics and gynecology patients and health maintenance organization enrollees found that women with a history of physical or sexual abuse had lower health functioning on all the subscales scales of the SF-36 (or the shorter SF-20) (18,19). A smaller study (N = 558) of women in the military also found associations between past violence and each of the eight subscales of the SF-36, but only reported results in terms of rape, physical assault, or both, with no distinction made as to whether these assaults were from an intimate partner or other perpetrator (20).

The association with poorer self-perceived general physical health is seen both in studies assessing current IPV (usually defined as occurring within the past year) (12,13,15) and in those assessing past or lifetime exposure to IPV (14,16). Similarly, the association persists when IPV is defined as including physical assaults (12), either physical or sexual (13,14,16), or psychological abuse alone (16). Interestingly, one study measuring IPV using the Conflict Tactics Scale (21) found an association between poorer general health and major verbal aggression, but not physical aggression (15). Very little prospective data examines causality of IPV exposure to subsequent physical health status. One small study of women exiting domestic violence shelters showed an improvement in general physical health over time (22).

Studies Assessing a Wide Array of Specific Symptoms

A few large cross-sectional studies of women from general or primary care populations have assessed the association between current or past IPV and a wide array of specific physical symptoms. In a study of 1,952 women seeking primary care, McCauley and colleagues found that current-year physical IPV was associated with 17 of 22 specific symptoms/conditions in bivariate analyses, but their final model only includes vaginal discharge, diarrhea, and broken bones, sprains or cuts, along with a high rating on any emotional symptom score (depression, anxiety, or somatization) and drug or alcohol abuse (23). A household survey of 1,155 Mexican-American women found that current-year physical or sexual IPV was associated with one or more symptoms from five of six symptoms groups: gastrointestinal (GI), cardiopulmonary, neurologic, sexual, and reproductive. There was a marginal association ($p = .06$) with the sixth group (any pain symptoms) (13).

Coker and colleagues found that a lifetime history of psychological IPV alone was associated with 11 of 23 conditions (disability preventing work, chronic neck or back pain, arthritis, migraines, other frequent headaches, sexually transmitted infections [STIs], chronic pelvic pain, stomach ulcer, gastric reflux, spastic colon, and frequent indigestion, constipation or diarrhea). Physical or sexual IPV was associated with 17 of 23 conditions (the above, plus stammering

or stuttering, problem seeing even with glasses, hearing loss, angina, other heart or circulatory problems, urinary tract infections (UTIs), and hysterectomy) (16). Campbell and associates found an association between past physical or sexual IPV and more frequent headache, back pain, vaginal infection, digestive problems, sexually transmitted diseases, vaginal bleeding, painful intercourse, pelvic pain, UTI, loss of appetite, and abdominal pain (14).

These studies tend to assess wide ranges of physical symptoms and conditions and find associations between IPV and the majority of them. It is difficult to determine whether IPV is more strongly associated with conditions that could be directly related to injury (for example, hearing loss), those that may be linked to a partner's other high-risk behaviors (for example, sexually transmitted diseases), conditions with presumed organic causes (for example, stomach ulcers), or those often believed to be functional (e.g., spastic colon).

Studies Looking at Overall Number or Severity of Symptoms

Several cross-sectional studies in primary care setting have assessed the association between IPV and the overall number of physical symptoms. McCauley and colleagues found that women experiencing current (within the past year) physical IPV had a greater number of physical symptoms than those who did not recently experience abuse. They further divided those with a current history of IPV into two groups based on the severity of physical assaults and found a dose–response relationship with the number of symptoms (mean 4.3 versus 5.3 versus 6.4 symptoms in women experiencing no, low-level, or severe physical abuse, respectively, $p < .001$) (24). Similarly, studies have found that women with past physical or sexual IPV also have an increased number of current chronic physical symptoms, even many years after the abuse has ended (14,19,25). Other studies have found that the frequency or severity of abuse was correlated with the severity and number of physical symptoms (26,27). The association between abuse and number of physical symptoms was also found in women who experienced emotional abuse without any physical abuse (28).

A few IPV studies have assessed severity of physical complaints using the Patient Health Questionnaire-15 (PHQ-15) (29). Although this scale assesses the severity of 15 symptoms that are often considered somatic, it does not assess whether a medical explanation is available for the symptoms. Women with current (18) or lifetime (30) IPV histories score higher on the PHQ-15 than do nonabused controls. A longitudinal study of 267 women recruited from eight healthcare settings found that women with ongoing IPV had increased severity of physical symptoms over time, as compared to women with no IPV history or those who only reported IPV at baseline (31).

Studies Assessing Symptom-Syndromes

Although clinicians are often taught that an association exists between IPV (or other forms of abuse) and symptom-based syndromes such as fibromyalgia, irritable bowel syndrome (IBS), or chronic pelvic pain, it is unclear if a specific relationship exists between IPV and these particular syndromes or if the increased prevalence of these conditions in abuse survivors is attributable to a greater reporting of physical symptoms in general. Moreover, some of the symptoms that are characteristic of these syndromes may arise from identifiable organic illness and not solely from a functional etiology.

A number of studies have found associations between IBS symptoms and lifetime physical abuse, sexual abuse, or emotional abuse, whether it started in childhood or adulthood (32–34). These studies also noted that abused patients had higher levels of pelvic pain, multiple somatic symptoms, and more lifetime surgeries (33), and higher levels of dyspepsia and heartburn (34). However, the same group of researchers, when studying 997 patients referred to a subspecialty gastroenterology clinic, found no difference in rates of abuse or type of abuse between patients with physician-confirmed organic GI disease versus functional GI disorders such as IBS or non-ulcer dyspepsia. Interestingly, patients with a history of childhood and adult abuse had higher rates of IBS-like *symptoms* than did nonabused patients, regardless of whether physicians had noted an organic GI disorder (35). Other smaller studies comparing patients with IBS who were referred to gastroenterology clinics to patients with organic GI disease or healthy controls have found an association between IBS and emotional abuse (36) or sexual abuse (37). A study designed to assess sexual abuse and chronic pelvic pain in gynecology patients also found an association between adult (but not childhood) sexual abuse and IBS (38). All of the these studies address lifetime experiences of abuse, without specifying if the abuse was perpetrated by an intimate partner. Moreover, little is known about the timing of the abuse and GI symptoms. One cross-sectional study including only patients with IBS noted that the IBS symptoms began on average 9 years after the onset of posttraumatic stress disorder (PTSD) (39).

Two small studies comparing patients with fibromyalgia to patients with rheumatoid arthritis found that those with fibromyalgia had higher lifetime prevalence rates of physical and sexual abuse (40,41), whereas another small study comparing fibromyalgia patients to a convenience sample of women without fibromyalgia found no significant association (but high rates of trauma, 52%–65%, in both groups) (42). Among patients with fibromyalgia, studies have found that those with a history of sexual or physical abuse had increased pain levels and higher rates of utilization for problems other than fibromyalgia (43), and those with symptoms of PTSD had greater levels of pain, emotional distress, life interference, and disability (44).

Schei and colleagues were able to demonstrate a significantly higher prevalence of chronic pelvic pain in 66 women who had been in physically abusive relationships within the past year, compared to 114 nonabused controls (45). Drossman and co-workers also showed an increased rate of pelvic pain in sexually or physically abused patients, as well as an overall increased rate of somatic complaints (33). Similarly, in a study of 581 nonpregnant gynecology patients, both childhood and adult sexual abuse were associated with pelvic pain, dyspareunia, a greater number of pelvic pain complaints, and a greater number of all pain syndromes (38). However, a small study comparing patients with chronic pelvic pain to patients with pain in other locations and healthy controls only found an association between pelvic pain and childhood physical abuse, not childhood sexual abuse or adult traumatization (46).

Studies' Adjustment for Non–Intimate Partner Violence Abuse

Despite a well-known association between IPV and other forms of violence (47–53), many studies looking at the association between IPV and physical symptoms are limited by a failure to account for other forms of violence. Several studies do differentiate between childhood and adult abuse, but do not indicate the relationship between the perpetrator and victim. These studies generally find that patients abused both as children and adults have a higher risk of having symptoms or greater number of symptoms than those abused only as children or only as adults (30,31,34,35,38,54). Similarly, a small study found that both childhood and adult abuse were independent predictors of fibromyalgia (41). Lesserman and associates did not find any difference in functional GI problems between women who had had a single traumatic event and those with more than one event, or between those whose trauma started in childhood or adulthood. However, they did not compare women who had been abused both as children and adults to those who experienced only one form of abuse (32). A study of 174 female primary care patients differentiated between physical and sexual IPV, child abuse, and community violence. In separate multivariate analyses, each of the six forms of violence was significantly associated with having six or more chronic physical symptoms, with odds ratios of similar magnitude. However, when looking at all forms of violence together, there was a strong dose–response relationship between the number of forms of violence experienced and the risk of six or more chronic physical symptoms (25).

Relationship Between Intimate Partner Violence and Health-seeking Behavior

Numerous studies find that IPV survivors have greater healthcare costs and utilization (55–58). Interestingly, much of that increased utilization appears to be attributed to physical, not mental health visits, and may be due to physical symptoms that are not directly linked to acute injury. A health maintenance organization study found that women with a history of abuse had a 92% increase in yearly costs, and that that increase was not driven by emergency department use (55). Furthermore, a random-digit dialing study of depressed women found that those with a history of abuse had an almost sixfold risk of seeking care for physical problems compared to depressed nonabused controls, whereas they were a third as likely to seek mental health care (59). Nicolaidis and colleagues found that, compared to nonabused controls, women with a history of IPV had *lower* odds and women with a history of child abuse had *higher* odds of receiving care from a mental health provider, after adjustment for severity of physical and depressive symptoms (30). Hastings and Kantor have also noted an association between IPV and increased numbers of surgeries overall and major surgeries in particular (60).

Multivariate Analyses of Conditions Predictive of Intimate Partner Violence

A few studies use multivariate analyses to look for clinical characteristics that predict whether a woman is currently in an abusive relationship. These studies often include both mental and physical health variables in the final models. In addition to demographic characteristics and five specific physical conditions, McCauley's model includes a high rating on any emotional symptom score (depression, anxiety, or somatization) and drug or alcohol abuse as independent predictors of IPV. The authors did not include overall number of physical symptoms as great colinearity existed between number of physical symptoms and high score on the somatization scale (23). Similarly, Tollestrup's model includes number of days respondent felt sad in past month, reported ability to handle stress, alcohol use, and general health (along with demographic characteristics) as independent predictors of IPV (15). In contrast, Weinbaum and colleagues found an association between IPV and poor physical health or pain-limiting activities when only adjusting for age, race, and ethnicity, but physical health and pain were not independent predictors in the full model, which included feeling overwhelmed, smoking, participation in Women, Infants, and Children (WIC—a federally funded supplemental nutrition program for pregnant women, new mothers, and children under age 5 years), and being out of work (12).

RELATIONSHIP BETWEEN INTIMATE PARTNER VIOLENCE, MENTAL HEALTH, AND PHYSICAL SYMPTOMS

Relationship Between Physical Symptoms and Mental Health

A large literature links depression to chronic pain (for a review, see [61]), and to the presence or severity of medically unexplained physical symptoms (2–5). Similarly, a number of studies have found a co-occurrence of PTSD and chronic pain symptoms. Such studies tend to look at the presence of PTSD, but do not differentiate as to whether the PTSD was caused by IPV or other traumatic experiences. When examining populations of chronic pain patients, the prevalence of PTSD was much higher than in the general population, particularly when the chronic pain occurred as a result of a traumatic injury. Studies have estimated anywhere from 10% to 54% of patients seeking care in specialty pain clinics meet criteria for a diagnosis of PTSD (62–65). Among patients with PTSD, there is a high prevalence of chronic pain (50–80%) as well as syndromes such as fibromyalgia (66). For example, one case-controlled study found that 21% of PTSD cases compared to 0% of controls met criteria for fibromyalgia syndrome (67). In addition to the high co-occurrence of the two conditions, there is evidence that patients with the co-occurring disorders have poorer coping skills, more intense pain, more affective distress from their pain, and greater disability than pain patients without PTSD or trauma (44,65,68,69).

Relationship Between Intimate Partner Violence, Physical Symptoms, and Mental Health

A well-known association exists between IPV and mental health issues such as depression, dysthymia, suicidality, generalized anxiety disorder, phobias, PTSD, and substance abuse (13,56,70–75). Similarly, as discussed earlier, a strong association exists between unexplained physical symptoms and mental health issues such as depression and PTSD. Still, most studies linking IPV and physical symptoms do not adjust for mental health.

Less is known about whether the relationship between past IPV and physical symptoms is independent of mental health conditions. In two small studies of primary care patients, Nicolaidis and associates found that a lifetime history of physical or sexual IPV was associated with risk of having six or more physical symptoms (25) or severity of physical symptoms (30), even after adjustment for mental health conditions.

THEORETICAL MODELS DESCRIBING THE RELATIONSHIPS AMONG INTIMATE PARTNER VIOLENCE, PHYSICAL SYMPTOMS, AND MENTAL HEALTH

Psychological Theories Relating Posttraumatic Stress Disorder and Physical Symptoms

Theoretical models often focus on a relationship between PTSD and chronic pain, but can also be applied to the relationship between IPV or other kinds of interpersonal violence and chronic physical symptoms. One theory for the development of these comorbidities is the *mutual maintenance model* suggested by Sharp and Harvey (76). In this model, seven factors may maintain the chronic symptoms of both PTSD and chronic pain: (1) Patients with these problems may focus their attention on threatening or painful stimuli, such that the symptoms are amplified; (2) anxiety sensitivity may increase their vulnerability to catastrophize minor symptoms; (3) symptoms may trigger memories of a traumatic event and then an arousal response; (4) avoidance may be adopted to minimize pain and disturbing thoughts from the trauma; (5) fatigue and lethargy may contribute; (6) generalized anxiety may contribute; and (7) paying attention to these symptoms may limit use of adaptive coping strategies.

Another important model proposed by Asmundson and colleagues is the *shared vulnerability model*. In this model, anxiety sensitivity is a predisposing factor in the development of both chronic pain and PTSD. Physical symptoms such as breathlessness would signal impending doom in a person with anxiety sensitivity. Someone may then avoid doing those daily activities that they fear may bring on physical symptoms or induce pain. This avoidance may then cause deconditioning, muscle tightness, or atrophy, all states that serve to maintain the pain over a long period of time (77,78).

Theories That Incorporate Physiological Factors

Other psychological theories incorporate the concept of physiological reactivity, which shows that standard stimuli result in increases in physiological measures such as heart rate and skin conductance (79). Thus, the increased physiological reactivity may impact perception of the symptoms. This increased physiological reactivity is incorporated in another summative theory, Keane and Barlow's *triple vulnerability model*. In this model, three predisposing conditions need to be in place to develop anxiety and PTSD: a generalized biological vulnerability, a generalized psychological vulnerability based on early experiences of control over salient events, and a specific psychological vulnerability in which there is a learned focus of anxiety in specific situations. This can be applied to the development of chronic pain in that pain sufferers perceive a lack of control over their pain and have negative affective associations with their pain experience. These reactions may cause avoidance of painful or difficult situations in daily life, which then promotes the psychological disturbances that lead to poorer coping mechanisms (62).

Alternatively, it is possible that violence causes lasting changes in the neuroendocrine system that chemically mediate an increase in symptoms. Although evidence is emerging for neuroendocrine abnormalities in patients with chronic mental or physical distress (80–87), little is known about the mechanisms linking violence to such changes.

It is possible that trauma induces an increased sensitivity in other organ systems. For example, Drossman has suggested that enhanced visceral sensitivity can stem from neural changes that occur as a result of childhood sexual exposure. This may then lead to a perception of abdominal or pelvic pain with amplification of nociceptor input despite a lack of pathological conditions (88,89). Drossman also suggests that patients with abuse histories have lower pain thresholds than those without these histories and may set lower standards for judging stimuli as painful. Other physiological theories include the increase in plasma cortisol among those with trauma and PTSD compared to those without trauma exposure (90,91).

Theories Relating the Experience of Battering to Physical Symptoms

Many of the these theories relate to PTSD, regardless of the type of trauma initiating the PTSD. It is possible, however, that the experience of living in an abusive relationship may affect the development of physical symptoms in ways that are different from other nonabusive traumatic experiences and unrelated to the presence of PTSD. Perpetrators of family violence classically berate their victims, isolate them socially, control their activities, and alternate between extreme displays of love and abuse (92,93). One can imagine that the nature of this abuse may contribute to the development of somatic complaints. Women are likely to have been told by their abuser that they are crazy or that the problem is all in their head. Moreover, survivors often feel that providers and others blame them for choosing to stay in an abusive relationship (92). An abuse survivor may be hesitant to accept a mental health diagnosis, may interpret it as proof that her provider thinks there is something wrong with her for getting

into an abusive relationship, or may be more likely to experience mental distress as physical symptoms. Similarly, the social isolation imposed by the batterer may inadvertently increase a woman's health-seeking behavior as she may have little opportunity for contact with people other than healthcare workers and less chance of receiving reassurance from family or friends. A woman's response to battering, such as her perceived ability to care for herself, may also mediate the relationship between abuse and health. Campbell and Soeken have tested a model that links severity of battering and self-care agency (measured using scales of self-esteem and perceived ability to care for self) to overall measures of physical and emotional health. They found both a direct relationship between severity of battering and health and an indirect relationship that is mediated by self-care agency as a protective factor (94).

TREATMENT ISSUES AND RECOMMENDATIONS

Clinical Issues in Treating Abuse Survivors with Physical Symptoms

Clinicians need to be aware of a number of special issues that may arise in treating abuse survivors for chronic pain or other physical symptoms. First, IPV survivors may have difficulty trusting a provider due to damage incurred as part of abusive relationships (95). Second, given their experiences of being controlled or intimidated by an abusive partner, survivors may be particularly sensitive to control issues in the physician–provider relationship (92). Finally, abuse survivors may be hesitant to disclose a history of abuse, as they may fear that such a disclosure would lead providers to believe their symptoms are all in their head or to undertreat their pain (96).

Recommendations for Assessing Violence in Patients with Physical Symptoms

One must consider the possibility of current or past abuse in anyone with chronic pain or unexplained physical symptoms, but especially those with multiple symptoms, symptoms that are not responding to treatment, or symptoms that are more severe than would be expected. When assessing for a history of violence in such patients, however, it is important to preface questions appropriately. Clinicians should make statements about how traumatic experiences often worsen the experience of pain or make physical symptoms more severe or harder to handle. Such statements, prior to any questions about abuse, allow the patient to understand that the clinician believes the symptoms and acknowledges their severity or impact. Clinicians should also clearly state that they don't believe the patient's symptoms are imagined. After such an introduction, then clinicians can proceed with assessing for violence using direct, nonjudgmental questions, as discussed elsewhere in this text.

Responding to Disclosure of Abuse in Patients with Chronic Pain or Unexplained Physical Symptoms

Regardless of the circumstances, any disclosure of current or past abuse must first be met with empathetic statements, a reminder that no one deserves to be abused, and an assessment for safety (25). Although no studies exist regarding the best response to disclosure of abuse in patients with chronic pain or unexplained physical symptoms, our clinical experience is that the following approach is helpful in such circumstances. First, the provider should show how impressed he or she is by the patient's strength and acknowledge how hard it must be (or must have been) to live through the experience. Even in a situation in which the patient continues to be romantically involved with an abusive partner, the provider must recognize that the patient has needed important skills and strengths to stay alive and keep herself and/or her children as safe as possible. During conversations that focus on coping with chronic pain or physical symptoms, the provider can then remind the patient of her strength and build on the fact that the patient can overcome great obstacles. The provider should thoroughly investigate the symptom's potential relationship to actual mechanisms of abuse. Even if there is no obvious connection to a mechanism of trauma, the provider should point out the association between abuse and the symptoms or syndrome the patient is experiencing, focusing on how abuse survivors have a greater likelihood of having the condition(s), increased pain, or more severe symptoms. It is important in these conversations to stress that the trauma history *compounds* the problem, not that it causes her to imagine it. The provider should also emphasize that no one fully understands

the reason for these epidemiologic associations, but that research is looking at possible trauma-induced changes to the body's chemistry. One should help a patient acknowledge the relationship between her symptoms and the abuse, but not force the issue if she does not agree. Next, one should assess for the presence of PTSD and treat if appropriate. Several treatments for PTSD such as antidepressants, clonidine, β-blockers, or cognitive-behavioral therapy may also be effective in improving pain control (97).

Moreover, one should explicitly talk about issues of control as they relate to the patient's experience with the batterer, to her experience with pain or other physical symptoms that she may feel control her life, and to the physician–patient relationship. Control issues can be difficult in any provider–patient relationship, but they are often greatly heightened for patients with chronic pain, especially concerning opioid prescribing and behavioral contracts. For abuse survivors, who may be more sensitive to control issues than other patients, this situation can be particularly difficult. As such, it is important that the provider acknowledges the issue, is explicit about what parts of the relationship he or she must control, and then offers as much control as possible to the patient. Our experience has been that patients respond well to this approach, especially when given the choice between two or three different treatments, dosing schedules, follow-up intervals, and the like.

General Principles for Treating Medically Unexplained Symptoms

Last, the provider should use many of the same principles of treating medically unexplained symptoms as they would for nonabuse patients. One should remember that three-quarters of medically unexplained symptoms resolve by 12 months without specific intervention (98). After routine testing for serious illness suggested by the presenting symptoms, reassurance and compassionate observation should be the next step. However, the practitioner faces a clinical challenge in treating the 25% of patients in whom the symptoms persist. Robert Smith and colleagues published a valuable review of the topic with a proposed treatment plan for such patients based on existing published evidence (99).

A central focus in treating patients with medically unexplained symptoms is the importance of promoting a healthy, strong, longitudinal patient–provider relationship. Thus, providers who may see the patients in an emergency department setting or a consultative setting, should refer the patient back to the continuity provider, whether that be in the primary care setting or a specialty setting, such as psychiatry, pain clinic, or the like. Furthermore, patients who seek out a variety of caregivers should develop a plan for the centrality of the continuity provider. For example, providers and patients should negotiate that the patient will see the primary care (or continuity) provider prior to getting a referral to any specialty consultations and after any emergency visit. Seeing such patients more frequently at first may be a way to address concerns, to develop trust, and to carry out the therapeutic intervention as noted below. Eventually, the visits can be spread out as the intervention takes effect and the patient improves in function and decreases in symptoms.

The way to foster the patient–provider relationship is to invoke a patient-centered interview method, which has been described in numerous texts (100,101). The patient-centered interview is the data-gathering, relational, and therapeutic activity that offers an opportunity to elicit and respond to emotional content (99). Smith developed an acronym, NURS, which reflects the response to patient expression of emotions: Name it, Understand it, Respect it and Support it.

Another way to improve the patient–provider relationship includes seeing the patient with positive regard. For example, a patient with borderline personality disorder and a history of severe childhood abuse may be seen as someone who inappropriately employs what was a successful coping mechanism for childhood. Providers should encourage patients to be responsible for their behaviors through negotiating expectations and limitations of the patient–provider relationship. Also, a provider should become aware of his own reactions to difficult patients with medically unexplained symptoms and trauma histories.

In addition to creating a strong patient–provider relationship, cognitive-behavior treatments (CBT) have been shown to be valuable for medically unexplained symptoms in all randomized trials and treatments reported in the multidisciplinary setting, including the psychiatric setting. The effectiveness has been somewhat limited in clinical trials because they have been run over a short term (10 weeks) for what are usually longstanding behavior patterns (102).

Four provider behaviors related to CBT should be employed regularly. They are:

- Setting achievable goals, both long- and short-term
- Achieving patient understanding and new ways of thinking about symptoms. This involves a thorough grasp of the patient explanatory model and by addressing the patient's main concerns (reassurance that no life-threatening condition exists; that no further testing is necessary; that the problem is real; explaining the mechanism of somatic diagnosis; the role that stress, depression, and PTSD play in the illness; that they are not crazy; that opioids and sedatives may aggravate the problem; and that cure is not likely but improvement in symptoms is)
- Obtaining a commitment from the patient to participate in treatment
- Negotiating a specific treatment plan (99)

In addition to the CBT noted earlier, it is important to discontinue addicting medications and treat concurrent substance use disorders.

IMPLICATIONS FOR POLICY, PRACTICE, AND RESEARCH

Policy

- Policy decisions about the need for IPV screening should take into account not only the availability of evidence-based interventions to decrease violence-related injury, but also the importance that information about violence may have in the management of chronic physical symptoms.

Practice

- Clinicians should consider the possibility that current or past violence is a contributing factor to the patient's presentation whenever treating patients with chronic pain, symptom syndromes, large numbers of physical symptoms, medically unexplained symptoms, or symptoms that are more severe or harder to treat than expected. It may be less helpful to base the decision to explore a violent history on whether or not the symptoms have an organic etiology.

- The clinician should make it clear to the patient that he is asking about trauma because it may be a factor in the exacerbation of pain or other physical symptoms, not because he believes the symptoms are imagined or psychosomatic.
- Knowledge of a patient's violent history may be used to strengthen the therapeutic relationship and to encourage the patient to apply already existing survival skills to symptom control. It may also highlight the need to pay extra attention to power and control dynamics.
- Assessing for and treating mental health issues related to IPV, such as depression, anxiety, PTSD, and substance abuse, may have beneficial effects on pain and physical symptoms.

Research

- Further research is needed to answer many questions about the relationship between IPV and chronic physical symptoms, including:
  - How does the association between violence and physical symptoms differ in relation to the type, duration, frequency, or severity of trauma; the relationship between the perpetrator and victim; or the existence of multiple lifetime victimizations?
  - How much of the relationship between IPV and physical symptoms is mediated by mental health issues such as depression, PTSD, or substance abuse?
  - Is there a causal relationship between IPV and physical symptoms (other than those directly linked to acute injury)? If so, what is the mechanism for the association?
  - How does a violent history influence the response to treatment for chronic pain or other physical symptoms?
  - What treatments are most effective for chronic pain or unexplained physical symptoms in survivors of IPV, and how do they differ from those used to treat nontraumatized patients?

References

1. Kroenke K. Studying symptoms: Sampling and measurement issues.[comment]. *Ann Intern Med.* 2001;134(9 Pt 2):844–853.

2. Kroenke K, Mangelsdorff AD. Common symptoms in ambulatory care: Incidence, evaluation, therapy, and outcome.[comment]. *Am J Med.* 1989; 86(3):262–266.

3. Katon W, Sullivan M, Walker E. Medical symptoms without identified pathology: Relationship to psychiatric disorders, childhood and adult trauma, and personality traits. *Ann Intern Med.* 2001;134(9): 917–925.

4. Kroenke K, Price RK. Symptoms in the community. Prevalence, classification, and psychiatric comorbidity. *Arch Intern Med.* 1993;153(21):2474–2480.

5. Kroenke K, Spitzer RL, Williams JB, et al. Physical symptoms in primary care. Predictors of psychiatric disorders and functional impairment. *Arch Fam Med.* 1994;3(9):774–779.

6. Aaron LA, Buchwald D. A Review of the evidence for overlap among unexplained clinical conditions. *Ann Intern Med.* 2001;134(9): 868–881.

7. Aaron LA, Burke MM, Buchwald D. Overlapping conditions among patients with chronic fatigue syndrome, fibromyalgia, and temporomandibular disorder.[comment]. *Arch Intern Med.* 2000;160(2): 221–227.

8. Escobar JI, Waitzkin H, Silver RC, et al. Abridged somatization: A study in primary care. *Psychosom Med.* 1998;60(4):466–472.

9. Kroenke K, Spitzer RL, deGruy FV, 3rd, et al. Multisomatoform disorder. An alternative to undifferentiated somatoform disorder for the somatizing patient in primary care.[comment]. *Arch Gen Psychiatry.* 1997;54(4):352–358.

10. Sharpe M, Carson A. Unexplained somatic symptoms, functional syndromes, and somatization: Do we need a paradigm shift?[comment]. *Ann Intern Med.* 2001;134(9 Pt 2):926–930.

11. Kroenke K, Harris L. Symptoms research: A fertile field. *Ann Intern Med.* 2001;134(9 Pt 2): 801–802.

12. Weinbaum Z, Stratton TL, Chavez G, et al. Female victims of intimate partner physical domestic violence (IPP-DV), California 1998. *Am J Prev Med.* 2001;21(4):313–319.

13. Lown EA, Vega WA. Intimate partner violence and health: Self-assessed health, chronic health, and somatic symptoms among Mexican American women. *Psychosom Med.* 2001;63(3):352–360.

14. Campbell J, Jones AS, Dienemann J, et al. Intimate partner violence and physical health consequences. *Arch Intern Med.* 2002;162(10):1157–1163.

15. Tollestrup K, Sklar D, Frost FJ, et al. Health indicators and intimate partner violence among women who are members of a managed care organization. *Prev Med.* 1999;29(5):431–440.

16. Coker AL, Smith PH, Bethea L, et al. Physical health consequences of physical and psychological intimate partner violence. *Arch Fam Med.* 2000;9(5): 451–457.

17. Ware JE, Snow K, Kosinski M, Gandek B. *SF-36 Health Survey. Manual and interpretation guide.* Boston, MA: The Health Institute, New England Medical Center, 1993.

18. Kovac SH, Klapow JC, Kroenke K, et al. Differing symptoms of abused versus nonabused women in obstetric-gynecology settings. *Am J Obstet Gynecol.* 2003;188(3):707–713.

19. Bonomi AE, Anderson ML, Rivara FP, Thompson RS. Health outcomes in women with physical and sexual intimate partner violence exposure. *J Womens Health.* 2007;16(7):987–997.

20. Sadler AG, Booth BM, Nielson D, Doebbeling BN. Health-related consequences of physical and sexual violence: women in the military. *Obstet Gynecol.* 2000;96(3):473–480.

21. Straus MA. Measuring intrafamily conflict and violence: The Conflict Tactics Scales. *J Marriage Fam.* 1979;41:75–88.

22. Sutherland C, Bybee D, Sullivan C. The long-term effects of battering on women's health. *Womens Health.* 1998;4(1):41–70.

23. McCauley J, Kern DE, Kolodner K, et al. The battering syndrome: Prevalence and clinical characteristics of domestic violence in primary care internal medicine practices. *Ann Intern Med.* 1995;123(10):737–746.

24. McCauley J, Kern DE, Kolodner K, et al. Relation of low-severity violence to women's health. *J Gen Intern Med.* 1998;13(10):687–691.

25. Nicolaidis C, Curry M, McFarland B, Gerrity M. Violence, mental health, and physical symptoms in an academic internal medicine practice. *J Gen Intern Med.* 2004;19(8):819–827.

26. Follingstad DR, Brennan AF, Hause ES, et al. Factors moderating physical and psychological symptoms of battered women. *J Fam Violence.* 1991; 6(1):81–95.

27. Eby K, Campbell JC, Sullivan C, Davidson W. Health effects of experiences of sexual violence for women with abusive partners. *Women's Health International.* 1995;16:563–576.

28. Porcerelli JH, West PA, Binienda J, Cogan R. Physical and psychological symptoms in emotionally abused and non-abused women. *J Am Board Fam Med.* 2006;19(2):201–204.

29. Kroenke K, Spitzer RL, Williams JB. The PHQ-15: Validity of a new measure for evaluating the severity of somatic symptoms. *Psychosom Med.* 2002; 64(2):258–266.

30. Nicolaidis C, McFarland B, Curry M, Gerrity M. Differences in physical and mental health symptoms and mental health utilization associated with intimate partner violence vs. child abuse. *Psychosomatics.* In press.

31. Gerber MR, Wittenberg E, Ganz ML, et al. Intimate partner violence exposure and change in women's physical symptoms over time. *J Gen Intern Med.* 2008;23(1):64–69.

32. Leserman J, Drossman DA, Li Z, et al. Sexual and physical abuse history in gastroenterology practice: How types of abuse impact health status. *Psychosom Med.* 1996;58(1):4–15.

33. Drossman DA, Leserman J, Nachman G, et al. Sexual and physical abuse in women with functional or organic GI disorders. *Ann Intern Med.* 1990;113(11):828–833.

34. Talley NJ, Fett SL, Zinsmeister AR, Melton LJ, 3rd. GI tract symptoms and self-reported abuse: A population-based study. *Gastroenterology.* 1994; 107(4):1040–1049.

35. Talley NJ, Fett SL, Zinsmeister AR. Self-reported abuse and GI disease in outpatients: Association with irritable bowel-type symptoms [see comments]. *Am J Gastroenterol.* 1995;90(3):366–371.

36. Ali A, Toner BB, Stuckless N, et al. Emotional abuse, self-blame, and self-silencing in women with irritable bowel syndrome. *Psychosom Med.* 2000;62(1):76–82.

37. Delvaux M, Denis P, Allemand H. Sexual abuse is more frequently reported by IBS patients than by patients with organic digestive diseases or controls. Results of a multicentre inquiry. French Club of Digestive Motility [see comments]. *Eur J Gastroenterol Hepatol.* 1997;9(4):345–352.

38. Jamieson DJ, Steege JF. The association of sexual abuse with pelvic pain complaints in a primary care population. *Am J Obstet Gynecol.* 1997;177(6): 1408–1412.

39. Irwin C, Falsetti SA, Lydiard RB, et al. Comorbidity of posttraumatic stress disorder and irritable bowel syndrome. *J Clin Psychiatry.* 1996;57(12):576–578.

40. Boisset-Pioro MH, Esdaile JM, Fitzcharles MA. Sexual and physical abuse in women with fibromyalgia syndrome. *Arthritis Rheum.* 1995; 38(2):235–241.

41. Walker EA, Keegan D, Gardner G, et al. Psychosocial factors in fibromyalgia compared with rheumatoid arthritis: II. Sexual, physical, and emotional abuse and neglect. *Psychosom Med.* 1997;59(6):572–577.

42. Taylor ML, Trotter DR, Csuka ME. The prevalence of sexual abuse in women with fibromyalgia. *Arthritis Rheum.* 1995;38(2):229–234.

43. Alexander RW, Bradley LA, Alarcon GS, et al. Sexual and physical abuse in women with fibromyalgia: Association with outpatient health care utilization and pain medication usage. *Arthritis Care Res.* 1998;11(2):102–115.

44. Sherman JJ, Turk DC, Okifuji A. Prevalence and impact of posttraumatic stress disorder-like symptoms on patients with fibromyalgia syndrome. *Clin J Pain.* 2000;16(2):127–134.

45. Schei B. Psycho-social factors in pelvic pain. A controlled study of women living in physically abusive relationships. *Acta Obstetricia et Gynecologica Scandinavica.* 1990;69(1):67–71.

46. Rapkin AJ, Kames LD, Darke LL, et al. History of physical and sexual abuse in women with chronic pelvic pain. *Obstet Gynecol.* 1990;76(1):92–96.

47. Doumas D, Margolin G, John RS. The intergenerational transmission of aggression across three generations. *J Fam Violence*. 1994;9(2):157–175.

48. Kalmuss D. The intergenerational transmission of marital aggression. *J Marriage Fam*. 1984;46(1):11–19.

49. Kwong MJ, Bartholomew K, Henderson AJZ, Trinke SJ. The intergenerational transmission of relationship violence. *J Fam Psychol*. 2003;17(3):288–301.

50. Mihalic SW, Elliott D. A social learning theory model of marital violence. *J Fam Violence*. 1997;12(1):21–47.

51. Smith JP, Williams JG. From abusive household to dating violence. *J Fam Violence*. 1992;7(2):153–165.

52. Stith SM, Rosen KH, Middleton KA, et al. The intergenerational transmission of spouse abuse: A meta-analysis. *J Marriage Fam*. 2000;62(3):640–654.

53. Coid J, Petruckevitch A, Feder G, et al. Relation between childhood sexual and physical abuse and risk of revictimisation in women: A cross-sectional survey. *Lancet*. 2001;358(9280):450–454.

54. McCauley J, Kern DE, Kolodner K, et al. Clinical characteristics of women with a history of childhood abuse: Unhealed wounds. *JAMA*. 1997;277(17):1362–1368.

55. Wisner CL, Gilmer TP, Saltzman LE, Zink TM. Intimate partner violence against women: Do victims cost health plans more? *J Fam Pract*. 1999;48(6):439–443.

56. Petersen R, Gazmararian J, Andersen Clark K. Partner violence: Implications for health and community settings. *Womens Health Issues*. 2001;11(2):116–125.

57. Ulrich YC, Cain KC, Sugg NK, et al. Medical care utilization patterns in women with diagnosed domestic violence. *Am J Prev Med*. 2003;24(1):9–15.

58. Kernic MA, Wolf ME, Holt VL. Rates and relative risk of hospital admission among women in violent intimate partner relationships. *Am J Public Health*. 2000;90(9):1416–1420.

59. Scholle SH, Rost KM, Golding JM. Physical abuse among depressed women. *J Gen Intern Med*. 1998;13(9):607–613.

60. Hastings DP, Kantor GK. Women's victimization history and surgical intervention. *AORN J*. 173–4 passim. 2003;77(1):163–168.

61. Bair MJ, Robinson RL, Katon W, Kroenke K. Depression and pain comorbidity: A literature review. *Arch Intern Med*. 2003;163(20):2433–2445.

62. Otis JD, Keane TM, Kerns RD. An examination of the relationship between chronic pain and post-traumatic stress disorder. *J Rehabil Res Dev*. 2003;40(5):397–405.

63. Beckham JC, Crawford AL, Feldman ME, et al. Chronic posttraumatic stress disorder and chronic pain in Vietnam combat veterans. *J Psychosom Res*. 1997;43(4):379–389.

64. Asmundson GJ, Norton GR, Allerdings MD, et al. Posttraumatic stress disorder and work-related injury. *J Anxiety Disord*. 1998;12(1):57–69.

65. Geisser ME, Roth RS, Bachman JE, Eckert TA. The relationship between symptoms of post-traumatic stress disorder and pain, affective disturbance and disability among patients with accident and non-accident related pain. *Pain*. 1996;66(2–3):207–214.

66. McFarlane AC, Atchison M, Rafalowicz E, Papay P. Physical symptoms in post-traumatic stress disorder. *J Psychosom Res*. 1994;38(7):715–726.

67. Amir M, Kaplan Z, Neumann L, et al. Posttraumatic stress disorder, tenderness and fibromyalgia. *J Psychosom Res*. 1997;42(6):607–613.

68. Smith MY, Egert J, Winkel G, Jacobson J. The impact of PTSD on pain experience in persons with HIV/AIDS. *Pain*. 2002;98(1–2):9–17.

69. Turk DC, Okifuji A. Perception of traumatic onset, compensation status, and physical findings: Impact on pain severity, emotional distress, and disability in chronic pain patients. *J Behav Med*. 1996;19(5):435–453.

70. Marais A, de Villiers PJ, Moller AT, Stein DJ. Domestic violence in patients visiting general practitioners: Prevalence, phenomenology, and association with psychopathology. *S Afr Med J*. 1999;89(6):635–640.

71. Hegarty K, Roberts G. How common is domestic violence against women? The definition of partner abuse in prevalence studies. *Aust N Z J Public Health*. 1998;22(1):49–54.

72. Golding JM. Intimate partner violence as a risk factor for mental disorders: A meta-analysis. *J Fam Violence*. 1999;14(2):99–132.

73. Thompson MP, Kaslow NJ, Kingree JB, et al. Partner abuse and posttraumatic stress disorder as risk factors for suicide attempts in a sample of low-income, inner-city women. *J Trauma Stress*. 1999;12(1):59–72.

74. Woods SJ. Prevalence and patterns of posttraumatic stress disorder in abused and postabused women. *Issues Ment Health Nurs*. 2000;21(3):309–324.

75. Brokaw J, Fullerton-Gleason L, Olson L, et al. Health status and intimate partner violence: A cross-sectional study. *Ann Emerg Med*. 2002;39(1):31–38.

76. Sharp TJ, Harvey AG. Chronic pain and posttraumatic stress disorder: Mutual maintenance? *Clin Psychol Rev*. 2001;21(6):857–877.

77. Asmundson GJ, Coons MJ, Taylor S, Katz J. PTSD and the experience of pain: Research and clinical implications of shared vulnerability and mutual maintenance models. *Can J Psychiatry*. 2002;47(10):930–937.

78. Asmundson GJ, Bonin MF, Frombach IK, Norton GR. Evidence of a disposition toward fearfulness and vulnerability to posttraumatic stress in dysfunctional pain patients. *Behav Res Ther*. 2000;38(8):801–812.

79. Carrey NJ, Butter HJ, Persinger MA, Bialik RJ. Physiological and cognitive correlates of child abuse.

J Am Acad Child Adolesc Psychiatry. 1995;34(8): 1067–1075.

80. Neeck G, Riedel W. Neuromediator and hormonal perturbations in fibromyalgia syndrome: Results of chronic stress? *Baillieres Clin Rheumatol.* 1994;8(4):763–775.

81. Crofford LJ, Engleberg NC, Demitrack MA. Neurohormonal perturbations in fibromyalgia. *Baillieres Clin Rheumatol.* 1996;10(2):365–378.

82. Bennett RM. Emerging concepts in the neurobiology of chronic pain: Evidence of abnormal sensory processing in fibromyalgia. *Mayo Clin Proc.* 1999;74(4):385–398.

83. Cannon JG, Angel JB, Abad LW, et al. Hormonal influences on stress-induced neutrophil mobilization in health and chronic fatigue syndrome. *J Clin Immunol.* 1998;18(4):291–298.

84. Clauw DJ, Chrousos GP. Chronic pain and fatigue syndromes: Overlapping clinical and neuroendocrine features and potential pathogenic mechanisms. *Neuroimmunomodulation.* 1997;4(3):134–153.

85. Demitrack MA, Crofford LJ. Evidence for and pathophysiologic implications of hypothalamic-pituitary-adrenal axis dysregulation in fibromyalgia and chronic fatigue syndrome. *Ann N Y Acad Sci.* 1998;840:684–697.

86. Pillemer SR, Bradley LA, Crofford LJ, et al. The neuroscience and endocrinology of fibromyalgia. *Arthritis Rheum.* 1997;40(11):1928–1939.

87. Weigent DA, Bradley LA, Blalock JE, Alarcon GS. Current concepts in the pathophysiology of abnormal pain perception in fibromyalgia. *Am J Med Sci.* 1998;315(6):405–412.

88. Drossman DA, Talley NJ, Leserman J, et al. Sexual and physical abuse and GI illness. Review and recommendations. *Ann Intern Med.* 1995;123(10): 782–794.

89. Drossman DA, Ringel Y, Vogt BA, et al. Alterations of brain activity associated with resolution of emotional distress and pain in a case of severe irritable bowel syndrome. *Gastroenterology.* 2003;124(3): 754–761.

90. Resnick HS, Yehuda R, Acierno R. Acute post-rape plasma cortisol, alcohol use, and PTSD symptom profile among recent rape victims. *Ann N Y Acad Sci.* 1997;821:433–436.

91. Resnick HS, Yehuda R, Pitman RK, Foy DW. Effect of previous trauma on acute plasma cortisol level following rape. *Am J Psychiatry.* 1995;152(11): 1675–1677.

92. Nicolaidis C. The Voices of Survivors documentary: Using patient narrative to educate physicians about domestic violence. *J Gen Intern Med.* 2002;17(2):117–124.

93. Campbell JC. "If I can't have you, no one can": Power and control in homicide of female partners. In: Radford J, Russel DEH, eds. *Femicide: The politics of woman killing.* Boston: Twayne, 1992.

94. Campbell JC, Soeken KL. Women's responses to battering: A test of the model. *Res Nurs Health.* 1999;22(1):49–58.

95. Battaglia TA, Finley E, Liebschutz JM. Survivors of intimate partner violence speak out: Trust in the patient-provider relationship. *J Gen Intern Med.* 2003;18(8):617–623.

96. Nicolaidis C, Gregg J, Galian H, et al. Health care beliefs and needs of depressed women with a history of intimate partner violence. *J Gen Intern Med.* 2006;21(Suppl 4).

97. Vieweg WV, Julius DA, Fernandez A, et al. Posttraumatic stress disorder: Clinical features, pathophysiology, and treatment. *Am J Med.* 2006; 119(5):383–390.

98. Khan AA, Khan A, Harezlak J, et al. Somatic symptoms in primary care: Etiology and outcome. *Psychosomatics.* 2003;44(6):471–478.

99. Smith RC, Lein C, Collins C, et al. Treating patients with medically unexplained symptoms in primary care. *J Gen Intern Med.* 2003;18(6): 478–489.

100. Smith R. Patient-centered interviewing: An evidence-based method. In: Stewart M, Weston WW, McWhinney IR, et al., eds. *Patient-centered medicine: Transforming the clinical method,* 2nd ed. Abington, UK: Radcliffe Publishing, 2001.

101. Stewart M, Brown J, Weston W, et al. *Patient-centered medicine: Transforming the clinical method.* Abington, UK: Radcliff Publishing, 2003.

102. Kroenke K, Swindle R. Cognitive-behavioral therapy for somatization and symptom syndromes: A critical review of controlled clinical trials. *Psychother Psychosom.* 2000;69(4):205–215.

Chapter 12

Mental Health Consequences of Intimate Partner Violence

Carole Warshaw, Phyllis Brashler, and Jessica Gil

KEY CONCEPTS

- Intimate partner violence (IPV) has been associated with a wide range of mental health consequences, including depression and post-traumatic stress disorder (PTSD).
- For many women, these issues resolve with increased safety and support, but others may benefit from additional resources and treatment.
- Survivors' experiences of mental health symptoms will vary based on a number of factors, including their own personal strengths and resources, the duration and severity of abuse, their experience of other lifetime trauma, and their access to services and social support.
- Women who are diagnosed with a mental illness are at greater risk for abuse and for developing PTSD.
- Stigma associated with mental illness reinforces abusers' abilities to manipulate mental health issues to control their partners, undermine them in custody battles, and discredit them with friends, family, and the courts.
- Advances in the fields of traumatic stress, child development, genetics, and neuroscience are generating new models for understanding the impact of early experience on subsequent health, mental health, and life trajectories, as well as the psychobiological impact of adult traumatic events. This emerging body of knowledge, particularly when grounded in survivor and advocacy perspectives, provides a more useful framework for understanding the range of mental health responses experienced by survivors of IPV.
- Training and practice environments that are both domestic violence (DV)- and trauma-informed can be developed to better meet the needs of survivors of IPV and other lifetime trauma.

The past 30 years have seen a substantial growth in research documenting the prevalence of intimate partner violence (IPV) and other lifetime trauma among women seen in health and mental health settings, as well as the range of mental health conditions associated with current and past abuse. More recently, advances in the fields of traumatic stress, child development, genetics, and neuroscience are generating new models for understanding the impact of early experience on subsequent health, mental health, and life trajectories, as well as the psychobiological impact of adult traumatic events. These, in turn, are changing our conceptual frameworks for understanding the effects of chronic interpersonal abuse across the lifespan, issues that research on IPV and mental health is only just beginning to reflect (1–9). This emerging body of knowledge, particularly when grounded in survivor and advocacy perspectives, provides a more useful framework for understanding the range of mental health responses experienced by survivors of IPV than do earlier approaches that failed to link social context with psychiatric symptoms and disorders.

This chapter reviews current research about the mental health consequences of IPV and other lifetime abuse and the intersection of IPV, lifetime trauma, and mental health. It also provides a critical perspective on the limits of these data for understanding women's experience of IPV and the concerns survivors have articulated about how these data are used and perceived. Finally, it offers a framework for understanding and responding to the traumatic effects of IPV and lifetime abuse and for addressing mental health issues in the context of IPV, including a number of issues not yet addressed by current research.

DOMESTIC VIOLENCE, TRAUMA, AND MENTAL HEALTH: FRAMING THE ISSUES

Addressing mental health in the context of ongoing IPV raises a number of issues for both survivors and practitioners. Domestic violence (DV) advocates and survivors have consistently voiced concerns about the ways mental health issues are used *against* battered women, not only by abusers but also by the systems in which women seek help (e.g., batterers using mental health issues to control their partners, undermine them in custody battles, and discredit them with friends, family, child protective services, and

the courts) (10,11). This has been due, in part, to the stigma associated with mental illness, historically gendered notions of psychopathology (a history of viewing women's responses to abuse in pathological terms), and a psychiatric diagnostic system that, historically, has not incorporated etiology or social context.

For survivors of IPV, abuse was often viewed as a reflection of victim "psychopathology," and symptoms were rarely seen as a *consequence* of being abused. Conscious of the need to create a public awareness that would hold abusers, not victims, accountable for their violence, advocates and survivors have been reluctant to frame women's responses to abuse in purely clinical terms. In addition, survivors of IPV were placed in greater jeopardy through their interactions with the mental health system (e.g., referrals to couples counseling when that was unsafe, involvement of batterers in treatment, use of mental health issues against women in custody battles) (12). These challenges have also been instrumental in reconfiguring clinical paradigms and underscoring the importance of framing victimization as a societal problem, not an attribute of the victim. As Brown suggests, we do not look for characteristics of other crime victims to understand why they have been victimized (13).

Over the past several decades, however, an overarching framework for understanding the impact of trauma on the human psyche has emerged through work with survivors of both civilian and combat trauma and through research on the cumulative effects of diverse childhood experiences and the developmental consequences of early abuse and neglect (7,14–22). Posttraumatic stress disorder as a diagnostic construct was initially developed to codify and formally bring attention to the disabling experiences of returning combat survivors (i.e., Da Costa's syndrome, combat neurosis, shell shock, battle fatigue) as well as survivors of sexual assault (rape trauma syndrome) and IPV (battered women's syndrome) (1,23–29). Ongoing debate continues within the traumatic stress field regarding whether the posttraumatic stress disorder (PTSD) diagnosis adequately captures the multiple domains that are affected by trauma, particularly when it is chronic, interpersonal, and/or begins early in life. The debate centers on whether the traumatic effects of abuse are best depicted by the diagnosis of PTSD in combination with common comorbidities (e.g., depression, anxiety, panic, substance abuse, eating disorders, somatization disorders, dissociative disorders, suicidality, etc.) or through the lens of *complex trauma* (i.e., disorders of extreme stress not otherwise specified [DESNOS], complex developmental trauma, developmental trauma disorder, posttraumatic personality disorder) originally described by Herman in 1992 and since validated by numerous other studies (8,30–32). These newer concepts attempt to address the effects of chronic interpersonal abuse not covered by the PTSD diagnosis and provide a more nuanced way of understanding the impact of trauma across the lifespan—effects that are mediated through the interactions of many other factors in addition to the traumatic experience itself (15). Only recently have tools been available to study the interactions between genes, individual environment, and broader social conditions. These tools have contributed to a more complex paradigm for examining the role of external social factors in the development of psychiatric symptoms and disorders (33). This has led to a significant shift in the ways mental health symptoms are conceptualized and to greater awareness of the role that abuse and violence play in the development of psychological distress and psychiatric morbidity. A DV advocacy perspective provides another critical piece of this equation—one that addresses the ongoing social realities that survivors face as they try to end the violence in their lives and deal with its traumatic effects.

INTIMATE PARTNER VIOLENCE AND LIFETIME TRAUMA

For many women, abuse by an adult partner is their first experience of victimization; for others, IPV occurs in the context of other lifetime trauma. A number of studies have begun to explore the link between histories of physical and sexual abuse in childhood and the experience of partner abuse as an adult. Women who are physically or sexually abused as children or who witness their mothers being abused appear to be at greater risk for victimization in adolescence and adulthood by both intimate and nonintimate perpetrators (34–41), and women who experience adolescent IPV are more likely to experience IPV as adults (42).

Studies of battered women in both clinical and shelter settings have found high rates of childhood abuse and childhood exposure to IPV. In a 2007 study by Kimerling and colleagues, women who experienced childhood physical or sexual abuse were almost six times more likely to experience adult physical or sexual victimization (43). Across studies, the average reported rates of childhood physical abuse and childhood sexual abuse among women in DV shelters or programs are 55.1% and 57.0%, respectively (44).

For women who have experienced multiple forms of victimization (e.g., childhood abuse; sexual assault; historical, cultural, or refugee trauma), adult partner abuse puts them at even greater risk for developing posttraumatic mental health conditions, including substance abuse (a common method of relieving pain and coping with anxiety, depression, and sleep disruption associated with current and/or past abuse). These conditions and coping strategies may, in turn, place them at risk for further abuse (29,45–53). The intersection between substance abuse and IPV is discussed in greater depth in another chapter in this text.

Socioeconomic factors can also expose women to victimization, which compounds their risk for developing the range of mental health sequelae noted earlier. For example, low-income women (those most likely to be seen in both IPV shelters and the public mental health system) have the highest risk of being victimized throughout their lives. In one study, the lifetime prevalence of severe physical or sexual assault among very-low-income women was found to be 84%; 63% of those studied had been physically assaulted as children, 40% had been sexually assaulted as children, and 60% had been physically assaulted by an intimate partner (54). Similarly, studies conducted in welfare-to-work programs have documented lifetime rates of intimate partner abuse ranging from 55% to 65% (55–58), as opposed to rates of 20% found in random population samples (59).

A body of clinical literature describes the retraumatizing effects of more subtle forms of social and cultural victimization (e.g., microtraumatization or insidious trauma) due to gender, race, ethnicity, sexual orientation, disability, and/or socioeconomic status (60–65). Thus, although IPV itself is associated with a wide range psychological consequences, women living in disenfranchised communities face multiple sources of stress in addition to violence, including social discrimination, poorer health status, and reduced access to critical resources, all of which can increase psychological distress (66,67). Again, many IPV survivors have experienced other forms of trauma, some of which may be ongoing, that can affect their responses to current IPV.

INTIMATE PARTNER VIOLENCE AND
MENTAL ILLNESS

Although most survivors of domestic abuse do not develop long-lasting psychiatric disabilities, mental illness appears to heighten women's risk for abuse (68,69). Poverty, homelessness, institutionalization, unsafe living conditions, and dependence on caregivers exacerbate these risks, leaving individuals with psychiatric disabilities vulnerable to victimization by a range of perpetrators—within families, on the streets, in institutional and residential settings, and by intimate or dating partners. For example, a study of homeless women diagnosed with a serious mental illness found that a significant majority had been abused by a partner (70% had suffered physical abuse, 30.4% sexual abuse) (70). Rates of physical or sexual abuse in adulthood by any perpetrator were 87% and 76%, respectively. Intimate partner violence itself is often a precipitant to homelessness (54,71,72). Moreover, IPV presents particular risks for individuals with serious mental illness. Exposure to ongoing abuse can exacerbate symptoms and precipitate mental health crises, making it more difficult to access resources and increasing abusers' control over their lives. Stigma associated with mental illness and clinicians' lack of knowledge about IPV reinforce abusers' abilities to manipulate mental health issues to control their partners, undermine them in custody battles, and discredit them with friends, family, and the courts. In a series of focus groups conducted in Chicago, DV advocates and survivors described a number of these tactics. For example, abusers use strategies such as threatening to commit and/or committing their partners to psychiatric institutions; forcing their partners to take overdoses, which are then presented as suicide attempts; and withholding psychotropic medications. Other examples include asserting that accusations of abuse are simply delusions, lying outright about their partners' behaviors, and rationalizing their own (e.g., claiming their partner "needed to be restrained"). This kind of manipulation not only increases an abuser's control over his partner, but also can have a chilling affect on a woman's ability to retain custody of her children, which is often one motivation behind her partner's behavior. Although this type of phenomenon cuts across cultures, immigrant women who are isolated and do not speak English are particularly vulnerable to this type of abuse (12).

Acute symptoms of mental illness can also heighten a woman's risk for victimization (68,69). Although psychiatric crises are often precipitated by recent trauma, for a woman experiencing symptoms of acute psychosis, clinicians may interpret accusations of victimization as delusions, thus leaving her vulnerable to further victimization. Women may be at particular risk for assault when experiencing cognitive or emotional difficulties associated with psychotic disorders (68). In addition, symptoms of severe trauma, such as dissociation or flashbacks, may also mimic psychotic disorders, heightening the potential for misdiagnosis and treatment that does not address underlying issues of abuse. Responses to previous trauma, such as dissociation or potentially risky coping strategies, may also increase a woman's vulnerability to abuse (73). Trauma or mental illness in childhood or adolescence can disrupt key developmental processes, leaving women without the skills they need to negotiate power and decision-making in relationships (74). When having to manage without these skills is compounded by abuse in adulthood, the likelihood of having legitimate rights respected in any relationship may become even more remote (30,75,76).

Prevalence of Intimate Partner Violence and Other Lifetime Trauma Among Women Seen in Mental Health Settings

On average, over half of women seen in a range of mental health settings either currently are or have been abused by an intimate partner, although rates vary widely among studies (29,75). As noted earlier, many have also experienced multiple forms of abuse throughout their lives, putting them at greater risk for a range of health and mental health sequelae and affecting their ability to mobilize resources necessary to achieve safety and stability (77–80). For example, studies across a variety of mental health settings have found significant rates of *lifetime abuse* among people living with serious mental illness, with those in inpatient facilities reporting the highest rates (53%–83%) (47,70,81–86).

Recent studies of adverse childhood experiences also demonstrate the prevalence of lifetime abuse among individuals who have a mental illness. A 2007 study of people diagnosed with schizophrenia found that 86% had experienced at least one adverse childhood event and 49% had experienced three or more (87). (In this study, adverse events included physical abuse, sexual abuse, parental mental illnesses, loss of a parent, parental separation or divorce, witnessing DV, and foster or kinship care.) The number of these events also predicted a range of adverse mental health outcomes (substance abuse, PTSD, length of hospitalization, suicidality, and poorer self-rated mental health, as well as functional status). Although no general population study uses the same definitions of adverse childhood events, a reasonable comparison can be made with the 1998 ACE study, which examined the prevalence of adverse childhood experiences within a large health maintenance organization population. It found that over half of the sample had experienced at least one category of adverse childhood experience, and approximately 25% reported experiencing two or more (1). In this study, the categories of adverse childhood experiences included physical, sexual, or psychological abuse; violence against mother; and living with household members who were substance abusers, mentally ill or suicidal, or ever imprisoned.

Although attention to victimization among people receiving public mental health services initially focused on the long-term effects of *childhood abuse*, rates of *adult victimization* by acquaintances, strangers, family members, and intimate partners appear to be equal or higher. In one study, over 70% of women admitted for a first psychotic episode had experienced at least one type of abuse, and 42% reported ongoing exposure (88). Only a few studies have specifically examined rates of adult partner, family member, or caretaker abuse among individuals with serious mental illnesses. In one inpatient study, 62% had been abused by a current or former spouse (81). Of the 64% of female inpatients who reported having been physically assaulted as adults in another study, more than half were living with the perpetrator at the time of hospitalization (84). In a third study, which looked at hospitalized patients (male and female) who had ongoing relationships with partners or family members, 62.8% reported a history of physical victimization by a partner, 45.8% reported physical abuse by a family member, and 29% reported having experienced domestic abuse within the past year (89). Yet, these issues are rarely attended to. Informal focus groups with women who self-identified as consumers of mental health services indicate that the majority had experienced DV and other forms of abuse, but few had been asked about those experiences. The majority

of women were also interested in receiving information about DV and about resources they could access in their communities (90). Without formal training and policies in place, abusive partners are often included in treatment planning, and safety issues go unaddressed.

Until recently, information about specific forms of violence against women, including childhood sexual abuse, sexual assault, and IPV, was often found in separate literatures. As a result, knowledge about the cumulative effects of lifetime exposure to trauma for adult survivors of IPV and the experiences of women from diverse communities has been limited. In general, studies examining the mental health impact of IPV are designed to assess for: (a) prevalence of specific psychiatric diagnoses among survivors of IPV and/or other lifetime trauma, (b) other effects of IPV for which there are validated measurements (e.g., self-esteem, internal versus external locus of control, functional status), and/or (c) additional factors associated with the frequency or severity of these conditions. Yet, methodological problems and lack of consistency across studies limit the generalizability of much of the currently available research. Measures are not standardized across studies nor are they culturally normed. And the majority of studies are cross-sectional in design and do not identify the timing of the assessment in relationship to recent crises. Moreover, the majority of studies have been conducted in clinical or shelter settings where rates of symptomatology are likely to be higher.

It is also important to keep in mind the limits of quantitative research for conveying survivors' actual experience. For example, although complex trauma models may ultimately prove to be a more accurate way to understand the multiple effects of chronic longstanding abuse, such as IPV, even diagnoses that specifically address traumatic events do not fully capture what living in a climate of fear does to a woman's psychological landscape or what a woman has to do to reconfigure her sense of identity, her belief in herself, her connections to others, and her relationship to a world that has betrayed her. Nor do they convey the unique intersection of strengths, supports, identities, and meanings that survivors carry with them as they traverse their lives.

Despite these limitations, over the past three decades, research documenting the effects of violence across the lifespan indicates that abuse, violence, and discrimination play key roles in many of the health and mental health problems experienced by women in the United States and throughout the world (1,25,26,28,91–93). Researchers have found that exposure to current and/or past abuse is a significant factor in the development and exacerbation of psychiatric disorders, increases the risk for revictimization, and influences the course of recovery from mental illness (87,94–104).

For many abuse survivors, symptoms abate with increased safety and social support, but for others this is not the case (91,105). Both random population studies and studies conducted in clinical settings indicate that victimization by an intimate partner places women at significantly higher risk for depression, anxiety, PTSD, somatization, medical problems, substance abuse, suicide attempts (whether or not they have suffered physical injury), and more generally for reporting unmet mental health needs (95,106–110). In a meta-analysis of mental health conditions experienced by survivors of IPV, the weighted mean prevalence across settings was 50% for depression, 61% for PTSD, and 20.3% for suicidality (44). Rates of depression were highest among women in IPV shelters (63.8%) and court-involved women (73.7%), PTSD rates were highest for women in shelters (66.9%) and drug treatment programs (58.1), and rates of suicide attempts were highest among women seen in psychiatric settings (53.6%). Somatoform disorders, eating disorders, and acute psychotic episodes have also been associated with both adult and childhood abuse.

DEPRESSION, INTIMATE PARTNER VIOLENCE, AND OTHER TRAUMA

Depression was one of the first mental health consequences of physical and/or sexual abuse to be identified in the research literature. Several factors seem to increase a woman's risk for depression, including perpetrator behavior and a history of multiple sexual victimizations. Women with histories of childhood sexual abuse and adult sexual assault show significantly higher rates of depression than do women in control groups, and these data have been extensively reviewed by Koss (111). Studies have found that the lifetime prevalence of major depressive disorder among women who have been sexual assaulted is at least twice that of women who have not, and may in fact be higher. One study of women seen in medical settings found that those who had been raped were three times as likely to experience depression as women who had not (112). This study also found that age at first assault was of particular significance. Women who experienced multiple victimizations, and who were first assaulted during childhood, were twice as likely to experience depression as women whose first victimization occurred as an adult. In addition, depression associated with PTSD may represent a distinct phenomenon. The numbing and feelings of deadness associated with PTSD are among the most difficult symptoms to eliminate, even when intrusion and hyperarousal have improved (20).

Intimate partner violence also increases women's risk for depression. Prevalence rates for depression among women abused by an intimate partner range from 35.7% to 63% (95). In one study of a random sample of women who belonged to a health maintenance organization, women who had experienced recent partner violence were 2.3 times as likely to report any depressive symptoms and 2.6 times as likely to report severe depressive symptoms as women who had not experienced any partner violence (113). A recent study of mothers who stayed at an emergency shelter for battered women found that mothers' mean scores for depression were far above the norm for the measure, with 67% scoring above the cutoff for clinical diagnosis (114). A third study by Hegarty and colleagues (114) looked at the association between depression and partner abuse among 1,257 consecutive women seen in primary care settings (115). Multivariate analysis indicated that women who were depressed were significantly more likely to have experienced some form of partner abuse. The strongest associations were for women who had experienced severe combined abuse and/or physical and emotional abuse or harassment. Fogarty and colleagues (116) examined the synergistic effects of childhood abuse (physical and sexual) and IPV on depression in a random population sample. Using data from the National Violence Against Women Survey (NVAW) (1995), they found rates of self-reported depressive symptoms in 35.7% of women reported IPV alone, 34.9% of women reporting only childhood abuse, and 50.2% of women reporting both—rates that were twice as high as those of women not reporting either type of violence (116).

Several studies of depression and IPV have suggested that frequency and severity of violence (117–119), psychological abuse (120,121), concomitant sexual violence (122) and lack of social support are associated with the severity of depressive symptoms, and may even be stronger predictors of depression than cultural and demographic factors or a prior history of mental illness (123,124). The study of maternal depression in an emergency shelter setting cited earlier also found higher rates of depression among women who reported more frequent sexual abuse by their partners (113).

For some women, symptoms of depression persist over time. One recent longitudinal, nationally representative study found that, among a community sample of married or cohabiting women, those who reported IPV were more likely to experience depressive symptoms 5 years later, suggesting that IPV places some women at greater risk for long-term mental health concerns (95). Bonomi and associates found that women with remote experiences of violence (experiences that occurred more than 5 years in the past) were more likely to report depressive symptoms than women who had never experienced partner violence. They also found that women with more recent experiences of violence reported more symptoms than women whose abuse experiences occurred in the past (125). In addition, experiencing ongoing abuse significantly affects the persistence of severe depressive symptoms (42). In a 14-year longitudinal study of the course of depression among adolescent mothers, findings indicated that women who had experienced IPV in both adolescence and adulthood had the highest mean depression scores (105). The authors suggest that exposure to IPV in adolescence may alter women's life trajectories, leading to both increased risk for adult IPV and for its mental health effects. For women who are able to leave the violent environment, however, symptoms are likely to decrease (126,127). In another study, the greatest reductions in rates of depression were found among women who had experienced physical/sexual and psychological abuse and for whom all three types of violence had ceased (128).

Although a handful of studies have looked at the distinct psychological effects of sexual assault in the context of IPV, research on post-rape depression may also be useful to examine. Although symptoms of anxiety predominate immediately after sexual assault, early signs of depression can be seen within a few hours. Women report sadness, apathy, and suicidal thoughts (112). Within a few weeks, moderate to severe depression may develop (43%–56%) and last up to 3 months according to some studies (129–132).

Other retrospective studies have found that post-rape depression may persist for many years (111,133). In their review of existing research, Koss and co-workers (2003) note that child sexual assault may have particularly long-lasting effects, and at least one study suggests that the impact of multiple victimizations may be cumulative (134,135).

Overall, depression appears to be a frequent consequence of IPV. Recency and severity of violence and cumulative burden of trauma, particularly sexual assault and childhood abuse, contribute to the development and severity of depression in this context. At the same time, cessation of exposure to IPV and social support are associated with a significant reduction in symptoms. However, with a few notable exceptions (136), most clinical depression studies do not factor in the role of current or past abuse, nor do current depression treatment guidelines include assessment or intervention for IPV.[1] Attention to the integration of these issues in future research and practice is warranted.

Co-occurrence of Depression and Posttraumatic Stress Disorder

More recent research on the mental health effects of IPV has begun to examine the relationship between depression and PTSD. Depression frequently co-occurs with PTSD and is increasingly viewed as a comorbid condition. Fifty percent of people who develop PTSD also develop major depressive disorder (MDD), and prior depression is associated with the development of PTSD following the experience of a traumatic event (137). Posttraumatic stress disorder has also been found to mediate the development of MDD in prospective studies of individuals following motor vehicle accidents and other non-IPV–related traumatic events, as well as among women who have been assaulted (138–142).

A number of studies have specifically examined the co-occurrence of PTSD and MDD among survivors of IPV, although the relationship between the two is not yet clear (143–145). For example, Pico-Alfonso and

---

[1] *Perinatal Depression: Prevalence, Screening Accuracy, and Screening Outcomes*, Structured Abstract. February 2005. Agency for Healthcare Research and Quality, Rockville, MD. http://www.ahrq.gov/clinic/tp/perideptp.htm

colleagues report low rates of PTSD among women experiencing IPV, but high rates of depression, particularly among women who had experienced sexual violence (122). In this study, only a small percentage of women experienced only PTSD. Most experienced symptoms of depression alone or depression plus PTSD. In another study of immigrant Latinas seen in a primary care clinic, current IPV was predictive of PTSD, but not depression. Again, in this sample, rates of MDD were high, but rates were not significantly different between women who reported IPV and those who did not. Women who met criteria for PTSD were 10 times more likely to have MDD (146). Finally, Nixon and colleagues found that, in a sample of women residing in a battered women's shelter, PTSD and MDD frequently co-occurred. Women with comorbid PTSD and MDD experienced greater symptom severity than those with either condition alone (147).

In sum, for women experiencing IPV, both PTSD and depression are common, and depression is frequently comorbid with PTSD. This raises questions about how to best frame the range of symptoms associated with interpersonal trauma (e.g., PTSD plus comorbidities versus complex trauma) and reflects a more general shift toward viewing symptoms from a dimensional (along a continuum) rather than categorical perspective (148). Additional research is needed to determine how these factors affect survivors' experience and their ability to access safety, as well as to determine optimal approaches to treatment, particularly in the context of ongoing IPV.

POSTTRAUMATIC STRESS DISORDER AND INTIMATE PARTNER VIOLENCE

Today, the vast majority of studies on the mental health effects of violence and abuse focus on PTSD. Posttraumatic stress disorder was the first diagnosis to incorporate the role of external events in the etiology of mental health symptoms and was initially viewed as the most appropriate diagnosis for women experiencing the range of psychological sequelae associated with sexual assault, battering, and childhood sexual abuse (28,149).

Diagnostic criteria for PTSD include *exposure* to an extreme traumatic stressor (experiencing, witnessing, or learning about actual or threatened death, serious injury, or threats to the physical integrity of oneself or others) AND *responding* with intense fear, helplessness, or horror (criterion A stressors), in addition to *symptoms* from each of three core categories. These categories include persistent: (a) *re-experiencing*: being flooded with dreams, memories, and flashbacks, and/or having intense physical and emotional responses to triggers (reminders) of the traumatic events; (b) *avoidance and numbing*: avoiding anything that reminds the individual of those experiences and/or feeling numb, shut down, or constricted emotionally; and (c) *symptoms of increased physiological arousal and hypervigilance* that affect sleep and concentration and cause irritability. Symptoms must persist for at least a month and cause significant distress and impairment. Survivors of IPV frequently experience additional layers of stress not captured by current diagnostic criteria for PTSD. In a review article on the association of chronic traumatization and PTSD in the context of IPV, Kaysen and colleagues propose the concept of "traumatic context" to account for common experiences of IPV survivors, such as the need to continually monitor for signs of danger, that do not reach the level of criterion A stressors, but nonetheless may contribute to PTSD symptoms (9).

To further complicate matters, a diagnosis of acute stress disorder (ASD) is used to describe symptoms that develop within the first month after exposure to a traumatic event and that last from 2 days to 4 weeks. Acute stress disorder symptoms overlap with those of PTSD but include a number of dissociative symptoms as well. Acute stress disorder is thought to be predictive of PTSD, but research on this question has been mixed. Some authors have argued that insufficient distinction exists between the two diagnoses, and that ASD really reflects early-onset PTSD (150,151). Although a number of studies have indicated that peritraumatic dissociation associated with ASD is one of the strongest predictors of PTSD, others have found that it is *persistent* rather than *peritraumatic* dissociation that is most predictive (152,153). These findings nonetheless have led to recommendations for early treatment interventions to prevent the development of chronic PTSD. Research on the applicability of these modalities in the presence of ongoing IPV, however, is virtually nonexistent. See Chapter 24 for a discussion of these issues.

Posttraumatic stress disorder affects twice as many women as men, resulting in lifetime prevalence rates of 10.4%–18.3% and 5.4%–10.2%, respectively (137,154–157). Gender differences appear to be related to the type of traumatic exposure women experience (158). Overall, women experience somewhat lower rates of traumatic events than men; however, women are more likely to experience those kinds of interpersonal assaults that carry the highest risks for PTSD such as rape, childhood sexual abuse, and DV (154). Rape is the traumatic event most often associated with PTSD among women (155,159), whereas for men, PTSD is more likely to be associated with physical assault or combat, particularly when it is high-stress (160). Childhood sexual abuse is also a significant risk factor for PTSD, accounting for almost a quarter of adult cases of PTSD among women. Women are more likely than men to develop PTSD subsequent to childhood sexual abuse and to develop PTSD following the experience of a nonassaultive trauma, if they have experienced assault in the past (154,161).

Some controversy still exists regarding these gender differences. A number of studies have found that, even when controlling for type of violence, women are still more likely to develop PTSD (162,163). In studies of individuals who experienced a similar traumatic event, including car accidents, natural disasters, physical trauma, and the terrorist attacks of 9/11, women developed PTSD at twice the rate of men, although other studies have not found evidence of these differences (164–166). Proposed mechanisms for these gender differences include women's younger age at first trauma exposure, stronger perceptions of loss of control, higher levels of distress at the time of the event, differences in cognitive appraisal of traumatic experience, insufficient social support, peritraumatic dissociation, and gender-specific psychobiological reactions to traumatic events (167,168). Another study conducted in a primary care setting, found preexisting trauma and previous psychiatric conditions, as well as gender, to be predictors of PTSD (169). Critiques of these studies note that collapsing traumatic events into "assaultive" and "nonassaultive" categories obscures the type of assault (sexual versus physical) and the relational context (intimate, caretaker, stranger; perceived versus actual loss of power). They also point out that lack of detailed questions about sexual assault may have led to underreporting in these studies. The debate in this arena raises questions for survivors of IPV, as well. For example, to what extent do these increased risks reflect physiological differences between women and men, the effects of gender socialization on responses to trauma and/or psychological distress, or to the types of violence women are more likely to be subjected

to (146)? More importantly, what are the implications for intervention and prevention (i.e., early treatment to prevent the development of PTSD, attention to integrating information about safety and social support into evidence-based PTSD treatment, prevention efforts to reduce the exposure of women and girls to gender-based violence)?

Rates of PTSD among women survivors of IPV are estimated to be between 33% and 84% with a weighted mean prevalence across studies of 61% (44,45,170–173). In the National Violence Against Women Study (a random population telephone survey of 8,000 women), 24% of those who reported IPV in the past year met criteria for PTSD (143). In other samples of women who reported recent IPV, rates of PTSD varied between 11.8% and 38% (91,122,145,172). And, among women using shelter services, prevalence rates of PTSD have been estimated to be as high as 75% (174). Although cross-sectional studies provide a window into symptoms that are present at a time of crisis, several longitudinal studies have begun to look at the course of PTSD among survivors of IPV. Mertin and colleagues (2001) found that while 42% of women in shelter met criteria for PTSD, only 14% did so 1 year later (175). In a 2005 community-based study of adolescents and young adults who had experienced IPV, PTSD remitted in 52% of the sample, whereas 48% showed no significant reduction of symptoms. Not surprisingly, respondents who developed chronic PTSD were more likely to have experienced additional traumatic event(s) during the 4-year follow-up period and to have higher rates of avoidant symptoms at baseline (176). Differences in these studies may also reflect differences between survivors who received shelter interventions and a community-based sample that did not. Other studies have found that approximately one-third of those who develop PTSD go on to develop a chronic course. For example, a study comparing women who were currently being abused to women who had been separated from an abusive partner for at least 2 years found that, whereas 74% of currently abused women experienced mild, moderate, or severe PTSD symptoms, 44% of women who were no longer being abused experienced comparable PTSD symptoms (177). In addition, lower levels of perceived social support have been associated with significantly higher rates of PTSD and depressive symptoms in women currently experiencing IPV. At the same time, PTSD numbing symptoms related to ongoing abuse can reduce a woman's ability to interact with others (40,178). Overall, it appears, as with depression, that social support and cessation of exposure to IPV are likely to contribute to improvement in PTSD for many women. For others, PTSD becomes chronic and requires more intensive treatment interventions, as well as linkages to community resources and support (179). Research is still needed that specifically examines which factors (including the natural course of PTSD) are most salient for particular women.

The sexual assault literature provides additional information on the course of PTSD that may also prove relevant to survivors of IPV, particularly if sexual violence is part of the picture. For example, immediately following sexual assault, up to 95% of women will develop symptoms of ASD (180,181). Distress seems to reach its peak at 3 weeks post-assault for victims of single-episode sexual assault in adulthood, and continue at this level for the next month (25,131,132,179). Although many symptoms may resolve after 3 months, residual fear, sexual difficulties, and problems with self-esteem can persist for 18 months or longer, and nearly 25% of survivors continue to be affected for several years (133,182–184). Other studies indicate that after 3 months, approximately one-half of adult sexual assault survivors will still meet criteria for PTSD, and many will continue to have PTSD for a year or longer (131,132,179,183,185). Post-rape recovery appears to be more difficult when assault occurs at an earlier age and when women experience greater fear of being injured or killed (182,186). Sexual assault by a known assailant appears to be as (187) or more devastating (188) than rape by a stranger, but women historically have been less likely to seek help or file police reports in this situation (189). The average time to PTSD remission ranges from 25 to 29 months (155, 159). In national studies, for 36%–42% of individuals, PTSD became a chronic condition (138,159,190). Posttraumatic stress disorder attributed to assaultive versus nonassaultive events is more likely to be chronic and last for almost three times as long. Further, women are more than twice as likely as men to develop chronic PTSD and to have PTSD symptoms for almost four times the duration (138).

From a more clinical perspective, women who have been assaulted develop responses similar to victims of other types of acute trauma: shock, confusion, horror, and helplessness, as well as dissociation, nightmares, flashbacks, numbing, avoidance, and hypervigilance (14,25). Flashbacks can be visual, auditory, olfactory, tactile, or somatic and may be triggered by a range of stimuli—subsequent abuse, hearing about someone else being assaulted, media portrayals of violence, sensory stimuli associated with the original traumatic experience(s), invasive medical procedures, or anniversaries of the trauma. They can also be cognitive (paranoid or suicidal thoughts), affective (feeling terrified or enraged), behavioral (cringing or fleeing), or relational (clinical interactions triggering abuse-related dynamics) (191).

The PTSD framework makes sense of the fluctuations trauma survivors experience between being flooded and needing to both dampen those feelings and remain vigilant to potential new dangers. Posttraumatic stress disorder may present as an extension of ASD, or it may develop after a period of dormancy (delayed PTSD). It may resolve on its own or with treatment, or it may take on a chronic form. The relative intensity of PTSD symptoms may vary over time. Although flashbacks are more prominent initially, avoidant symptoms may predominate later in the course. This symptom progression may make trauma-engendered fears less accessible to change, and thus painfully constrict women's lives, particularly in the arenas of intimacy, sexuality, and the ability to move freely in the world. Avoidant PTSD responses may also prevent a woman from taking action on her own behalf, because the emotional costs might be too great (e.g., not pursuing legal action, not obtaining needed medical procedures). The hypervigilance associated with PTSD can also constrain a woman's sense of freedom and safety. It is these adaptations that appear to have the most profound and potentially harmful long-term effects (192).

For women who are still in danger, the stress is not "post," the trauma is ongoing, and symptoms may be an adaptive response to danger. The development of PTSD, however, can make it more difficult to mobilize resources, putting women at even greater risk for being isolated and controlled by an abusive partner. In addition, many women continue to be traumatized after they have left an abusive relationship—through stalking, prolonged divorce or custody hearings, visitation, and retraumatization by the legal or other systems.

Association of Posttraumatic Stress Disorder with Particular Forms of Intimate Partner Violence

Posttraumatic stress disorder among survivors of intimate partner abuse has been correlated with the severity of the abuse, a history of repeated abuse (148) and/ or childhood victimization (45), the presence of sexual assault (143,193–196), degree of psychological abuse, and stalking (121,197–199). The more types of intimate partner abuse (physical, psychological, or sexual) a survivor experiences, the greater her risk for developing PTSD (91,122,136,170).

Sexual and psychological abuse both appear to contribute independently to the development of PTSD. Psychological abuse is what women who are being abused often describe as the most emotionally debilitating aspect of their experiences.[2] This may relate both to the psychological wounds abusers inflict and survivors carry, and to the chronic stress of having to continually monitor for signs of danger (193). Specific components of psychological abuse, such as behaviors designed to induce feelings of shame or guilt, may also contribute to these responses (200). It is not just a batterer's words or acts, but also the intentions, perceptions, and feelings that are communicated by the abuser and experienced by the person being victimized that carry such long-term effects (192,201).

A number of studies have indicated that psychological abuse is as or more predictive of low self-esteem, depression, and PTSD than physical abuse and, at least in some couples, predicts future physical and/or sexual violence (121,122,197,198,202,203). In one study, psychological abuse was found to be the best predictor (37) of PTSD in abused women, although psychological abuse in conjunction with physical abuse carried a higher risk than psychological abuse alone (121). A second study by this author found no difference between the effects of psychological abuse versus psychological/physical abuse on the development of PTSD, although in this sample, PTSD rarely occurred alone (it was more likely to co-occur with depression) (122). In another study of women whose partners were in batterer treatment, certain types of psychological abuse predicted PTSD above that associated with physical violence

(what the authors referred to as "denigration and restrictive engulfment"), although the authors speculated this might have been an artifact of other categories (e.g., psychological dominance and intimidation) not being statistically distinguishable from the actual physical abuse participants experienced.

Basile, using data from the National Violence Against Women (NVAW) survey, found that in their multivariate analysis, physical and psychological violence were related to PTSD risk (sexual violence was associated in the bivariate analysis) (196). The authors speculated that this may have been an artifact of the small sample of women who reported sexual violence in their current relationship. McFarlane, on the other hand, reported a greater number of PTSD symptoms among women who had been sexually assaulted in the context of IPV (155,159,204). The likelihood of having more than four symptoms (the proxy for a PTSD diagnosis) in this context was only higher among the White women in their sample. However, adult victims of sexual assault (particularly completed rape) represent the largest single group of trauma victims affected by PTSD, a finding confirmed in the national comorbidity study and the 1996 Detroit Area Survey of Trauma (188). In a recent study by Temple and colleagues, PTSD risk was further increased if the perpetrator was a woman's partner rather than a stranger (195). Overall, this research suggests that all forms of IPV appear to place women at risk for PTSD, and the more types of IPV experienced, the greater the risk (78,155,205,206). Psychological abuse and sexual violence appear to carry independent risks.

Although questions remain about the role of specific types of intimate partner abuse in the development of PTSD, existing data suggest that the number and type of traumatic events, in general, does affect an individual's risk for developing PTSD. Epidemiologic studies examining *single-event trauma* found that episodic assaultive traumatic events including rape, sexual assault, physical assault, or being robbed, mugged, shot, or stabbed were associated with higher rates of PTSD than nonassaultive events (78,155,159,205,206). In addition, experiencing *multiple* traumatic events places women at even greater risk for developing PTSD, particularly if the trauma is ongoing (e.g., IPV and childhood abuse) (78,177, 193,207–211).

Longitudinal and cross-sectional studies of chronic and often escalating trauma, including IPV and childhood physical or sexual abuse, have shown that

---

[2] Psychological abuse often takes the form of verbal intimidation and threats, ridicule and humiliation, destruction of property, threats to significant others, stalking and monitoring a woman's activities, and controlling her access to money, personal items, and contact with friends, family, and children. Accusations about sexual infidelity can be particularly humiliating. Emotional withdrawal, threats of abandonment, and threats to harm or take away the children are also used as tactics of control.

duration and severity of abuse also increase PTSD risk (155,159,176). The experience of trauma at a young age is a well-acknowledged risk factor for the development PTSD in adulthood (212). In a study of over 3,000 women, a 23-fold increase in adult PTSD was reported among those who had experienced all three forms of child abuse—physical, sexual, and psychological (45,167,213,214). Similarly, women who experience IPV are more likely to have histories of childhood abuse, thus increasing the risk for PTSD in this group (205, 215–218). Mental illness and conditions associated with severe childhood abuse (dissociative spectrum disorders, complex trauma/DESNOS, substance use disorders) contribute to these risks, as well.

Posttraumatic Stress Disorder and Comorbid Conditions

Posttraumatic stress disorder is associated with increased rates of psychiatric and medical comorbidity, service use, and disability as well as greater healthcare costs, more so for women than for men (155,159,219). Over 80% of people with PTSD develop at least one additional psychiatric disorder, most commonly major depression (as discussed earlier), as well as generalized anxiety disorder, panic disorder, and alcohol/substance abuse and dependence (155,159). Alcohol and other substance use are also often comorbid with PTSD (155,220–222). Posttraumatic stress disorder symptoms appear to precede the use of drugs and alcohol among women but not among men, suggesting their use as self-medication for women (223–226). Women in violent relationships also report increased problem drinking and substance abuse, yet the temporal relationship to IPV or PTSD symptoms has not been well described (227). In one study of women on methadone, use of cocaine increased their risk for IPV at 6-month follow-up (226). In another sample of women who had experienced partner violence, problem drinking was related to revictimization (228). Alcohol use was related to higher rates of depression among African-American women in violent relationships; however, no relation to PTSD symptoms was investigated (229). Although use of substances may increase women's risk for IPV, coercion by an abusive partner may also increase women's risk for drug and alcohol use. The occurrence of PTSD, depression, and other comorbid conditions has important implications for prevention and treatment. These considerations are discussed at greater length in another chapter in this text.

Posttraumatic Stress Disorder and Suicide

Women in violent relationships are at increased risk for suicide, and this risk is compounded by the presence of PTSD (230). Over 90% of women hospitalized following a suicide attempt reported current severe IPV (91,145). In community samples, 23% of women experiencing IPV reported a past suicide attempt versus 3% without a history of IPV, and 36.8% of IPV survivors seriously considered suicide (122). In another study, suicidal thoughts and attempts were higher among IPV survivors experiencing both psychological and physical abuse than among women who experienced psychological abuse alone. This relationship was thought to be related in part to the presence of PTSD and depression (231). Further, comorbid PTSD and depression appears to confer a higher risk than either disorder alone (91,232–235). In fact, the prevalence of suicidal ideation and suicide attempts is significantly higher among women who are battered by their partners (196,236), women who are victims of marital rape and/or sexual assault (77,237–239), and women who have been sexually abused as children (108). A study by Kaslow reported that African-American women who attempted suicide were 2.5 times more likely to have experienced physical abuse and 2.8 times more likely to have experienced emotional abuse by an intimate partner than demographically similar women who had not been abused (240). In addition, according to a 2003 Washington State Fatality Review, 13% of women who committed suicide had a court-documented history of domestic abuse (241). Other states are reporting similar IPV fatality review findings (242).

THE NEUROBIOLOGY OF TRAUMA

Advances in research on the neurobiology of trauma have led to greater understanding of the links between biology, behavior, and psychological distress. Initial research in this area focused on PTSD among Vietnam veterans in Veterans Administration (VA) hospitals. As van der Kolk has described, people with PTSD develop "profound and persistent alterations in physiologic reactivity and stress hormone secretion, making it difficult to properly evaluate sensory stimuli and respond with appropriate levels of physiologic and neurohormonal arousal" (243).

A number of psychophysiological models have been posited to explain PTSD. These include noradrenergic dysregulation (increased sensitivity and reactivity of the sympathetic nervous system under stress), disturbances of serotonergic activity (stress resilience, sleep regulation, impulse control, conditioned avoidance, and aggression and mood), and kindling (lowering of the excitability threshold after repeated electrical stimulation).

After traumatic exposure, limbic nuclei (areas of the brain responsible for regulating emotions and fear) become sensitized, leading to excessive responsivity and increased startle and arousal responses—core features of PTSD that often persist after other symptoms resolve. Activation of the amygdala is postulated to mediate the autonomic stimulation that results from exposure to trauma, transforming sensory input into physiologic signals that, in turn, produce and modulate emotional responses. Neuroimaging studies suggest that alterations to the hippocampus, amygdala, anterior cingulate, and medial prefrontal cortex directly correlate with symptoms of PTSD (244). More specifically, emotional dysregulation is associated with reduced cortical inhibition of limbic circuitry and imbalances in γ-aminobutyric acid (GABA)-aminergic and glutaminergic transmission. Some authors postulate that PTSD may best be viewed as a failure to regain physiological homeostasis after a normal response to trauma (245).

In animal models, stress reduces brain plasticity, flexibility, and new learning by increasing activity in the amygdala (increasing dendritic branching or arborization), reducing hippocampal neurogenesis, and decreasing levels of brain-derived neurotrophic factor (BDNF), a substance critical to buffering against stress and adapting to change (9,246,247). Other studies have found that PTSD treatment can counter these effects (248).

In addition, people with PTSD may exhibit alternation in basal levels of the key stress hormones (including cortisol), as well as enhanced reactivity and negative feedback inhibition of the hypothalamic-pituitary-adrenal axis (HPA)—a pattern that appears to be distinct from that found in depression and from acute and chronic stress among individuals who do not have PTSD (9). Adaptations to chronic stress result in reduced resting glucocorticoid levels, decreased secretion in response to subsequent stress, and increased concentration of glucocorticoid receptors in the hippocampus (9).

Reduced levels of basal cortisol were a consistent finding in samples of combat males with PTSD (249). However, when women—and specifically abused women—were studied, this pattern was not replicated. One small study specifically conducted with DV survivors (chronic nature, frequent comorbidity with depression) found similar results: negative feedback inhibition of the HPA axis occurred among survivors who had PTSD alone, and less cortisol suppression occurred among those who had both depression and PTSD (250,251). In several other studies of IPV survivors, IPV was associated with lower cortisol levels but not to PTSD symptoms, suggesting that HPA axis alterations were a consequence of abuse and not PTSD (100,252). In contrast, two additional studies reported that PTSD symptoms were related to cortisol in abused women. Research also indicates that HPA axis hyperreactivity among women exposed to early childhood abuse causes increased adrenocorticotropic hormone (ACTH) and cortisol responses to stress. These changes in corticotropin releasing factor (CRF) may predispose women to the development of subsequent mood and anxiety disorders (242).

Several studies examined neurological differences among adults who were abused as children, and found that such abuse affects the development of the limbic system and cerebral cortex, particularly the left hemisphere (253), as well as connecting structures such as the corpus callosum, which is utilized to process, interpret, and integrate sensory data (2,254). Early life stress can affect brain development in ways that increase one's vulnerability to developing PTSD as an adult. Postulated mechanisms include accelerated loss of neurons (255), delays in myelination (2), abnormalities in pruning of neurons (201), or reduced levels of brain growth factors including BDNF (4). Functional magnetic resonance imaging (fMRI) studies have utilized a variety of symptom-provocation techniques (e.g., script-driven trauma imagery) to examine differences in responses between subjects with PTSD and controls (256,257). Bremner and colleagues used this technology to examine functional alterations in brain activity among women with histories of childhood sexual abuse, reporting decreased activity in the hippocampus and anterior cingulate cortex and increased activity in the dorsal lateral prefrontal cortex, posterior cingulate, and amygdala, following recall of a traumatic event (9). In another set of studies, Lanius and colleagues examined two different subtypes of trauma response—one primarily characterized by hyperarousal and the other by dissociation. Their findings supported the concept of PTSD as a disorder of affect regulation. People who experience intrusive reexperiencing and hyperarousal activate different neural circuitry than those who experience more numbing and dissociation. One involves the reduced cortical inhibitory control over limbic fear circuitry discussed earlier. The other involves enhanced suppression of fear/arousal responses (increased cortical and reduced limbic activation compared to controls). The authors postulate that survival in the context of ongoing abuse may involve either mechanism—hypervigilance to signs of danger versus psychic numbing when other options are not available (4).

Hippocampal volume has also been reported to be reduced in women who have experienced severe childhood sexual abuse (258). These findings are similar to those of combat veterans with PTSD. Although initially thought to be a consequence of trauma (stress-induced cortisol production causing neurotoxicity), additional research has led to the view of reduced hippocampal volume as a potential risk factor for the development of psychiatric complications following exposure (242). Interestingly, the authors found no differences in memory testing between abused and nonabused groups. They speculate that these data may be better conceptualized as a dysfunction within the systems that monitor and regulate access to memory in emotionally charged contexts, potentially interfering with the processing of new stimuli (259). A study specifically focused on adult survivors of IPV found no differences in hippocampal volume from controls. Other differences were correlated with severity of childhood physical abuse, not current IPV or PTSD (260). In addition, subjects with PTSD exposed to scripts of their traumatic experiences show decreased activity in the speech areas of the left hemisphere (Broca's) necessary for the cognitive labeling and sequencing of experience. This may explain the difficulty some trauma survivors have in processing the initial trauma and subsequent triggering events, and in describing their experiences in a coherent narrative form (261). Reductions in verbal declarative memory but not differences in IQ have been found among survivors of childhood sexual abuse with PTSD as compared to childhood sexual abuse survivors without PTSD and women who had not experienced abuse (8,32,262).

COMPLEX POSTTRAUMATIC STRESS DISORDER OR DISORDERS OF EXTREME STRESS NOT OTHERWISE SPECIFIED

Although the PTSD diagnosis captures many of the psychophysiological responses to adult single-event assault, important dimensions of the impact of ongoing abuse and violence are not addressed by this diagnostic construct. The frequency of comorbidity associated with PTSD, in fact, has led to notion that "comorbidity" is a misnomer, masking a more complex form of PTSD that can develop when people have been abused over long periods of time—one that includes both axis I and axis II sequelae of abuse (8,32,235,262,263). Childhood abuse and entrapment in an abusive partner relationship are qualitatively different from many other types of trauma. As a number of authors describe, these acts are premeditated, ongoing, and most often perpetrated by someone whom the victim is attached to and dependent upon (192). There is often denial and distortion on the part of abuser, and the victim is coerced or threatened to maintain secrecy (8). When abuse occurs during childhood, it has the potential to disrupt neurobiological and social development. *Complex posttraumatic stress disorder* or DESNOS is not officially listed as a diagnosis in the *Diagnostic and Statistical Manual of Mental Disorders* (DSM-IV-TR), although it is contained in the International Classifications of Disease (ICD). The symptoms that comprise DESNOS are listed as associated features of PTSD. DSM-IV field trials indicate that this construct is internally consistent and reliable and distinguishes early- from later-onset trauma (8,14,202,264). Women who are severely abused by a partner may also experience more complex posttraumatic responses, particularly if they were abused in childhood as well. For a more detailed discussion of complex trauma in relation to IPV, see the Chapter 24.

DEVELOPING A MORE COMPLEX TRAUMA FRAMEWORK

The developmental impact of prolonged exposure to abuse by a caretaker, or the effect of intimate partner abuse on a woman's sense of herself, go far beyond what are described by current psychiatric nosology—even by diagnoses that specifically address traumatic events. The effects of abuse in childhood and/or adulthood can affect women's experiences of themselves and others throughout their lives. As noted earlier, many women who have been victimized do not develop psychiatric disorders, but few are unaffected by those experiences. *Trauma theory* provides a framework for understanding symptoms as psychophysiological survival strategies used to adapt to potentially life-shattering situations. It also allows for a more balanced approach to treatment—one that focuses on resilience and strength, as well as on psychological harm (8). For example, trauma theory has reframed borderline symptomatology adaptations to early trauma. Without a trauma framework, it is difficult to make therapeutic sense of the feelings and behaviors that can make life so stormy for survivors of severe abuse. Children who are abused or neglected and who don't have other forms of support are more likely to develop neurophysiological changes than children who are not—changes that can affect their subsequent emotional and physical functioning, including difficulty in recognizing, regulating, and integrating emotions and allowing themselves to be comforted by others (i.e., being able to use relationships appropriately to help them manage internal states), particularly when trust has repeatedly been betrayed (11,265).

Work with survivors of IPV has led to somewhat similar perspectives on viewing symptoms as both adaptations and survival strategies. For example, many women initially attempt to remedy their situations themselves, by talking, seeking help, fighting back, trying to change the conditions either that they perceive or are told cause the abuse. When those attempts fail, they may retreat into a mode that appears more passive and "compliant," but which may actually reflect how they have learned to reduce their immediate danger. When those tactics no longer work, they may learn to dissociate from feelings that have become unbearable, perceiving that even if they can't change what is happening outside of them—or face increasing danger or death if they try to leave—they can at least try to change their own responses and "leave the situation" emotionally. For some women, substance abuse becomes another way of either "coping" or "leaving." For those who become increasingly isolated from outside resources, suicide, or very rarely homicide, may seem like the only way to end the abuse (30).

Even a trauma framework, however, defines an overwhelming response to "minor" stimuli as part of a disorder. Viewing this heightened sensitivity as pathological rather than as a reflection of acute social awareness runs the risk of discounting the experiences that allow a survivor to recognize the kinds of behaviors and attitudes that are potentially dangerous before they reach more serious levels. The risk of purely clinical models is in defining the problem as being "in the patient," who then becomes the focus of intervention, particularly when this occurs at the expense of attending to issues such as immediate safety and support or to broader system and societal change.

CONCLUSION: MENTAL HEALTH APPROACHES TO INTIMATE PARTNER VIOLENCE—COMBINING TRAUMA AND ADVOCACY PERSPECTIVES

Trauma theory has evolved in ways that now make it a more useful framework for understanding the impact of chronic abuse, including IPV. Although trauma models are not a substitute for advocacy-based approaches that help survivors achieve freedom and safety and work to end IPV, trauma theory can enhance clinical work by increasing understanding of the psychological consequences of abuse and how trauma affects both IPV survivors (and their children) and the clinicians and systems that serve them. Trauma theory provides a framework for understanding the mental health effects of abuse and violence in a way that normalizes human responses to trauma and recognizes the role of external events in the generation of mental health symptoms.

Not only does a trauma framework help destigmatize vulnerability that stems from responses to earlier trauma, it also provides a more nuanced developmental understanding of how individuals come to be who and where they are in their lives that reflects the complex interplay of neurobiology, relationships, environment/social conditions, and experience. A trauma model also fits with peer support recovery approaches (i.e., if the harm occurs in a relationship, then healing often takes place through relationships as well; people can develop new skills to address the capacities that were disrupted or derailed). Both trauma models and advocacy perspectives recognize the resilience and strength of survivors in dealing with both individual abuse and social disenfranchisement.

Trauma models also offer guidance on creating services that are sensitive to the experiences of survivors of chronic abuse and that incorporate an understanding of how those experiences can affect one's ability to regulate emotions, process information, and attend to one's surroundings. They provide tools for responding skillfully and empathically to individuals for whom trust is a critical issue, without having one's own reactions interfere. Trauma-informed service environments offer emotional as well as physical safety and are consistent with DV advocacy and mental health peer support models in their focus on empowerment, collaboration, and choice. They are also designed to ensure that services themselves do not retraumatize survivors and that they provide strategies to attend to the impact on clinicians.

Adapting trauma theory to create more comprehensive and attuned practice environments and treatment models holds promise for creating services that are more responsive to survivors' experiences and needs. Although existing trauma models need to be adapted and reframed to address the particular issues faced by survivors of IPV, ongoing exploration is necessary to address the applicability of these models for a diverse range of communities and to develop alternate models for healing that may be more community-based. Whether it is partnering with IPV programs in ways that enhance their ability to respond to trauma-related mental health issues, or ensuring that survivors are able to access culturally relevant, trauma-specific mental health care, issues of philosophy, resources, training, and collaboration are vitally important.

IMPLICATIONS FOR POLICY, PRACTICE, AND RESEARCH

Policy

- Policies need to be developed and implemented within the private and publicly funded mental health systems that incorporate attention to ongoing IPV and other lifetime trauma, including routine assessment, attending to physical and emotional safety, and supporting the use of treatment models that are culture, trauma, and IPV-informed.

- Policy initiatives on peripartum depression should include assessment and intervention for current and past abuse.
- State and federal policies should address the needs of people living with mental illness who may be at greater risk for experiencing violence and abuse.

Practice

- Standards of mental health training and practice should incorporate an understanding of the role of abuse and violence in the development of psychiatric symptoms and disorders, as well as the ways abusers use mental health issues to control and undermine their partners.
- Attention to the specific issues faced by survivors of ongoing IPV should be incorporated into professional mental health training and practice, including initiatives to create trauma-informed services.
- Treatment for the mental health effects of IPV should incorporate recognition of the complexities of survivors' lives and the need to develop flexible, multimodal approaches to addressing trauma in the context of ongoing IPV.

Research

- Researchers examining the mental health effects of IPV should incorporate an understanding of IPV as a social condition with a range of mental health effects, and should be cognizant of the ways decontextualized approaches can promote stigma and reinforce the ability of abusers and public systems to use mental health issues against survivors of IPV.
- A need exists to develop and utilize standardized measures that better reflect survivors' experience and that are both culturally relevant and culturally normed, taking care to contextualize findings, to not overgeneralize from women in crisis, and to examine the range of survivors' responses, not just the mean. In designing research, potential consequences to survivors should always be kept in mind.
- Research on mental health and IPV should begin to integrate newer findings from the fields of child development and neuroscience in ways that help destigmatize the psychophysiological consequences of abuse

and violence and promote both safety and recovery.

- Research is needed to examine the interactions between ongoing abuse and a range of mental health effects and their implications for both treatment and advocacy interventions. This should include survivors of IPV who are also experiencing other coexisting psychiatric conditions and chronic mental illness.
- Research should also be designed to examine the range of factors that affect survivors' experience and their ability to access safety, as well as to determine optimal approaches to treatment, particularly in the context of ongoing IPV.

References

1. Felitti VJ, Anda RF, Nordenberg D, et al. Relationship of childhood abuse and household dysfunction to many of the leading causes of death in adults. The Adverse Childhood Experiences (ACE) Study. *Am J Prev Med*. 1998;14(4):245–258.

2. De Bellis MD, Van Dillen T. Childhood post-traumatic stress disorder: An overview. *Child Adolesc Psychiatr Clin N Am*. 2005;14(4):745–772, ix.

3. Classen CC, Pain C, Field NP, Woods P. Post-traumatic personality disorder: A reformulation of complex posttraumatic stress disorder and borderline personality disorder. *Psychiatr Clin North Am*. 2006;29(1):87–112, viii-ix.

4. Lanius RA, Bluhm R, Lanius U, Pain C. A review of neuroimaging studies in PTSD: Heterogeneity of response to symptom provocation. *J Psychiatr Res*. 2006;40(8):709–729.

5. Lyons-Ruth K, Dutra L, Schuder MR, Bianchi I. From infant attachment disorganization to adult dissociation: Relational adaptations or traumatic experiences? *Psychiatr Clin North Am*. 2006; 29(1):63–86, viii.

6. McEwen BS. Protective and damaging effects of stress mediators: Central role of the brain. *Dialogues Clin Neurosci*. 2006;8(4):367–381.

7. Nemeroff CB. Neurobiological consequences of childhood trauma. *J Clin Psychiatry*. 2004;65 (Suppl 1):18–28.

8. van der Kolk BA, Roth S, Pelcovitz D, et al. Disorders of extreme stress: The empirical foundation of a complex adaptation to trauma. *J Trauma Stress*. 2005;18(5):389–399.

9. Yehuda R. Advances in understanding neuroendocrine alterations in PTSD and their therapeutic implications. *Ann N Y Acad Sci*. 2006; 1071: 137–166.

10. Warshaw C, Gugenheim AM, Moroney G, Barnes H. Fragmented services, unmet needs: Building collaboration between the mental health and domestic violence communities. *Health Aff (Millwood)*. 2003;22(5):230–234.

11. Warshaw C, Pease T, Markham DW, et al. *Access to advocacy: Serving women with psychiatric disabilities in domestic violence settings*. Chicago: Domestic Violence & Mental Health Policy Initiative, 2007.

12. Warshaw C, Moroney G, Barnes H. *Report on mental health issues and service needs in Chicago-area domestic violence programs*. Chicago: Domestic Violence & Mental Health Policy Initiative, 2003.

13. Brown LS. Not outside the range: One feminist perspective on psychic trauma. In: Caruth C, ed. *Trauma: Explorations in memory*. Baltimore: Johns Hopkins University Press;1995:100–112.

14. Herman JL. *Trauma and recovery: The aftermath of violence: Domestic abuse to political terror*. New York: Basic Books, 1992.

15. Anda RF, Felitti VJ, Bremner JD, et al. The enduring effects of abuse and related adverse experiences in childhood: A convergence of evidence from neurobiology and epidemiology. *Eur Arch Psychiatry Clin Neurosci*. 2006;256(3):174–186.

16. Putnam FW. Dissociative phenomena. In: Tasman A, Goldfinger S, eds. *Review of psychiatry*, Vol. 10. Washington, DC: American Psychiatric Association Press, 1991:145–160.

17. Schore AN. Dysregulation of the right brain: A fundamental mechanism of traumatic attachment and the psychopathogenesis of posttraumatic stress disorder. *Aust N Z J Psychiatry*. 2002;36(1):9–30.

18. Shonkoff J, Phillips D. *From neurons to neighborhoods: The science of early childhood development*. Washington, DC: National Academies Press, 1997.

19. Teicher MH, Andersen SL, Polcari A, et al. Developmental neurobiology of childhood stress and trauma. *Psychiatr Clin North Am*. 2002;25(2): 397–426, vii-viii.

20. van der Kolk B, McFarlane A, Weisaeth C, eds. *Traumatic stress: The effects of overwhelming experience on mind, body, and society*. New York: Guilford, 1996.

21. Bloom S. *Creating sanctuary: Toward an evolution of sane societies*. New York: Routledge, 1997.

22. Horowitz MJ. *Stress response syndromes*, 2nd ed. Northvale, NJ: Jason Aronson, 1986.

23. Burgess AW, Holmstrom LL. Rape trauma syndrome. *Am J Psychiatry*. 1974;131(9):981–986.

24. Walker LE. *The battered woman syndrome*. New York: Springer, 1984.

25. Crowell NA, Burgess AW. Prevention and intervention. In: Crowell NA, Burgess AW, eds. *Understanding violence against women*. Washington, DC: National Academy Press;1996:93–141.

26. Garcia-Moreno C. WHO *multi-country study on women's health and domestic violence against women: Initial results on prevalence, health outcomes, and women's responses*. Geneva: World Health Organization, 2005.

27. Heise LL, Pitanguy J, Germain A. *Violence against women: The hidden burden.* Washington, DC: The World Bank;1994:255.

28. Koss MP, Goodman LA, Browne L, et al. *No safe haven: Male violence against women at home, at work, and in the community.* Washington, DC: American Psychological Association, 1994.

29. Mowbray CT, Oyserman D, Saunders D, Rueda-Riedle A. Women with severe mental disorders: Issues and service needs. In: Levin BL, Blanch AK, Jennings A, eds. *Women's mental health services: A public health perspective.* Thousand Oaks, CA: Sage;1998:175–200.

30. Harris M, Fallot RD, eds. *Using trauma theory to design service systems.* San Francisco: Jossey-Bass, 2001.

31. Herman JL. Complex PTSD: A syndrome in survivors of prolonged and repeated trauma. *J Trauma Stress.* 1992;5:377–391.

32. Roth S, Newman E, Pelcovitz D, et al. Complex PTSD in victims exposed to sexual and physical abuse: Results from the DSM-IV Field Trial for Posttraumatic Stress Disorder. *J Trauma Stress.* 1997;10(4):539–555.

33. Weaver IC, La Plante P, Weaver S, et al. Early environmental regulation of hippocampal glucocorticoid receptor gene expression: Characterization of intracellular mediators and potential genomic target sites. *Mol Cell Endocrinol.* 2001;185 (1–2):205–218.

34. Lang AJ, Stein MB, Kennedy CM, Foy DW. Adult psychopathology and intimate partner violence among survivors of childhood maltreatment. *J Interpers Violence.* 2004;19(10):1102–1118.

35. Stermac L, Reist D, Addison M, Miller G. Childhood risk factors for women's sexual revictimization. *J Interpers Violence.* 2002;17(6):647–670.

36. Wenzel SL, Tucker JS, Elliott MN, et al. Physical violence against impoverished women: A longitudinal analysis of risk and protective factors. *Womens Health Issues.* 2004;14(5):144–154.

37. Bensley L, Van Eenwyk J, Wynkoop Simmons K. Childhood family violence history and women's risk for intimate partner violence and poor health. *Am J Prev Med.* 2003;25(1):38–44.

38. Classen CC, Palesh OG, Aggarwal R. Sexual revictimization: A review of the empirical literature. *Trauma Violence Abuse.* 2005;6(2):103–129.

39. Cloitre M, Tardiff K, Marzuk PM, et al. Childhood abuse and subsequent sexual assault among female inpatients. *J Trauma Stress.* 1996;9(3):473–482.

40. Coker AL, Watkins KW, Smith PH, Brandt HM. Social support reduces the impact of partner violence on health: Application of structural equation models. *Prev Med.* 2003;37(3):259–267.

41. Desai S, Arias I, Thompson MP, Basile KC. Childhood victimization and subsequent adult revictimization assessed in a nationally representative sample of women and men. *Violence Vict.* 2002;17(6):639–653.

42. Lindhorst T, Oxford M. The long-term effects of intimate partner violence on adolescent mothers' depressive symptoms. *Soc Sci Med.* 2008;66(6):1322–1333.

43. Kimerling R, Alvarez J, Pavao J, et al. Epidemiology and consequences of women's revictimization. *Womens Health Issues.* 2007;17(2):101–106.

44. Golding JM. Unpublished manuscript. Chicago: Domestic Violence and Mental Health Policy Initiative, 2000.

45. Astin MC, Ogland-Hand SM, Coleman EM, Foy DS. Posttraumatic stress disorder and childhood abuse in battered women: Comparisons with maritally distressed women. *J Consult Clin Psychol.* 1995;63(2):308–312.

46. Briere J, Runtz M. Symptomatology associated with childhood sexual victimization in a nonclinical adult sample. *Child Abuse Negl.* 1988;12(1):51–59.

47. Bryer JB, Nelson BA, Miller JB, Krol PA. Childhood sexual and physical abuse as factors in adult psychiatric illness. *Am J Psychiatry.* 1987;144(11): 1426–1430.

48. Burstow B. Toward a radical understanding of trauma and trauma work. *Violence Against Women.* 2003;9(11):1293–1317.

49. Danieli Y, ed. *International handbook of multigenerational legacies of trauma.* New York: Plenum Press, 1998.

50. Duran B, Duran E, Yellow-Horse Braveheart M. Native Americans and the trauma of history. In: Thornton R, ed. *Studying Native America: Problems and prospects in Native American Studies.* Madison: University of Wisconsin Press, 1998.

51. Epstein JN, Saunders BE, Kilpatrick DG. Predicting PTSD in women with a history of childhood rape. *J Trauma Stress.* 1997;10(4):573–588.

52. Langeland W, Hartgers C. Child sexual and physical abuse and alcoholism: A review. *J Stud Alcohol.* 1998;59(3):336–348.

53. Wilsnack SC, Vogeltanz ND, Klassen AD, Harris TR. Childhood sexual abuse and women's substance abuse: national survey findings. *J Stud Alcohol.* 1997;58(3):264–271.

54. Bassuk EL, Buckner JC, Weinreb LF, et al. Homelessness in female-headed families: Childhood and adult risk and protective factors. *Am J Public Health.* 1997;87(2):241–248.

55. Browne A. Family violence and homelessness: The relevance of trauma histories in the lives of homeless women. *Am J Orthopsychiatry.* 1993;63(3): 370–384.

56. Allard MA, Albelda R, Colten ME, Costenza C. *In harm's way? Domestic violence, AFDC receipt, and welfare reform in Massachusetts.* Boston: University of Massachusetts, McCormack Institute, 1997.

57. Lloyd S. *The effects of violence on women's employment.* Chicago: Joint Center for Poverty Research, 1996.

58. Raphael J. *Domestic violence: Telling the untold welfare-to-work story.* Chicago, IL: Taylor Institute, 1995.

59. Tjaden P, Thoennes N. Prevalence and consequences of male-to-female and female-to-male intimate partner violence as measured by the National Violence Against Women Survey. *Violence Against Women.* 2000;6(2):142–161.

60. Brown LS, Root MP, eds. *Diversity and complexity in feminist therapy.* New York: Haworth, 1990.

61. Espin OM, Gawelek MA. Women's diversity: Ethnicity, race, class, and gender in theories of feminist psychology. In: Ballou M, Brown LS, eds. *Personality and psychopathology: Feminist reappraisals.* New York: Guilford;1992:88–107.

62. Greene B. African American women. In: Comas-Diaz L, Greene B, eds. *Women of color: Integrating ethnic and gender identities in psychotherapy.* New York: Guilford;1994:10–29.

63. Krieger N. Inequality, diversity, and health: Thoughts on "race/ethnicity" and "gender." *J Am Med Womens Assoc.* 1996;51(4):133–136.

64. Root MP. Women of color and traumatic stress in "domestic captivity": Gender and race as disempowering statuses. In: Marella A, Friedman M, Gerrity E, Scuffled R, eds. *Ethnocultural aspects of posttraumatic stress disorder: Issues, research and clinical applications.* Washington, DC: American Psychological Association, 1996.

65. Weskott M. *The feminist legacy of Karen Horney.* New Haven: Yale University Press, 1986.

66. Ruzek SB, Olesen VL, Clarke A, eds. *Women's health: Complexities and differences.* Columbus: Ohio State University Press, 1997.

67. Warshaw C. Women and violence. In: Stotland NL, Stewart DE, eds. *Psychological aspects of women's health care: The interface between psychiatry and obstetrics and gynecology,* 2nd ed. Washington, DC: American Psychiatric Press;2001: 477–548.

68. Briere J, Woo R, McRae B, et al. Lifetime victimization history, demographics, and clinical status in female psychiatric emergency room patients. *J Nerv Ment Dis.* 1997;185(2):95–101.

69. Goodman LA, Dutton MA, Harris M. The relationship between violence dimensions and symptom severity among homeless, mentally ill women. *J Trauma Stress.* 1997;10(1):51–70.

70. Goodman LA, Salyers MP, Mueser KT, et al. Recent victimization in women and men with severe mental illness: Prevalence and correlates. *J Trauma Stress.* 2001;14(4):615–632.

71. Caton CL, Shrout PE, Dominguez B, et al. Risk factors for homelessness among women with schizophrenia. *Am J Public Health.* 1995;85 (8 Pt 1):1153–1156.

72. Shinn M, Weitzman BC, Stojanovic D, et al. Predictors of homelessness among families in New York City: From shelter request to housing stability. *Am J Public Health.* 1998;88(11):1651–1657.

73. Alexander MJ, Muenzenmaier K. Trauma, addiction, and recovery: Addressing public health epidemics among women with severe mental illness. In: Levin BL, Blanch AK, Jennings A, eds. *Women's mental health services: A public health perspective.* Thousand Oaks, CA: Sage;1998:215–239.

74. Carmen EH. Inner-city community mental health: The interplay of abuse and race in chronic mentally ill women. In: Willie CV, Rieker PP, Kramer BM, eds. *Mental health, racism and sexism.* Pittsburgh, PA: University of Pittsburgh;1995:217–236.

75. Friedman SH, Loue S. Incidence and prevalence of intimate partner violence by and against women with severe mental illness. *J Womens Health (Larchmt).* 2007;16(4):471–480.

76. Gearon JS, Bellack AS. Women with schizophrenia and co-occurring substance use disorders: An increased risk for violent victimization and HIV. *Community Ment Health J.* 1999;35(5):401–419.

77. Gladstone GL, Parker GB, Mitchell PB, et al. Implications of childhood trauma for depressed women: An analysis of pathways from childhood sexual abuse to deliberate self-harm and revictimization. *Am J Psychiatry.* 2004;161(8):1417–1425.

78. Mezey G, Bacchus L, Bewley S, White S. Domestic violence, lifetime trauma and psychological health of childbearing women. *BJOG.* 2005;112(2): 197–204.

79. Ramos BM, Carlson BE, McNutt L-A. Lifetime abuse, mental health, and African American women. *J Fam Violence.* 2004;19(3):153–164.

80. Renner LM, Slack KS. Intimate partner violence and child maltreatment: Understanding intra- and intergenerational connections. *Child Abuse Negl.* 2006;30(6):599–617.

81. Carmen EH, Rieker PP, Mills T. Victims of violence and psychiatric illness. *Am J Psychiatry.* 1984;141(3):378–383.

82. Craine LS, Henson CE, Colliver JA, MacLean DG. Prevalence of a history of sexual abuse among female psychiatric patients in a state hospital system. *Hosp Community Psychiatry.* 1988;39(3): 300–304.

83. Cusack KJ, Grubaugh AL, Knapp RG, Frueh BC. Unrecognized trauma and PTSD among public mental health consumers with chronic and severe mental illness. *Community Ment Health J.* 2006;42(5):487–500.

84. Jacobson A, Richardson B. Assault experiences of 100 psychiatric inpatients: Evidence of the need for routine inquiry. *Am J Psychiatry.* 1987;144(7): 908–913.

85. Lipschitz DS, Kaplan ML, Sorkenn JB, et al. Prevalence and characteristics of physical and sexual abuse among psychiatric outpatients. *Psychiatr Serv.* 1996;47(2):189–191.

86. Lombardo S, Pohl R. Sexual abuse history of women treated in a psychiatric outpatient clinic. *Psychiatr Serv.* 1997;48(4):534–536.

87. Rosenberg SD, Lu W, Mueser KT, et al. Correlates of adverse childhood events among adults with schizophrenia spectrum disorders. *Psychiatr Serv.* 2007;58(2):245–253.

88. Neria Y, Bromet EJ, Sievers S, et al. Trauma exposure and posttraumatic stress disorder in psychosis: Findings from a first-admission cohort. *J Consult Clin Psychol.* 2002;70(1):246–251.

89. Cascardi M, Mueser KT, DeGiralomo J, Murrin M. Physical aggression against psychiatric inpatients by family members and partners. *Psychiatr Serv.* 1996;47(5):531–533.

90. Sajdak L. Personal communication. 2005.

91. Coker AL, Davis KE, Arias I, et al. Physical and mental health effects of intimate partner violence for men and women. *Am J Prev Med.* 2002;23(4):260–268.

92. Mueser KT, Rosenberg SD, Goodman LA, Trumbetta SL. Trauma, PTSD, and the course of severe mental illness: An interactive model. *Schizophr Res.* 2002;53(1–2):123–143.

93. Plichta SB, Falik M. Prevalence of violence and its implications for women's health. *Womens Health Issues.* 2001;11(3):244–258.

94. Bebbington PE, Bhugra D, Brugha T, et al. Psychosis, victimisation and childhood disadvantage: Evidence from the second British National Survey of Psychiatric Morbidity. *Br J Psychiatry.* 2004;185:220–226.

95. Bonomi AE, Thompson RS, Anderson M, et al. Intimate partner violence and women's physical, mental, and social functioning. *Am J Prev Med.* 2006;30(6):458–466.

96. Chapman DP, Whitfield CL, Felitti VJ, et al. Adverse childhood experiences and the risk of depressive disorders in adulthood. *J Affect Disord.* 2004;82(2):217–225.

97. Dube SR, Anda RF, Whitfield CL, et al. Long-term consequences of childhood sexual abuse by gender of victim. *Am J Prev Med.* 2005;28(5):430–438.

98. Edwards VJ, Holden GW, Felitti VJ, Anda RF. Relationship between multiple forms of childhood maltreatment and adult mental health in community respondents: Results from the adverse childhood experiences study. *Am J Psychiatry.* 2003;160(8):1453–1460.

99. Garno JL, Goldberg JF, Ramirez PM, Ritzler BA. Impact of childhood abuse on the clinical course of bipolar disorder. *Br J Psychiatry.* 2005;186:121–125.

100. Heim C, Nemeroff CB. The role of childhood trauma in the neurobiology of mood and anxiety disorders: Preclinical and clinical studies. *Biol Psychiatry.* 2001;49(12):1023–1039.

101. Kessler RC, Chiu WT, Demler O, et al. Prevalence, severity, and comorbidity of 12-month DSM-IV disorders in the National Comorbidity Survey Replication. *Arch Gen Psychiatry.* 2005;62(6):617–627.

102. Logan TK, Shannon L, Cole J, Walker R. The impact of differential patterns of physical violence and stalking on mental health and help-seeking among women with protective orders. *Violence Against Women.* 2006;12(9):866–886.

103. McCauley J, Kern DE, Kolodner K, et al. Clinical characteristics of women with a history of childhood abuse: unhealed wounds. *JAMA.* 1997;277(17):1362–1368.

104. Read J, Perry BD, Moskowitz A, Connolly J. The contribution of early traumatic events to schizophrenia in some patients: A traumagenic neurodevelopmental model. *Psychiatry.* 2001;64(4):319–345.

105. Kernic MA, Holt VL, Stoner JA, et al. Resolution of depression among victims of intimate partner violence: is cessation of violence enough? *Violence Vict.* 2003;18(2):115–129.

106. Graffunder CM, Noonan RK, Cox P, Wheaton J. Through a public health lens. Preventing violence against women: An update from the US Centers for Disease Control and Prevention. *J Womens Health (Larchmt).* 2004;13(1):5–16.

107. Lipsky S, Caetano R. Impact of intimate partner violence on unmet need for mental health care: Results from the NSDUH. *Psychiatr Serv.* 2007;58(6):822–829.

108. Kaslow NJ, Thompson MP, Okun A, et al. Risk and protective factors for suicidal behavior in abused African American women. *J Consult Clin Psychol.* 2002;70(2):311–319.

109. Kovac SH, Klapow JC, Kroenke K, et al. Differing symptoms of abused versus nonabused women in obstetric-gynecology settings. *Am J Obstet Gynecol.* 2003;188(3):707–713.

110. McCauley J, Kern DE, Kolodner K, et al. Relation of low-severity violence to women's health. *J Gen Intern Med.* 1998;13(10):687–691.

111. Koss MP, Bailey JA, Yuan NP, et al. Depression and PTSD in survivors of male violence: Research and training initiatives to facilitate recovery. *Psychol Women Q.* 2003;27(2):130–142.

112. Dickinson LM, deGruy FV, 3rd, Dickinson WP, Candib LM. Health-related quality of life and symptom profiles of female survivors of sexual abuse. *Arch Fam Med.* 1999;8(1):35–43.

113. Jarvis KL, Gordon EE, Novaco RW. Psychological distress of children and mothers in domestic violence emergency shelters. *J Fam Violence.* 2005;20(6):389–402.

114. Hegarty K, Gunn J, Chondros P, Small R. Association between depression and abuse by partners of women attending general practice: Descriptive, cross sectional survey. *BMJ.* 2004;328(7440):621–624.

115. Zlotnick C, Johnson DM, Kohn R. Intimate partner violence and long-term psychosocial functioning in a national sample of American women. *J Interpers Violence.* 2006;21(2):262–275.

116. Fogarty CT, Fredman L, Heeren TC, Liebschutz J. Synergistic effects of child abuse and intimate partner violence on depressive symptoms in women. *Prev Med.* 2008;46(5):463–469.

117. Campbell JC, Kub J, Belknap RA, Templin TN. Predictors of depression in battered women. *Violence Against Women.* 1997;3(3):271–293.

118. Cascardi M, O'Leary KD, Schlee KA. Co-occurrence and correlates of posttraumatic stress disorder and major depression in physically abused women. *J Fam Violence*. 1999;14(3):227–249.

119. Dienemann J, Boyle E, Baker D, et al. Intimate partner abuse among women diagnosed with depression. *Issues Ment Health Nurs*. 2000;21(5):499–513.

120. Koopman C, Ismailji T, Palesh O, et al. Relationships of depression to child and adult abuse and bodily pain among women who have experienced intimate partner violence. *J Interpers Violence*. 2007;22(4):438–455.

121. Pico-Alfonso MA. Psychological intimate partner violence: The major predictor of posttraumatic stress disorder in abused women. *Neurosci Biobehav Rev*. 2005;29(1):181–193.

122. Pico-Alfonso MA, Garcia-Linares MI, Celda-Navarro N, et al. The impact of physical, psychological, and sexual intimate male partner violence on women's mental health: Depressive symptoms, posttraumatic stress disorder, state anxiety, and suicide. *J Womens Health (Larchmt)*. 2006;15(5):599–611.

123. Kocot T, Goodman LA. The roles of coping and social support in battered women's mental health. *Violence Against Women*. 2003;9(3):323–346.

124. Mitchell MD, Hargrove GL, Collins MH, et al. Coping variables that mediate the relation between intimate partner violence and mental health outcomes among low-income, African American women. *J Clin Psychol*. 2006;62(12):1503–1520.

125. Campbell JC, Soeken KL. Women's responses to battering over time: An analysis of change. *J Interpers Violence*. 1999;14(1):21–40.

126. Astin MC, Lawrence KJ, Foy DW. Posttraumatic stress disorder among battered women: Risk and resiliency factors. *Violence Vict*. 1993;8(1):17–28.

127. Campbell R, Sullivan CM, Davidson WS. Women who use domestic violence shelters: Changes in depression over time. *Psychol Women Q*. 1996;19(2):237–255.

128. Ruch LO, Amedeo SR, Leon JJ, Gartrell JW. Repeated sexual victimization and trauma change during the acute phase of the sexual assault trauma syndrome. *Women Health*. 1991;17(1):1–19.

129. Frank E, Stewart BD. Depressive symptoms in rape victims. A revisit. *J Affect Disord*. 1984;7(1):77–85.

130. Neville HA, Heppner MJ. Contextualizing rape: Reviewing sequelae and proposing a culturally inclusive ecological model of sexual assault recovery. *Appl Prev Psychol*. 1999;8:41–62.

131. Rothbaum B, Foa EB, Riggs SA. A prospective examination of post-traumatic stress disorder in rape victims. *J Trauma Stress*. 1992;5:455–475.

132. Rothbaum BO, Foa EB. Symptoms of posttraumatic stress disorder and duration of symptoms. In: Davidson JR, Foa EB, eds. *Posttraumatic Stress Disorder: DSM-IV and beyond*. Washington, DC: American Psychiatric Association Press;1993:23–26.

133. Resick PA. The psychological impact of rape. *J Interpers Violence*. 1993;8(2):223–255.

134. Brett K, Barfield, W., Williams, C. Prevalence of self-reported postpartum depressive symptoms:17 states, 2004–2005. *MMWR*. 2008 57(14):361–366.

135. Nemeroff CBH, Thase ME, Klein DN, et al. Differential responses to psychotherapy versus pharmacotherapy in patients with chronic forms of major depression and childhood trauma. *Proc Natl Acad Sci*. 2003;100(24):14293–14296.

136. Fedovskiy K, Higgins S, Paranjape A. Intimate partner violence: How does it impact major depressive disorder and post traumatic stress disorder among immigrant Latinas? *J Immigr Minor Health*. 2008;10(1):45–51.

137. Hapke U, Schumann A, Rumpf HJ, et al. Posttraumatic stress disorder: The role of trauma, preexisting psychiatric disorders, and gender. *Eur Arch Psychiatry Clin Neurosci*. 2006;256(5):299–306.

138. Breslau N, Davis GC, Peterson EL, Schultz LR. A second look at comorbidity in victims of trauma: The posttraumatic stress disorder-major depression connection. *Biol Psychiatry*. 2000;48(9):902–909.

139. Galea S, Vlahov D, Tracy M, et al. Hispanic ethnicity and posttraumatic stress disorder after a disaster: Evidence from a general population survey after September 11, 2001. *Ann Epidemiol*. 2004;14(8):520–531.

140. O'Campo P, Kub J, Woods A, et al. Depression, PTSD, and comorbidity related to intimate partner violence in civilian and military women. *Brief Treat Crisis Interv*. 2006;6(2):99–110.

141. O'Donnell ML, Creamer M, Pattison P, Atkin C. Psychiatric morbidity following injury. *Am J Psychiatry*. 2004;161(3):507–514.

142. Shalev AY, Freedman S. PTSD following terrorist attacks: A prospective evaluation. *Am J Psychiatry*. 2005;162(6):1188–1191.

143. Coker AL, Weston R, Creson DL, et al. PTSD symptoms among men and women survivors of |intimate partner violence: The role of risk and protective factors. *Violence Vict*. 2005;20(6):625–643.

144. Lipsky S, Field CA, Caetano R, Larkin GL. Posttraumatic stress disorder symptomatology and comorbid depressive symptoms among abused women referred from emergency department care. *Violence Vict*. 2005;20(6):645–659.

145. Seedat S, Stein MB, Forde DR. Association between physical partner violence, posttraumatic stress, childhood trauma, and suicide attempts in a community sample of women. *Violence Vict*. 2005;20(1):87–98.

146. Nixon RDV, Resick PA, Nishith P. An exploration of comorbid depression among female victims of intimate partner violence with posttraumatic stress disorder. *J Affect Disord*. 2004;82(2):315–320.

147. First MB. *A research agenda for DSM-V: Summary of the DSM-V Preplanning White Papers*: APPI, 2002.

148. Kaysen D, Resick PA, Wise D. Living in danger: The impact of chronic traumatization and the traumatic context on posttraumatic stress disorder. *Trauma Violence Abuse.* 2003;4(3):247–264.

149. Chalk RA, King PA. *Violence in families: Assessing prevention and treatment programs.* Washington, DC: National Academies Press, 1998.

150. Birmes P, Brunet A, Carreras D, et al. The predictive power of peritraumatic dissociation and acute stress symptoms for posttraumatic stress symptoms: A three-month prospective study. *Am J Psychiatry.* 2003;160(7):1337–1339.

151. Brewin CR, Andrews B, Rose S. Diagnostic overlap between acute stress disorder and PTSD in victims of violent crime. *Am J Psychiatry.* 2003;160(4): 783–785.

152. Briere J, Scott C, Weathers F. Peritraumatic and persistent dissociation in the presumed etiology of PTSD. *Am J Psychiatry.* 2005;162(12):2295–2301.

153. Ozer EJ, Best SR, Lipsey TL, Weiss DS. Predictors of posttraumatic stress disorder and symptoms in adults: A meta-analysis. *Psychol Bull.* 2003;129(1):52–73.

154. Breslau N, Davis GC, Andreski P, et al. Sex differences in posttraumatic stress disorder. *Arch Gen Psychiatry.* 1997;54(11):1044–1048.

155. Kessler RC, Sonnega A, Bromet E, et al. Posttraumatic stress disorder in the national comorbidity survey. *Arch Gen Psychiatry.* 1995;52(12): 1048–1060.

156. Olff M, Langeland W, Draijer N, Gersons BP. Gender differences in posttraumatic stress disorder. *Psychol Bull.* 2007;133(2):183–204.

157. Stein MB, Walker JR, Forde DR. Gender differences in susceptibility to posttraumatic stress disorder. *Behav Res Ther.* 2000;38(6):619–628.

158. Turner JB, Turse NA, Dohrenwend BP. Circumstances of service and gender differences in war-related PTSD: Findings from the National Vietnam Veteran Readjustment Study. *J Trauma Stress.* 2007;20(4):643–649.

159. Breslau N, Kessler RC, Chilcoat HD, et al. Trauma and posttraumatic stress disorder in the community: The 1996 Detroit Area Survey of Trauma. *Arch Gen Psychiatry.* 1998;55(7):626–632.

160. Liebschutz J, Saitz R, Brower V, et al. PTSD in urban primary care: High prevalence and low physician recognition. *J Gen Intern Med.* 2007; 22(6):719–726.

161. Walker JL, Carey PD, Mohr N, et al. Gender differences in the prevalence of childhood sexual abuse and in the development of pediatric PTSD. *Arch Womens Ment Health.* 2004;7(2):111–121.

162. Breslau N AJ. Gender differences in the sensitivity to posttraumatic stress disorder: An epidemiological study of urban young adults. *J Abnorm Psychol.* 2007;116(3):607–611.

163. Perkonigg A, Kessler RC, Storz S, Wittchen HU. Traumatic events and post-traumatic stress disorder in the community: Prevalence, risk factors and comorbidity. *Acta Psychiatr Scand.* 2000; 101(1):46–59.

164. Baker CK, Norris FH, Diaz DM, et al. Violence and PTSD in Mexico: Gender and regional differences. *Soc Psychiatry Psychiatr Epidemiol.* 2005;40(7): 519–528.

165. Holbrook TL, Hoyt DB, Stein MB, Sieber WJ. Gender differences in long-term posttraumatic stress disorder outcomes after major trauma: Women are at higher risk of adverse outcomes than men. *J Trauma.* 2002;53(5):882–888.

166. Pulcino T, Galea S, Ahern J, et al. Posttraumatic stress in women after the September 11 terrorist attacks in New York City. *J Womens Health (Larchmt).* 2003;12(8):809–820.

167. Seedat S, Stein DJ, Carey PD. Post-traumatic stress disorder in women: Epidemiological and treatment issues. *CNS Drugs.* 2005;19(5):411–427.

168. Tolin DF, Foa EB. Sex differences in trauma and posttraumatic stress disorder: A quantitative review of 25 years of research. *Psychol Bull.* 2006;132(6): 959–992.

169. Cortina LM, Kubiak SP. Gender and posttraumatic stress: Sexual violence as an explanation for women's increased risk. *J Abnorm Psychol.* 2006;115(4): 753–759.

170. Dutton MA, Goodman LA, Bennett L. Court-involved battered women's responses to violence: The role of psychological, physical, and sexual abuse. *Violence Vict.* 1999;14(1):89–104.

171. Kemp A, Rawlings EI, Green BL. Post-traumatic stress disorder (PTSD) in battered women: A shelter sample. *J Trauma Stress.* 1991;4(1): 137–148.

172. Kubany ES, McKenzie WF, Owens JA, et al. PTSD among women survivors of domestic violence in Hawaii. *Hawaii Med J.* 1996;55(9):164–165.

173. Woods SJ, Wineman NM. Trauma, posttraumatic stress disorder symptom clusters, and physical health symptoms in postabused women. *Arch Psychiatr Nurs.* 2004;18(1):26–34.

174. Mertin P, Mohr PB. A follow-up study of posttraumatic stress disorder, anxiety, and depression in Australian victims of domestic violence. *Violence Vict.* 2001;16:645–654.

175. Woods SJ. Prevalence and patterns of posttraumatic stress disorder in abused and postabused women. *Issues Ment Health Nurs.* 2000;21(3):309–324.

176. Perkonigg A, Pfister H, Stein MB, et al. Longitudinal course of posttraumatic stress disorder and posttraumatic stress disorder symptoms in a community sample of adolescents and young adults. *Am J Psychiatry.* 2005;162(7):1320–1327.

177. Krause ED, Kaltman S, Goodman L, Dutton MA. Role of distinct PTSD symptoms in intimate partner reabuse: A prospective study. *J Trauma Stress.* 2006;19(4):507–516.

178. Glass N, Perrin N, Campbell JC, Soeken K. The protective role of tangible support on posttraumatic stress disorder symptoms in urban

women survivors of violence. *Res Nurs Health.* 2007;30(5):558–568.

179. Resnick H, Acierno R, Waldrop AE, et al. Randomized controlled evaluation of an early intervention to prevent post-rape psychopathology. *Behav Res Ther.* 2007;45(10):2432–2447.

180. Katz BL. The psychological impact of stranger versus nonstranger rape on victims' recovery. In: Parrot A, Bechhofer L, eds. *Acquaintance rape: The hidden crime.* New York: John Wiley;1991:251–269.

181. Koss MP, Dinero TE, Seibel C, Cox S. Stranger and acquaintance rape: Are there differences in the victim's experience? *Psychol Women Qy.* 1988;12(1):1–24.

182. Hanson RK. The psychological impact of sexual assault on women and children: A review. *Ann Sex Res.* 1990;3(2):187–232.

183. Resick PA. Psychological effects of victimization: Implications for the criminal justice system. *Crime Delinq.* 1987;33:468.

184. Ullman SE, Filipas HH, Townsend SM, Starzynski LL. Trauma exposure, posttraumatic stress disorder and problem drinking in sexual assault survivors. *J Stud Alcohol.* 2005;66(5):610–619.

185. Filipas HH, Ullman SE. Child sexual abuse, coping responses, self-blame, posttraumatic stress disorder, and adult sexual revictimization. *J Interpers Violence.* 2006;21(5):652–672.

186. Kilpatrick DG, Saunders BE, Veronen LJ, et al. Criminal victimization: Lifetime prevalence, reporting to police, and psychological impact. *Crime Delinq.* 1987;33.

187. Golding JM, Siegel JM, Sorenson SB, et al. Social support sources following sexual assault. *J Community Psychol.* 1989;17(1):92–107.

188. Temple JR, Weston R, Rodriguez BF, Marshall LL. Differing effects of partner and nonpartner sexual assault on women's mental health. *Violence Against Women.* 2007;13(3):285–297.

189. Elliott DM, Briere J. Transference and countertransference. In: Classen CC, Yalom I, eds. *Treating women molested in childhood.* San Francisco: Jossey Bass;1995:187–226.

190. Kessler RC. Posttraumatic stress disorder: The burden to the individual and to society. *J Clin Psychiatry.* 2000;61(Suppl 5):4–12; discussion 13–14.

191. Norris FH, Kaniasty K. Psychological distress following criminal victimization in the general population: Cross-sectional, longitudinal, and prospective analyses. *J Consult Clin Psychol.* 1994;62(1): 111–123.

192. Rieker P, Carmen EH. The victim-to-patient process: The disconfirmation and transformation of abuse. *Am J Orthopsychiatry.* 1986;56(3):360–370.

193. Basile KC, Arias I, Desai S, Thompson MP. The differential association of intimate partner physical, sexual, psychological, and stalking violence and posttraumatic stress symptoms in a nationally representative sample of women. *J Trauma Stress.* 2004;17(5):413–421.

194. Bennice JA, Resick PA, Mechanic M, Astin M. The relative effects of intimate partner physical and sexual violence on post-traumatic stress disorder symptomatology. *Violence Vict.* 2003;18(1):87–94.

195. Cole J, Logan TK, Shannon L. Intimate sexual victimization among women with protective orders: Types and associations of physical and mental health problems. *Violence Vict.* 2005;20(6):695–715.

196. McFarlane J, Malecha A, Watson K, et al. Intimate partner sexual assault against women: Frequency, health consequences, and treatment outcomes. *Obstet Gynecol.* 2005;105(1):99–108.

197. Arias I, Pape KT. Psychological abuse: Implications for adjustment and commitment to leave violent partners. *Violence Vict.* 1999;14(1):55–67.

198. Coker AL, Smith PH, McKeown RE, King MJ. Frequency and correlates of intimate partner violence by type: Physical, sexual, and psychological battering. *Am J Public Health.* 2000;90(4):553–559.

199. Mechanic MB, Uhlmansiek MH, Weaver TL, Resick PA. The impact of severe stalking experienced by acutely battered women: An examination of violence, psychological symptoms and strategic responding. *Violence Vict.* 2000;15(4):443–458.

200. Street AE, Arias I. Psychological abuse and posttraumatic stress disorder in battered women: Examining the roles of shame and guilt. *Violence Vict.* 2001;16(1):65–78.

201. Smith PH, Earp JA, DeVellis R. Measuring battering: Development of the Women's Experience With Battering (WEB) Scale. *Women's Health: Research on Gender, Behavior, and Policy.* 1995;1(4):273–288.

202. Dutton MA, Kaltman S, Goodman LA, et al. Patterns of intimate partner violence: Correlates and outcomes. *Violence Vict.* 2005;20(5):483–497.

203. Sackett LA, Saunders DG. The impact of different forms of psychological abuse on battered women. *Violence Vict.* 1999;14(1):105–117.

204. Foa EB, Rothbaum BO, Riggs DS, Murdock TB. Treatment of posttraumatic stress disorder in rape victims: A comparison between cognitive-behavioral procedures and counseling. *J Consult Clin Psychol.* 1991;59(5):715–723.

205. Breslau N. Gender differences in trauma and posttraumatic stress disorder. *J Gend Specif Med.* 2002;5(1):34–40.

206. Breslau N, Chilcoat HD, Kessler RC, Davis GC. Previous exposure to trauma and PTSD effects of subsequent trauma: Results from the Detroit Area Survey of Trauma. *Am J Psychiatry.* 1999;156(6): 902–907.

207. Campbell JC, Webster D, Koziol-McLain J, et al. Assessing risk factors for intimate partner homicide. *Natl Instit Justice J.* 2003;250:14–19.

208. Kaplow JB, Dodge KA, Amaya-Jackson L, Saxe GN. Pathways to PTSD, part II: Sexually abused children. *Am J Psychiatry.* 2005;162(7):1305–1310.

209. Noll JG. Does childhood sexual abuse set in motion a cycle of violence against women? What we know

209. and what we need to learn. *J Interpers Violence.* 2005;20(4):455–462.

210. Varma D, Chandra PS, Thomas T, Carey MP. Intimate partner violence and sexual coercion among pregnant women in India: Relationship with depression and post-traumatic stress disorder. *J Affect Disord.* 2007;102(1–3):227–235.

211. Woods AB, Page GG, O'Campo P, et al. The mediation effect of posttraumatic stress disorder symptoms on the relationship of intimate partner violence and IFN-gamma levels. *Am J Community Psychol.* 2005;36(1–2):159–175.

212. Schneider R, Baumrind N, Kimerling R. Exposure to child abuse and risk for mental health problems in women. *Violence Vict.* 2007;22(5):620–631.

213. Bradley R, Schwartz AC, Kaslow NJ. Posttraumatic stress disorder symptoms among low-income, African American women with a history of intimate partner violence and suicidal behaviors: Self-esteem, social support, and religious coping. *J Trauma Stress.* 2005;18(6):685–696.

214. O'Keefe M. Posttraumatic stress disorder among incarcerated battered women: A comparison of battered women who killed their abusers and those incarcerated for other offenses. *J Trauma Stress.* 1998;11(1):71–85.

215. Solomon SD, Davidson JR. Trauma: Prevalence, impairment, service use, and cost. *J Clin Psychiatry.* 1997;58(Suppl 9):5–11.

216. Walker EA, Katon W, Russo J, et al. Health care costs associated with posttraumatic stress disorder symptoms in women. *Arch Gen Psychiatry.* 2003;60(4):369–374.

217. Kimerling R. An investigation of sex differences in nonpsychiatric morbidity associated with posttraumatic stress disorder. *J Am Med Womens Assoc.* 2004;59(1):43–47.

218. Dobie DJ, Kivlahan DR, Maynard C, et al. Posttraumatic stress disorder in female veterans: Association with self-reported health problems and functional impairment. *Arch Intern Med.* 2004;164(4):394–400.

219. Creamer M, Burgess P, McFarlane AC. Posttraumatic stress disorder: Findings from the Australian National Survey of Mental Health and Well-being. *Psychol Med.* 2001;31(7):1237–1247.

220. Reynolds M, Mezey G, Chapman M, et al. Comorbid post-traumatic stress disorder in a substance misusing clinical population. *Drug Alcohol Depend.* 2005;77(3):251–258.

221. Milliken CS, Auchterlonie JL, Hoge CW. Longitudinal assessment of mental health problems among active and reserve component soldiers returning from the Iraq war. *JAMA.* 2007;298(18):2141–2148.

222. Chilcoat HD, Breslau N. Investigations of causal pathways between PTSD and drug use disorders. *Addict Behav.* 1998;23(6):827–840.

223. Carbone-Lopez K, Kruttschnitt C, Macmillan R. Patterns of intimate partner violence and their associations with physical health, psychological distress, and substance use. *Public Health Rep.* 2006;121(4):382–392.

224. Weinsheimer RL, Schermer CR, Malcoe LH, et al. Severe intimate partner violence and alcohol use among female trauma patients. *J Trauma.* 2005;58(1):22–29.

225. El-Bassel N, Gilbert L, Witte S, et al. Intimate partner violence and substance abuse among minority women receiving care from an inner-city emergency department. *Women's Health Issues.* 2003;13(1):16–22.

226. White HR, Chen PH. Problem drinking and intimate partner violence. *J Stud Alcohol.* 2002;63(2):205–214.

227. El-Bassel N, Gilbert L, Wu E, et al. Relationship between drug abuse and intimate partner violence: A longitudinal study among women receiving methadone. *Am J Public Health.* 2005;95(3):465–470.

228. Paranjape A, Heron S, Thompson M, et al. Are alcohol problems linked with an increase in depressive symptoms in abused, inner-city African American women? *Womens Health Issues.* 2007;17(1):37–43.

229. Sareen J, Cox BJ, Stein MB, et al. Physical and mental comorbidity, disability, and suicidal behavior associated with posttraumatic stress disorder in a large community sample. *Psychosom Med.* 2007;69(3):242–248.

230. Heru AM, Stuart GL, Rainey S, et al. Prevalence and severity of intimate partner violence and associations with family functioning and alcohol abuse in psychiatric inpatients with suicidal intent. *J Clin Psychiatry.* 2006;67(1):23–29.

231. Oquendo M, Brent DA, Birmaher B, et al. Posttraumatic stress disorder comorbid with major depression: Factors mediating the association with suicidal behavior. *Am J Psychiatry.* 2005;162(3):560–566.

232. Sato-DiLorenzo A, Sharps PW. Dangerous intimate partner relationships and women's mental health and health behaviors. *Issues Ment Health Nurs.* 2007;28(8):837–848.

233. Sansone RA, Chu JA, Wiederman MW. Suicide attempts and domestic violence among women psychiatric inpatients. *Intern J Psychiatry Clin Pract.* 2007;11(2):163–166.

234. Thompson MP, Kaslow NJ, Kingree JB. Risk factors for suicide attempts among African American women experiencing recent intimate partner violence. *Violence Vict.* 2002;17(3):283–295.

235. Stark E, Flitcraft A. Killing the beast within: Woman battering and female suicidality. *Int J Health Serv.* 1995;25(1):43–64.

236. Weaver TL, Allen JA, Hopper E, et al. Mediators of suicidal ideation within a sheltered sample of raped and battered women. *Health Care Women Int.* 2007;28(5):478–489.

237. Talbot NL, Duberstein PR, Cox C, et al. Preliminary report on childhood sexual abuse, suicidal ideation, and suicide attempts among middle-aged and older depressed women. *Am J Geriatr Psychiatry.* 2004;12(5):536–538.

238. Anderson PL, Tiro JA, Price AW, et al. Additive impact of childhood emotional, physical, and sexual abuse on suicide attempts among low-income African American women. *Suicide Life Threat Behav.* 2002;32(2):131–138.

239. Briere J, Runtz M. Suicidal thoughts and behaviors in former sexual abuse victims. *Can J Behav Sci.* 1986;18:413–423.

240. Mitchell C. Personal communication; 2007.

241. Starr K, Fawcett J. *If I had one more day: Findings and recommendations from the Washington State Domestic Violence Fatality Review 2006.* Washington State Coalition Against Domestic Violence, 2006.

242. van der Kolk BA. The psychobiology of posttraumatic stress disorder. *J Clin Psychiatry.* 1997;58 (Suppl 9):16–24.

243. Davidson JR, van der Kolk B E. The psychopharmacological treatment of posttraumatic stress disorder. In: van der Kolk BE, Weisaeth L, eds. *Traumatic stress: The effects of overwhelming experience on mind, body, and society.* New York, NY: Guilford Press, 1996.

244. Yehuda R, LeDoux J. Response variation following trauma: A translational neuroscience approach to understanding PTSD. *Neuron.* 2007; 56(1):19–32.

245. Charney DS. Life stress, genes, and depression: Multiple pathways lead to increased risk and new opportunities for intervention. *Sci STKE.* 2004:225.

246. Yehuda R, Kahana B, Binder-Byrnes K, et al. Lower urinary cortisol excretion in Holocaust survivors with posttraumatic stress disorder. *Am J Psychiatry.* 1995;152:982–986.

247. Yehuda R, McFarlane A, eds. Psychobiology of posttraumatic stress disorder. *Ann N Y Acad Sci.* 1997; 821.

248. Bremner JD, Elzinga B, Schmahl C, Vermetten E. Structural and functional plasticity of the human brain in posttraumatic stress disorder. *Prog Brain Res.* 2008;167:171–186.

249. Griffin MG, Resick PA, Yehuda R. Enhanced cortisol suppression following dexamethasone administration in domestic violence survivors. *Am J Psychiatry.* 2005;162(6):1192–1199.

250. Pico-Alfonso MA, Garcia-Linares MI, Celda-Navarro N, et al. Changes in cortisol and dehydroepiandrosterone in women victims of physical and psychological intimate partner violence. *Biol Psychiatry.* 2004;56(4):233–240.

251. Seedat S, Stein MB, Kennedy CM, Hauger RL. Plasma cortisol and neuropeptide Y in female victims of intimate partner violence. *Psychoneuroendocrinology.* 2003;28(6):796–808.

252. Heim C, Newport DJ, Heit S, et al. Pituitary-adrenal and autonomic responses to stress in women after sexual and physical abuse in childhood. *JAMA.* 2000;284(5):592–597.

253. Cicchetti D, Blender JA. A multiple-levels-of-analysis perspective on resilience: Implications for the developing brain, neural plasticity, and preventive interventions. *Ann N Y Acad Sci.* 2006;1094: 248–258.

254. Sapolsky RM, Romero LM, Munck AU. How do glucocorticoids influence stress responses? Integrating permissive, suppressive, stimulatory, and preparative actions. *Endocr Rev.* 2000;21(1):55–89.

255. Dunlop SA, Archer MA, Quinlivan JA, et al. Repeated prenatal corticosteroids delay myelination in the ovine central nervous system. *J Matern Fetal Med.* 1997;6(6):309–313.

256. Bremner JD, Mletzko T, Welter S, et al. Effects of phenytoin on memory, cognition and brain structure in post-traumatic stress disorder: A pilot study. *J Psychopharmacol.* 2005;19(2):159–165.

257. Bremner JD, Vythilingam M, Vermetten E, et al. MRI and PET study of deficits in hippocampal structure and function in women with childhood sexual abuse and posttraumatic stress disorder. *Am J Psychiatry.* 2003;160(5):924–932.

258. Stein MB, Koverola C, Hanna AC, et al. Hippocampal volume in women victimized by child sexual abuse. *Psychol Med.* 1997;27:951–959.

259. Fennema-Notestine C, Stein MB, Kennedy CM, et al. Brain morphometry in female victims of intimate partner violence with and without posttraumatic stress disorder. *Biol Psychiatry* 2003;53(7):632.

260. Bremner JD, Vermetten E, Afzal N, Vythilingam M. Deficits in verbal declarative memory function in women with childhood sexual abuse-related posttraumatic stress disorder. *J Nerv Ment Dis.* 2004;192(10):643–649.

261. Pitman RK SL, Rauch SL. Investigating the pathogenesis of posttraumatic stress disorder with neuroimaging. *J Clin Psychiatry.* 2001;62(Suppl 17): 47–54.

262. van der Kolk BA, Courtois CA. Editorial comments: Complex developmental trauma. *J Trauma Stress.* 2005;18(5):385–388.

263. Carmen EH. Victim to patient to survivor processes: Clinical perspectives. Paper presented at: Dare to vision: Shaping the national agenda for women, abuse, and mental health services, Holyoke, Massachusetts, 1994.

264. Gondolf EW, Fisher ER. *Battered women as survivors: An alternate to treating learned helplessness.* Lexington, MA: Lexington Books, 1988.

265. Dutton MA. *Empowering and healing the battered woman: A model for assessment and intervention.* New York: Springer, 1992.

Chapter 13

Substance Abuse in Intimate Partner Violence

Carol B. Cunradi

KEY CONCEPTS

- Alcohol and substance abuse are very prevalent in society, especially among males and young adults. In 2003, approximately half of all Americans 12 years of age or older were current drinkers, and nearly one in 10 were current drug users.
- The etiologic role of alcohol in the occurrence of intimate partner violence (IPV) has not yet been established. However, high rates of hazardous drinking have been noted among perpetrators and victims of IPV; high rates of IPV perpetration and victimization have been found in individuals who drink at hazardous levels.
- Studies have shown that alcohol and drug use are associated with the level of severity of IPV and injury.
- Alcohol is neither necessary for IPV to occur, nor is it a sufficient cause for IPV. However, alcohol contributes to the occurrence of violence in some situations. This may be due to the effect of alcohol on cognitive processes, altering the relationship between normative beliefs regarding IPV and the occurrence of IPV.
- Research has shown that heavy drinking by the perpetrator is a contributing cause of IPV. In addition, childhood exposure to abuse and household dysfunction is associated with an increased risk of IPV and alcohol and other substance abuse during adulthood. Further, behavioral couples therapy may have a role in decreasing rates of IPV and alcohol abuse in some situations.

The association between intimate partner violence (IPV) and substance abuse has been noted for over 30 years. For example, shortly after the "discovery" of battered women in the 1970s and the subsequent recognition of domestic violence as a social problem (1,2), numerous case reports and studies based on clinical samples of battered wives highlighted the role of alcohol use, drunkenness, or drinking during the event on the part of the perpetrator (3–6), the victim (7), or both (8,9). Since that time, a large body of research has been devoted toward increasing understandings of the factors that underlie the association between male and female alcohol and other drug (AOD) use and the elevated risk of IPV. This chapter summarizes recent findings on IPV and substance use on the part of both partners and also addresses substance use prevalence in the general population, as well as theoretical conceptualization of the AOD–IPV relationship, recent advances in AOD–IPV research, and implications for policy, practice, and research.

SUBSTANCE USE PREVALENCE IN THE UNITED STATES

Before reviewing the literature on substance abuse and IPV, it is important to understand the estimated prevalence of substance use in the U.S. general household population. Based on results from the 2003 National Survey on Drug Use and Health (10) approximately half of all Americans aged 12 or older were current drinkers of alcohol (had at least one drink in the past 30 days). Among those aged 18 years of age and older, 62.4% of males were current drinkers, compared to 46% of females. The highest prevalence of both binge drinking (had five or more drinks on the same occasion at least once in the past 30 days) and heavy drinking (had five or more drinks on the same occasion on at least 5 different days in the past 30 days) occurred among young adults aged 18 to 25, with the peak rate for both measures occurring at age 21. For young adults in this age group, the rate of binge drinking was 41.6%, and the rate of heavy alcohol use was 15.1%.

Alcohol use disorders (i.e., alcohol abuse and dependence) have tremendous costs not only to the individual and his or her family, but also for employers, communities, healthcare systems, and society at large (11–14). In the *Diagnostic and Statistical Manual of Mental Health Disorders* (DSM-IV), alcohol abuse and dependence (15) are defined as maladaptive patterns of drinking, leading to clinically significant impairment or distress (16). Based on data from the National Epidemiologic Survey on Alcohol and Related Conditions (16), the 12-month prevalence of DSM-IV alcohol abuse among those 18 years and

older in the U.S. general population during 2001–2002 is estimated at 6.93% among males and 2.55% among females. The highest rates were seen among men (9.35%) and women (4.57%) in the 18–29-year-old age range. In terms of the 12-month prevalence of DSM-IV alcohol dependence, the rate among men was found to be 5.42%; among women, the rate was 2.32%. Again, the highest rates were seen among men (13.00%) and women (5.52%) in the 18–29-year-old age range.

Regarding illicit drug use, 8.2% of the population aged 12 years of age or older were current drug users (used an illicit drug at least once in the past month) in 2003 (10). Marijuana was the most commonly used illicit drug; it was used by 75.2% of current drug users. About 45.4% of current drug users used illicit drugs other than marijuana or hashish, either with or without using marijuana. Illicit drug use peaks during the late teenage years and early adulthood. For example, 19.2% of 16–17-year-olds were current drug users, as were 23.3% of 18–20-year-olds and 18.3% of 21–25-year-olds. In general, rates of current illicit drug use were higher among males (10%) than females (6.5%), except for rates of nonmedical use of prescription-type psychotherapeutics, which were similar for males (2.7%) and females (2.6%).

ALCOHOL PROBLEMS AND INTIMATE PARTNER VIOLENCE RISK

Although the precise etiologic role of alcohol in the occurrence of IPV has not been established, considerable empirical evidence suggests that alcohol use often precedes or accompanies acts of marital aggression, especially on the part of the male (17). Elevated rates of hazardous drinking-related behaviors (e.g., heavy drinking) are often found among both IPV victims and perpetrators; elevated rates of IPV perpetration and victimization are often found among those who engage in hazardous drinking behavior. For example, past-year prevalence of male-to-female IPV among married or cohabiting men in the U.S. household population has been estimated at between 12% and 14% (18,19). Among men seeking treatment for alcoholism, the pretreatment year prevalence of IPV has been estimated at upwards of 50% (20–22). Nevertheless, it is clear that acute alcohol consumption (e.g., hazardous drinking or intoxication) is neither necessary for IPV to occur nor a sufficient cause of IPV (23–25).

Table 13.1 Bivariate Analysis of Intimate Partner Violence (IPV) and Alcohol-Related Problems

Associations between male alcohol-related problems and partner violence					
White (*n* = 555)		Black (*n* = 358)		Hispanic (*n* = 527)	
Alcohol Problems *n* = 78	No Alcohol Problems *n* = 477	Alcohol Problems *n* = 71	No Alcohol Problems *n* = 287	Alcohol Problems *n* = 126	No Alcohol Problems *n* = 401
MFPV 28%	9%	56%	14%	27%	14%
No MFPV 72%	91%	44%	86%	73%	86%
Chi-sq 8.20**		15.93****		7.41**	
FMPV 31%	13%	58%	23%	35%	17%
No FMPV 69%	87%	42%	77%	65%	83%
Chi-sq 10.17***		13.28%		14.74****	
Associations between female alcohol-related problems and partner violence					
White (*n* = 555)		Black (*n* = 358)		Hispanic (*n* = 527)	
Alcohol Problems *n* = 33	No Alcohol Problems *n* = 522	Alcohol Problems *n* = 29	No Alcohol Problems *n* = 329	Alcohol Problems *n* = 34	No Alcohol Problems *n* = 493
MFPV 36%	10%	61%	20%	14%	17%
No MFPV 64%	90%	39%	80%	86%	83%
Chi-sq 6.21*		6.94**		0.20#	
FMPV 50%	13%	70%	27%	37%	20%
No FMPV 50%	87%	30%	73%	63%	80%
Chi-sq 7.91**		11.14***		2.43#	

*$p < .05$; **$p < .01$; ***$p < .005$; ****$p < .001$; # not significant

FMPV, female-to-male partner violence;

MFPV, male-to-femle partner violence.

Reprinted with permission from Cunradi et al. Alcohol-related problems and intimate partner violence among White, Black, and Hispanic couples in the U.S. *Alcohol Clini Experim Res*, 1999; 23(9):1492–1501.

Cunradi and colleagues (26) analyzed the bivariate association between past-year IPV and alcohol-related problems (i.e., alcohol dependence symptoms and drinking-related social consequences) among a national household sample of White, Black and Hispanic married or cohabiting couples who participated in the 1995 National Study of Couples (27). Findings from the Cunradi study (26) are summarized in Table 13.1

These data highlight a number of important findings. First, men tend to report more alcohol-related problems than do women, both in terms of alcohol dependence symptoms and drinking-related social consequences. Second, there appear to be significant racial/ethnic differences in rates of male alcohol-related problems, but not female alcohol-related problems. Third, higher rates of male-to-female partner violence (MFPV) and female-to-male partner violence (FMPV) are found among couples who report male alcohol-related problems compared to couples who did not report male alcohol-related problems. Fourth, higher rates of MFPV and FMPV are found among White and Black couples who report female alcohol-related problems compared to those who did not report female alcohol-related problems; no differences were found among Hispanic couples. Finally, it is important to point out that most of the men and women in this study who were categorized with alcohol-related problems did not meet the criteria for DSM-IV alcohol dependence (15); rather, they may have exhibited only one alcohol dependence symptom or had only one alcohol-related social consequence.

Additional multivariate logistic regression analysis of these cross-sectional data indicated that past-year male and female alcohol-related problems were associated with increased risk of MFPV among Black couples, but not among White or Hispanic couples. Male alcohol-related problems were associated with FMPV among White, Black, and Hispanic couples; female alcohol-related problems were associated with FMPV among White and Black couples, but not Hispanic couples. Past 12-month alcohol-related problems may be related to IPV through several pathways. First, it is likely that couples experiencing drinking-related social consequences or alcohol dependence symptoms have higher levels of marital discord, fights, and verbal aggression, which would place them at risk for IPV. For example, in an analysis of problem domains in the 1984 National Alcohol Survey, Hilton (1991) found that belligerence and problems with their spouse were related (phi = .31). Second, recent alcohol-related problems may serve as a marker for couples whose drinking behaviors and interpersonal relationships have gotten out of control. For example, one or both partner's loss of control or lack of restraint around drinking may similarly manifest in interpersonal exchanges, resulting in aggression or violence.

ALCOHOL, DRUGS, AND INTIMATE PARTNER VIOLENCE SEVERITY

Numerous studies indicate that alcohol and drug use are associated with level of IPV severity (i.e., potential for injury). The following sections examine AOD use and IPV severity among community samples and clinical samples. This distinction is important because, in general, longitudinal research suggests that severity and chronicity of IPV is greater among clinical samples (28).

Community Samples

Leonard and Quigley (25), in an analysis of young newlyweds, found that husband drinking (by husband's report) was significantly associated with IPV severity, although the effect was reduced when adjusted for wife drinking. Wife drinking was not significantly associated with severe versus moderate

IPV. Magdol and coworkers (29) analyzed a sample of 21-year-old New Zealander men and women involved in dating or cohabiting relationships. Their findings indicate that perpetrators and victims of severe IPV reported more symptoms of alcohol dependence and used more types of illicit drugs than those who did not experience severe IPV. In an analysis of a large sample of White male Army personnel, Pan and colleagues (30) found that alcohol problems distinguished men who engaged in nonsevere and severe IPV from men who reported no physical aggression. Drug problems were associated with increased risk of severe IPV, but were not associated with nonsevere IPV. Among a community-based sample of 724 women ages 18–30, Testa and colleagues (31) found that women's hard drug use, but not heavy episodic drinking, was associated with increased likelihood of experiencing moderate and severe IPV in ongoing relationships. Male alcohol and drug use was not assessed. Cunradi and colleagues (32) found that past-year male and female alcohol-related problems were associated with increased risk of moderate and severe male IPV among a national household-based sample of married and cohabiting couples. In addition, female drug use, but not male drug use, was also associated with these outcomes. The null finding on male drug use is somewhat unexpected given both the empirical literature (33,34) and the proposed causal pathways linking certain opiates, especially cocaine, with aggressive and violent behavior. Women drug users who experienced severe male IPV may also have higher rates of other mental health disorders that could contribute to their elevated risk observed in this study. For example, rates of comorbid psychiatric disorders, particularly antisocial personality disorder, are higher among women with substance abuse/dependence than men (35).

Clinical Samples

Coker and associates (36), in a family practice clinic setting, found that women whose male partners had drug or alcohol problems, or who reported that both they and their partner had a drug or alcohol problem, were at increased risk for IPV, including physical, sexual, and psychological abuse. Results from two case-control studies among women presenting at hospital emergency departments indicate that the male partner's problem drinking and drug use were significantly associated with risk of IPV injury (37,38). In one study (37), women's positive urinalysis test results for cocaine and alcohol were independently associated with increased risk for IPV injury after adjustment for other covariates. Miller (39) compared IPV rates among samples of women in drug treatment, battered women's shelters, and the community, matched to the treatment and shelter samples' neighborhoods. She found that women in the community sample who used drugs had lower rates of severe IPV than women in drug treatment, but higher rates of severe IPV than non–drug using women in the community sample. In one of the few longitudinal studies of drug abuse and IPV based on a sample of urban, low-income women in methadone maintenance treatment, El-Bassel and colleagues (40) found that women who reported frequent crack use or marijuana at wave 2 were more likely than non–drug using women to report IPV at wave 3. Additionally, women who reported IPV at wave 2 were more likely than women who did not report IPV to indicate frequent heroin use at wave 3. Taken together, these studies support the association between men's (and to a lesser extent, women's) drug and alcohol use as risk factors for severe IPV.

THEORETICAL CONCEPTUALIZATION OF THE ALCOHOL AND OTHER DRUG–INTIMATE PARTNER VIOLENCE RELATIONSHIPS

Expectations about the consequences of drinking behavior are critical social and cultural determinants of alcohol's role in IPV. According to deviance disavowal and social learning models, alcohol may lead to violence because drinking alcohol is a "discriminative cue" that aggressive and other non-normative behavior would be unlikely to be socially punished (41,42). Such expectancies are often intermingled with drinking and violence more generally; in this case, drinking might be seen as an acceptable excuse for violent behavior. Although neither a "necessary or sufficient" cause of IPV, it is clear that acute alcohol use contributes to the occurrence of IPV for some people under some circumstances (43). One theoretical explanation for the seemingly disparate outcomes vis-à-vis alcohol and IPV is that alcohol's effects are cognitively mediated. In other words, alcohol may pharmacologically alter cognitive processes, which can result in a range of behaviors (44). Disinhibition models of drinking, for example, further suggest that

alcohol's pharmacological effects may cause individuals to resort to inappropriate means of conflict resolution (e.g., shifting from psychological to physical aggression) (45). These scenarios suggest that alcohol may moderate the relationship between IPV normative beliefs (e.g., perceived peer approval of IPV; perceived involvement in IPV by family, friends, and coworkers) and the occurrence of IPV. That is, couples may be differentially prone to IPV as related to, say, socioeconomic status, but the manifestation of IPV may increase in the context of alcohol use. Specific patterns of use (e.g., heavy drinking), rather than alcohol use per se, appear to matter most in the occurrence of IPV (46).

Evidence for the moderating role of alcohol in its association between IPV normative beliefs and IPV occurrence is found in the 1985 National Family Violence Survey (41). Rates of husband-to-wife IPV varied as a function of male occupational status (i.e., blue-collar or white-collar), approval of marital aggression, and drinking. Blue-collar men who approved of marital aggression and were binge drinkers had the highest rate of IPV. Blue- and white-collar men who disapproved of marital aggression and were abstainers had the lowest rates of IPV. The findings indicate a three-way interaction between occupational status, attitudes toward marital aggression, and alcohol (41). The relationship between drinking type and norms differed by occupational status (i.e., blue-collar versus white-collar). It should also be noted that drinking problems, as well as drug use (e.g., prescription pain killers, tranquilizers, and sleeping pills), may be an *outcome* of IPV, particularly among victims. Detailed, temporally ordered information on the drinking and drug use behavior of each spouse/partner in the couple is needed, to disentangle the role of substance use in relation to the occurrence of IPV.

RECENT ADVANCES IN ALCOHOL AND OTHER DRUG–INTIMATE PARTNER VIOLENCE RESEARCH

Conceptual Advances

Refined understandings of IPV typology in relation to substance use has been a key conceptual advance. Johnson (47) argues that at least two distinct types of IPV occur: *common couple violence* and *patriarchal terrorism*. The former is theorized to characterize the type of situational outbursts that may occur between couples, typically in the course of conflict. Common couple violence can be bidirectional (i.e., male-to-female or female-to-male), and usually involves "moderate" acts (e.g., pushing, shoving, grabbing, slapping), although escalation to more severe episodes (e.g., hitting with fist, kicking) is possible. Patriarchal terrorism is characterized by a pattern of more severe violence typically associated with terms such as "wife beating" and "battered women." It involves the systematic use of violence, as well as other control tactics, such as threats, isolation, and economic dependency. Theoretically, the distal and proximal correlates of IPV are thought to differ based on male batterer typology (48,49). Understanding IPV typology in relation to substance use is important for implementation of public policy and intervention strategies (47). For example, Holtzworth-Munroe and Stuart's typology describes family-only batterers, thought to engage in the least IPV; dysphoric or borderline batterers, thought to engage in more moderate to severe IPV; and generally violent and antisocial batterers, thought to engage in moderate to severe IPV and high levels of extrafamilial violence. This third group was also thought most likely to exhibit antisocial personality disorder (50). Fals-Stewart and colleagues (51) found that the occurrence of IPV among the most violent men with antisocial personality disorder was not related to drinking, but that drinking may increase the severity of the violent episode. In terms of treatment, couples experiencing common couple violence with or without AOD use may be amenable to relationship counseling. In the case of patriarchal terrorism, however, relationship counseling may be contraindicated due to fear and safety concerns on the part of the female victim (52).

Empirical Advances

Significant empirical advances in the epidemiology of substance use and IPV have been accomplished through longitudinal study design, especially studies that follow both members of the dyad over time. Longitudinal assessment of AOD use by each partner in relation to the occurrence of IPV allows researchers to draw conclusions about the temporal ordering of factors and provides insight into causality. In particular, use of calendar-based diary methods, such as the Timeline Followback Spousal Violence Interview, has allowed the daily patterns and frequency of IPV

to be reliably measured (53). To date, research using longitudinal study design suggests that men's heavy drinking is a contributing cause of IPV (51,54–56). An important caveat is that even sophisticated longitudinal modeling of the AOD–IPV association has the potential to be biased by spurious variables or through model mis-specification (43).

Important empirical advances have also been made regarding the intergenerational transmission of family violence. Over 15 years ago, Widom (57) analyzed research reports published between 1970 and 1986, and determined that there were not enough data to conclude that exposure to childhood violence increases the risk for intergenerational transmission of violence. More recent research, however, provides evidence that childhood exposure to physical or other forms of abuse and household dysfunction is associated with increased risk of IPV, as well as AOD use, during adulthood. Using multigroup path analysis, Schafer and colleagues (58) found that impulsivity, alcohol problems, and childhood physical abuse were differentially associated with risk of IPV as a function of race/ethnicity among a national sample of Black, White, and Hispanic couples. Data from the Adverse Childhood Experiences (ACE) study (59) also provides strong evidence pointing to the intergenerational transmission of violence. In this study, the relationship of childhood physical or sexual abuse or growing up with a battered mother, and risk of being an adult victim or perpetrator of IPV, was assessed among a cohort of 8,629 participants enrolled in a large health maintenance organization (HMO). The results indicated that each of the three violent childhood experiences increased the risk of IPV victimization or perpetration twofold. Additionally, among participants who reported all three types of violent childhood experiences, the risk of victimization and perpetration was increased 3.5-fold for women and 3.8-fold for men (60). As Ehrensaft and colleagues (61) point out, however, childhood maltreatment per se may not be a necessary precondition for adult IPV. Rather, growing up with exposure to a hostile, maladaptive parenting style may be sufficient to put individuals at risk for IPV later in life.

Intervention and Treatment

One of the most promising treatment advances in reducing the joint occurrence of AOD and IPV among male abusers and their female partners is behavioral couples therapy (BCT) (22). Because male alcoholics seeking treatment have high (e.g., 50%–60%) rates of pretreatment IPV prevalence (62), addressing the occurrence of IPV during BCT alcoholism treatment is a pragmatic necessity. The BCT treatment program, attended conjointly by alcoholic males and their female partners, typically consists of approximately 20 weekly therapy sessions over a 5–6 month period. The alcoholic partner, in conjunction with active support from his spouse, enters into a Sobriety Contract to promote sobriety, engagement in positive couple and family activities, and training in communication and negotiation skills. Based on longitudinal follow-up of 303 married or cohabiting male alcoholics who underwent BCT, O'Farrell and associates (63) reported significant reductions in IPV in the first and second year after BCT from the year before BCT. Their analysis indicated that greater BCT treatment involvement was related to lower violence after BCT; this association was mediated by reduced problem drinking and enhanced relationship functioning (63). Integrating AOD–IPV treatment may hold the most promise for effectively reducing the joint occurrence of heavy drinking and partner violence (64).

IMPLICATIONS FOR POLICY, PRACTICE, AND RESEARCH

Policy

- Effecting polices aimed at environmental prevention of AOD–IPV is a largely unexplored area, but one that holds much potential. For example, workplace-based prevention efforts that focus on policy changes, such as automatic employee assistance program (EAP) referral for those engaging in IPV, company-based security measures aimed at enforcing restraining orders barring violent spouses from the worksite, expedited legal assistance for IPV victims, and periodic workshops to train supervisors and co-workers how to recognize and respond to signs of IPV, should be implemented.
- Another arena for environmental prevention of AOD–IPV problems is neighborhood-based interventions. Impoverished neighborhoods have been found to have high rates of substance use problems and IPV, even after statistically adjusting for the household income of individual residents (65,66). Exploring the factors that underlie the elevated risk for IPV in such neighborhoods could provide the basis for environmental prevention of IPV and related problems.
- Environmental interventions may also have an impact on changing IPV normative beliefs (i.e., group social norms). In turn, altering the social norms around the acceptability of IPV may result in lowered IPV occurrence among some segments of the household population.

Practice

- The evidence pointing to the intergenerational transmission of violence suggests that conducting primary prevention among families may result in lowered occurrence of IPV. Specifically, this includes reducing levels of what Felitti and colleagues (59) characterize as adverse childhood events: physical, sexual, or emotional abuse during childhood; exposure to IPV in the home; parental AOD problems, and other forms of family dysfunction that children are exposed to. Affecting this type of primary prevention would likely involve a large expenditure of resources to ensure an impact at the population level. Given the preponderance of data from the ACE study (60,67–70), however, it appears that such an investment would result in lowered rates of IPV, alcohol problems, smoking, and reduction of other health and social problems. The cost–benefit ratio for such an effort would be of inestimable value.

Research

- Research over the past few decades has demonstrated that AOD use is associated with IPV. Nevertheless, substance use in itself is not a sufficient cause or trigger of IPV. As Leonard (43) points out, it is clear that alcohol contributes to IPV in some people under some circumstances. For example, research indicates that alcohol is unlikely to predict violence among those who have very low hostile motivations (71,72). Personality factors, such as antisocial personality disorder, may moderate the association between drinking and male-to-female IPV (51).

- Future AOD–IPV research should focus on the particular circumstances under which AOD use appears to influence the occurrence of IPV, and among which types of individuals.
- Research should continue to explore the factors that moderate the AOD–IPV relationship.

References

1. Martin D. *Battered wives*. San Francisco: Glide, 1976.
2. Gelles RJ. Violence in the American family. In: Martin JP, ed. *Violence and the family*. Chichester: John Wiley & Sons;1978:169.
3. Gayford J. Battered wives: A preliminary survey of 100 cases. *Br Med J*. 1975;1:194–197.
4. Gelles RJ. *The violent home: A study of physical aggression between husbands and wives*. Beverly Hills, CA: Sage, 1972.
5. Pagelow M. *Woman-battering: Victims and their experiences*. Beverly Hills, CA: Sage, 1981.
6. Walker LE. The battered woman syndrome study. In: Finkelhor D, Gelles RJ, Hotaling GT, Straus MA, eds. *The dark side of families*. Beverly Hills, CA: Sage;1983:31–48.
7. Eberle P. Alcohol abusers and non-users: A discriminate analysis of differences between two subgroups of batterers. *J Health Soc Behav*. 1982; 23:260–271.
8. Coleman K, Weinman M, Hsi B. Factors affecting conjugal violence. *J Psychol*. 1980;105:197–202.
9. Telch C, Lindquist C. Violent versus nonviolent couples: A comparison of patterns. *Psychotherapy*. 1984;21:242–248.
10. Substance Abuse and Mental Health Services Administration. *Results from the 2003 National Survey on Drug Use and Health: National Findings*. Rockville, MD: Office of Applied Studies; 2004. NSDUH Series H-25, DHHS Publication No. SMA 04-3964.
11. Goetzel RZ, Hawkins K, Ozminkowski RJ. The health and productivity cost burden of the "top 10" physical and mental conditions affecting six large US employers in 1999. *J Occup Environ Med*. 2003;45:5–14.
12. Roy-Byrne PP, Stang P, Wittchen HU, et al. Lifetime panic-depression comorbidity in the National Comorbidity Survey: Association with symptoms. *Br J Psychiatry*. 2000;176:229–235.
13. Sanderson K, Andrews G. Prevalence and severity of mental health disability and relationship to diagnosis. *Psychiatr Serv*. 2002;53:80–86.
14. Stewart WF, Ricci JA, Chee E, et al. Cost of lost productive work time among US workers with depression. *JAMA*. 2003;289:3134–3144.
15. American Psychiatric Association. *Diagnostic and statistical manual of mental disorders*, 4th ed. Washington, DC: American Psychiatric Association, 1994.
16. Grant BF, Dawson DA, Stinson FS, et al. The 12-month prevalence and trends in DSM-IV alcohol abuse and dependence: United States 1991–1992 and 2001–2002. *Drug Alcohol Depend*. 2004;74: 223–234.
17. Leonard KE. Drinking patterns and intoxication in marital violence: Review, critique, and future directions for research. In: Martin SE, ed. *Alcohol and interpersonal violence: Fostering multidisciplinary perspectives*. Rockville, MD: NIAAA Research Monograph No. 24, NIH Pub. No. 93-3496, National Institutes of Health; 1993:253–280.
18. Schafer J, Caetano R, Clark CL. Rates of intimate partner violence in the United States. *Am J Public Health*. 1998;88(11):1702–1704.
19. Straus MA, Gelles RJ. How violent are American families? Estimates from the National Family Violence Resurvey and other studies. In: Straus MA, Gelles RJ, eds. *Physical violence in American families: Risk factors and adaptations to violence in 8/145 families*. New Brunswick, NJ: Transaction Publishers;1990:95–112.
20. Chermack ST, Fuller BE, Blow FC. Predictors of expressed partner and non-partner violence among patients in substance abuse treatment. *Drug Alcohol Depend*. 2000;58:43–54.
21. Murphy CM, O'Farrell TJ. Factors associated with marital aggression in male alcoholics. *J Fam Psychol*. 1994;8:321–335.
22. O'Farrell TJ, Murphy CM. Marital violence before and after alcoholism treatment. *J Consult Clin Psychol*. 1995;63:256–262.
23. Gelles R. *Intimate violence in families*. Thousand Oaks, CA: Sage, 1997.
24. Lee WV, Weinstein SP. How far have we come? A critical review of the research on men who batter. In: Galanter M, ed. *Recent developments in alcoholism*, Vol. 13. Alcohol and violence: Epidemiology, neurobiology, psychology, family issues. New York: Plenum Press;1997:337–356.
25. Leonard KE, Quigley BM. Drinking and marital aggression in newlyweds: An event-based analysis of drinking and the occurrence of husband marital aggression. *J Stud Alcohol*. 1999;60:537–545.
26. Cunradi CB, Caetano R, Clark CL, Schafer J. Alcohol-related problems and intimate partner violence among white, black, and Hispanic couples in the US. *Alcohol Clin Exp Res*. 1999;23(9): 1492–1501.
27. Caetano R, Cunradi CB, Schafer J, Clark CL. Intimate partner violence and drinking among white, black and Hispanic couples in the US. *J Subst Abuse*. 2000;11(2):123–138.
28. Caetano R, Field CA, Ramisetty-Mikler S, McGrath C. The 5-year course of intimate partner violence

among white, black, and Hispanic couples in the United States. *J Interpers Violence.* 2005;20(9):1039–1057.

29. Magdol L, Moffitt TE, Caspi A, et al. Gender differences in partner violence in a birth cohort of 21 year olds: Bridging the gap between clinical and epidemiological approaches. *J Consult Clinical Psych.* 1997;65(1):68–78.

30. Pan H, Neidig P, O'Leary K. Predicting mild and severe husband-to-wife physical aggression. *J Consult Clin Psych.* 1994;62:975–981.

31. Testa M, Livingston JA, Leonard KE. Women's substance use and experiences of intimate partner violence: A longitudinal investigation among a community sample. *Addict Behav.* 2003;28:1649–1664.

32. Cunradi CB, Caetano R, Schafer J. Alcohol-related problems, drug use, and male intimate partner violence severity among US couples. *Alcohol Clin Exp Res.* 2002;26(4):493–500.

33. Budd R. Cocaine abuse and violent death. *Am J Drug Alcohol Abuse.* 1989;15:375–382.

34. Inciardi J, Pottieger A. Crack-cocaine use and street crime. *J Drug Issues.* 1994;24:273–292.

35. Merikangas KR, Stevens DE. Substance abuse among women: Familial factors and comorbidity. In: Wetherington CL, Roman AB, eds. *Drug addiction research and the health of women.* Rockville, MD: US Department of Health and Human Services, National Institutes of Health, National Institute on Drug Abuse;1998:245–269.

36. Coker A, Smith P, McKeown R, King M. Frequency and correlates of intimate partner violence by type: Physical, sexual, and psychological battering. *Am J Public Health.* 2000;90(4):553–559.

37. Grisso J, Schwarz D, Hirschinger N, et al. Violent injuries among women in an urban area. *N Engl J Med.* 1999;341:1899–1905.

38. Kyriacou D, Anglin D, Taliaferro T, et al. Risk factors for injury to women from domestic violence. *N Engl J Med.* 1999;341:1892–1898.

39. Miller BA. Partner violence experiences and women's drug use: Exploring the connections. In: Wetherington CL, Roman AB, eds. *Drug addiction research and the health of women.* Rockville, MD: US Department of Health and Human Services, National Institutes of Health;1998:407–416.

40. El-Bassel N, Gilbert L, Wu E, et al. Relationship between drug abuse and intimate partner violence: A longitudinal study among women receiving methadone. *Am J Public Health.* 2005;95(3):465–470.

41. Kaufman Kantor G, Straus MA. The 'drunken bum' theory of wife beating. In: Straus M, Gelles R, eds. *Physical violence in American families.* New Brunswick: Transaction, 1990.

42. Graham K, Leonard KE, Room R, et al. Current directions in research on understanding and preventing intoxicated aggression. *Addiction.* 1998;93(5):659–676.

43. Leonard KE. Alcohol and intimate partner violence: When can we say that heavy drinking is a contributing cause of violence? *Addiction.* 2005;100:422–425.

44. Sayette MA. Cognitive theory and research. In: Leonard KE, Blane HT, eds. *Psychological theories of drinking and alcoholism,* 2nd ed. New York: The Guilford Press;1999:247–291.

45. Warneke LB. Benzodiazepines: Abuse and new use. *Can J Psychiatry.* 1991;36:194–205.

46. O'Leary KD, Schumacher JA. The association between alcohol use and intimate partner violence: Linear effect, threshold effect, or both? *Addict Behav.* 2003;28:1575–1585.

47. Johnson MP. Patriarchal terrorism and common couple violence: Two forms of violence against women. *J Marriage Fam.* 1995;57:283–294.

48. Holtzworth-Munroe A, Stuart GL. Typologies of batterers: Three subtypes and the differences among them. *Psychol Bull.* 1994;116(3):476–497.

49. Holtzworth-Munroe A, Meehan JC, Herron K, et al. Testing the Holtzworth-Munroe and Stuart (1994) batterer typology. *J Consult Clin Psychol.* 2000;68(6):1000–1019.

50. Holtzworth-Munroe A, Meehan JC. Typologies of men who are maritally violent: Scientific and clinical implications. *J Interpers Violence.* 2004;19(12):1369–1389.

51. Fals-Stewart W, Leonard KE, Birchler GR. The occurrence of male-to-female intimate partner violence on days of men's drinking: The moderating effects of antisocial personality disorder. *J Consult Clin Psychol.* 2005;73(2):239–248.

52. Downs WR, Miller BA. Treating dual problems of partner violence and substance abuse. In: Wekerle C, Wall A-M, eds. *The violence and addiction equation.* New York: Brunner-Routledge; 2002:254–274.

53. Fals-Stewart W, Birchler GR, Kelley ML. The Timeline Followback Spousal Violence Interview to assess physical aggression between intimate partners: Reliability and validity. *J Fam Violence.* 2003;18(3):131–142.

54. Fals-Stewart W. The occurrence of intimate partner violence on days of alcohol consumption: A longitudinal diary study. *J Consult Clin Psychol.* 2003;71:41–52.

55. Fals-Stewart W, Golden J, Schumacher JA. Intimate partner violence and substance use: A longitudinal day-to-day examination. *Addict Behav.* 2003;28:1555–1574.

56. O'Farrell TJ, Fals-Stewart W, Murphy M, Murphy CM. Partner violence before and after individual based alcoholism treatment for male alcoholic patients. *J Consult Clin Psychol.* 2003;71:92–102.

57. Widom CS. Does violence beget violence? A critical examination of the literature. *Psychol Bull.* 1989;106:3–28.

58. Schafer J, Caetano R, Cunradi CB. A path model of risk factors for intimate partner violence among couples in the United States. *J Interpers Violence.* 2004;19(2):127–142.

59. Felitti VJ, Anda RF, Nordenberg D, et al. Relationship of childhood abuse and household dysfunction to many of the leading causes of death in adults: The Adverse Childhood Experiences (ACE) Study. *Am J Prev Med.* 1998;14(4):245–258.

60. Whitfield CL, Anda RF, Dube SR, Felitti VJ. Violence childhood experiences and the risk of intimate partner violence in adults: Assessment in a large Health Maintenance Organization. *J Interpers Violence.* 2003;18(2):166–185.

61. Ehrensaft MK, Cohen P, Brown J, et al. Intergenerational transmission of partner violence: A 20-year prospective study. *J Consult Clin Psychol.* 2003;71(4):741–753.

62. Murphy CM, O'Farrell TJ. Marital violence among alcoholics. *Curr Dir Psychol Sci.* 1996;5:183–186.

63. O'Farrell TJ, Murphy CM, Stephan SH, et al. Partner violence before and after couples-based alcoholism treatment for male alcoholic patients: The role of treatment involvement and abstinence. *J Consult Clin Psychol.* 2004;72(2):202–217.

64. Stuart GL. Improving violence intervention outcomes by integrating alcohol treatment. *J Interpers Violence.* 2005;20(4):388–393.

65. O'Campo P, Gielen A, Faden R, et al. Violence by male partners against women during the childbearing year: A contextual analysis. *Am J Public Health.* 1995;85(8):1092–1097.

66. Cunradi CB, Caetano R, Clark C, Schafer J. Neighborhood poverty as a predictor of intimate partner violence among white, black, and Hispanic couples in the United States: A multilevel analysis. *Ann Epidemiol.* 2000;10(5):297–308.

67. Anda RF, Croft JB, Felitti VJ, et al. Adverse childhood experiences and smoking during adolescence and adulthood. *JAMA.* 1999;282: 1652–1658.

68. Dube SR, Anda RF, Felitti VJ, et al. Childhood abuse, household dysfunction, and the risk of attempted suicide throughout the lifespan: Findings from the adverse childhood experiences study. *JAMA.* 2001;286:3089–3096.

69. Dube SR, Anda RF, Felitti VJ, et al. Adverse childhood experiences and personal alcohol abuse as an adult. *Addict Behav.* 2002;27(5):713–725.

70. Hillis SD, Anda RF, Felitti VJ, Marchbanks PA. Adverse childhood experiences and sexual risk behaviors in women: A retrospective cohort study. *Fam Plan Perspect.* 2001;33:206–211.

71. Jacob T, Leonard KE, Haber JR. Family interactions of alcoholics as related to alcoholism type and drinking condition. *Alcohol Clin Exp Res.* 2001; 25:835–843.

72. Giancola P. Alcohol-related aggression in men and women: The influence of dispositional aggressivity. *J Stud Alcohol.* 2002;63:696–708.

Chapter 14

Traumatic Brain Injury and Intimate Partner Violence

Sharon R. Wilson

KEY CONCEPTS

- The mechanisms of injury in intimate partner violence (IPV) must be identified and documented.
- Clinical symptoms and sequelae exhibited by victims with mild, moderate, and severe traumatic brain injury (TBI) are varied.
- Etiology and prevalence of TBI in the general population and in IPV victims is an area for further research.
- Identification of the primary, secondary, and tertiary clinical manifestations of TBI frequently sustained by IPV victims is key to treatment.
- Understanding "second impact syndrome," its etiology, and clinical significance in IPV is key to preventing further brain injury.
- The significance of tertiary injury manifestations in TBI assault patients, including clinical presentations and common misdiagnoses, cannot be underestimated.

- Diagnostic strategies must include early detection, screening, neuropsychological evaluations, and rehabilitation for TBI in IPV victims.

Head injuries are a devastating and often undiagnosed consequence of intimate partner violence (IPV). Assaults to the head and face are the most frequently occurring IPV injury (1–12). Head and facial assaults frequently result in traumatic brain injury (TBI) (5,11,13,14). The Brain Injury Association of America defines TBI as "an insult to the brain, not of a degenerative or congenital nature, but caused by an external physical force, that may produce a diminished or altered state of consciousness, which results in an impairment of cognitive abilities or physical functioning" (15). The Brain Injury Association's definition further states, "Traumatic brain injury can also result in the disturbance of behavioral or emotional functioning. The resultant impairments may be temporary or permanent and cause partial or total functional disability or psychosocial maladjustment" (15).

Traumatic brain injury is a recognized public health problem and a significant cause of death and disability in the United States and worldwide (16–20). The Centers for Disease Control and Prevention (CDC 2003) reported TBI as the fifth leading cause of death in the United States. An estimated 1.5 million individuals sustain a TBI each year, resulting in 50,000 deaths and up to 90,000 survivors with long-term disability (16,21). During times of war, these numbers all increase.

GENERAL CLASSIFICATIONS OF TRAUMATIC BRAIN INJURY

Traumatic brain injury can be classified as *open* or *closed* head injury. Open head injury may occur as a result of direct, blunt, or penetrating force impacting the head and resulting in skull fracture. Direct brain injury may result from the object or bone fragments. Open injury in IPV may result from penetration by knives, bullets, screwdrivers, hammers, or ice picks. Closed head injury results from blunt impact forceful enough to move the brain within the skull without sustaining an open fracture. Rapid acceleration and deceleration mechanisms, such as severe shaking also result in closed injury. Open and closed head injuries result from nonviolent mechanisms such as motor vehicle accidents (MVAs), falls, and sports-related events.

Clinically, head injuries are categorized as severe, moderate, or mild. The category or severity of injury is dependent upon the type (direct or indirect) and intensity of force. Severity has been measured using coma scores, loss of consciousness (LOC), post-traumatic amnesia (PTA), or type of pathology. The Glasgow Coma Scale (GCS), Glasgow Coma Scale-Extended (GCS-E), Glasgow Outcome Scale (GOS), the Glasgow Outcome Scale-Extended (GOSE), and the Functional Status Examination (FSE) are examples of tools used to measure severity and clinical outcome of TBI based on specific neurologic, cognitive, behavioral, social, and family relationship findings (16,20,22–27). The GCS-E and the GOSE were developed to more accurately assess patients with mild TBI, the most common IPV brain injury. The GCS-E, GOS, and GOSE scores can be obtained at the time of injury and from days to months post injury (20,23,27). The FSE assesses change in functional status following TBI in relation to everyday functioning (28).

Severe Traumatic Brain Injury

Severity of TBI is measured by a score of function and/or duration of PTA (Table 14.1). Severe TBI victims have a postresuscitative GCS of 8 or less (scale of 1–15) within 48 hours of injury (25,29,30). The GCS-E defines a set of behavioral landmarks that fix the duration of PTA and codes an additional digit (scale 7–1) to the GCS; consequently GCS-E can not be scored for severe TBI victims at the time of injury. Severe TBI victims will have GOS scores of 3 or less (scale 5–1) or GOSE scores of 4 or less (scale 8–1) (20). Studies have shown PTA to be the best single predictor for all severities of

Table 14.1 Defining Severity of Traumatic Brain Injury (TBI)

Degree of Severity	Functioning Scores	Duration of Posttraumatic Amnesia (PTA)
Severe	GCS < 8 (post-resus.) GOS < 3 GOSE < 4	PTA > 1 week
Moderate	GCS = 9–12 GOS = 4 GOSE = 5–6	PTA up to 1 day
Mild • Amnesia • +/- LOC • Negative neuroimaging	GCS = 13–15	PTA < 24 hours

GCS, Glasgow Coma Scale; GOS, Glasgow Outcome Scale;

GOSE, Glasgow Outcome Scale Extended;

LOC, Loss of Consciousness.

TBI (27,31,32). Posttraumatic amnesia beyond 1 week is considered severe injury. The traditional use of LOC as a primary measure of injury severity has limitations. Loss of consciousness may be associated with specific early deficits but does not necessarily imply severity of TBI (32,33). Open head injuries are considered severe regardless of coma score, duration of LOC, or occurrence of PTA (15,34,35). Intracranial contusion, laceration, hematoma, hemorrhage, or diffuse axonal injuries (DAI) are categorized as severe TBI (25,36).

Morbidity and mortality rates for victims with severe brain injury are poor, with a reported 7% chance of moderate disability and a 40% mortality rate (37,38). Kraus and colleagues conducted a prospective examination of gender as an independent predictor of survival following severe and moderate TBI of 795 patients (652 males, 143 females) at two Level 1 trauma centers in Los Angeles, California over a 3.5-year period. The GOS was used to measure long-term outcome. The authors found mortality 1.28 times higher in females than in males, with the greatest difference (2.14) found in post-discharge deaths. After controlling for age, GCS, blunt versus penetrating injury, and presence of multiple traumas, females were 1.75 times more likely to die of their TBI (95% confidence interval [CI] 1.09−2.82). Females were 1.57 times more likely to experience poor outcomes such as severe disability or persistent vegetative states (36).

Severe TBI is diagnosed both clinically and with computed tomography (CT) scan and magnetic resonance imaging (MRI). Healthcare professionals may be more attuned to high-risk behaviors in men resulting in severe head injury and not expect a severe degree of injury in women (7). Blunt impact is the most common mechanism of injury in IPV assault-related TBI but penetrating brain injury secondary to firearms is the most lethal (39,40). The findings of Kraus and colleagues and other investigators suggest that, even though women may sustain fewer severe and moderate TBI compared to men, they have a higher mortality rate and poorer outcome following brain injury (16,36,41). Slewa-Younan and co-workers conducted a retrospective examination of 54 women with moderate to severe TBI admitted for inpatient rehabilitation. The authors examined differences by gender on various measures of injury severity and outcome after rehabilitation in an age- and education-matched sample of patients with TBI. Their study revealed greater severity of injury in men and no significant gender differences in outcome measures or in non–central nervous system (CNS)-associated injuries (42).

Moderate Traumatic Brain Injury

Moderate TBI has been defined as a postresuscitative GCS of 9–12, GOS of 4, GOSE of 5–6, or PTA up to 1 day (15,20,23,29,30,32,35,43,44). It is seldom possible to score amnesia in victims with a GCS of 12 or less; however, the GCS-E can be utilized to track amnesia through the patient's recovery once the GCS reaches 13 (23). Neuroimaging studies (CT and MRI) are used to detect traumatic brain lesions. Victims with moderate TBI may have a wide variety of clinical presentations, including an altered level of consciousness, confusion, somnolence, seizures, vomiting, headache, double vision, amnesia, and focal neurologic deficits (16,20,25,32,36,41). An initial non-contrast CT scan of the head should be performed when victims exhibit any of these clinical symptoms (45,46). Approximately 10% of all head injury patients are diagnosed with a moderate brain injury (23,43,47). The absence of CT abnormalities does not guarantee a good outcome, and the presence of abnormalities does not necessarily reflect long-term disability (45). MRI is more sensitive and specific than CT in the evaluation of cerebral contusions, small nonhemorrhagic lesions, and detection of DAI (19,45). Victims with moderate TBI are hospitalized for appropriate neurosurgical evaluation, intervention, and rehabilitation. The 5-point GOS is commonly used to assess clinical outcomes of moderate to severely brain-injured patients. The 5 categories of the GOS are as follows: 5 = good recovery, 4 = moderate disability, 3 = severe disability, 2 = vegetative state, and 1 = death (20).

Mild Traumatic Brain Injury

Mild TBI, also referred to as concussion or "the silent epidemic" is frequently undiagnosed or misdiagnosed and is one of the most common forms of neurologic disorder (15,48–50). It has been estimated that mild TBI accounts for 90% of new cases of medically diagnosed head injuries in the United States each year (27,51). Mild TBI has been defined as a traumatically induced physiological disruption of brain function characterized by any alteration of mental status at time of injury, anterograde or retrograde amnesia, with or without brief LOC, GCS score of 13 to 15, negative neuroimaging, and PTA of less than 24 hours

(25,26,32,34,35). Mild TBI victims who do not sustain LOC may not seek acute medical care. When a mild TBI victim does present for medical care, her GCS score is frequently normal (15) and she may not be thoroughly assessed. Consequently, patients are discharged from emergency departments or other clinical settings without appropriate follow-up to address complex cognitive symptoms or their potential rehabilitative needs (27). Cognitive and behavioral symptoms of mild TBI cover a wide spectrum and are often transient, occurring within the days immediately following injury. Presentations may include complaints of dizziness, disorientation, amnesia, headache, LOC, confusion, nausea, vomiting, somnolence, emotional lability, fatigue, depression, anxiety, visual disturbance, noise sensitivity, benign positional vertigo, gait disturbance, attention deficits, poor memory, poor concentration, slowed thought process, and neurologic deficits (15,22,25,26,33,34,49,52–57). Following mild TBI, 25%–35% of patients report postconcussion symptoms (PCS) such as headache, dizziness, and concentration and memory problems 6 months after injury (48). Symptoms of posttraumatic stress disorder (PTSD) such as irritability, anger, difficulty with concentration, and event amnesia have been reported in MVA and IPV victims with mild TBI (11,58).

The GCS-E and GOSE are reported in the literature as severity and outcome indexes more sensitive to the nuances and complexities of mild TBI (Figure 14.1) (16,20,23,27). Because of the large number of mild TBI victims with GCS scores of 15, the supplementary

GCS-E coding may aide in the acute assessment and provide important prognostic information regarding symptom severity and recovery (23,27).

The GOSE is an extension of the original 5-point GOS and is thought to exceed the validity of the GOS in mild to moderate TBI (24); it has been found to be more sensitive to change at 3-month and 6-month assessments (20). Kirkness and colleagues utilized the GOSE as one of the measures to assess gender and age differences in the post-injury course of patients 3 months and 6 months following TBI (16). The authors found a significant relationship between gender and age with respect to functional outcome at 6 months post TBI when controlling initial injury severity. Women 30 years and older had significantly poorer outcome as measured by the GOSE ($p = .031$) than men or younger women. Women 30 years and older also had a different rate of recovery, showing no improvement between 3 and 6 months post injury.

The 8 categories of the GOSE are: 8 = upper good recovery, 7 = lower good recovery, 6 = upper moderate disability, 5 = lower moderate disability, 4 = upper severe disability, 3 = lower severe disability, 2 = persistent vegetative state, and 1 = dead (16,20,24). "Good recovery" refers to the ability to participate in normal social life and return to work if desired (dizziness and headache may still be present). "Moderate disability" refers to the ability to be independent in personal care, travel by public transport, and work in a sheltered setting (independent but disabled). "Severe disability" refers to dependence on another person for

7 = No amnesia: victim can remember impact of injury

6 = Amnesia for 30 min or less: victim regained consciousness while at scene of injury

5 = Amnesia of ½ hour to 3 hours: victim remembers being placed in ambulance or
car, ride to hospital, arriving in emergency department (ED)
or admission to ward, etc.

4 = Amnesia for 3–24 hours: duration determined by content of memory (an event in
ED, on the ward or a procedure)

3 = Amnesia for 1–7 days

2 = Amnesia for 8–30 days

1 = Amnesia for 31–90 days

0 = Amnesia for > 3 months

X = Cannot be scored: inappropriate or unintelligible responses, unconscious,
intubated, facial fractures, etc.

Figure 14.1 Amnesia scores of the Glasgow Coma Scale - Extended (GCS-E).

some activities every day. "Persistent vegetative state" is no response to commands or intelligible speech and no evidence of behaviorally meaningful activity (16).

Along with impairments in physical functioning, mild TBI affects a wide range of somatic, cognitive, visual, and affective symptoms. Many of these symptoms are unrecognized and not appropriately addressed in acute care environments. The standard of care is often limited to reassurance, discharge instructions, and medications. The opportunity for referral and early intervention is frequently lost. Familiarity with clinical tools more sensitive to subtle presentations of mild TBI may prevent premature discharge from acute care settings and allow better treatment and follow-up.

PREVALENCE OF TRAUMATIC BRAIN INJURY IN GENERAL POPULATION AND IN INTIMATE PARTNER VIOLENCE

Head trauma is an underestimated cause of chronic disability. An estimated 5.3 million Americans currently live with disabilities secondary to brain injury (59). Conservative estimates place the incidence of TBI at 100 per 100,000 patient population, a prevalence of 2.5 to 6.5 million (60). An emergency department-based study conducted by Boswell and co-workers reported 41% of their sample population had sustained a TBI (61). At least 1 million people with TBI are treated and released from emergency departments yearly (59). Mild TBI remains one of the most prevalent neurologic disorders, with an estimated incidence of 100–300 per 100,000 hospital treated patients (62).

Underestimation of the number of head injury victims with TBI has been attributed to imprecise information gathering, misdiagnosis, underreporting, lack of recognition of late-developing neurologic and endocrine symptoms, and failure to recognize the range of traumatic injury–related dysfunctions (18,30,55,63–66). Traumatic brain injury predominantly affects young men, with the risk of brain injury in men twice that of women (26,59,60,67). The three leading causes of TBI are motor vehicle collisions, violence, and falls. Motor vehicle collisions are the leading cause of TBI, accounting for 50%–70% (35,59,68,69). Violence, mostly from firearms, has surpassed motor vehicle collisions as the leading cause of death related to TBI (67). More than 50,000 people die each year as a result of TBI (16,59,67).

The incidence of head injury sustained by IPV victims during the course of their abuse is unknown (5). Women seeking medical attention for head, neck, and facial injuries are 7.5 times more likely to be victims of IPV than women with injuries limited to other locations (9). An estimated 36% of IPV victims sustain injuries to the head, neck, or face (9,12). These assaults can result in TBI, one of the most undiagnosed, prevalent, and serious consequences of IPV (1). Women are more likely to incur an IPV-related head injury at home and are more likely to die from an assault-related head injury than are men (70). Investigators examining IPV victims residing in and out of emergency shelters found 74%–77% had symptoms consistent with TBI (5,11). Rates of severe head injury were higher in sheltered women than nonsheltered women (11). Some male batterers avoid striking victims in the face to avoid detection. Instead, blows are delivered to the back of the head (71). A history of TBI is often undocumented in medical records of IPV victims. Loss of consciousness may not be reported because of PTA or a cognitive impairment associated with the brain injury. Nondisclosure is consistent with the tendency to hide or minimize patterns of abuse when seeking emergency treatment (72,73). As a result, many IPV brain injuries are unrecognized and prevalence is underestimated. Wadman and Muelleman's examination of emergency department use by IPV homicide victims found TBI the most frequently documented injury prior to the victim's IPV homicide (40).

CLINICAL MANIFESTATIONS OF TRAUMATIC BRAIN INJURY

Clinical manifestations of TBI can be classified as primary, secondary, or tertiary injuries (25,34,74). Primary brain injury is damage sustained by the victim at the time of assault. This includes concussion, contusion, axonal injury, hemorrhage, hematoma, and skull fracture. Secondary brain injury is the delayed manifestations of the primary injury. This includes subsequent development of cerebral edema, ischemia, cerebral hemorrhage, or herniation syndrome. Tertiary describes delayed or long-term manifestations of the victim's primary and secondary TBI and includes seizures, infections, stress, and the complex myriad of PCS and PTSD symptoms.

BRAIN INJURIES

Concussion

Concussions or mild TBIs are the most common brain injuries and are a major public health concern, affecting approximately 128 per 100,000 persons in the United States yearly (15,18,27,48,75). Even though there is no universal agreement on the definition or grading of concussion, it can be defined as a temporary and brief interruption of neurologic function caused by nonpenetrating blunt trauma to the head or by rapid acceleration, deceleration, or rotation of the head (25,33,75,76). The prefrontal cortex, temporal lobes (inferior and medial), and junction of the upper midbrain and thalamus are injured during mild TBI or concussion (19,45,75,77). When the victim's head sustains a direct blow or is subject to acceleration or deceleration forces, the brain rotates within the skull, resulting in focal damage from the anterior and middle cranial fossae or a shearing strain of neuronal axons (45,75,77,78). Intimate partner violence victims with injury in these regions of the brain may have emotional complaints and impairments of attention, information processing, and recent verbal memory (45,79).

Numerous grading systems have been developed to grade the severity of concussion based on LOC, non-LOC, and PTA. The brief LOC that may occur with concussive injury has been attributed to rotational force exerted at the upper midbrain–thalamus junction disrupting the functioning of the reticular neurons that maintain alertness (75). The etiology of PTA is unknown, but its duration has been considered the best indicator of TBI severity and the most dependable marker of outcome (16,23,27,31). The American Academy of Neurology (AAN) Practice Parameter Grading System for Concussion (80) is a 3-point scale used to evaluate severity of concussion and establish guidelines for the management of sport-related concussions (31,32,75,80). The AAN grading system is as follows: Grade 1: transient confusion, no LOC, resolution of concussion symptoms and mental status abnormalities in less than 15 minutes; Grade 2: transient confusion, no LOC, concussion symptoms or mental status abnormalities of greater than 15 minutes; Grade 3: any LOC, either brief (seconds) or prolonged (minutes).

Gender differences in concussive injury or mild TBI have been examined in athletics. A meta-analysis of 39 studies involving 1,463 cases of mild TBI and 1,191 control cases by Belanger and colleagues found the overall effect of concussion in athletes is comparable with that found for nonathletes sustaining mild TBI, with delayed memory, executive functions and language, and cognitive functions most affected (21). Some mechanisms of concussive injury in women's soccer parallel IPV mechanisms, such as impact against a solid object (goal post, ground), impact against a person (elbow, knee, head), or repeated impacts to the head (heading the ball). Gender differences found in mild TBI secondary to soccer are consistent with those reported in other investigations (16,41,42,52).

Covassin and associates' cohort study of collegiate athletes compared gender differences regarding the incidence of concussion in six sports during the 1997–2000 academic years (81). Data was collected using the NCAA Injury Surveillance System (ISS) that included recorded injury data from men's and women's sports. Women soccer players sustained a significantly greater number of concussions than other women athletes (seven times risk of softball; two times risk of lacrosse) and significantly more concussions than male cohorts (7% of all male game injury; 11.4% of all female game injury). In an earlier study of a single season of Canadian university soccer, Delaney and co-workers found women soccer players were more than 2.5 times as likely to have sustained a concussion than were men soccer players ($p < .05$) (82). Ellemberg and colleagues assessed cognitive functioning after a first concussion in female soccer players, 6–8 months post injury compared to age-matched teammates without history of concussion (18). The concussed athletes had normal short- and long-term verbal memory, attention, and simple reaction time. However, the authors found persistent impairments up to 8 months post-injury. Concussed athletes remained less accurate on the task of executive planning and significantly slower on cognitive functions related to cognitive processing speed (decision making, inhibition, and flexibility) (18).

A GCS of 14–15 and a negative CT scan are two of the defining features of concussion or mild TBI (19,26,33,45,75,76). CT without contrast is indicated for LOC, severe or prolonged altered mental status, PTA, or neurologic signs (19,26,45,75). Less than 10% of patients will develop cerebral hemorrhage or cerebral edema as secondary injuries, and less than 2% will require neurosurgical intervention (75).

In a recent study, Nygren de Boussard and colleagues reviewed 100,784 patients admitted for concussion over a 10-year period and found 127 (0.13%) readmitted for delayed intracranial complications (17).

Postconcussive symptoms are hallmarks of a tertiary injury sustained in the majority of mild TBI or concussed patients, with a wide range of sometimes disabling symptoms often reported during the first week after injury (26,33,75,76). Postconcussive symptoms may be transient or long-term, with an estimated 40%–80% of patients with mild TBI diagnosed with PCS (26,83,84). Per the International Classification of Disease, 10th Revision, the criteria for PCS are:

1. Interval between head trauma with LOC and onset of symptoms is less than or equal to 4 weeks.
2. Symptoms in at least three of the following categories: (a) headache, dizziness, fatigue, noise intolerance; (b) irritability, depression, anxiety, emotional lability; (c) subjective concentration, memory, or intellectual difficulties without neuropsychological evidence of marked impairment; (d) insomnia; (e) reduced alcohol tolerance; (f) preoccupation with above symptoms and fear of brain damage with hypochondrial concern and adoption of sick role (75).

A wide range (24%–60%) of mild TBI patients report persistent symptoms at 3 months with 10%–15% reporting symptoms for more than a year post-injury (52,66). Symptoms established for more than a few weeks may persist for months and resist treatment (75). The majority (approximately 85%) of individuals diagnosed with mild TBI and PCS will be asymptomatic 1 year post-injury (66).

Identified risks for PCS suggest that women who are victims of IPV are at greater risk for developing neurobehavioral sequelae (71). These risks are: (a) women are more prone to PCS after head injury (85), (b) IPV victims with mild TBI secondary to an assault have a significantly worse PCS than those with other mechanisms of injury, (c) assault victims with PCS have poorer vocational outcomes (84), and (d) repeat concussions increase the likelihood of developing persistent PCS (60,64,81,82,86).

Posttraumatic stress disorder is a tertiary injury experienced by mild TBI victims (11,58,87). Posttraumatic stress disorder is a common mental health sequelae of mild TBI (17%–33%) and IPV (64%) (87,88). Findings of numerous studies suggest that women have higher probabilities of PTSD following a traumatic event than men, with women twice as likely to develop the disorder (58,88–91). Features characteristic of PTSD include reexperiencing the traumatic event, emotional numbness or avoidance, and increased arousal (87,88,90,91). Diagnosis requires persistence of symptoms for more than 1 month and clinically significant impairment in at least one major life domain (91). Bryant and Harvey's investigation of the relationship between PCS and PTSD in mild TBI found that postconcussive symptoms were more evident in patients with PTSD. The authors theorize that PCS may be mediated by an interaction of neurologic and psychological factors after mild TBI (87). Valera and Berenbaum's study of IPV victims with TBI found victims with greater levels of partner abuse severity had higher levels of PTSD symptom severity (11).

Cerebral Contusion

Contusion is a more serious TBI sustained by IPV victims. Contusions typically result from direct impact, and are bruises on the cortical surface of the brain produced when parenchymal blood vessels are damaged. Vascular damage results in scattered areas of petechial hemorrhage and edema (19,44,45). Intimate partner violence victims sustaining a single impact may have multiple contused areas. Contusions opposite the side of impact are *contrecoup injuries*.

Neuroimaging with non-contrast CT and MRI can diagnose contusions during the immediate, post-assault period. However, CT scan remains the gold standard for acute imaging and management of injured patients (17,19,44,45). MRI has greater sensitivity and specificity than CT and is commonly used to further evaluate moderate and severe TBI. Small contusions without areas of hemorrhage may be difficult to identify on CT scan immediately post-injury. MRI is superior to CT for the initial detection and accurate definition of contusions (45). An IPV victim with contusion may experience a brief, unreported LOC that delays diagnosis. Despite the brief duration of LOC, tertiary manifestations such as post-assault confusion and obtundation may be prolonged and associated with neurologic deficits. Post-injury neurologic problems include seizure, increased intracranial pressure, focal neurologic deficits, and PCS (15,34,44,71,85).

Intimate partner violence victims with significant contusions may have an uneventful recovery.

Victims subjected to recurrent injury or who have a history of alcohol abuse have a higher incidence of hemorrhage into the contusion. Substance abuse is highly associated with IPV and TBI, with 35%–50% of TBI patients reported to have alcohol intoxication (15,30,60,71). An examination of the long-term consequences of IPV found 16% of woman in violent relationships abuse alcohol (92). Increased hemorrhage and edema of the contusion may cause a local mass effect requiring neurosurgical decompression to prevent ischemia and infarction.

Diffuse Axonal Injury

Diffuse axonal injury (DAI) is the result of shear–strain forces on the brain. Low-rigidity neurons at the superficial gray–white junction and deeper structures such as the brainstem are susceptible to rotational acceleration/deceleration forces. Sufficient injury from the stretching or tearing of axons extending from neuron cell bodies results in nerve cell death (45,75,78). A wide spectrum of axonal injury occurs in TBI, and virtually all head injuries have some degree of axonal injury (93). Intimate partner violence victims may present anywhere within this spectrum. Direct impact trauma, such as a blow to the head or violent shaking, are common IPV mechanisms of injury associated with DAI (11,15,35,94).

Victims with persistent traumatic coma, not secondary to ischemia or mass lesion, are usually diagnosed with DAI (25). The onset of coma is at the time of injury and lasts for 6 or more hours. No early clinical predictors exist to differentiate mild, moderate, or severe DAI. Initial CT is usually negative and should be followed by MRI when the patient's clinical condition allows (19,45,74). MRI has been successful in the detection and characterization of DAI. Lesions usually spare the cortex, appearing as numerous, small, and deep in the white matter and brainstem (19,45).

Severity of DAI is classified as mild, moderate, or severe based on clinical course. Victims with severe DAI remain comatose for extended periods, exhibiting persistent brainstem and autonomic dysfunction. Severe DAI is frequently associated with intracranial injuries, and victims rarely survive. Motor vehicle collision is the most common mechanism of injury (15,25).

Moderate DAI is most common and secondary to falls, motor vehicle collisions, assaults, or violent shaking. The resulting coma lasts more than 24 hours,

and victims will have severe PTA with persistent moderate to severe cognitive deficits. Approximately 25% die from complications associated with their prolonged coma (25).

Mild DAI can result from assaults, shaking, falls, or motor vehicle collisions. The duration of coma is 6–24 hours. Victims may exhibit persistent PCS and/ or mild permanent disabilities, with approximately 15% dying from infection or associated intracranial injury (25).

Intimate partner violence assault-related DAI is most frequently due to a forceful blow to the head or severe shaking resulting in a shearing brain injury (11,15,94,95). Violent shaking as a mechanism of IPV injury is frequently overlooked. Women with the "shaken adult syndrome" have the diagnostic triad of retinal hemorrhages, subdural hematoma, and patterned bruising of the shoulders and upper chest that is associated with the "shaken baby syndrome" (94–97). The DAI may be mild, moderate, or severe. Jackson and colleagues' study of IPV victims found 68% reported having been severely shaken by their partner, with a frequency ranging from one episode to more than 20 episodes. A history of severe shaking at any time within 5 years correlated with higher symptom severities (5).

The first reported case of fatal shaken adult syndrome was documented post mortem in an adult Palestinian male who died under Israeli police interrogation (95). The victim was shaken over a 12-hour period before collapsing. Autopsy concluded death to be the result of brain injury due to rotational acceleration of the head without direct impact. Histopathological examination disclosed DAI and retinal hemorrhages. Shaking as a means of torture has been recognized and widely debated (95,98,99). Shaking, as a mechanism of TBI in IPV is underrecognized, and the diagnosis frequently delayed or missed (71). Consequently, IPV-related shaken adult syndrome is underreported in the literature, and its prevalence, morbidity, and mortality are not well defined.

Epidural Hematoma

Epidural hematoma (EDH) is categorized as a severe TBI caused by forceful direct impact resulting in a deformity of the skull. An EDH forms between the skull's inner table and the dura, and is present in 0.5% of head injuries (15,25,34,74,100).

Most EDHs (80%) are secondary to blunt trauma in the temporoparietal region of the skull resulting in fracture across the middle meningeal artery or a dural sinus (15,25,34,74,100).

Victims complain of severe headache, nausea, vomiting, and dizziness. Thirty percent of victims with EDH present with the classic posttraumatic decreased LOC followed by a lucid interval (25,34). The survival rate is nearly 100% for individuals whose injury is rapidly diagnosed and hematoma evacuated. The survival rate of EDH with associated coma is approximately 80% with rapid diagnosis and treatment (25,34). Noncontrast CT is the best diagnostic imaging study. The most common location is the temporal region, where the EDH appears biconvex with the margins stopping at the cranial sutures. Approximately 20% of EDHs have blood in the subdural space (100).

Subdural Hematoma

Subdural hematoma (SDH) is usually the result of forceful acceleration–deceleration injury and consists of blood clots between the dura and the brain resulting from the tearing of bridging veins with rapid head movement (25,34,74,100). These SDHs tend to be large and primarily located in the frontal and parietal regions. Approximately 10%–15% are bilateral, and 50% are associated with other intracranial injuries. The mortality rate of SDH with concurrent intracranial injury is 60%–90%, whereas an isolated SDH mortality rate is less than 20% (100). Subdural hematoma occurs in 30% of head injuries and is more common than EDH (25).

Intimate partner violence assaults involving shaking, punching, or impacting the head against an object may result in an SDH. The slow venous bleeding may delay development of clinical signs and symptoms, resulting in more extensive brain injury from prolonged compression. Victims with SDH may present with a wide spectrum of primary, secondary, and tertiary manifestations, ranging from coma to subtle personality changes (74). An SDH with LOC at the time of injury has a poor prognosis because of the presumed concurrent DAI (25).

Clinically, SDHs are classified as acute, subacute, and chronic. Victims with acute SDH are symptomatic within 24 hours of injury and often have a decreased LOC. Fifty to seventy percent have a posttraumatic lucid period followed by a decline in mental status. Neurologic deficits and signs of brain herniation may be present (25). Subacute SDHs become symptomatic 24 hours to 2 weeks post-injury. Victims may present with headache, altered mental status, muscle weakness, or paralysis. Chronic SDHs do not become symptomatic until 2 or more weeks post-injury. Chronic SDH may initially be small and asymptomatic. Recurrent bleeding eventually expands the hematoma, which becomes symptomatic. Clinical presentation may be subtle and nonspecific, with some victims unwilling or unable to disclose a history of trauma. Chronic SDH has an estimated overall mortality rate of 10% (25).

Noncontrast CT is the acute diagnostic imaging study of choice for SDHs (25,45,74,100). MRI is more sensitive than CT and is extremely helpful in the detection of small subacute and chronic SDHs (45,74,100). Evacuation is the treatment for acute and subacute SDH. Symptomatic chronic SDH require surgical evacuation, with up to 75% having a good outcome.

Traumatic Subarachnoid Hemorrhage

Traumatic subarachnoid hemorrhage (SAH) is present with most moderate to severe head injuries. It is defined as blood within the cerebrospinal fluid (CSF) and meningeal intima from superficial brain contusions or lacerations of small vessels crossing the subarachnoid space (25,74,100). Assault victims with SAH typically have altered mental status and complaints of severe headache with photophobia. Diagnosis is by noncontrast CT that detects over 90% of all SAH bleeds within the initial 24 hours (100). Blood is seen within the basilar cisterns at the interhemispheric fissures and sulci. Traumatic brain injury victims with associated traumatic SAH have worse outcomes than those without associated SAH (25). Posttraumatic cerebral vasospasm is a frequent complication that can can cause cerebral ischemia and lead to disability.

Intracerebral Hematoma

Intimate partner violence victims with blunt head trauma may incur an intracerebral hematoma (ICH) deep within the brain tissue. This injury is secondary to shearing acceleration–deceleration force injury to small, deep arterioles resulting in petechial hemorrhages that join to form the hematoma (25). The majority (85%) of ICHs are located in the frontal and temporal lobes. More than 50% of those injured have an LOC at time of injury. Clinical course is dependent on size, location, persistent bleeding, severity of impact, and coexisting intracranial and extracranial lesions (19,25). Intracerebral hematoma associated with concurrent intracranial lesions and cerebral edema may herniate; ICH is diagnosed by noncontrast CT (45,74,100). Emergent surgical decompression may be required, with a mortality rate of approximately 45% for those unconscious at the time of surgery (25).

Penetrating Traumatic Brain Injury

Intimate partner violence victims sustain penetrating brain injury from either impalement or firearms. Penetration occurs from the impact of a bullet, knife, or other sharp object that forces hair, skin, bone, and fragments from the object into the brain (15). Sorenson and Wiebs examined weapons in the lives of IPV victims residing in emergency shelters and found impalement weapons included scissors, screwdrivers, and knives (101). The authors reported approximately 37% of victims reported a firearm had been used to hurt, scare, or intimidate. The most commonly reported weapons to inflict penetrating injury were screwdrivers (36.8%), knives (34.4%), handguns (32.1%), long guns (13.9%), and machetes (9.4%) (101).

The most common penetrating head injury seen in the United States is a gunshot wound (GSW) to the head, with up to 76% of victims dying at the scene (15,25). Wadman and Muelleman's study of IPV homicide reported firearm injuries (52.9%) as the leading mechanism of death, with the head as the most common site (78%) of lethal GSWs (40). In another study, close-proximity GSW to the head or neck was found to be the cause of death in a majority (74%) of IPV homicides (39).

Penetrating GSWs to the head are produced with moderate- to high-velocity projectiles discharged at close range. The bullet may bounce off the opposite inner table of the skull and ricochet within the brain, or may stop within the brain. Ricochet within the skull widens the area of injury. "Through and through" injuries include the effects of penetration and additional shearing, stretching, and rupture of brain tissue (102). The morbidity and mortality from GSW to the head is dependent on the bullet's intracranial path, speed of entry, size, and type. Extremely high mortality rates are associated with bullets that cross the midline, pass through ventricles, or lodge in the posterior fossa (25). Large or fragmented bullets usually result in fatal injury. Gunshot wound is the single

most frequent cause of death from TBI, with firearms accounting for more than 50% of IPV homicides (15). Clinical evaluation of a victim with a GSW to the head focuses on the GCS and pupillary response. A GCS of less than 5 has a mortality rate of nearly 100%. A GCS of more than 8 with reactive pupils has an approximate 25% mortality rate (103). CT scan is the neuroimaging study of choice for GSWs.

Skull Fractures

Fractures of the skull from IPV assaults are caused by forceful direct impact mechanisms of injury. Victims with skull fractures may not have an associated severe underlying TBI. Fractures usually start at the point of maximum impact and clinically may be difficult to diagnose. CT with bone windows will detect and define the extent of most skull fractures (74,100).

Skull fractures are described as linear, comminuted, diastatic, or depressed. They involve the calvarium and/or the base of the skull. *Linear skull fractures* are the most common and most often associated with EDH (25,34,74,100). *Comminuted skull fractures* are multiple linear fractures radiating from the point of impact and are usually the result of a more severe mechanism. *Diastatic skull fracture* features disruption of the coronal or lamboid sutures of the skull.

Depressed skull fracture results from the force of impact moving the fractured piece of bone inward toward the brain, and is usually secondary to direct impact injury from weapons such as hammers or baseball bats. Victims with depressed skull fractures usually have significant underlying TBI and major complications (15,25,34,74,100).

Basilar skull fractures are at the base of the skull and linear, usually extending through the temporal bone, with resultant hemotympanum (25). Basilar skull fractures require considerable blunt force, and IPV victims should be evaluated for TBI and other associated injury and sequelae (25,74). Clinical signs consistent with basilar skull fracture include hemotympanum, rhinorrhea, otorrhea, retroauricular hematoma, or periorbital ecchymosis and should have further evaluation (44,74). A noncontrast CT should be obtained to detect underlying brain injury or hemorrhage (74).

Approximately 41% of IPV victims in the Sorenson and Wiebs study reported hammers used as a weapon during IPV assault (101). Other authors have reported kicking, head banging, and punching as mechanisms of injury resulting in skull fractures (1,8,104).

SECOND IMPACT SYNDROME

Catastrophic deterioration from diffuse cerebral edema following mild TBI is a rare, delayed posttraumatic complication that may result in death or persistent vegetative state. A specific form of cerebral edema resulting from repeated minor head injury has been proposed as an etiology (64). This *second impact syndrome* (SIS) or *recurrent TBI* has long been described in pediatric, sport, and IPV literature (23,40,65, 105–110). Second impact syndrome has been defined as occurring when an individual who has sustained an initial head injury, most often a concussion, sustains a second head injury before symptoms associated with the first have fully resolved (15,106).

Women with IPV-related TBI are at significant risk for SIS (40,109). The second injury may occur days to weeks after the first injury. Following the first TBI, the risk for a second is three times greater. Following a second injury, the risk for a third TBI is eight times greater (59,82). Valera's 2003 study of brain injury in IPV victims found 74% had sustained some type of TBI secondary to violence from their partner and that 51% had sustained multiple TBIs from recurrent IPV assaults (11). The chronic nature of IPV leads to multiple recurrent physical injuries having immediate and long-term consequences for the victim. The sequelae of recurrent mild TBI or SIS have a broad spectrum, ranging from complete resolution of symptoms to death. Sport- and IPV-related studies examining the impact of concussions and SIS in female athletes and IPV victims have shown the occurrence of one or more TBI results in increased risk for recurrent injury, prolonged recovery, and more severe neuropsychological deficits (18,81,82,111). Undetected recurrent head injuries may represent missed opportunities for intervention and protection from poor cognitive outcomes and potentially lethal IPV assault. The studies of war-related TBI and SIS will certainly contribute to our understanding of this important health problem.

TERTIARY BRAIN INJURIES AND THEIR SIGNIFICANCE IN INTIMATE PARTNER VIOLENCE

Victims often endure repeated undisclosed or undetected IPV assaults to the head and face. Consequently, the sequelae of their TBI are often misdiagnosed (60).

Victims of IPV endure the same mechanisms of injury, report the same constellation of symptoms, and experience the same rates of recovery as patients and victims with mild TBI from other mechanisms (13,14,18,81,82,86,112–114). Research has examined the interrelationship between IPV and TBI (5,11,71). Corrigan and associates screened women who presented to emergency departments for health issues associated with IPV. The authors found 30% of the women had at least one assault-related LOC and 67% had residual potentially TBI-related symptoms consistent with PCS (71). Victims of IPV frequently report difficulty with concentration, memory, headache, depression, and anxiety (5,11,71,115–117). Victims also report problems with confusion, judgment, problem-solving, and decision-making (118–120). The diagnosis of borderline personality, PTSD, or depression is frequently given to women with mild TBI and PCS (115,119). In the absence of accurate diagnosis and treatment, the victim's constellation of symptoms can result in long-term physical and cognitive disability. The ability to resume normal or baseline function within the family, socially, or at work may be limited. The victim's ability to plan for the safety of herself and her children may be severely handicapped.

Although many head-injured IPV victims report symptoms consistent with moderate to severe TBI, the repeated concussive and subconcussive injuries most commonly result in mild TBI (11). Somatic complaints, cognitive deficits, and emotional symptoms can appear weeks to months following assault (1,121). Valera found that only 25% of women with an IPV-related head injury sought medical care (11). A high index of suspicion is required to make the diagnosis of mild TBI, especially in IPV-related assaults. Traumatic brain injury does not require LOC and is often not diagnosed even in the presence of clinical signs, including LOC (115). The diagnosis may be overlooked because of other more severe traumatic injuries that may have altered neurologic function. The victim's cognitive impairment may be attributed to the "emotional" component of the assault or to the presence of alcohol and/or drugs. Patients evaluated for mild TBI typically have GCS of 14–15, normal imaging, and nonfocal neurologic examinations. An estimated 22%–35% of women presenting to emergency departments for medical care are there because of IPV (122). Yet, only 1%–6% of women cared for in the emergency department are diagnosed with IPV-related injuries or complaints (40,109). Consequently, the percentage of women with IPV-related TBI is underdiagnosed and underreported.

Recurrent mild TBI has been extensively studied in men's and women's athletics with the development of specific strategies for rapid assessment, treatment, protective equipment, and regulations for participation (15,18,31–33,76,81,82,86,110). Despite the demonstrated similarities in mechanisms and impairments with IPV-related mild TBI, protective measures to prevent further abuse and recurrent head injury for IPV victims have not been as extensively studied and are rarely implemented (7,115,123).

TREATMENT STRATEGIES

There is no "cure" for TBI. Prevention, education, early detection, and appropriate referral are interventions that play significant roles in treating victims with TBI. Traumatic brain injury is a hidden consequence and additional danger faced by IPV victims. Early utilization of the GCS-E, GOSE, FSE, or the multifaceted concussion-assessment batteries described by Broglio and colleagues are a small sample of evaluation tools that may be of benefit (124). Early identification of mild TBI, early recognition of prolonged PCS, and early intervention can minimize the development of long-term somatic, cognitive, and behavioral consequences endured by IPV and other mild TBI victims (20,21,41,47,51,55,125,126). Somatic consequences reported by IPV victims include chronic headache, nausea, dizziness, seizure, insomnia, and somnolence (115,127). The most sensitive cognitive deficits following mild TBI are impairments of working memory processes such as speed of information processing, attention, and recent verbal and recent visual memory (79). Intimate partner violence victims complain of easy distractibility, confusion, disorientation, and difficulty with concentration, memory, and judgment (115). These victims may exhibit difficulty processing complex information, developing plans, and executing goals (7). Long-term behavioral consequences include increased irritability, anxiety, depression, mania, increased risk-taking, and high-risk behavior (115). Failure to appropriately diagnose and treat PCS worsens psychogenic

impairment and results in less favorable vocational outcomes (128,129).

Routine screening of IPV victims for TBI has been recommended by some authors (5,7,130). Screening should include direct questions regarding the onset, frequency, and duration of blows to the head and face, severe shaking, or LOC (5). Additionally, victims should be evaluated for symptoms consistent with PCS. Victims are considered at risk when a history of head injury is reported, and they experience three or more PCS symptoms interfere with their daily functioning at least once a day (5). Victims with a history of repetitive assaults to the head or repetitive shaking who report headaches, dizziness, or LOC are at higher risk for TBI. Those with positive screens for mild TBI should be referred for neuropsychological assessment. Cognitive recovery may precede or follow resolution of clinical symptoms, and the assessment of cognitive function is an important post-injury intervention (21,33,76).

Rehabilitation neuropsychology places a positive focus on diagnosis and treatment. The philosophy is that victims with neuropsychological impairments (a) can benefit from treatment, (b) have strengths and weaknesses, and (c) have varying levels of impairment in several areas (115). Neuropsychological evaluation and treatment provide information on the victim's strengths and weaknesses to facilitate rehabilitation. Victims are often relieved to learn that some of their symptoms are secondary to neurologic rather than psychologic etiologies. Some researchers believe this form of psychotherapy is the best approach to use with victims who have sustained brain injuries (1). Neuropsychological therapy does not place the impetus for change solely on the victim, but involves considerable direction from the therapist (1).

Assuring that victims receive appropriate treatment may be critical to their survival (40,131). Therapists working with IPV victims often assume the role of protector by frequently reassessing each victim's safety. Clinicians, therapists, family, and friends have been frustrated with victims who return to violent relationships despite intervention efforts (132). Knowledge and understanding of the symptom complex and impairments associated with TBI allows this behavior to be viewed with less frustration and managed more effectively. Prevention of recurrent head injury and safety planning should be addressed for each IPV victim.

IMPLICATIONS FOR POLICY, PRACTICE, AND RESEARCH

Policy

- Intimate partner violence advocates and health-care providers should be trained to screen for post-TBI symptoms and initiate medical referrals for further assessment when screens are positive.
- Training programs on IPV for mental health and substance abuse professionals should include assessment for TBI.
- Public health education regarding undiagnosed TBI might bring more hidden victims to the attention of healthcare providers.

Practice

- Mild TBI should be considered in the differential diagnosis of IPV victims who present with chronic, vague complaints such as fatigue, dizziness, depression, or difficulties with concentration or judgment.
- Education of IPV victims after TBI should include discussion of the dangers of recurrent head injury or SIS.
- Traumatic brain injury victims should receive early referral for neurologic and rehabilitation neuropsychological assessment and intervention.
- Coroners should seek information about prior IPV in TBI victims.

Research

- Additional research is needed to examine the rates of TBI in victims of IPV assaults and examine the impact these brain injuries have on the victim's cognitive functioning.
- Studies examining long-term consequences of persistent PCS and PTSD of IPV victims will be valuable.
- Long-term investigations of the associations between TBI, specific neuropsychological functions, and psychopathology among IPV victims are needed. This research would aid clinicians and other professionals working with IPV victims to better understand the long-term effects of TBI.
- Further attention should be given to preinjury substance abuse, depression, or other psychological issues that could overlap or confound the victim's symptom complex.

- The question of why women experience worse outcomes than men after TBI, including higher mortality rates, remains unanswered despite numerous investigations. Theories evoking mechanisms of injury, hormone-related gender differences in recovery of brain function, and gender differences in head–neck musculature and stabilization have been put forth (41,133).
- Existence of a complex relationship between number and frequency of brain injuries, severity of partner abuse, resultant cognitive functioning, and psychosocial pathology has been theorized (11). Research designed to better define these relationships and their effect on IPV victim outcomes may be of benefit.

References

1. Banks M, Ackerman RJ. Head and brain injuries experienced by African American women victims of intimate partner violence. *Women Ther.* 2002;25:133–143.
2. Berrios D, Grady D. Domestic violence: Risk factors and outcomes. *West J Med.* 1991;155:133–135.
3. Crandall M, Nathens HB, Rivara FB. Injury patterns among female trauma patients: Recognizing intentional injury. *J Trauma.* 2004;57:42–45.
4. Fanslow J, Norton RN, Spinola CG. Indicators of assault related injuries among women presenting to the emergency department. *Ann Emerg Med.* 1998;32:341–348.
5. Jackson H, Philip E, Nutter RL, Diller L. Traumatic brain injury: A hidden consequence for battered women. *Prof Psychol Res Pr.* 2002;33:39–45.
6. Le B, Dierks EJ, Veeck BA, et al. Maxillofacial injuries associated with domestic violence. *J Oral Maxillofac Surg.* 2001;59:1277–1283.
7. Monahan K, O'Leary KD. Head injury and battered women: An initial inquiry. *Health Soc Work.* 1999;24:269–278.
8. Muelleman R, Lenaghan PA, Pakieser RA. Battered women: Injury locations and types. *Ann Emerg Med.* 1996;28:486–491.
9. Perciaccante V, Ochs HA, Dodson TB. Head, neck, and facial injuries as markers of domestic violence in women. *J Oral Maxillofac Surg.* 1999;57:760–762.
10. Shepard J, Shetland M, Pearce NX, et al. Pattern, severity and etiology of injuries in victims of assault. *J R Soc Med.* 1990;83:75–78.
11. Valera E, Berenbaum H. Brain injury in battered women. *J Consult Clin Psychol.* 2003;71:797–804.
12. Varvaro F, Lasko DL. Physical abuse as a cause of injury in women: Information for orthopaedic nurses. *Orthop Nurs.* 1993;12:37–41.

13. Oche H, Neuenschwander MC, Dodson TB. Are head, neck and facial injuries markers of domestic violence. *J Am Dent Assoc*. 1996;127:757–761.

14. Walker L. Post traumatic stress disorder in women: Diagnosis and treatment of battered woman syndrome. *Psychotherapy*. 1991;28:21–29.

15. American Brain Injury Association (ABIA). Types of Brain Injury. At http://www.biausa.org. Accessed 2/2/2004.

16. Kirkness C, Burr RL, Mitchell PH, Newell DW. Is there a sex difference in the course following traumatic brain injury? *Biol Res Nurs*. 2004;5(4):299–310.

17. Nygren de Boussard C, Bellocco R, Geijerstam JL, et al. Delayed intracranial complications after concussion. *J Trauma*. 2006;61:577–581.

18. Ellemberg D, Leclerc S, Couture S, Daigle C. Prolonged neuropsychological impairments following a first concussion in female university soccer athletes. *Clin J Sport Med*. 2007;17:369–374.

19. Kurca E, Sivak S, Kucera P. Impaired cognitive functions in mild traumatic brain injury patients with normal and pathologic magnetic resonance imaging. *Neuroradiology*. 2006;48:661–669.

20. Yang C, Tu YK, Hua MS, Huang SJ. The association between the postconcussion symptoms and clinical outcomes for patients with mild traumatic brain injury. *J Trauma*. 2007;62:657–663.

21. Belanger H, Curtiss G, Demery JA, et al. Factors moderating neuropsychological outcomes following mild traumatic brain injury: A meta-analysis. *J Int Neuropsychol Soc*. 2005;11:215–227.

22. Wilson J, Pettigrew LE, Teasdale GM. Emotional and cognitive consequences of head injury in relation to the Glasgow Outcome Scale. *J Neurol Neurosurg Psychiatry*. 2000;69:204–209.

23. Nell V, Yates DW, Kruger J. An extended Glasgow Coma Scale (GCS-E) with enhanced sensitivity to mild brain injury. *Arch Phys Med Rehab*. 2000;81:614–617.

24. Levin H, Boake C, Song J, et al. Validity and sensitivity to change of the extended Glasgow Outcome Scale in mild to moderate traumatic brain injury. *J Neurotrauma*. 2001;18:575–584.

25. Heegaard W, Biros MH. Trauma system injuries: Head. In: Marx J, Hockberger RS, Walls RM, ed. *Rosen's emergency medicine concepts and clinical practice*, 6th ed. Philadelphia: Mosby Publishing, 2006.

26. Sheedy J, Gina G, Donnelly J, Faux S. Emergency department assessment of mild traumatic brain injury and prediction of post-concussive symptoms at one month post injury. *J Clin Exp Neuropsychol*. 2006;28(5):755–772.

27. Drake A, McDonald EC, Magnus NE, et al. Utility of Glasgow Coma Scale: Extended in symptom prediction following mild traumatic brain injury. *Brain Inj*. 2006;20(5):469–475.

28. Dikmen S, Machamer J, Miller B, et al. Functional status examination: A new instrument for assessing outcome in traumatic brain injury. *J Neurotrauma*. 2001;18:127–140.

29. Teasdale G, Jennett B. Assessment of coma and impaired consciousness: A practical scale. *Lancet*. 1974;2:81–84.

30. Sperry J, Gentilello LM, Minei JP, et al. Waiting for the patient to "sober up": effect of alcohol intoxication on Glasgow Coma Scale score of brain injured patients. *J Trauma*. 2006;61:1305–1311.

31. Cantu R. Posttraumatic retrograde and anterograde amnesia: Pathophysiology and implications in grading and safe return to play. *J Athl Train*. 2001;36(3):244–248.

32. Kelly J. Loss of consciousness: Pathophysiology and implications in grading and safe return to play. *J Athl Train*. 2001;36(3):249–252.

33. Aubry M, Cantu R, Dvorak J, et al. Summary and agreement statement of the first International Conference on Concussion in Sport, Vienna. *Br J Sports Med*. 2001;36:6–10.

34. Narayan R. Closed head injury. In: Rengachary S, Wilkins RH, eds. *Principles of neurosurgery*. London: Wolfe Publishing, 1994.

35. Novack T. *Introduction to brain injury: Facts and stats*. Birmingham: UAB–TBIMS, 2000.

36. Kraus J, Peek-Asa C, McArthur D. The independent effect of gender on outcomes following traumatic brain injury: A preliminary investigation. *Neurosurg Focus*. 2000;8(1):1–7.

37. Krause J. Epidemiology of head injury. In: Cooper P, ed. *Head injury*, 3rd ed. Baltimore: Willams and Wilkins, 1963.

38. Marshall L, Gautelle T, Klauber MR, et al. The outcome of severe closed head injury. *J Neurosurg*. 1991;75:S28.

39. Arbuckle J, Olson L, Howard M, et al. Safe at home? Domestic violence homicides among women in New Mexico. *Ann of Emerg Med*. 1996;27:210–215.

40. Wadman M, Muelleman RL. Domestic violence homicides: ED use before victimization. *Am J Emerg Med*. 1999;17:689–691.

41. Farace E, Alves WM. Do women fare worse: A meta-analysis of gender differences in traumatic brain injury outcome. *J Neurosurg*. 2000;93:539–545.

42. Slewa-Younan S, Green AM, Baguley IJ, et al. Sex differences in injury severity and outcome measures after traumatic brain injury. *Arch Phys Med Rehabil*. 2004;85:376–379.

43. Colohan A, Oyesiku NM. Moderate head injury: An overview. *J Neurotrauma*. 1992;9(S1):52–59.

44. Biros M, Heegaard W. Trauma system injuries: Head. In: Marx J, Hockberger RS, Walls RM, eds. *Rosen's emergency medicine concepts and clinical practice*. St. Louis: Mosby Publishing, 2002.

45. Johnston K, Pito A, Chankowsky J, Chen JK. New frontiers in diagnostic imaging in concussive head injury. *Clin J Sport Med*. 2001;11:166–175.

46. Livingston D, Lavery RF, Passannante MR, et al. Emergency department discharge of patients with a negative cranial computed tomography scan after minimal head injury. *Ann Surg.* 2000;232: 126–132.

47. Romer C, von Holst H, Gururaj G, et al. *Prevention, critical care and rehabilitation of neurotrauma: Perspectives and future strategies.* Stockholm: Karolinska Institute, 1995.

48. Raskin S, Mateer C. *Neuropsychological management of mild traumatic brain injury.* New York: Oxford University Press, 2000.

49. Committee on Mild Traumatic Brain Injury (ACoRM). Definition of mild traumatic brain injury. *J Head Trauma Rehabil.* 1993;8:48–59.

50. Goldstein M. Traumatic brain injury: A silent epidemic. *Ann Neurol.* 1990;27:327.

51. Thornhill S, Teasdale G, Murray G, et al. Disability in young people and adults one year after head injury: Prospective cohort study. *BMJ.* 2000; 320:1631–1635.

52. Lundin A, DeBoussard C, Edman G, Borg J. Symptoms and disability until 3 months after mild TBI. *Brain Inj.* 2006;20(8):759–806.

53. Parker T, Osternig LR, van Donkelaar P, Chou LS. Gait stability following concussion. *Med Sci Sports Exerc.* 2006;38(6):1032–1040.

54. Iverson G. Misdiagnosis of the persistent postconcussion syndrome in patients with depression. *Arch Clin Neuropsychol.* 2006;21:303–310.

55. Stulemeiger M, van der Werf S, Bleijenberg G, et al. Recovery from mild traumatic brain injury: A focus on fatigue. *J Neurol.* 2006;253(8):1041–1047.

56. Halterman C, Langan J, Drew A, et al. Tracking the recovery of visuospatial attention deficits in mild traumatic brain injury. *Brain.* 2006;129:747–753.

57. Catena R, van Donkelaar P, Chou LS. Altered balance control following concussion is better detected with an attention test during gait. *Gait Posture.* 2007;25:406–411.

58. Hickling E, Gillen R, Blanchard EB, et al. Traumatic brain injury and posttraumatic stress disorder: A preliminary investigation of neuropsychological test results of PTSD secondary to motor vehicle accidents. *Brain Inj.* 1998;12(4):265–274.

59. Society BI. Traumatic Brain Injury. At http://www.bisociety.org. Accessed 5/1/2004.

60. NIH. Rehabilitation of persons with traumatic brain injury. *JAMA.* 1999;282:974–983.

61. Boswell J, McErlean M, Verdile VP. Prevalence of traumatic brain injury in an ED population. *Am J Emer Med.* 2002;20(3):177–180.

62. Cassidy J, Carroll LJ, Peloso PM, et al. Incidence, risk factors and prevention of mild traumatic brain injury: Results of the WHO collaborative centre task force on mild traumatic brain injury. *J Rehabil Med.* 2004;43:S28 -S60.

63. Parker R. Enhancing information gathering after mild head injury in the acute and chronic phase. *J Neurolog Ortho Med and Surg.* 1995;16: 8118–8125.

64. McCrory P, Berkovic SF. Second impact syndrome. *Neurology.* 1998;50:677–683.

65. Matser J, Kessels AH, Jordan BD, et al. Chronic traumatic brain injury in professional soccer players. *Neurology.* 1998;51:791–796.

66. Mulhern S, McMillan TM. Knowledge and expectation of postconcussion symptoms in the general population. *J Psychosom Res.* 2006;61: 439–445.

67. MMWR Surveillance Summaries. Surveillance for traumatic brain deaths: United States: 1989–1998. 2002.

68. Bernstein D. Recovering from mild head injury. *Brain Inj.* 1999;13:151–172.

69. Centers for Disease Control and Prevention. *Injury Fact Book.* Washington DC: Author, 2001.

70. Gilthorpe M, Wilson RC, Moles DR, Bedi R. Variations in admissions to hospital for head injury and assault to the head. Part 1: Age and gender. *Br J Oral Maxillofac Surg.* 1999;37(4):294–300.

71. Corrigan J, Wolfe M, Mysiw JW, et al. Early identification of mild traumatic brain injury in female victims of domestic violence. *Am J Obstet Gynecol.* 2003;188:S71–S76.

72. Saltzman L, Fingerhut LA, Raud MR, et al. Building data systems for monitoring and responding to violence against women: Recommendations from a workshop. *MMWR Morb Mortal Wkly.* 2000;49:1–16.

73. Sosin D, Sniezek JE, Thurman DJ. Incidence of mild and moderate brain injury in the United States. *Brain Inj.* 1996;10:47–54.

74. Huddle D, Glazer M, Chaney DB. Emergency imaging of the brain. In: Schwartz D, Reisdorff EJ, eds. *Emergency radiology.* New York: McGraw-Hill, 2000.

75. Ropper A, Gorson KC. Concussion. *N Engl J Med.* 2007;356:166–172.

76. McCrory P, Johnston K, Meeuwisse W, et al. Summary and agreement statement of the 2nd International Conference on Concussion in Sport, Prague 2004. *Br J Sports Med.* 2005;39:196–204.

77. McAllister T, Sparling M, Flashman L, Saykin A. Neuroimaging findings in mild traumatic brain injury. *J Clin Exp Neuropsychol.* 2001;3:775–791.

78. Bigler E. Neuropsychological results and neuropathological findings at autopsy in a case of mild traumatic brain injury. *J Int Neuropsychol Soc.* 2004;10:794–806.

79. McAllister T, Flashman L, Sparling M, Saykin A. Working memory deficits after traumatic brain injury: Catecholaminergic mechanisms and prospects for treatment: A review. *Brain Inj.* 2004;18:331–350.

80. Kelly J, Rosenberg JH. The diagnosis and management of concussion in sports. *Neurology.* 1997;48:575–580.

81. Covassin T, Swanik CB, Sachs ML. Sex differences and the incidence of concussions among collegiate athletes. *J Athl Train.* 2003;38:238–244.

82. Delaney J, Lacroix VJ, Leclerc S, Johnston KM. Concussions among university football and soccer players. *Clin J Sport Med.* 2002; 12:331–338.

83. Bazarian J, McClung J, Shah MN, Cheng YT, et al. Mild traumatic brain injury in the United States, 1998–2000. *Brain Inj.* 2005;19:85–91.

84. Hanlon R, Demery JA, Martinovich Z. Effects of acute injury characteristics on neuropsychological status and vocational outcome following mild traumatic brain injury. *Brain Inj.* 1999;13:873–888.

85. Bazarian J, Wong T, Harris M, et al. Epidemiology and predictors of post-concussive syndrome after minor head injury in an emergency population. *Brain Inj.* 1999;13:173–183.

86. Slobounov S, Slobounov E, Sebastianelli W, et al. Differential rate of recovery in athletes after first and second concussion episodes. *Neurosurgery.* 2007;61:338–344.

87. Bryant R, Harvey AG. Postconcussive symptoms and posttraumatic stress disorder after mild traumatic brain injury. *J Nerv Ment Dis.* 1999;187(5): 302–305.

88. Pico-Alfonso M. Psychological intimate partner violence: The major predictor of posttraumatic stress disorder in abused women. *Neurosci Biobehav Rev.* 2005;29:181–193.

89. Breslau N, Kessler R, Chilcoat H, et al. Trauma and posttraumatic stress disorder in the community. The 1996 Detroit area survey of trauma. *Arch Gen Psychiatry.* 1998;55:627–632.

90. Baker C, Norris FH, Diaz DM, et al. Violence and PTSD in Mexico: gender and regional differences. *Soc Psychiatry Psychiatr Epidemiol.* 2005;40: 519–528.

91. Cortina L, Kubiak SP. Gender and posttraumatic stress: Sexual violence as an explanation for women's increased risk. *Abnorm Psych.* 2006; 115(4):753–759.

92. McCauley S, Kern DZ, Kolodner K, et al. The "battering syndrome": Prevalence and clinical characteristics of domestic violence in primary care internal medicine practices. *Ann Intern Med.* 1995;123:737–746.

93. Geddes J, Whitwell HZ. Shaken adult syndrome revisited. *Am J Forensic Med Pathol.* 2003;24: 310–311.

94. Carrigan T, Walker E, Barnes S. Domestic violence: The shaken adult syndrome. *J Accid Emerg Med.* 2000;17:138–139.

95. Pounder D. Shaken adult syndrome. *Am J Forensic Med Pathol.* 1997;18(4):321–324.

96. Case M, Braham MA, Handy TC, et al. Position paper on fatal abusive head injuries in infants and young children. *Am J Forensic Med Pathol.* 2001;22:112–122.

97. Leadbeatter S, James R. The shaken infant syndrome: Shaking alone may not be responsible for damage. *BMJ.* 1995;310:1600.

98. Amnesty International. *Israel and the occupied territories: Death by shaking: The case of 'Abd al-Samad Harizat.* London: Amnesty International. 1995.

99. Physicians for Human Rights. *Israel and the occupied territories: Shaking as a form of torture: Death in custody of 'Abd al-Samad Harizat.* Boston: Author, 1995.

100. Castillo M, Harris JH. Imaging of skull and brain emergencies. In: Harris J, Harris WH, ed. *The radiology of emergency medicine,* 4th ed. Philadelphia: Lippincott Williams and Wilkins, 2000.

101. Sorenson S, Wiebs DJ. Weapons in the lives of battered women. *Am J Public Health.* 2004; 94(8):1412–1417.

102. Brumback R. *Oklahoma notes: Neurology and clinical neuroscience,* 2nd ed. New York: Springer, 1996.

103. Ward J, Chisholm AH, Prince VT, et al. Penetrating head injury. *Crit Care Nurs Q.* 1994; 17(1):79.

104. Olson L, Anctil C, Fullerton L, et al. Increasing emergency physician recognition of domestic violence. *Ann Emerg Med.* 1996;27:741–746.

105. Cantu R. Second impact syndrome: Immediate management. *Phys Sportsmed.* 1992;20:55–66.

106. Cantu R, Voy R. Second impact syndrome: A risk in any contact sport. *Phys Sportsmed.* 1995;23:27–34.

107. CDC. Sports-related recurrent brain injuries: United States. *MMWR.* 1997;46:224–227.

108. Collins M, Grindel SH, Lovell MR, et al. Relationship between concussion and neuropsychological performance in college football players. *JAMA.* 1999;282:964–970.

109. Greenfeld L, Rand MR, Craven D, et al. *Violence by intimates: Analysis of data on crimes by current or former spouses, boyfriends and girlfriends.* Vol. NCJ—167237. Washington, DC: National Institute of Justice; 1998.

110. Iverson G, Gaetz M, Lovell MR, Collins MW. Cumulative effects of concussion in amateur athletes. *Brain Inj.* 2004;18:433–443.

111. Gronwall D. Minor head injury. *Neuropsychology.* 1991;5:253–265.

112. Dutton M. *Empowering and healing the battered woman: A model for assessment and intervention.* New York: Springer, 1992.

113. McGrath E, Keita GP, Strickland BR, Russo NF. *Women and depression: Risk factors and treatment issues.* Washington DC: American Psychological Association, 1990.

114. Walker L. *The abused woman: A survivor therapy approach.* New York: Newbridge Communications, 1994.

115. Ackerman R, Banks ME. Assessment, treatment, and rehabilitation for interpersonal violence

victims: Women sustaining head injuries. *Women Ther.* 2003;26:343–363.

116. Alexander M. Mild traumatic brain injury: Pathophysiology, natural history and clinical management. *Neurology.* 1995;45:1253–1260.

117. Cicerone K, Kalmar K. Persistent post-concussion syndrome: The structure of subjective complaints after mild traumatic brain injury. *J Head Trauma Rehabil.* 1995;10:1–17.

118. Browne A. Violence against women by male partners: Prevalence, outcomes and policy implications. *Am Psychol.* 1993;48:1077–1087.

119. Gelles R, Straus MA. The medical and psychological costs of family violence. In: Straus M, Gelles RJ, eds. *Physical violence in American families: Risk factors and adaptations to violence in 8,145 families.* New Brunswick, NJ: Transaction Books, 1990.

120. Sato R, Heiby IM. Correlates of depressive symptoms among battered women. *J Fam Violence.* 1992;7:229–245.

121. Diaz-Olavarrista C, Campbell J. Domestic violence against patients with chronic neurologic disorders. *Arch Neurol.* 1999;56:681–685.

122. Hadley S. Working with battered women in the emergency department: A model program. *J Emerg Nurs.* 1992;18:18.

123. Tjaden P, Thoennes N. Extent, nature and consequences of intimate partner violence: Findings from the national violence against women survey. Vol. NCJ-181867. Washington DC: US Department of Justice, Bureau of Justice Statistics, 2000.

124. Broglio S, Macciocchi SN, Ferrara MS. Sensitivity of the concussion assessment battery. *Neurosurgery.* 2007;60(6):1050–1057.

125. Kelly R. The post-traumatic syndrome, an iatrogenic disease. *Forensic Sci.* 1975;6:17–24.

126. Andersson E, Emanuelson I, Bjorklund R, Stalhammar DA. Mild traumatic brain injuries: The impact of early intervention on late sequelae. A randomized control study. *Acta Neurochir.* 2007;149:151–160.

127. Raskin S. The relationship between sexual abuse and mild traumatic brain injury. *Brain Inj.* 1997;11:587–603.

128. Lawler K, Terregino CA. Guidelines for evaluation and education of adult patients with mild traumatic brain injuries in an acute care hospital setting. *J Head Trauma Rehabil.* 1996;11:18–28.

129. Paniak C, Toller-Lobe G, Reynolds S, et al. A randomized trial of two treatments for mild traumatic brain injury: 1 year follow-up. *Brain Inj.* 2000;14:219–226.

130. Banks M, Ackerman RJ. *Post-assault traumatic brain injury interview and checklist manual.* Akron, OH: ABackans Diversified Computer Processing, Inc, 1997.

131. Gordon W, Brown M, Sliwinski M, et al. The enigma of "hidden" traumatic brain injury. *J Head Trauma Rehabil.* 1998;13:39–56.

132. Loseke D. *The battered woman and shelters: The social construction of wife abuse.* Albany: State University of New York Press, 1992.

133. Tierney R, Sitler MR, Swanik CB, et al. Gender differences in head-neck segment dynamic stabilization during head acceleration. *Med Sci Sports Exerc.* 2005;37(2):272–279.

Chapter 15

Maxillofacial Injuries in Intimate Partner Violence

Sharon R. Wilson, Thomas B. Dodson, and Leslie R. Halpern

KEY CONCEPTS

- A paucity of evidence-based data exists with respect to the epidemiology and mechanisms of maxillofacial injuries associated with victims of intimate partner violence (IPV).
- Specific clinical approaches aid the healthcare provider in the identification of victims of IPV who present with maxillofacial injuries, including physical examinations and imaging and diagnostic surveys using head, neck, and facial injury location as a risk predictor.
- Using maxillofacial injuries as a sole risk predictor for an IPV-related injury etiology has statistical limitations and pitfalls; however, using these tools can increase the sensitivity and specificity of this risk predictor.
- Significant skills for educating healthcare providers to identify victims of IPV using maxillofacial injuries and how this predictor can be used for mandatory reporting, early intervention, and eradication of IPV are now being tested across the country.

Broadly defined, intimate partner violence (IPV) includes the physical, sexual, and psychological abuse of adults in intimate relationships. In this country, IPV is a serious threat to the public health (1,2). Over 2.5 million women are abused annually, and 30%–50% of female homicides were perpetrated by former or current intimate partners (3,4). A stated objective of the Public Health Service's Healthy People 2010 Program strongly encourages that emergency departments and the disciplines of medicine, surgery, and dentistry become more efficient in diagnosing and managing victims of IPV (4,5). Although interventions may prevent future IPV-related injuries, they cannot be initiated until the diagnosis is made (2,4–9).

Injury assessment may lead to earlier recognition of IPV; however, it is both difficult and challenging because of a lack of standardized methods (4). No obvious clinical characteristics of this disease process exist, and there is often a mismatch of injury and diagnosis. The clinical standard for identifying IPV-related injury and other nonverifiable injuries is subject self-report through either a spontaneous or a prompted disclosure. Other studies have suggested useful, but ambiguous, criteria for identifying victims of IPV seen in the emergency department and outpatient clinical setting (6,7,9).

Studies have shown that the strongest predictor of IPV is the frequency rather than the severity of injuries. When interviewed in the emergency department, only 1%–6% of women are diagnosed as being assaulted by their intimate sexual partners. Trauma to the head, face, shoulders, breast, abdomen, and extremities are often documented, but the victim's report of injury is incompatible or inconsistent with the mechanism or location of injury (7,10–12). Common traumatic injuries are associated with IPV (Table 15.1). Therefore, when these injuries are present, they should alert the clinician to the possibility of IPV, and all IPV assault victims should be assessed for other associated injuries.

Although facial injuries account for a large number of emergency department visits, there appear to be few reports detailing the etiology and pattern of maxillofacial injuries in victims of an IPV-related injury (9,11,13,14). The purpose of this chapter is to present evidence-based data that support the use of maxillofacial injuries as a prime predictor variable in identifying victims of IPV. The specific aims of this chapter are to discuss the epidemiology of maxillofacial injuries associated with IPV; mechanisms of head, neck, and facial injury etiology; and clinical workups using maxillofacial injuries as a predictor to more expediently identify victims of IPV. The advantages and limitations of these approaches will be addressed, as well

as efforts to educate providers on maxillofacial injuries as a clinical risk indicator for IPV.

PREVALENCE OF MAXILLOFACIAL INJURIES IN INTIMATE PARTNER VIOLENCE

As with IPV assaults in general, the prevalence of maxillofacial IPV injuries is not well defined and is most likely underestimated. Although facial injuries account for a large number of emergency department visits, there seem to be few reports detailing the cause and pattern of facial injuries in women who frequent the emergency department/clinical setting. In addition, there has been a paucity of well-designed epidemiologic studies to more precisely measure the observational evidence-based data (Table 15.2).

Motor vehicle collisions and interpersonal assaults have been recognized as two of the primary mechanisms by which maxillofacial fractures occur (15–26). Etiology is dependent upon the population studied. Injury sustained during interpersonal assaults account for 5%–59% of facial injuries (25,27–29). Assault and interpersonal violence have been documented as frequent etiologies of facial fractures in adults younger than 50 years of age (22,25,28,29). An Australian study of 2,581 patients with radiographic evidence of facial fractures found 1,135 were secondary to interpersonal violence, 286 secondary to motor vehicle accident (MVA), and the remainder resulted from a variety of mechanisms. The majority of victims were male, and

Table 15.1 Common Traumatic Injuries Associated with Intimate Partner Violence (IPV)		
Central Injuries	Repetitive Injuries	Injury Characteristics/Patterns
Head, neck, face Breast Abdomen Chest Back Genitals	Frequent visits to the emergency department for trauma/accidents Radiographic documentation of prior fractures Injuries at different stages of healing	Patterned injuries due to blunt force from object or body part of assailant Thermal burn patterns from hot liquid splash, dip, or cigarette burns Human bite marks Punch contusions Fingertip imprints/contusions Spiral wrist fractures Maxillofacial fractures

Adapted with permission from Feldman MD, Swenson SL, Moreno-John GA. Patient management after acute intimate partner violence or sexual assault. In: *Violence against women: A physician's guide to identification and management.* Liebschutz JM, Frayne SM, Saxe GN, eds. Philadelphia, American College of Physicians, 2003.

Table 15.2 Frequency Estimates of Maxillofacial Injuries in Victims of Intimate Partner Violence (IPV)*

Author	Study Design	Dataset Origin	Age (range)	n (%)	Sex	Injury*
Zacharides et al. (1990)	Retrospective	Chart review	16–62	51 (9)	F	H, N, F
Fisher et al. (1990)	Cross-sectional	Chart review	10–78	23 (20)	F	H, N, F
Berrios and Grady (1991)	Retrospective	Chart review	16–66	149 (68)	F	H, N, F
Ochs et al. (1996)	Cross-sectional	Cohort	18–51	15 (94)	F	H, N, F
Muelleman et al. (1996)	Cross-sectional	Cohort	19–65	121 (51)	F	H, N, F
Hartzell (1996)	Retrospective	Chart review	15–63	7 (30)	F	Ocular
Huang et al. (1998)	Retrospective	Chart review	15–45	109 (36)	F	H, N, F
Perciaccante et al. (1999)	Cross-sectional	Cohort	24–56	34 (31)	F	H, N, F
Greene et al. (1999)	Retrospective	Chart review	32 (Mean)	29 (22)	F	H, N, F
Le et al. (2002)	Retrospective	Chart review	15–71	85 (30)	F	H, N, F
Crandall et al. (2004)	Cross-sectional	Chart review	16–65	145 (72)	F	H, N, F
Halpern, Dodson (2006)	RCT	Cohort	27–64	63 (31)	F	H, N, F

* Anatomic location of injury

RCT, Random controlled trial; H, head; N, Neck; F, Face.

the most frequently sustained injury was mandible fracture(s). Alcohol use was involved in 87% of these assault-related injuries (30). The most frequently injured are 15 to 45 years in age (11,13,24,26,31–33). Figure 15.1 depicts the anatomic areas of the maxillofacial skeleton most often targeted.

Reports from emergency department visits indicate that, more than 75% of the time, women who presented with facial trauma had concomitant injuries within the oral cavity, especially in young adults (20,34). Oral manifestations of sexually transmitted diseases (STDs), difficulty sitting or walking, fear of the reclined position of the dental chair, and an inordinate fear of the dental exam may indicate a history of IPV (34). A prospective study by Leathers and co-workers examined 203 adult patients seeking treatment at King/Drew Medical Center in Los Angeles. In this study a disproportionate number of women who presented with oral trauma (more than 38%) reported their injuries resulted from IPV (35).

A retrospective study of facial trauma in women by Huang in 1998 showed there was often inadequate documentation regarding the circumstances of the facial injury (11). Huang concluded this indicates IPV may be severely underreported in maxillofacial injuries in women. Case series reports indicate that 67% of women with facial injuries had been assaulted by a husband or boyfriend, with 68% of battered women

in another study sustaining 45% of injuries to the mid face (15,26). A study by Ochs and co-workers showed an extremely high incidence of head, neck, and facial injuries in victims of IPV (23). In their study, 94.4% of victims who identified IPV as the cause of their injuries had head, neck, and facial injuries. Nearly 35% of injured women in this study who presented to the emergency department for treatment of injuries were victims of IPV. In this same study, if a woman had a head, neck, or facial injury, she was 11.8 times more likely to be a victim of IPV than were women who had other types of injuries. In the absence of head, neck, or facial injury, it was unlikely that the patient was a victim of IPV.

A study by Perciaccante and colleagues evaluated head, neck, and facial injuries as markers of IPV in women (9). This study sampled 100 injured women, 34 of whom were victims of IPV with concomitant head, neck, and facial injuries. Of the 100 injured women, 58 had head, neck, and facial injuries, and 31 of those were victims of IPV. A woman who had head, neck, and facial injuries was 7.5 times more likely to be a victim of IPV than a woman who had other injuries. This was a sensitive but not very specific indicator of IPV; however, the authors concluded that women presenting to the emergency department for non-MVA injury be considered at high risk for IPV.

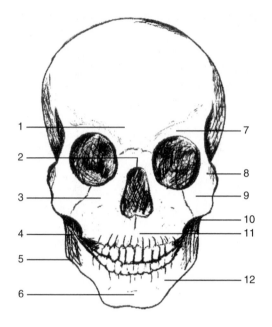

1	Frontal Bone	7	Superior Orbit
2	Nasal Orbit Ethmold	8	Lateral Wall of Orbit
3	Maxilla	9	Zygoma
4	Ramus of Mandible	10	Subconydlar Area of Mandible
5	Angle of Mandible	11	Premaxilla/Dentoalveolar Area of Mandible
6	Symphysis of Mandible	12	Parasymphysis of Mandible

Figure 15.1 Anatomical locations of maxillofacial fractures.

A study by Greene and colleagues in 1999 drew conclusions similar to those of some of the studies previously mentioned (19). One-third of female blunt assault facial trauma patients were subjects of IPV. Le and colleagues performed a retrospective review in 2001 of patients treated for IPV injuries. Eighty-one percent presented with maxillofacial injuries in which the middle third of the face was the most commonly injured area (69%). Facial fractures occurred in 30%, and most of the facial fractures (40%) were nasal fractures.

Dutton and Strachen examined the motives of men who committed IPV and interpersonal violence assaults against women seen in the ED (36). They concluded possible motives to be the need for power and the maintenance of gender roles in the assailant's relationships. The authors theorize that assaults to the face and head reinforce the assailant's dominance and control by leaving visible wounds as reminders of their power (36). The residual effect of injury—scars, facial

asymmetries, damage to dentition, loss of masticatory function, and psychological wounds—persist as painful reminders of the abuse.

DESCRIPTION OF MAXILLOFACIAL INJURIES ASSOCIATED WITH INTIMATE PARTNER VIOLENCE

Research that examines mechanisms of injury in IPV victims provides healthcare providers an understanding of the location and severity of trauma that patients experience at the hands of their perpetrators (37). The most frequently reported maxillofacial injuries secondary to IPV assaults are contusions, abrasions, lacerations, and facial fractures (9,11,13,15,19,23,24,26,31, 38–42). Less frequently reported injuries include hyphemas, ruptured globes, and fractured or subluxated teeth (43,44). Unusual injuries such as ptosis secondary to a hairline fracture of the superior orbit and facial palsy secondary to blunt trauma to the side of the face have also been reported (44,45).

Blunt trauma is the most common mechanism of injury, with hands and fists the most frequent weapons (13,21,26,36,40). Other weapons include feet, bottles, pipes, and sticks (13,21). Victims are typically assaulted by slaps, punches, or being pushed against an object. Intimate partner violence maxillofacial injuries range from simple, soft tissue contusions and abrasions that require little or no intervention to fractures requiring hospital admission and surgical repair. Assessment must include airway, breathing, circulation, cervical spine, and neurologic evaluations.

Soft Tissue Injuries

Contusions and Abrasions

Contusions and abrasions with associated soft tissue swelling and tenderness are the most frequently occurring IPV maxillofacial injury (13,21,24,36,39). Injuries are frequently multiple in nature and found in any facial anatomic location. Le and colleagues found contusions to be the most common (61%) maxillofacial injury (13). Petridou reported a 43% predictive value for IPV among women in a Greek ambulatory care setting who presented with contusion and swelling of the lips (24). Muelleman and co-workers found facial contusions to be the most common injury type among battered women, with a sensitivity of 40.5% but low predictive value (21). Of note is their finding that the presence of at least one of 12 other identified specific injury types (e.g., tympanic membrane rupture, upper extremity abrasion, abdominal contusion) increased the sensitivity of facial contusions to 81.4% as a predictor for IPV (21).

Maxillofacial ecchymosis, swelling, and tenderness can be associated with underlying facial fractures and should be examined carefully for crepitus or boney deformity. Computed tomography (CT) scans should be obtained when soft tissue injuries limit the reliability of the clinical examination, plain radiography reveals a fracture, or there is a high index of suspicion despite negative films (16,18).

Lacerations

Intimate partner violence assault-related maxillofacial lacerations result from blunt trauma (9,13,21, 38,42,43,46). Maxillofacial lacerations have been reported in 13.5% and 17% of IPV patients (13,21). Le conducted a retrospective review of 236 emergency department patients treated for IPV injuries over a 5-year period. Fists were the most common weapon, and 17% of patients who sustained facial lacerations had injuries severe enough to require suture repair (13). Sixty-nine percent of lacerations involved the middle third of the face, whereas lacerations of the upper and lower third of the face were 13% and 19%, respectively.

As stated earlier, victims sustaining complex facial lacerations must be carefully evaluated for underlying fractures, intra-oral injury, and other associated injuries to the head, neck, chest, abdomen, or extremities. Life-threatening injuries are addressed prior to facial laceration repair. Maxillofacial trauma is usually associated with other traumatic injuries (9,11,13,17,21,23,26,31, 39,43,47). Muelleman's finding that battered women had greater odds of presenting with 12 specific injury types than nonbattered controls reinforces the importance of questioning and carefully examining women with maxillofacial injury for associated injuries (21).

Ocular Injuries

Ocular injuries secondary to IPV occur by differing mechanisms including strangulation, shaking, scratching, punching, or direct impact with blunt or penetrating objects (15,40,45,46,48–52). Berrios and Grady found 45% of IPV victims were specifically struck in the eyes (15). Soft tissue injury, contusions, abrasions, and lacerations are the most frequently reported ocular injury in IPV assaults (13,15,21,43). Additional ocular injuries sustained by IPV victims include subconjunctival hemorrhage, retinal tears, traumatic iritis, ruptured globes, and ptosis from direct impact (43). Conjunctival petechiae from strangulation and retinal tears from shaking have also been reported (16,48–52).

Hard Tissue Injuries: Fractures

When discussing fractures, the face can be divided anatomically into upper, middle, and lower thirds. The upper third consists of the frontal bone, frontal sinus, and supraorbital rim. The middle third includes nasal bones, orbits, maxilla, and zygoma. The mandible comprises the lower third of the face.

When examining the occurrences of maxillofacial fractures secondary to IPV trauma 28%–44% are nasal,

15%–76% mandibular, and 27% midface (27,29,32). Isolated fractures of the zygoma and orbital rim occur less frequently (11,15,40,53,54). Studies examining maxillofacial fractures in IPV assaults report a wide range of occurrences, 3%–51%. Many studies are retrospective reviews or case series from varying clinical settings. The majority of facial fractures reported from IPV assaults are nasal, mandibular, orbital, and maxillary.

Upper Third Fractures

Frontal sinus and supraorbital rim fractures (upper third fractures) occur when victims sustain a forceful blow to the head. Supraorbital rim fractures typically involve the frontal sinus (16,18,55). Victims of IPV with supraorbital rim fractures may have decreased forehead sensation due to supraorbital nerve injury. Approximately 70% of victims will have sustained a loss of consciousness (LOC) and 28% will have associated facial fractures (16,18,55).

Huang and associates, in their study of maxillofacial injuries in women admitted for facial trauma, found 4.6% of female assault victims were diagnosed with frontal sinus fractures (11). Le and colleagues' retrospective review of emergency department IPV assault victims found a 1% occurrence of supraorbital rim fractures and no frontal sinus fractures (13).

Because of the frontal sinus' thick anterior wall and thin posterior wall, assault victims with frontal sinus fractures require CT evaluation of the posterior sinus wall for associated fracture (55); 75% of victims with frontal sinus fractures will have posterior wall involvement. These victims have a presumed dural tear and require hospitalization (16,29,55).

Middle Third Fractures

The anatomical location of the nose makes it the most common site of facial trauma. Nasal fractures (middle third fractures) typically displace in the direction of the blow. Clinically, nasal fractures may be associated with epistaxis, edema, tenderness, deformity, or septal hematoma. Le and colleagues found nasal fracture to be the most common midface fracture (40%) in female IPV assaults (13). Nasal fractures were the most frequently occurring fracture in isolation and in conjunction with other maxillofacial fractures. Other studies of assault-related maxillofacial injuries in IPV have reported lower occurrences (11,12). Huang and

associates' retrospective chart review of all patients admitted to a trauma center with facial bone fractures found 35% of women sustained facial fractures secondary to assault, with 17.4% being nasal (11). Fisher and colleagues reviewed a small sample of rape and IPV victims and found 21.9% sustained nasal fractures (12). Other studies have reported lower occurrences (2% and 3%) of nasal fractures from IPV assault (21,26).

The diagnosis of simple nasal fracture is clinical. Epistaxis is typically minimal and unless gross deformity is present, victims are given analgesics, instructed to apply ice, and to return for reevaluation in 5–7 days (16). Due to the often minor clinical presentation and simple treatment regimen, many IPV victims with nasal injury may not seek medical care. The prevalence of this fracture in IPV assault is most likely underestimated.

Orbital fractures (middle third fractures) in IPV assault are most frequently the result of closed-fist punches (15,40,43,56). The reported occurrence of orbital fractures in IPV assaults range from 7% to 35% (11,13,40,43,56). Orbital fractures are classified as involving the orbital rim, orbital walls, and orbital floor or as a component of midface fractures (16).

The orbital floor or "blow-out" fracture is the most common and most frequently reported orbit fracture in IPV assaults (11,13,16,18,40). Blow-out fractures involve the floor (weakest area) and medial wall of the orbit. Two mechanisms of injury have been proposed. One mechanism proposes direct impact to the inferior rim causing the orbital floor to buckle and fracture (16). A second mechanism involves hydraulic transmission of the force from a punch through the globe to the floor and walls of the orbit (16,18). The floor is weaker than the walls and globe and subsequently fractures.

Victims with blow-out fractures may have several indicative clinical signs including periorbital edema, impaired ocular motion, infraorbital hypoesthesia, or diplopia. Enophthalmos may be associated with large orbital floor fractures if the orbital contents herniate into the maxillary sinus (16,18). Associated ocular injuries may include subconjunctival hemorrhage, hyphema, retrobulbar hemorrhage, vitreous hemorrhage, retinal detachment, ruptured globe, orbital emphysema, and optic nerve injury (16,18,40,43).

Hartzell and colleagues' retrospective study examined the frequency of orbital fractures secondary to sexual assault or IPV and found that 35% of women sustained orbit fractures as a direct result of their assault (40). Orbital floor fractures secondary to IPV assault comprised 50% of reported fractures (40). Other authors who studied maxillofacial injury in IPV assault victims found lower occurrences of orbit fractures. Le and colleagues report a 22% total occurrence of orbital fractures, with 17% occurrence of orbital floor fractures (13). Similarly, Huang and colleagues report 16.5% orbital floor fractures, and Beck and colleagues, 14% orbital fractures (11,43). Goldberg and associates found the lowest (7.3%) occurrence of orbital fractures, but attributes his findings to under-reporting of IPV-related assaults (56).

The accuracy of plain radiography to diagnosis orbital floor fractures varies. Historically, the most useful have been the occipitomental (Waters), the occipitofrontal (Coldwell), and two oblique orbital views (46). Helical CT of the face is commonly used to evaluate victims with severe facial trauma or altered LOC whose physical examination is of limited value (57,58). Victims who sustain symptomatic orbital floor fractures require careful follow-up by surgical and/or ophthalmology consultants.

Fracture of the maxilla, also a middle third fracture, has a variable rate of occurrence in IPV facial assaults, ranging from 0% to 11% in some studies (11,13,26,40,43). Maxillary fractures are rarely isolated (16). Victims with maxillary fractures may have extensive soft tissue trauma, swelling, midface mobility, cerebrospinal fluid rhinorrhea, malocclusion, and hypesthesias. Maxillary fractures are commonly classified as LeFort I, II, III. LeFort II and III fractures frequently occur in combination. A LeFort I fracture involves the maxilla at the level of the nasal fossa. LeFort II involves the maxilla, nasal bone, and medial aspects of the orbits. LeFort III involves the maxilla, zygoma, nasal bones, ethmoid bones, vomer, and lesser bones of the cranial base (16,18). LeFort III fracture is commonly referred to as *craniofacial disjunction*, and victims with severely displaced LeFort fractures may have a flattened "smash face" appearance.

Quadrapod or zygomatico-maxillary complex (ZMC) fractures are the most common fracture involving the maxilla. The ZMC refers to the articulation of the zygoma with the frontal, maxillary, temporal, and sphenoid bones forming the zygomatic arch, lateral orbital wall, inferior orbit rim, and orbital floor (16). Victims sustaining blunt trauma to the zygoma will typically sustain fractures to these weaker structures and the walls of the maxillary sinus. Le and colleagues

report a 17% occurrence of ZMC fractures in IPV assault victims (13). Zachariades and colleagues found a 10% occurrence of ZMC fracture and 2% occurrence of LeFort III fracture (26). Assaulted women with maxillofacial trauma in Huang's study sustained multiple ZMC fractures, including 23% zygoma, 12% maxilla, 3% vomer, 1% palate, and 16.5% orbital floor fractures (11).

Traditionally, the initial radiographic diagnosis of isolated maxillary, LeFort, and ZMC fractures has been accomplished with occipitomental (Waters), occipitofrontal (Coldwell), lateral, and submental vertical ("bucket handle") views (18). Helical CT of the face is the study of choice for defining complex facial fractures involving the orbits, the ZMC, and LeFort fractures (57–59).

Emergent care of IPV victims with these fractures entails airway and cervical spine protection. The presence of CSF rhinorrhea or intracranial air on radiographic studies is indicative of an open skull fracture. Hospitalization and prophylactic antibiotics are indicated (16,60).

The zygoma is a dense midface bone that sustains two common fractures: (a) depression of the malar eminence and (b) depression of the zygomatic arch. As noted earlier, trauma to the zygoma usually fractures the weaker articulations and the maxillary sinus rather than the zygoma itself (18). Victims with tripod or ZMC fracture may have asymmetrical facial flattening, edema, ecchymosis, malocclusion, facial nerve injury, and "dish face" deformity. Zygomatic arch fracture is associated with a palpable boney defect over the arch, facial asymmetry, edema, and trismus (18). Le and colleagues found a 3% occurrence of isolated IPV assault-related zygoma arch fractures (13). Malar eminence and zygomatic arch fractures do not require hospitalization. Medically, they are treated with pain medication and given surgical referral for possible reduction and fixation (16).

Lower Third Fractures

Mandibular (lower third) fractures are the third most common fracture, with nasal and zygomatic fractures occurring more frequently (16,18,22,29,32). In IPV assaults, mandible fractures along with nasal fractures are one of the two most common fractures (11,13,26,61). The mandible is a strong ring-like structure that typically requires forceful direct impact to fracture (16,18,32). Multiple fractures may occur from a single blow, and may occur distant from the point of impact (11,13,26). Clinically, mandible fractures are associated with deviation of the chin toward the fracture, pain, malocclusion, inability to open the mouth, intraoral ecchymosis, gingival laceration, oral hematoma, or dental trauma.

Mandibular fractures secondary to IPV assaults have rates of occurrence ranging from 12% to 47% (11–13,26). The majority of injuries reported in these studies occurred in the victim's home, by known assailants. Injuries were secondary to blunt force, with fists being the most frequently used weapon. Other weapons include bottles, sticks, pipes, and feet (13,26).

Huang and co-workers reviewed the cases of 307 women admitted to an inpatient service identified as having maxillofacial injuries. The authors found that, of the 109 identified assault victims, 51 (47%) sustained mandibular fractures (11). Zachariades and colleagues interviewed and reviewed the records of 546 women treated with facial injuries over a 2.5-year period (26). The authors found approximately 9% of injuries were secondary to violence exerted by men. Of these, 51% of the assaulted patients sustained maxillofacial fractures with 39% of those fractures being mandibular (26). Le and colleagues found 70 of 236 (30%) emergency department IPV patients sustained a total of 85 fractures to the face (13). Twenty-seven fractures (32%) were isolated mandible fractures. The majority of mandible fractures were single, but two victims had double fractures and one victim had four fractures. Mandible fractures were most frequently of the condyle or the angle, followed by fractures of the body. Bilateral coronoid process fractures secondary to IPV assault have been reported (61).

Greene and associates' epidemiologic study of facial injury in female blunt assault cases found a 32% occurrence of IPV assaults in admitted patients (19). The majority (78%) of women were admitted for the treatment of facial fractures, with mandible fractures constituting 57%. Operative treatment with rigid internal fixation was required for 37.4%. Female patients had less fracture severity than their male counterparts and were better candidates for closed reduction and arch bars (19).

Mandible fractures are typically diagnosed with dental panoramic or mandibular radiographs. CT may be required to diagnose fractured condyles (16,18). Intimate partner violence assault victims with mandible fractures are frequently hospitalized and may require open or closed surgical repair. Victims with open mandible fractures are treated with intravenous antibiotics. Complications occur in 15%–20% of patients, and range from infections such as abscess and osteomyelitis to permanent malocclusions (16).

DIAGNOSTIC TOOLS/SURVEYS THAT INCLUDE MAXILLOFACIAL INJURIES AS RISK FACTORS

Intimate partner violence assault literature supports head, neck, and face injury as potential clinical markers (9,15–26,61,62) of IPV. Initial studies to develop a IPV diagnostic protocol using injury location were conducted over a decade ago at Grady Memorial Hospital (GMH) in Atlanta, Georgia. Grady is a Level I trauma center serving a medically indigent population composed predominately of African Americans who reside in Fulton and DeKalb counties in Georgia. Demographics consisted of 88% African American, 7.6% Caucasian, 3.6% Hispanic, and 0.5% Asian. Ochs and co-workers reported the initial finding based on a sample 127 male and female subjects who presented to the emergency department for evaluation and management of nonverifiable injuries (23). The age distribution of the population was 36.5 ± 14.4 years. The prevalence of IPV in this setting was 30%. Injury location was determined by physical examination and grouped into "head-neck-face" (HNF) or other. Subject self-reports were used to determine injury etiology. Intimate partner violence victims were defined as those who reported that their injuries were due to assaults by their intimate partners. The results of this study suggested that injuries localized to the HNF region were associated with an increased risk for injury due to IPV (relative risk [RR] = 11.8; 95% confidence interval [CI] = 1.65,85.8, p = .01). In this clinical setting, HNF injuries as markers of IPV had high sensitivity (94%), but poor specificity (45%).

The results also suggested, consistent with other studies, that women were much more likely than men to be victims of IPV. The low specificity (45%) prompted a second cross-sectional analysis of the same subject population, but the sample was limited to females (9). The purposes of this second investigation were: (a) to confirm the findings of the first study and (b) to identify other risk factors for IPV that may improve specificity. The sample consisted of 100 women. The prevalence of IPV was 34%. Head-neck-facial injuries were associated with an increased risk for injuries due to IPV (RR = 7.5,95% CI = 2, 22.9, $p < .001$). Age was identified as a confounding variable, as it was associated with both injury and location and injury etiology. After controlling for age, injury location was still associated with IPV ($p < .002$). The results suggested that younger women with HNF trauma were more likely to be victims of IPV than older women with injuries to non-HNF locations (chest, abdomen, extremities). When both injury location and age were included in the model, the combined sensitivity and specificity of these two predictors was 91% and 59%, respectively.

In an effort to enhance the specificity of HNF injuries as objective markers for IPV, a third preliminary study was conducted in which two screening instruments were added: (a) short Woman Abuse Screening Tool (short-WAST) (63,64), and (b) Partner Violence Screen (PVS) (65). The preliminary study consisted of 100 female subjects presenting for evaluation and treatment of injuries in the GMH emergency department. The presence of HNF injuries was significantly associated with injury etiology of IPV (RR = 5.9, $p < .001$). A positive response to either the WAST or PVS was associated with IPV etiology. By combining injury location and the WAST or PVS score, a logistic model with 90% sensitivity and 93% specificity suggested that the combination of injury location and response to either the short-WAST or PVS produced valid and reliable model for predicting IPV (66). A recent study by Perciaccante and colleagues combined injury location and the short-WAST to produce a more accurate model for predicting IPV than either modality alone or injury location and the PVS score (67). The short-WAST tool appears to show greater specificity than the PVS. In a validated model dataset, injury location and short-WAST score combined was statistically associated with an increased risk of IPV ($p < .05$).

The preliminary studies cited here were set in an inner city emergency department located in a major metropolitan city in the American South. The sample was composed of medically indigent, predominately Black (>90%) females. Although the problems of IPV span cultural, socioeconomic, and geographic barriers, it was not clear that the markers of IPV that were identified would be generally applicable in different geographic or clinical settings. The preliminary results presented here, however, provided a foundation to assess the generalizability of the proposed IPV diagnostic protocol by implementing the protocol in a geographic setting with a subject population that

contrasts markedly with the setting and sample used in the preliminary studies.

Halpern and colleagues (2005, 2006) tested the external validity of the protocol using the two variables of injury location and a verbal questionnaire associated with IPV-related injuries from the preliminary studies just stated (Figure 15.2) (62,68). By comparing two hospitals that differ by geographic location, socioeconomic status, and healthcare cost, their results suggest that clinicians can use injury location in conjunction with the PVS score to stratify (that is, as high or low) the risk of self-report of IPV-related injuries. In addition, further studies have determined that in terms of detecting women with IPV-related injuries, the investigators' proposed diagnostic protocol is 40 times more likely to report an IPV-related injury as compared with 11 times more likely with the standard operating procedure of the emergency department (OR; $p = .01$). The sensitivity of the diagnostic protocol was superior to standard operating procedures, but specificities were equivalent (69).

Other studies have identified age, race, income, education, and social history as risk factors for IPV-related injuries (4,10,62,70). A recent study developed a predictive model utilizing HNF injury location and responses to a verbal questionnaire to stratify risk of self-report of IPV-related injury etiology. This risk was modified by other variables of age and race and tested in a predictive model for goodness of fit using an independent set of patients compared with the model. The authors concluded that injury location, positive responses to the questionnaire, and age can significantly facilitate early diagnosis of IPV (62).

LIMITATIONS OF SURVEYS/ DIAGNOSTIC PROTOCOLS USING MAXILLOFACIAL INJURIES AS RISK PREDICTORS

Much controversy centers on whether routine screenings for IPV should be performed in healthcare settings. The United States Preventive Services Task Force in 2004 found insufficient evidence to recommend for or against routine screening of women for IPV (71). A systematic review was published in June of 2006 to answer the question, "Should health professionals screen women for IPV?" Some of the papers in this review suggested that women respondents were often accepting of screening in the healthcare setting, but that health

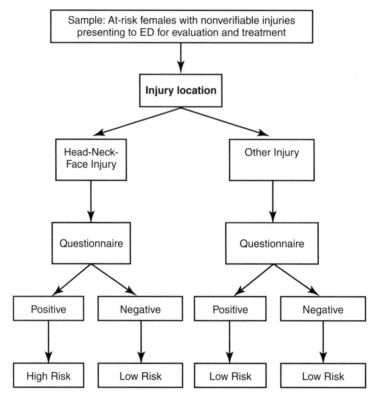

Figure 15.2 Diagnostic protocol for intimate partner violence. Adapted from Halpern LR, Perciccante V, Hayes C, et al. A protocol to diagnose intimate partner violence in the emergency department. *J Trauma.* 2006;60(5):1101–1105.

professionals were frequently not in favor of screening. Several studies showed that when screening was used, a greater proportion of abused women were identified. Overall, little evidence was found in this review to suggest a dynamic impact on improved diagnosis with the routine use of screening. The conclusion of this systematic review, therefore, was that universal implementation of screening programs in healthcare settings cannot be justified. A systematic review was published in the Cochran Database of Systematic Reviews in 2005 regarding IPV screening and intervention programs for adults who had dental or facial injuries. The authors found no eligible randomized controlled trials on this topic. They concluded that "there is no evidence to support or refute the effectiveness of screening and intervention programs detecting and supporting victims of IPV with dental or facial injuries"(72).

Individual studies suggest the value of screening for violence and abuse. A study performed using office-based screening questionnaires suggested that there was a significant increase in the ability to identify families exposed to violence and abuse, to provide appropriate referral information (71). Taliaferro has written a review article on the topic of screening and identification of violence and abuse. She emphasized the need to assess risk versus benefit of such screening to individual patients. Although anecdotal evidence suggests the benefits of screening, there are potential risks to such questionnaires (73). Some of the limitations that often challenge assessment of screening tools are:

1. *Selection bias.* Women who are recruited from the emergency department in one metropolitan hospital may represent one extreme population in both the degree of abuse and socioeconomic characteristics than the population demographics of other hospital and clinical settings. The implementation of these diagnostic protocols in multiple clinical settings can control for selection bias. Translation issues for those who speak English as a second language can be carefully controlled by the use of bilingual interpreters, as has been identified in other studies (4,74,75).

2. *Misclassification.* Measuring the outcome variable (injury etiology) at one point in time and relying on subject self-report may result in misclassification. Clearly, subject report of injury as the standard for diagnosis runs the risk of misclassification, most commonly a false negative (i.e., subject denies injury is due to IPV and reports a different injury etiology such as a fall). There are two major types of misclassification, false positives and false negatives. In this setting, a false positive would be defined as a subject who reported she was injured due to IPV, when in fact her injury etiology was something other than IPV. False-positive errors occur rarely (62,63,65). A false-negative would be defined as a subject who reported an injury due to some other etiology, when in fact it was due to IPV. This error occurs more commonly (41,76). The net effect of having predominately one type of misclassification error (false negative >> false positives) results in an underestimation of the true sensitivity and should have minimal effect on the specificity estimate.

3. *Limitations of the diagnostic protocol.* The hallmark of a successful diagnostic protocol is to have excellent sensitivity, specificity, positive predictive value (PPV), and negative predictive values (NPV). It is therefore critical to set rigorous levels of these statistical criteria because of complications due to false positives or false negatives. For example, a false positive (innocent spouse accused of assault) can result in serious legal and social consequences. Alternatively, a false negative (guilty spouse not accused of assault) can result in repeated injuries and death to the victim. A high false-negative rate can also occur because questions regarding verbal abuse and nonphysical aggression are not included in the questionnaire. It is likely that more victims can be identified if indicators of both physical and nonphysical violence are used in the protocol. With respect to positive and negative predictive values, these are used most often to determine how successful a clinical outcome can be by identifying a disease with a diagnostic tool. The higher the PPV, it is believed, the better the clinical outcome. The studies that utilize injury location are characterized by high PPV and NPV when compared with the standard operating procedures of the emergency departments that they were compared with (67,75).

4. *Reproducibility and generalizability.* It is not clear that the results obtained in one clinical setting of this study can be applicable to other clinical settings, such as the private office or private community hospitals in the suburbs. The results obtained in two clinical settings that are markedly different in terms of their geographic and socioeconomic variables, as shown earlier, suggest that a diagnostic protocol using maxillofacial injuries and a questionnaire may be valuable in a variety of clinical settings. Other studies would include continued testing in different clinical settings to determine if the findings are repeatable. For instance, the protocol will be translated into different languages to allow early interventional strategies that will deter future battering of these and other future victims. Specifically, future studies should involve comparisons of ethnic differences in IPV prevalence rates in order to determine whether a sensitive approach to cultural diversity can maximize identification rates of victims. Furthermore, since prevalence rates range from 5% to 35% in most emergency departments, and one in four women who frequent the emergency department are victims of IPV, a closer analysis on differences in subject presentation with respect to chief complaint may also provide for a greater capture of victims of violence.

EDUCATING CLINICIANS WHO ADDRESS ORAL AND MAXILLOFACIAL TRAUMA

In 2006, the American Dental Association (ADA) news ran a commentary summarizing the importance of increasing the dental community's education, understanding, and obligation to recognize the signs and symptoms of family violence (34,77). The ADA Principles of Ethics and Code of Professional Conduct states that "Dentists shall be obliged to become familiar with the signs of abuse and neglect and to report suspected cases to the proper authorities consistent with state laws."

The American Association of Oral and Maxillofacial Surgeons (AAOMS) states, in accordance with the ADA and American College of Surgeons, that "Surgeons are encouraged to take a leadership role in communities, hospitals, and medical schools in preventing and treating intimate partner violence" (4). Dentists are in a unique position to help victims within the community setting since one-half to two-thirds of adults visit the dentist annually (34,78). Facial bruising, fracture of bones in various stages of healing, finger marks on the face and neck, burns, oro-facial injuries such as torn frenulums, lip lacerations, loose teeth, and multiple fractures of teeth and dental neglect are all within clear view. Oral manifestations of STDs, fearfulness of the dental examination, difficulty sitting or walking, and fear of the reclined position of the chair all should be considered as signs and symptoms of possible prior sexual abuse (71).

Educators in oral health have taken a variety of major steps to provide the knowledge base for dentists regarding these stumbling blocks (77):

> The Prevent Abuse and Neglect through Dental Awareness (PANDA) coalition was started in Missouri in 1992, and Lynn Douglas Mouden, DDS, MPH was one of its co-founders. The original PANDA coalition was comprised of the Missouri Dental Association and Delta Dental Plan of Missouri, as well as, the Missouri Division of Family Services and the Missouri Bureau of Dental Health. As of March 2008, 46 states have replicated Missouri's program along with international coalitions in Romania, Guam, Peru, Canada, Finland, Israel, Mexico, and Brazil, as well as within the USPHS Indian Health Service and the U.S. Army Dental Command worldwide. PANDA educational programs include information on the history of family violence in our society, clinical examples of confirmed family violence, and discussions of legal and liability issues involved in reporting child maltreatment and appropriate interventions for adult victims of family violence. While originally intended for dental audiences, the PANDA education programs are also presented for physicians, nurses, teachers, day care workers, and anyone that has an interest in preventing family violence.

A recent study tested the efficacy of an educational and behavioral change intervention designed to help dentists overcome their reluctance to identify and treat victims of IPV and to effect positive changes in dentists' knowledge, attitudes, and behaviors with respect to caring for patients who experience IPV (78). Results suggest that the intervention effectively improved dentists' intentions to practice Ask, Validate, Document, Refer (ADVR) intervention (78). The AVDR tutorial provides a concrete intervention that can be applied within the scope of the dental practice. In addition, the ability to use computer technology as an integral tool in the educational arena provides a great stride forward in educational training of healthcare providers to identify victims of IPV.

IMPLICATIONS FOR POLICY, PRACTICE, AND RESEARCH

Policy

- Training in specialties such as emergency medicine, surgery, and dentistry should institute mandatory instruction that links injury patterns with the most common etiologies of IPV- related injuries seen.

Practice

- Intimate partner violence should be included in the differential diagnosis of all female patients with maxillofacial injury.
- Maxillofacial assault victims should have a detailed injury history documented that includes mechanism of injury, weapon, relationship to assailant, location of assault, description of injury, associated injuries, and history of prior assault.
- Patients with head and facial injury should be educated regarding the increased risk associated with recurrent injuries and often co-occurring traumatic brain injury (TBI).
- All injured female patients should receive educational information and referrals for IPV counseling, including bedside danger assessment and safety planning prior to discharge.

Research

- Prospective clinical studies are needed to further examine the sensitivity and specificity of maxillofacial and other injury types as clinical markers for IPV assault.
- Attention should be given to the use of clinical markers and patient profile data as indicators for a more extensive IPV evaluation. The development of systemized IPV evaluation criteria could be a valuable adjunct to screening in some clinical settings.
- Research to investigate the relationship between severity (contusion versus fracture) of maxillofacial assault injury and IPV lethality are needed. This research could serve to expand the utility of facial injury as a clinical marker for IPV and better define the victim's potential risk.
- Studies that examine the association between IPV assault maxillofacial injury and TBI will aid healthcare providers and other

professionals working with IPV victims to make appropriate counseling and rehabilitation referrals.

- Authors have theorized that male batterers target the woman's face to leave visible marks that exert his dominance over the woman and in the relationship (36). Research to examine the short- and long-term psychosocial consequences of maxillofacial battery will be valuable.

References

1. Watts C, Zimmerman, C. Violence against women: Global scope and magnitude. *Lancet.* 2002; 359:1232–1237.
2. Haywood Y, Haile-Mariam, T. Violence against women. *Emergency Med Clinics N Amer.* 1999; 17(3):603–614.
3. Chiodo G, Tilden, VP, Limandri, BJ, et al. Addressing family violence among dental subjects: Assessment and intervention. *J Am Dent Assoc.* 1994;125:69–75.
4. Melnick D, Maio RF, Blow E, et al. Prevalence of domestic violence and associated factors among women on a trauma service. *J Trauma.* 2002; 53(1):33–37.
5. Hathaway J, Mucci LA, Silveman JG, et al. Health status and health care use of Massachusetts women reporting partner abuse. *Am J Prev Med.* 2000;19(4):302–307.
6. Knudson M, Vassar MJ, Straus EM, et al. Surgeons and injury prevention: What you don't know can hurt you. *J Am Coll Surg.* 2001;193(2):119–124.
7. Senn D, McDowell JD, Alder ME. Dentistry's role in the recognition and reporting of domestic violence, abuse and neglect. *Dent Clin North Amer.* 2001;45(2):343–363.
8. Zillmer D. Domestic violence: The role of the orthopedic surgeon in identification and treatment. *J Am Acad Orthop Surg.* 2000;8(2):91–96.
9. Perciaccante V, Ochs HA, Dodson TB. Head, neck and facial injuries as markers of domestic violence in women. *J Oral Maxillofac Surg.* 1999;57(7): 760–762.
10. Spedding R, McWilliams M, McNicholl BP, Dearden CH. Markers for domestic violence in women. *J Acad Emerg Med.* 1999;16(6):400–402.
11. Huang V, Moore C, Bohrer P, Thaller SR. Maxillofacial injuries in women. *Ann Plast Surg.* 1998;41:482–484.
12. Fisher E, Kraus H, Lewis VL. Assaulted women: Maxillofacial injuries in rape and domestic violence. *Plast Reconstr Surg.* 1994;86(1):161–162.
13. Le B, Dierks SJ, Veeck BA, et al. Maxillofacial injuries associated with domestic violence. *J Oral Maxillofac Surg.* 2001;59:1279–1283.
14. Monahan K, O'Leary KD. Head injury and battered women: An initial inquiry. *Health Soc Work.* 1999;24(4):269–278.
15. Berrios D, Grady D. Domestic violence: Risk factors and outcomes. *West J Med.* 1991;155:133–135.
16. Cantril S. Rosen's emergency medicine concepts and clinical practice. In: Marx J, Hockberger RS, Walls RM, eds. *Trauma system injuries—face.* St. Louis: Mosby; 2002.
17. Centers for Disease Control and Prevention. Prevalence of intimate partner violence and injuries. *MMWR Morb Mortal Wkly Rep.* 2000;49: 589–592.
18. Flores C, Schwartz DT. Facial radiology. In: Schwartz D, Reisdorff EJ, eds. *Emergency radiology.* New York: McGraw-Hill; 2000.
19. Greene D, Maas CS, Carvalo G, Raven, R. Epidemiology of facial injury in female blunt assault trauma cases. *Arch Facial Plast Surg.* 1999; 1(4):288–291.
20. McDowell J. Forensic dentistry. Recognizing the signs and symptoms of domestic violence: A guide for dentists. *J Okla Dent Assoc.* 1997;88(2):21–28.
21. Muelleman R, Lenaghan PA, Pakieser RA. Battered women: Injury location and types. *Ann Emerg Med.* 1996;28:486–492.
22. Nakhgevany K, LiBassi M, Esposito B. Facial trauma in motor vehicle accidents: Etiological factors. *Am J Emer Med.* 1994;12:160.
23. Ochs H, Neuenschwande MC, Dodson TB. Are head, neck and facial injuries markers of domestic violence? *J Am Dent Assoc.* 1996;127(6):757–761.
24. Petridou E, Browns A, Lichter E, et al. What distinguishes unintentional injuries from injuries due to intimate partner violence: A study in Greek ambulatory care settings. *Inj Prev.* 2002;8: 197–201.
25. Telfer M, Jones GM, Shepherd JP. Trends in the aetiology of maxillofacial fractures in the United Kingdom (1977–1989). *Br J Oral Maxillofac Surg.* 1991;29:250–255.
26. Zachariades N, Koumoura F, Konsolaki-Agouridaki E. Facial trauma in women resulting from violence by men. *J Oral Maxillofac Surg.* 1990;48(12): 1250–1253.
27. Hussain K, Wijetunge DB, Grubnic S, Jackson IT. A comprehensive analysis of craniofacial trauma. *J Trauma.* 1994;36:34.
28. Hutchison I, Magennis P, Shepherd J, Brown A. The BAOMS United Kingdom survey of facial injuries part 1: Aetiology and the association with alcohol. *Br J Oral Maxillofac Surg.* 1998;36:4–14.
29. Tanaka N, Tomitsuka K, Shionoya K, et al. Aetiology of maxillofacial fracture. *Br J Oral Maxillofac Surg.* 1994;32:19–23.
30. Lee K, Snape L, Steenberg LJ, et al. Comparison between interpersonal violence and motor vehicle accidents in the aetiology of maxillofacial fractures. *Austral J Surg.* 2007;77:695–698.

31. Crandall M, Nathens AB, Rivava FP. Injury pattern among female trauma patients: Recognizing intentional injury. *J Trauma.* 2004;57:42–45.

32. Haug R, Prather J, Indresano AT. An epidemiologic survey of facial fractures and concomitant injuries. *J Oral Maxillofac Surg.* 1990;48:926.

33. Gilthorpe M, Wilson RC, Moles DR, Bedi R. Variation in admissions to hospitals for head injury and assault to the head. Part 1: Age and gender. *Br J Oral Maxillofac Surg.* 1999;37(4):294–300.

34. Kenney J. Domestic violence: A complex healthcare issue for dentistry today. *Forensic Science International.* 2006:S121–S125.

35. Leathers R, Shetty V, Black E, et al. Orofacial injury profiles and patterns of care in an inner-city hospital. *Int J Oral Biol.* 1998;23(1):53–58.

36. Dutton D, Strachan CE. Motivational needs for power and spouse-specific assertiveness in assaultive and non-assaultive men. *Violence Vict.* 1987;2: 145–156.

37. Sherdian D, Nash KR. Acute injury patterns in intimate partner violence. *Trauma Violence Abuse.* 2007:281–289.

38. Craven D. *Female victims of crime.* Washington DC: US Department of Justice; 1996.

39. Fanslow J, Norton RN, Spinola CG. Indicators of assault-related injuries among women presenting to the emergency department. *Ann Emerg Med.* 1998;32:341–348.

40. Hartzell K, Botek AA, Goldberg KH. Orbital fractures in women due to sexual assault and domestic violence. *Ophthalmology.* 1996;103(6):953–957.

41. Shepherd J, Gaylord JJ, Leslie IJ, Scully C. Female victims of assault. *J Craniomaxillofac Surg.* 1988;16:233–237.

42. Shepherd J, Shapland M, Pearce NX, et al. Pattern, severity and aetiology of injuries in victims of assault. *J R Soc Med.* 1990;83:75–78.

43. Beck S, Freitag SL, Singer N. Ocular injuries in battered women. *Ophthalmology.* 1996;103(7): 997–998.

44. Simo R, Jones NS. Extratemporal facial nerve paralysis after blunt trauma. *J Trauma.* 1996; 40(2):306–307.

45. Molitor L. A 26-year-old women with unexplained ptosis. *J Emerg Nurs.* 1999;25:430.

46. Sorenson S, Wiebs OJ. Weapon in the lives of battered women. *Am J Public Health.* 2004; 94(8):1414–1417.

47. Grisso J, Wishner AR, Schwartz DF, et al. A population based study of injuries in inner-city women. *Am J Epidemiol.* 1991;134:59.

48. Carrigan T, Walker E, Barnes S. Domestic violence: The shaken adult syndrome. *J Accid Emerg Med.* 2000;17:138–139.

49. Funk M, Schuppel J. Strangulation injuries. *Wisc Med J.* 2003;102(3):41–45.

50. Hawley D, McClane GE, Strack GB. A review of 300 attempted strangulation cases, part III: Injuries in fatal cases. *J Emerg Med.* 2001;21:317–329.

51. McClane G, Strack GB, Hawley D. A review of 300 attempted strangulation cases, part II: Clinical evaluation of the surviving victim. *J Emerg Med.* 2001;21:311–315.

52. Purvin V. Unilateral headache and ptosis in a 30-year-old woman. *Surv Opthalmol.* 1997;42(2): 163–168.

53. Covington D, Wainsright DJ, Teichgraeber JF, Parks DH. Changing patterns in the epidemiology and treatment of zygoma fractures: 10-year review. *J Trauma.* 1994;37:243.

54. Ellis E, El-Atter A, Moos KF. An analysis of 2,067 cases of zygomatico-orbital fracture. *J Oral Maxillofac Surg.* 1985;43:417–428.

55. Wallis A, Donald PJ. Frontal sinus fractures: A review of 72 cases. *Laryngoscope.* 1988;98:593.

56. Goldberg S, McRill CM, Bruno CR, et al. Orbital fractures due to domestic violence: An epidemiologic study. *Orbit.* 2000;19(3):143–154.

57. Rehm C, Ross SE. Diagnosis of unsuspected facial fractures on routine head computerized tomographic scans in the unconscious multiply injured patient. *J Oral Maxillofac Surg.* 1995; 53:522.

58. Rhea J, Rao PM, Noveline RA. Helical CT and three-dimensional CT of facial and orbital injury. *Radiol Clin North Am.* 1999;37:489.

59. Russell J, Davidson MJ, Daly BD, Corrigan AM. Computed tomography in the diagnosis of maxillofacial trauma. *Br J Oral Maxillofac Trauma.* 1990;28:287.

60. Clemenza J, Kaltman SK, Diamond DL. Craniofacial trauma and cerebrospinal fluid leakage: A retrospective clinical study. *J Oral Maxillofac Surg.* 1995;53:1004.

61. Philip M, Sivarajasingan V, Shepherd J. Bilateral reflex fracture of the coronoid process of the mandible. A case report. *Int J Oral Maxillofac Surg.* 1999;28(3):195–196.

62. Halpern L, Dodson TB. A predictive model for diagnosing victims of intimate partner violence. *JADA.* 2006;137:604–609.

63. Brown J, Lent B, Brett P. Development of the woman abuse screening tool for use in family practice. *Fam Med.* 1996;28:422–428.

64. Brown J, Schmidt G, Lent B, Sas G, Lemelin J. Screening for violence against women. Validation and feasibility studies of a French screening tool. *Can Fam Physician.* 2001;47:988–995.

65. Feldhaus K, McLain J, Amsbury HL. Accuracy of three brief screening questions for detecting partner violence in the emergency department. *JAMA.* 1997;277(17):439–441.

66. Carey J, Dodson TB. Predicting domestic violence based on injury location and screening questions. *J Oral Maxillofac Surg.* 1999:42–43.

67. Perciaccante V, Carey JW, Dodson TB. Injury location and woman's abuse screening: Tool scores as markers for intimate partner violence (IPV). *J Dental Research.* 2002;81:A-492.

68. Halpern L, Susarla S, Dodson TB. Injury location and screening questionnaires as markers for intimate partner violence. *J Oral Maxillofac Surg.* 2005;63(9):1255–1261.

69. Halpern L, Parry B, Hayward G, Peak D, Dodson TB. A new protocol versus standard emergency department protocol to diagnoses intimate partner violence. *AAOMS 89th Annual Meeting.* Honolulu, Hawaii; 2007.

70. Lipsky S, Caetano R, Field CA, Barzargan S. Violence-related injury and intimate partner violence in an urban emergency department. *J Trauma.* 2004;57(2):352–359.

71. Zeitler D. The abused female oral and maxillofacial surgery patient: Treatment approaches for identification and management. *Oral Maxillofac Clin North Am.* 2007;19:259–263.

72. Coulthard P, Yong SL, Adamson L, et al. Domestic violence screening and intervention programmes for adults with dental or facial injury. *Cochrane Database Syst Rev.* 2004;2:CD004486.

73. Taliaferro E. Screening and identification of intimate partner violence. *Clin Fam Pract.* 2003;5(1):89–100.

74. Brown J, Schmidt G, Lent B, Sas G. Application of the woman abuse screening tool (WAST and WAST-short) in the family practice setting. *J Fam Pract.* 2000;49:896–903.

75. Halpern L, Perciaccante VJ, Hayes C, et al. A protocol to diagnose intimate partner violence in the emergency room setting. *J Trauma.* 2006;60(5):1101–1105.

76. Abbott J, Johnson R, Koziol-Mclain J, et al. Domestic violence against women: Incidence and prevalence in an emergency department population. *JAMA.* 1995;273:1763–1767.

77. Mouden LD, Family violence prevention: Dentistry's attitude and responsibilities. *Quintessence Int.* 29(7):452-454,1998.

78. Hsieh N, Herzig K, Gansky S, et al. Changing dentist's knowledge, attitudes and behavior regarding domestic violence through an interactive multimedia tutorial. *JADA.* 2006;137(5):596–603.

79. Fenton S, Bouquot J, Unkel J. Orofacial considerations for pediatric, adult, and elderly victims of abuse. *Emerg Med Clin North Am.* 2000;18(3):601–617.

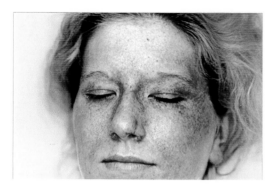

Plate 1 Scattered facial petechiae. *Forensic photograph courtesy of Nancy Housel, RN and with consent of the victim.*

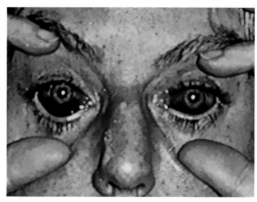

Plate 2 Subconjunctival hemorrhages. *Forensic photograph courtesy of San Diego Police Department.*

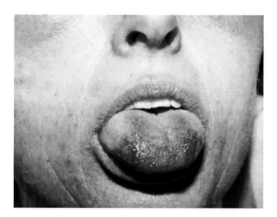

Plate 3 Tongue swelling. *Forensic photograph courtesy of San Diego Police Department.*

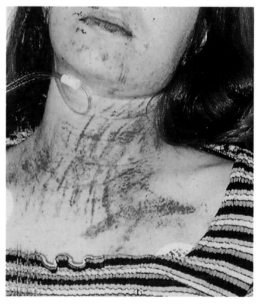

Plate 4 Self-excoriations during strangulation. *Forensic photograph courtesy of Mono County District Attorney's Office and the consent of the victim.*

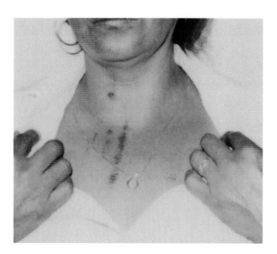

Plate 5 Self-excoriations to neck during strangulation. *Forensic photograph courtesy of San Diego Police Department.*

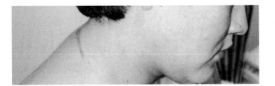

Plate 6 Ligature mark to posterior neck. *Forensic photograph courtesy of Diana Cummings, RN and with consent of the victim.*

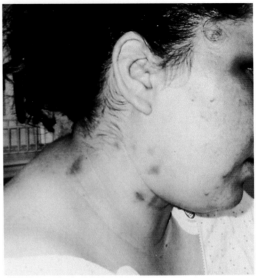

Plate 7 Fingertip contusions to lateral neck. *Forensic photograph courtesy of Diana Cummings, RN and with consent of the victim.*

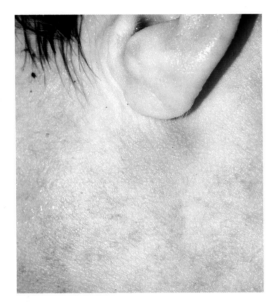

Plate 8 Thumb-tip contusion to mastoid process. *Forensic photograph courtesy of Dean Hawley, MD.*

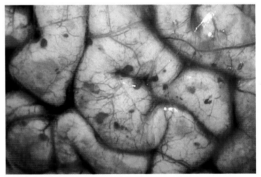

Plate 9 Petechiae in the cerebral arachnoid. *Postmortem forensic photograph courtesy of Dean Hawley, MD.*

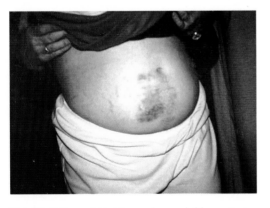

Plate 10 Patterned, bluish-purple punch-like contusion to the lower abdomen with circular knuckle impressions consistent with an upper-cut punch to the abdomen. (Notice the upward ecchymotic spread consistent with the patient being forced to lay supine immediately after being punched.) *Forensic photography courtesy of Dan Sheridan, RN, PhD.*

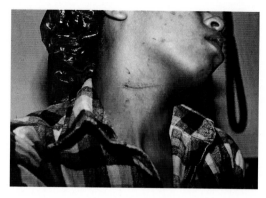

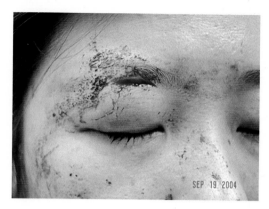

Plate 11 Two fingernail scratch-like abrasions to the lateral neck self inflicted in attempt to remove assailant's hands and/or inflicted by her assailant during a reported manual strangulation. *Forensic photography courtesy of Dan Sheridan, RN, PhD.*

Plate 12 Right eyebrow laceration from blunt force trauma. *Forensic photography courtesy of Dan Sheridan, RN, PhD.*

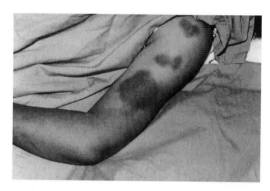

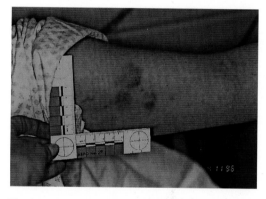

Plate 13 Multiple patterned contusions to the upper lateral arm consistent with history of being punched with a fist several times.*Forensic photography courtesy of Dan Sheridan, RN, PhD.*

Plate 14 Patterned thumb/fingertip like bruises to upper arm with history of being grabbed during assault. *Forensic photography courtesy of Dan Sheridan, RN, PhD.*

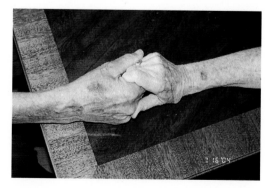

Plate 15 Nonabuse Ecchymoses in elderly. Ecchymoses, nonabuse-related lesions, to the arms and hands of an elderly couple. Tissue and blood vessel fragility common in old age can lead to bruising attributed to everyday activities. *Forensic photography courtesy of Dan Sheridan, RN, PhD.*

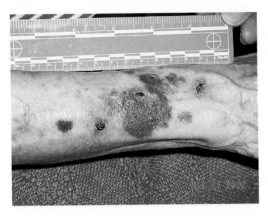

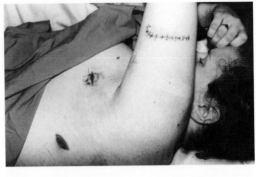

Plate 16 Ecchymoses with minor skin tearing (partial avulsions) to the arm. If the elderly patient is relatively active, such an injury could be unintentional and sustained during routine activities of daily living. However, if the patient requires total care, these same injuries should prompt further assessment for excessive force or physical abuse. *Forensic photography courtesy of Dan Sheridan, RN, PhD.*

Plate 17 Patient stated the assailant attacked her with a knife and cut her left arm and then stabbed her in the chest. She has three sharp force injuries: one to the arm, now repaired, one to the lower chest from the assault, left open and a therapeutic incision to upper chest, now partially closed, after chest tube insertion. *Forensic photography courtesy of Dan Sheridan, RN, PhD.*

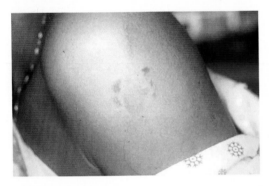

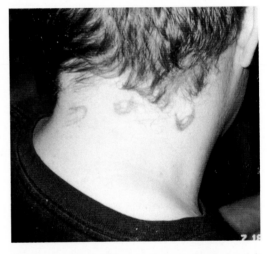

Plate 18 Bite injury to left upper arm. For forensic documentation, additional photos should be close up, at right angles with a right-angle ruler next to the wound. *Forensic photography courtesy of Dan Sheridan, RN, PhD.*

Plate 19 Patterned Burns from a "super-heated" cigarette lighter. This patient has three, reddish-colored patterned burns to the posterior neck consistent with the shape of a disposable cigarette lighter that was "super-heated" and then pressed against the skin. (It is not known if the lighter was heated three separate times or if the lighter was heated once and pressed quickly, three times, against the skin.) *Forensic photography courtesy of Dan Sheridan, RN, PhD.*

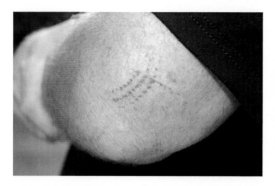

Plate 20 Patterned contusion (baseball seams) to Elbow. Patient struck by fast, pitched ball during a sporting event. (This is an image of a nonintentional injury, but baseballs have also been thrown with intent to injure, either in a baseball game or during an intimate partner physical assault.) *Forensic photography courtesy of Dan Sheridan, RN, PhD.*

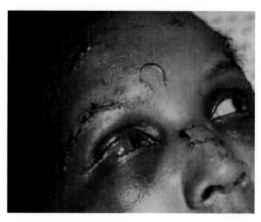

Plate 21 Patterned abrasion (finger ring) to forehead. Punch injury with patterned, ring-shaped abrasion to mid forehead. Other injuries to face include bilateral periorbital ecchymoses. *Forensic photography courtesy of Dan Sheridan, RN, PhD.*

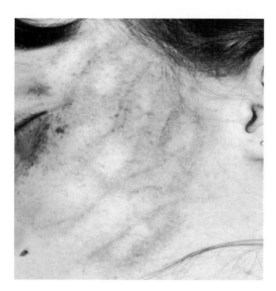

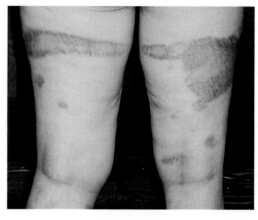

Plate 23 Horizontal patterned bruise with central clearing that extends across both legs. This injury pattern is consistent with being struck with a solid object, in this case a cane. There are other bruises in various stages of healing. *Forensic photography courtesy of Dan Sheridan, RN, PhD.*

Plate 22 Bruising to the face with parallel raised welts and central clearing consistent with the strike of an open hand. The outline of the fingers, including the flexor creases is clearly evident. *Forensic photography courtesy of Dan Sheridan, RN, PhD.*

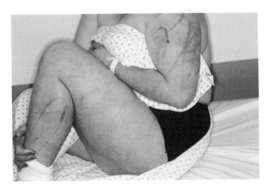

Plate 24 Patterned bruising, "loop-cord" injury. Multiple reddish-colored, looped, cord-like bruises in a pattern consistent with patient's history of laying on her right side, in a curled defensive posture while being whipped with a looped telephone cord. *Forensic photography courtesy of Dan Sheridan, RN, PhD.*

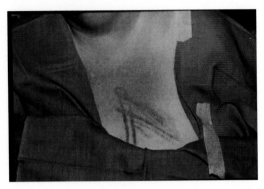

Plate 25 Parallel "train track" abrasions are consistent with a zipper abrading the skin. Patient said she was wearing a zippered heavy cotton pull-over shirt and her boyfriend grabbed her by the front of the shirt and shoved her against the wall, forcing the zipper up and then down against the skin. *Forensic photography courtesy of Dan Sheridan, RN, PhD.*

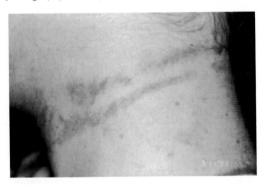

Plate 26 Patterned abrasion (ligature marks) to neck. Two circumferential ligature marks to the neck, the lower one newer than the upper one, secondary to being brighter red and having more intact margins.*Forensic photography courtesy of Dan Sheridan, RN, PhD.*

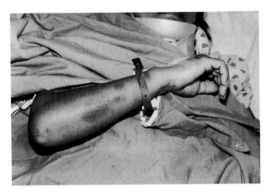

Plate 27 Mid forearm bruises consistent with defensive posturing of holding arm up to protect face and anterior neck/chest. *Forensic photography courtesy of Dan Sheridan, RN, PhD.*

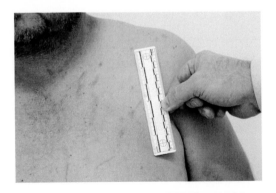

Plate 28 Suspect exam reveals linear abrasions to chest. Long, linear, fan-patterned abrasions are consistent with claw marks that could be sustained in a fight or as a victim struggles to defend or escape. *Forensic photos courtesy of the Office of the District Attorney, Placer County, CA.*

Chapter 16

Strangulation in Intimate Partner Violence

Ellen Taliaferro, Dean Hawley, George McClane, and Gael Strack

---

KEY CONCEPTS

- Strangulation is a common form of intimate partner violence (IPV) assault often over-looked or minimized by victims as well as professionals.
- Strangulation survivors who appear to be stable can harbor insidious injuries associated with high morbidity and mortality if not recognized and treated in a timely fashion.
- *Strangulation* is the correct term to use for manual and ligature strangulation, but lay persons may still use the word *choking*.
- The pathophysiology of strangulation assault or death usually is asphyxiation produced not by airway compromise, but by vascular compromise in the neck.
- Survivors of strangulation assault can manifest a variety of signs and symptoms.
- Strangulation assault should be meticulously assessed and documented, as these medical records are likely to be used in criminal proceedings.
- Strangulation assault victims should be considered for hospital admission for observation, and require careful instructions regarding postdischarge care and follow-up.

Strangulation, a common form of intimate partner violence (IPV) assault, is one of three major types of intentionally inflicted neck trauma: blunt impact trauma, penetrating injuries, and strangulation. Strangulation, like the other two forms of neck trauma, can result in laryngotracheal injuries, digestive tract injuries, vascular injuries, and neurologic insult.

Neck trauma presents a challenge to clinicians because stable-appearing patients can harbor insidi-ous injuries associated with high morbidity and mortality if not recognized and treated in a timely fashion. Patients with neck injury can have numerous signs and symptoms, but most are nonspecific, which makes diagnostic strategies difficult, especially in the stable-appearing patient. For instance, blunt vascular injuries are rare but represent some of the most under-diagnosed injuries associated with neck trauma (1).

BACKGROUND

Healthcare awareness that manual strangulation is a common form of IPV assault has lagged behind the awareness of the social services and IPV victim advocacy community, which has known for a long time that strangulation is a common means of IPV assault. Medical literature describing victims who survive strangulation is scant. The majority of articles on strangulation are found in the forensic literature, describing the postmortem findings on autopsy (2).

Until the 1980s, a distinct dearth of medical litera-ture addressed manual strangulation and its sequelae in surviving victims. In 1983, Stanley and Hanson published an article, "Manual Strangulation Injuries of the Larynx," in the Archives of Otolaryngology (3). The following year, Iserson published a review article, "Strangulation: A Review of Ligature, Manual, and Postural Neck Compression Injuries," in the Annals of Emergency Medicine (4).

The first hint that manual strangulation injuries in surviving patients were underreported appeared in 1985 when Line and colleagues published, "Stran-gulation: A Full Spectrum of Blunt Neck Trauma." These authors noted that although strangulation represents an important form of blunt neck trauma, "discussion of strangulation injuries has been infre-quent." They reviewed the records of 112 nonsurvi-vors and 59 survivors. The records of the 59 survivors represented patients who had been admitted to Los Angeles County – University of Southern California Medical Center over an 11-year study period. These authors pointed out that their study population was not a true indication of the incidence of strangula-tion. They noted that a large number of patients had been seen in the minor trauma area of the main emergency department, complaining of being stran-gled. However, these patients were judged to be asymptomatic and had not been referred to the oto-laryngology service (5).

Other authors in the 1980s also commented on the paucity of literature addressing strangulation sur-vivors. Most studies of manual strangulation and case reports were found in the forensic literature, reported by forensic pathologists. This began to change in the 1990s, when Strack, McClane, and Hawley reported on 300 strangulation cases selected from domestic vio-lence (DV), elder abuse, and child abuse cases on file with the San Diego City (California) Attorney's Office, Domestic Violence Unit. This study, prompted by the deaths of two teenage girls in 1995, highlighted the issue of strangulation as a common form of IPV assault (6).

DEFINITION OF STRANGULATION

The term *strangulation* is a general one. The Merri-am-Webster online dictionary defines the term stran-gulation as "excessive or pathological constriction or compression of a bodily tube (as a blood vessel or a loop of intestine) that interrupts its ability to act as a passage"(7). Strangulation of the "bodily tubes" of the neck causes asphyxia, which Merriam-Webster defines as a lack of oxygen or excess of carbon dioxide in the body that is usually caused by interruption of breathing and that causes unconsciousness (8). Stran-gulation is only one of several causes of homicide by asphyxia. Other well-known causes include drowning, carbon monoxide poisoning, and smothering (9).

The terms *strangulation, choking,* and *suffocation* are often confused, yet they all lead to asphyxia. In strangulation, external compression of the neck can impede oxygen transport by preventing blood flow to or from the brain or due to direct airway compres-sion. Choking refers to an object in the retropharynx or upper airway that impedes oxygen intake during inspiration and can occur accidentally or intention-ally. Suffocation refers to obstruction of the airway at the nose and mouth and can also occur accidentally or intentionally. Therefore, the term "strangulation" should always be used to specifically denote external neck compression. Reserve the term "choking" for internal airway blockage (2). When the victim, perpe-trator, or witness uses the term choking to imply being strangled, document their statement with quotation marks. Professionals working in this field should always use the word strangulation when referring to external compression of the neck.

Intentional Strangulation

Confusion regarding intentional strangulation arises when the forms of strangulation, such as hanging, ligature strangulation, and manual strangulation, are interchanged, as has happened often in past literature.

There are three forms of strangulation: hanging, ligature strangulation, and manual strangulation. According to one study on IPV strangulation, 97% occurs manually and only 3% of IPV strangulation is done with a ligature (6).

Hanging is caused by a ligature around the neck, *suspending the body against the pull of gravity*. Forms of hanging need to be further distinguished. An *accidental hanging* occurs when, for example, a child gets his neck tangled in a window blind cord or crib clothing and then falls partially out of the crib, thus resulting in neck suspension. This is different from the injury of *positional asphyxia*, when an infant's chest or abdomen is compressed by crib slats or bedding. In hospitals or other situations in which neck restraint is used to subdue violent or demented individuals deemed to be dangerous to self or others, an inflicted form of positional asphyxiation can occur by the same mechanism as seen in pediatric accidental hanging. *Intentional hanging* further separates into two other forms of hanging: *judicial hanging* (as in the carrying out of a death sentence) and *suicidal/homicidal hanging* not mandated by the law.

Other considerations regarding hanging depend on how far the body falls before being suspended by a neck ligature, and knot placement. *Full-suspension hanging* results when the individual is freely suspended with no part of the body touching the ground or floor. In contrast, *partial-suspension hanging* refers to a partial suspension of the victim's body with some body part still in contact with the ground. Partial-suspension hanging can occur while lying flat in bed. A partial-suspension hanging can be created as a postmortem injury by an assailant attempting to disguise a homicide.

There is considerable misunderstanding about neck injury in hanging, including the notion that radical displaced fractures occur. Folklore regarding judicial hangings include allegedly formalized, even statute-mandated procedures that vary and sometimes describe drop height, rope diameter, and weights, where the purpose seems to be affecting death due to central nervous system trauma rather than asphyxiation (10).

Ligature knot location further divides hanging into typical and atypical categories. *Typical hanging* refers to the knot being posterior and midline directly under the occiput, which leads to a higher likelihood of complete arterial occlusion. *Atypical hanging* refers to all other forms of knot placement (2).

Ligature strangulation is caused by a ligature around the neck where the body is *not* suspended against the pull of gravity. As with hanging, ligature strangulation can be intentional or accidental. Intentional ligature strangulation in IPV frequently employs belts, ropes, and phone cords.[1] A section on nonintentional strangulation follows in this chapter.

Manual strangulation, in current times, results when the assailant's hand or hands are used to neck compression. The definition of manual strangulation can also encompass use of a forearm, knee, foot, or other body part to apply pressure across the victim's neck. Sometimes the perpetrator brings about asphyxiation by pinning the victim against the wall or floor and applying pressure with the forearm or other body part across the neck. In the past, many literature reports of manual strangulation focused on a now abandoned practice of many police agencies: the "carotid restraint hold," "*shime waza*," or "the sleeper hold"—a form of restraint used to subdue a suspect. This maneuver often leaves no external marks on the body. The practice has been restricted or abandoned by law enforcement, as many suspects have died—not the intent of the restraining police officer (10).

Nonintentional Strangulation

Gowens and colleagues report a case of a student who sustained laryngeal rupture and a carotid injury from having her scarf caught in the spokes of a cycle-powered rickshaw. Although respiratory arrest ensued, the patient was successfully resuscitated. Findings included massive edema and subcutaneous emphysema of the neck, a fractured hyoid bone, seizure activity, carotid stenosis, and hemiparesis (11). Accidental strangulation from a scarf being caught in the spokes of a moving wheel was widely publicized in 1927 following the death of famous dancer Isadora Duncan in Nice, France. Duncan was riding in an open-topped, two-seater Buggatti sports car when the fringe of her long scarf caught in the car's rear wheel. Her head was dragged to the side and she died from strangulation (12). Subsequently, death by accidental strangulation from having a scarf caught in moving wheel spokes has been designated as the "Isadora Duncan syndrome." This form of accidental strangulation is also reported in India and Southeast Asia, where women

---

[1] Some experts will refer to both hanging and garroting as "ligature strangulation." In hanging, the force on the neck is from the weight of the victim's body and in garroting the force is caused by a pulling of the perpetrator or other mechanical force.

wear cloths around their neck and use cycle-powered rickshaws to travel short distances (13).

Therapeutic Strangulation

A thousand years ago, ocular surgeons were challenged to obtain enough pain relief to make their surgical procedures possible. They used a number of substances ranging from opium to alcohol. Sometimes they employed selective asphyxia by compressing the carotid vessels in the neck to obtain temporary relief of pain while they performed their surgical procedures (14).

EPIDEMIOLOGY

The overall true incidence of manual strangulation is unknown. This is due in part to the fact that strangulation statistics are often simply reported as "strangulation" as opposed to hanging, ligature strangulation, and manual strangulation. In addition, some strangulation deaths are simply reported as "asphyxiation" deaths.

The most reliable data comes from the Federal Bureau of Investigation (FBI) Uniform Crime Reporting Program. This program has been administrated by the FBI since 1930. It is a nationwide, cooperative, statistical effort by more than 17,000 city, county, and state law enforcement agencies voluntarily reporting data on crimes brought to their attention. During 2002, the reported statistics cover 94.3% of the United States population in metropolitan statistical areas, 89.9% of the population in cities outside metropolitan areas, and 89.5% in rural counties. In 2002, the Uniform Crime Reporting Program reported 143 deaths due to strangulation. Another 103 deaths are reported as simply asphyxiation. Combined, these deaths represent 1.75% of all the total number of 14,054 murder victims reported in 2002. Death by strangulation accounted for 1.01% of all violent deaths in 2002 (15).

Reports of the incidence of strangulation appearing in the lay press can be quite misleading. For instance, Peelo and colleagues investigated the reporting of 2,685 homicides in England and Wales in three national newspapers: The *Times*, the *Mail*, and the *Mirror* in a 4-year period from 1993 to 1997. They found that the most common methods of homicide reported were a sharp instrument (33.3%), followed by hitting and kicking (24.1%), and strangulation/suffocation (13%). These authors report that all three newspapers enhanced reporting rates for strangulation and suffocation cases, shooting, neglect, and arson and burning cases. Below average reporting of homicide occurred in all three newspapers for hitting and kicking cases, poisoning, and for those cases in which the victim was pushed (or caused to fall) (16).

DiMaio reports, "Homicides due to asphyxia are relatively uncommon"(17) in a review of the files of Bexar County, San Antonio, Texas from January 1, 1985 through December 31, 1998. In a conversation in January 2005, he noted that a total of 133 cases were found, accounting for 3.41% of all homicides (hit-and-run accidents and excited delirium cases were included in the total number of homicides) (Table 16.1).

The incidence of strangulation in IPV that is reported in the literature ranges from 10% to 68%. Based on a previous study of women in a primary care setting, Campbell reports that 10%–44% of abused women report strangulation and blows to the head resulting in loss of consciousness (LOC). Wilbur and colleagues interviewed 62 women in DV shelters and found that 68% of these women had been strangled by an intimate partner (18,19). In 1991, Berrios and Grady reported the results of their review of data from standardized interviews with 218 women who presented to the San Francisco General Hospital emergency department with injuries due to DV. In this patient population, "choking" or strangulation was reported in 23% of the patients (20). The victims reported being "choked" by their partner's hands (97%) or with a ligature (3%). When victims described being choked by their partner's hands (manual strangulation), they indicated that the suspect used one hand, two hands, an arm, or a "choke hold." Some women stated that they were strangled on the ground, bed, or sofa while being straddled by the suspect. Some stated that they were strangled while pinned against a wall. In some cases, the women reported that they were lifted off the ground during the strangulation. Most of the police reports simply indicated that the suspect "choked" the victim, without providing any further detail as to the method of strangulation (6). When a ligature was used to strangle the victim, the suspects used objects such as electrical cords, mops, belts, ropes, towels, turtleneck sweaters, bras, or bathing suit tops. In one case, the victim reported that her boyfriend put a plastic bag over her head and tried to suffocate her (6).

Table 16.1 Homicide by Asphyxia (Review of 133 Cases)		
Means of Asphyxia	N	Notes
Ligature strangulation	48	• 21 male and 27 female • Petechiae present in 86% of cases*

Manual strangulation	41	27 females
		  • 14 were victims of rape
		  • 10 were victims of domestic violence
		  • 1 was incurred during a robbery
		  • 2 were victims in which no motive was identified
		14 males
		  • 5 secondary to robbery/burglary
		  • 2 secondary to personal disputes
		  • 1 secondary to a homosexual dispute
		  • 1 secondary to drugs
		  • 5 were victims in which no motive was identified
		Petechiae present in 89% of cases of bodies not in advanced stages of decomposition.

Suffocation	26	
Choking	5	
Combined methods	9	
Drowning	3	
Hanging	1	

PATHOPHYSIOLOGY

Violent manual strangulation or ligature strangulation initially produces severe pain and panic. If the force of the external pressure applied to the neck continues or increases, unconsciousness ensues and can result in brain death (Figure 16.1).

External force applied to the neck that is strong enough to compress the jugular veins produces venous congestion that results in stasis of the cerebral blood flow. Stronger force compresses the carotid arteries, stops arterial blood flow, and impedes oxygen delivery to the brain. Either or both processes lead to reduced oxygen to the brain and unconsciousness. As the struggling victim loses consciousness, the strap muscles in the neck relax, leaving the vessels under them completely unprotected. When unconsciousness negates the protective layer of the voluntarily controlled laryngeal strap muscles, then the same amount of applied external force can cause complete arterial occlusion. Oxygen deprivation ensues, as does the risk of brain injury or death (1).

In general, the immediate pathophysiological sequence of events in survivors of IPV strangulation assault stem from compression of neck vessels. Otolaryngologists Stanley and Hanson note, "Manual strangulation injures are infrequently encountered by the otolaryngologist because the force required to produce the injury is usually successful in producing acute asphyxia and death" (21).

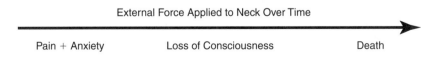

External Force Applied to Neck Over Time

Pain + Anxiety   Loss of Consciousness   Death

Figure 16.1 Sequencing of fatal strangulation.

Regardless of how asphyxia occurs, the decreased blood flow in the brain produces anoxic encephalopathy. As the brain cells are not equally sensitive to the loss of oxygenation, brain cell death may occur at different rates. Nerve cells in the hippocampus and dentate nucleus and the Purkinje cells of the cerebellum are more susceptible to anoxia than the cortical nerve and glial cells. Thus anoxic encephalopathy can result in clinical "brain death," in which the brain is essentially lost while the heart and other critical internal organs can be maintained by medical life support, but with no hope for meaningful recovery.

If the victim survives, complications may include persistent vegetative coma, cerebral edema, and herniation of the brain. Brain herniation occurs when the brain becomes severely swollen due to the accumulation of cell injury and cell death secondary to hypoxia. The brain then begins to herniate or push through the opening in the bottom of the skull into the spinal canal. In those patients who do eventually recover consciousness, lifelong brain damage may be observed (10).

IMMEDIATE DEATH CAUSED BY MANUAL STRANGULATION

Two mechanisms are put forth in the pathological literature to explain immediate death caused by strangulation: asphyxia stemming from compression of arteries, veins, or airway in the neck; or reflex cardiac arrest (22,23).

Asphyxia from manual compression resulting in immediate death can occur from one or more of the following mechanisms:

- Occlusion of the jugular veins causes blood to back up into the cranial vault and results in stasis of blood in the brain that causes unconsciousness, depressed respiration, and subsequent asphyxia.
- Carotid artery occlusion prevents the blood flow to the brain.
- Pressure obstruction of the larynx cuts off airflow to the lungs (10).

Only slight pressure applied to the neck will fully or partially obstruct the veins that return blood flow from the brain. The resulting backing up of the blood in the brain produces a passive congestion of blood in the vessels of the brain. More force is needed to

occlude the carotid arteries, and quite a bit of force is required to occlude or collapse the airway.

Although much agreement exists to support vascular collapse and occlusion as a mechanism of asphyxia, the literature is not so clear on how common brain death is when caused by reflex cardiac arrest. Hawley and colleagues state that reflex cardiac arrest via vagus nerve overstimulation resulting in profound bradycardia and cardiac arrest due to the carotid body reflex is very uncommon as a cause of death from manual strangulation. This assertion is based on the fact that, whereas reflex cardiac dysrhythmia can be reproducibly demonstrated in humans, the force must be applied over a very localized and specific anatomic area (10).

CLINICAL FINDINGS IN SURVIVORS OF STRANGULATION

As with other forms of neck trauma, patients who have survived strangulation can have a variety of signs and symptoms. Victims who do have signs and symptoms often have nonspecific and often vague ones, making evaluation difficult and challenging. The largest series of strangulation survivors to date consists of 300 cases reported by Strack and co-workers. Of these 300 cases, 67% of the victims had no symptoms at all. Of the remaining survivors, 18% had pain only; 7% had other symptoms (raspy voice, coughing, sore throat, nausea, vomiting, vomiting blood, ear pain, headaches, LOC, and lightheadedness); 5% had breathing difficulty; and 2% had difficulty swallowing (6).

The usual signs of neck trauma in the form of skin discoloration or markings were not present at all in 50% of the victims. Of the other 50% of victims, only 15% of the documented cases had a photograph of sufficient quality to be used in court as physical evidence of strangulation. Twelve percent of the cases were so minor that photographs were not even taken, and 23% of the cases had photographs that were not of sufficient quality to be useful as physical evidence (6).

Of note, some or all of these patients may develop symptoms in the future. Wilbur and colleagues (19) interviewed 62 women seen in a specialized IPV clinic or shelter and determined that 42 (68%) of them had a history of having been strangled one or more times. When questioned about symptoms that occurred within 2 weeks of the strangulation event, these 42 patients reported several diverse symptoms ranging from general symptoms of dizziness and LOC to symptoms related to specific systems. These are summarized in Table 16.2.

INITIAL CLINICAL ASSESSMENT

The evaluation of the strangled victim is a process tailored by three circumstances: patient stability, time since the strangulation assault occurred, and focused evaluation of the five common pathologic outcomes: laryngotracheal injuries, digestive tract injuries, vascular injuries, neurological system injuries, and orthopedic injuries.

The Stable Patient

Most patients seen in the emergency department with a history of a recent IPV strangulation assault will be stable and ambulatory (6). As with all trauma patients a quick ABCD review for proper Airway, Breathing, Circulation, and Disability (neurologic functioning) begins the examination, followed by patient history and physical examination. Cervical spine protection should be applied in any complaint of neck pain or neurologic complaint until injury has been assessed.

Good documentation of patient symptoms at the time of presentation sets the stage for good evidence collection as well as determining baseline status. All visible findings should be documented by charting (narrative), using body maps (diagrammatic), and obtaining photos (photodocumentation). If possible, tape record the victim to provide a baseline capture of voice strength and status. Measure the neck size with a tape measure and record (19).

Note that petechiae may be present and range from isolated or a few petechiae, as seen in Figure 16.2 (Plate 1), to multiple petechiae that are so pronounced that subconjunctival hemorrhages appear, as noted in Figure 16.3 (Plate 2). Check for intraoral findings such as tongue swelling, bite injuries, and intraoral petechiae. Figure 16.4 (Plate 3) shows tongue swelling, which can occur from strangulation. Fingernail markings may also be present. Linear and vertical scratches often reflect self-defense injury inflicted by the victim as she struggles to free the perpetrator's hands from her neck (Figures 16.5 and 16.6; Plates 4 and 5). When a ligature of some type is used, the marking can appear anteriorly, or, as seen in Figure 16.7 (Plate 6),

posteriorly. Figure 16.8 (Plate 7) and Figure 16.9 (Plate 8) show fingertip contusions on the neck and in the mastoid area. Usually a single contusion to the lateral neck or mastoid area is correlated with the grasping pressure of the perpetrator's thumb during one-hand frontal strangulation assault.

The Unstable Patient

For the unstable patient, a fast ABCD evaluation and stabilization process begins the procedure. A cervical fracture should be assumed in the unstable strangulation survivor, and cervical spine immobilization should be maintained until cervical spine fracture or dislocation can be ruled out.

Laryngeal injuries account for less than 1% of all trauma injuries (1). Both vascular and laryngeal injuries can compromise the airway in the unstable patient. Securing the airway is of prime concern. Orotracheal rapid sequence intubation (RSI) is considered safe and appropriate in the strangled survivor but should be done by an experienced and trained health provider. Relative contraindications to RSI are massive facial trauma or suspected major laryngeal injury. Controversy arises when the airway is unstable, a laryngoskeletal fracture is evident on a computed tomography (CT) scan, or laryngeal mucosa disruption is noted. In these cases, airway management is obtained by alternate means of control such as fiberoptic intubation under sedation and local anesthesia or tracheostomy (24).

Fortunately, although strangulation can result in laryngotracheal trauma (25), in general the estimated incidence of laryngotracheal trauma from all forms of neck trauma is rare, accounting for an estimated 1:15,000 to 1:43,000 visits to emergency rooms. However, these injuries are potentially lethal, carrying a mortality rate of approximately 20% (24). Suspect the presence of laryngotrauma when these symptoms and signs are present: hoarseness, tenderness, subcutaneous emphysema, respiratory distress, dysphagia, hemoptysis, stridor, inability to tolerate the supine position, dysphonia, or aphonia. Overall, the signs and symptoms can range from a surprising lack of clinical signs to any of those listed. One series of 30 patients found a significant correlation between the symptoms of hemoptysis and stridor and the severity of the laryngotracheal injury (24).

Aerodigestive tract injuries are seen in less than 1% of patients admitted to the hospital after any form blunt trauma to the neck (26). Such injuries are

Table 16.2 Signs and Symptoms Post Strangulation (appear or persisted within 2-week observation period)

System	Symptom	Sign
HEENT	Vision change	Petechiae (slight vs. florid)
	Ringing in ears (tinnitus)	Red marks on the neck
	Sore throat	Fingernail marks on neck
	Voice change	Vision changes
	Difficulty swallowing (dysphagia)	Voice changes
	Neck pain	Ptosis
		Facial droop
		Headache
		Tongue swelling or evidence of self-mastication in mouth
		Facial swelling
		Neck swelling
		Nose bleed
Respiratory	Difficulty breathing	Stridor
	Chest pain	Hoarseness
		Subcutaneous emphysema
		Respiratory distress
		Hemoptysis
		Inability to tolerate the supine position
		Dysphonia or aphonia
Gastrointestinal	Heartburn/acid reflux	Vomited
	Dysphagia	
Gynecological	Pain in pregnant abdomen	Vaginal bleeding
		Miscarriage
Genitourinary		Urinary incontinence
Skin		Scratches on the neck
		Petechiae
		Red linear marks
		Ligature marks
Neurological	Dizziness	Mental status changes
	Weakness	Loss of sensation
	Reports loss of consciousness	Loss of consciousness
	Headache	Eyelid droop (ptosis)
		Facial droop
		Extremity weakness or paralysis
		Aphasia or difficulty speaking
Psychiatric	Memory problems	
	Depression	
	Suicidal ideation	
	Insomnia	
	Nightmares	
	Anxiety	
Musculoskeletal	Neck or back pain	Cervical spine tenderness
		Thoracic cage tenderness
		Shoulder or clavicular tenderness

HEENT, head, eyes, ears, nose, throat exam.

Adapted from Strack GB, McClane GE, Hawley DA. A review of 300 attempted strangulation cases part 1: Criminal legal issues. *J Emerg Med.* 2001;21(3):303–309.

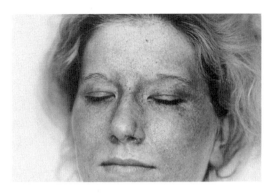

Figure 16.2 Scattered facial petechiae. *Forensic photograph courtesy of Nancy Housel, RN and with consent of the victim.*

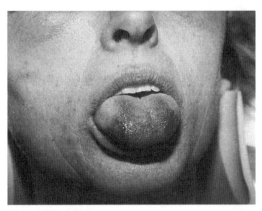

Figure 16.4 Tongue swelling. *Forensic photograph courtesy of San Diego Police Department.*

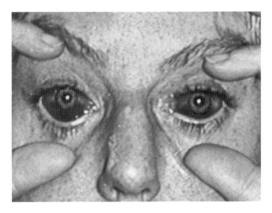

Figure 16.3 Subconjunctival hemorrhages. *Forensic photograph courtesy of San Diego Police Department.*

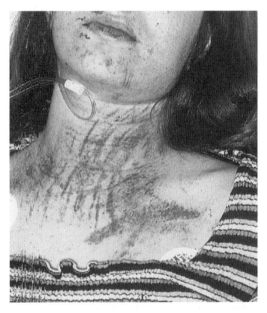

Figure 16.5 Self-excoriations to neck during strangulation. *Forensic photograph courtesy of Mono County District Attorney's Office and the consent of the victim.*

suggested by the presence of cervical subcutaneous emphysema (can be seen radiographically 95% of the time) and crepitus.

Early diagnosis and treatment of these injuries is critical because the mortality rate of unrecognized injury has been reported to be as high as 92%. Evaluation consists of chest and lateral neck radiographs, flexible nasopharyngoscopy or laryngoscopy, direct laryngoscopy, and esophagoscopy (27).

"Fractures of the upper thyroid horns are a frequent finding after a variety of neck injuries—resulting from a direct mechanical trauma, e.g. compression of the neck in manual strangulation or ligature strangulation, from blunt injuries (falls or blows against the neck), and sometimes from indirect trauma (whiplash-injuries)" (28). Browning and Whittet reported on five

cases of an anatomical variation in which the tip of the cornu turned medially and caused an indentation into the pharynx, causing pain and globus sensation (a feeling of something in the throat in the absence of obvious pathological findings). Resection of these abnormalities led to resolution of the symptoms experienced by the patients. In addition to the reported cases involving anatomical variations, it is known that such variations result from neck trauma, in particular

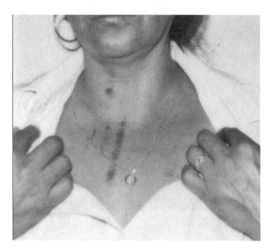

Figure 16.6 Self-excoriations to neck during strangulation. *Forensic photograph courtesy of San Diego Police Department.*

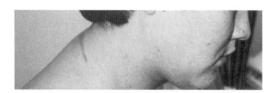

Figure 16.7 Ligature mark to posterior neck. *Forensic photograph courtesy of Diana Cummings, RN and with consent of the victim.*

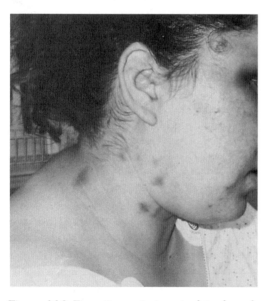

Figure 16.8 Fingertip contusions to lateral neck. *Forensic photograph courtesy of Diana Cummings, RN and with consent of the victim.*

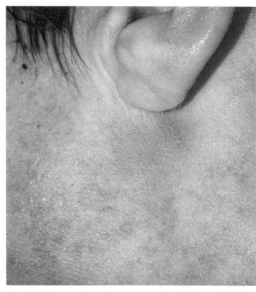

Figure 16.9 Thumb-tip contusion to mastoid process. *Forensic photograph courtesy of Dean Hawley, MD.*

strangulation, which is perpetrated manually from the front of the victim. The likelihood of a fracture resulting from such an assault is related to increasing age, as the cartilage calcifies with time. Similar fractures can also result from manipulation of the larynx to facilitate endotracheal intubation (29).

Reports of carotid artery dissection resulting from IPV exist in the medical literature (30). As early as 1980, the true incidence of spontaneous carotid dissection was unknown. Once considered rare, increased awareness, combined with noninvasive evaluation by ultrasonography and MRI, has shown a more frequent occurrence (31). Milligan and Anderson reported two cases of women of reproductive age who had suffered strokes. Neither was taking oral contraceptives and no causal factors were discovered during the assessment of these patients except that the radiological findings were characteristic of traumatic internal carotid artery occlusion. At first, both patients denied a history of trauma but further inquiry uncovered a history of strangulation during an IPV assault by each patient's husband (32). In 1993, Vanezis and colleagues reported a case of carotid artery thrombosis following manual strangulation (33). As a result, some authors, such as Malek and colleagues, propose that there is a real danger of delayed stroke in women who have sustained strangulation assaults (30).

CLINICAL MANAGEMENT

McClane and associates recommend this overall initial management approach (2):

- *Pulse oximetry.* A simple, noninvasive, fingertip transducer that measures a patient's oxygen saturation utilizing infrared technology; this is the first step in evaluating a patient with mental status changes that may be secondary to hypoxemia.
- *Chest radiographs.* Provides rapid diagnosis of pulmonary edema, pneumonia, or aspiration
- *Nasal radiographs.* Provides ancillary evaluation for the strangled patient presenting with hemoptysis (because of nasal fracture)
- *Soft-tissue neck radiographs.* For evaluation of subcutaneous (SC) emphysema within the soft tissues because of fractured larynx; may also demonstrate tracheal deviation because of edema or hematoma
- *Cervical spine radiographs.* The lateral view may reveal a fractured hyoid bone
- *Axial CT scan.* Provides detailed cross-sectional evaluation of neck structures
- *Magnetic resonance imaging (MRI) scan.* Provides comprehensive evaluation of soft tissues of the neck
- *Carotid Doppler ultrasound.* Critical in patients with neurologic lateralizing signs (i.e., stroke)
- *Pharyngoscopy.* Simple bedside maneuver that may reveal pharyngeal petechiae, edema, or other findings caused by strangulation
- *Indirect laryngoscopy.* Simple bedside maneuver using a mirror and headlamp. After anesthetizing the retropharynx, the dental mirror is placed against the soft palate and angled downward, so that the vocal cords can be visualized opening with inspiration and closing with vocalization.
- *Direct fiberoptic laryngobronchoscopy.* Vocal cord and tracheal evaluation in patients with dyspnea, dysphonia, aphonia, or odynophagia (2); this technique offers an advantage over indirect exam in that photos of the internal injuries can be obtained.

Serial examinations are critical, with special emphasis on the patient's mental status as well as evidence of airway or vascular compromise. Decompensation of the previously stable patient is suggested by dyspnea, dysphonia, expanding hematoma, carotid bruit, cerebral ischemia, or unresponsive shock (1).

MEDICAL FORENSIC EXAMINATION AND DOCUMENTATION

In strangulation survivors, it serves to capture data necessary for prosecution, and this can make the difference between the perpetrator being charged with a misdemeanor or a felony. In California, a misdemeanor conviction for a DV case has a maximum sentence of 1 year in local jail and no more than a $10,000 fine. A felony conviction for a DV case, on the other hand, carries a higher sentence including prison terms of 2 years or more (6,34).

The forensic examination takes time and training to be done right. If at all possible, a physician, physician's assistant, a nurse practitioner, or a nurse who is trained in forensic documentation should do the data collection and documentation. Forensic documentation should consist of charting, the use of body maps, and the use of photo documentation of visible findings. Tape record the patient's voice to establish a baseline of vocal competency. Measure neck size with a tape measure, being sure to note landmarks used when obtaining the measurement.

The state of California Office of Emergency Services has produced a Forensic Medical Report: Domestic Violence Examination, form OES 502 (35). This form also has detailed documentation of the history and physical examination of victims of DV and was created through a consensus process including health professionals, forensic experts, prosecuting attorneys, and DV advocates. It is designed as a tool to aid in the examination and documentation of findings in IPV victims and can be used whole or in part. Table 16.3 is a modification of OES 502 that includes information noted on different pages of the form that is useful for strangulation cases.

It is important to discern and document in the medical record the mental status of these patients, as well as to clearly describe their perceptions of the strangulation event itself. Documentation of the patient's emotional demeanor is especially useful and relevant to the courts if these cases go forward for prosecution.

Among those patients who are strangled to the point of unconsciousness or near-syncope, the vast majority report thinking that, at some point during the strangulation, they were going to die. Strangulation victims in IPV are nearly always female, and the perpetrators are nearly always male. Normal gender differences result in the victim being usually outweighed as well

Table 16.3 Forensic Documentation Form				
Description of Strangulation Event:				
One Hand		Two Hands		Forearm
Frontal Assault		Frontal Assault		Frontal Assault
Rear Assault		Rear Assault		Rear Assault
☐ If ligature used, describe:				
☐ Photodocumentation done: (include images of front, back, sides of neck and face, eyes, ears, nose per routine plus macro images of any findings)				
☐ Audio or audiovideo recording of victim's voice				

Adapted with permission from California OES 502: Forensic Medical Examination of Domestic Violence (www.calmtc.org).

as overpowered by the batterer. When asked to break down the stream-of-consciousness that they experienced during the strangulation, victims characteristically and consistently describe four distinct stages, as described by McClane in 2001 (2). In the *Denial* stage, victims of strangulation describe an out-of-body experience, frequently making such statements such as "I couldn't believe that it was happening," or "it was like I was watching what was happening to me on television." In the *Realization* stage, victims perceive the frightening reality as intense neck pain, and terror become hyperacute. In the *Primal* stage, realization yields to visceral, mammalian instincts: Vigorous struggle often ensues in the victim's primal attempt to preserve airway and life. In the last stage of *Resignation*, victims rapidly tire, and begin to resign themselves to dying. Statements such as, "I began to say my prayers," or "I knew then that this was it," are frequent. Commonly, victims relate that their final thoughts are related to their children's welfare in their absence, even when their children were grown (2).

STRANGULATION FATALITIES

Although it is possible to learn much about strangulation assaults in survivors by using pattern recognition and forensic examination, it is no coincidence that the best medical evidence of strangulation is derived from postmortem examination (autopsy) of the body. Autopsy provides the opportunity to examine injuries that occur under the skin, as well as the ability to track the force vector that produced the injuries (10).

Victim Evaluation at Autopsy for Death Occurring at the Scene, Before Medical Intervention

In addition to external neck markings, strangulation usually produces evidence of asphyxiation, recognized as pinpoint hemorrhages (petechiae) in the skin, conjunctiva of the eyes, and in the deep internal organs. Figure 16.10 (Plate 9) shows petechiae seen in the cerebral arachnoid. Petechiae are nonspecific findings that can develop from any cause of asphyxia including strangulation, hanging, drowning, sudden infant death syndrome, aspiration of gastric contents, profound depressant drug intoxication, and some natural diseases. The presence of petechiae does not prove strangulation, and the absence of petechiae does not disprove strangulation. Prompt fatal strangulation by carotid obstruction will usually not produce petechiae. At autopsy, a common place to find petechiae is the undersurface of the scalp. The internal mucosal lining of the larynx may show petechiae (10). Petechiae may be very difficult to recognize in the skin of darkly pigmented people (10).

Fingernail marks, superficially incised curvilinear abrasions, might be observed singly or in sets. In rare cases, all four fingers will mark the skin in a single pattern. Fingernail marks are rarely associated with the assailant's hands, but commonly associated with the victim's own fingers, as she struggles to pry the assailant's grasp off her neck. Finger touch pad contusions are caused by the assailant's grasp. The thumb generates more pressure per surface area than the other fingers, so singular thumb impression contusions are found more often than contusions showing the

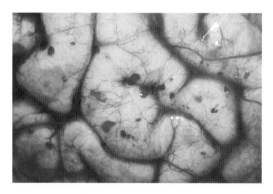

Figure 16.10 Petechiae in the cerebral arachnoid. *Postmortem forensic photograph courtesy of Dean Hawley, MD.*

complete hand grasp. Ligature abrasions follow a predictable pattern of horizontal circumscription about the neck; distinguishable from the marks left by suicidal hanging, in which a suspension point causes the ligature furrow to rise toward one ear.

In addition to petechiae, one may also (rarely) find interstitial free air in the lung or mediastinum (36,37).

Even in fatal cases, there may be no external evidence of injury. In some of these cases, injuries may become apparent by the next day, as the skin begins to dry and become more transparent. In these cases, police homicide investigators are posed a difficult problem: a victim found dead, without external evidence of trauma. If no suspicion of DV is developed during the scene investigation, there may be little or no suspicion of criminal harm when the victim presents for autopsy examination (10).

A high index of suspicion must be maintained in these cases. Otherwise, the autopsy will be conducted to rule out drug overdose, and the injury of strangulation will not be found until the neck dissection is carried out, ordinarily at the end of the case. Therefore, photographs and trace evidence collections will not have been made from the undisturbed body, and the prosecutor will be left without essential evidence (10).

Ultimately, a medical opinion of strangulation as the mechanism of neck injury will be based on a complete examination of the patient's neck, either at autopsy or by radiography, to detect superficial and deep injuries fitting a pattern that supports the diagnosis. Autopsy examination of the neck includes complete dissection, with removal of the larynx including the hyoid bone, and preferably with the tongue attached. The superficial and deep musculature must be individually examined for contusion hemorrhage. The laryngeal skeleton is then exposed to examine for fracture. Finally, the cervical spine is opened and examined for injury (10).

The larynx (the "voice box") separates the trachea and the superior portion of the aerodigestive tract. Its skeleton is composed of four distinct entities: hyoid bone, thyroid cartilage, cricoid cartilage, and arytenoid cartilage. A fracture of the hyoid bone in strangulation is often reported to be common, but it is actually only found in a minority (at most one-third) of all fatalities (10).

As mentioned in the section regarding orthopedic injuries, fractures of the upper thyroid horns are a frequent finding after a variety of neck injuries, including strangulation. In an in-lab experimental measurement study mean weight resulting in injury of the horn was 3 kg (men: 3.3 kg, women: 2.6 kg). The location of the fractures occurred, in nearly all cases, at the base of the horn. The amount of weight required to cause an injury was dependent on the degree of ossification, with the highest rate of fractures found in cases with incomplete ossification; in cases without ossification, specimens often remained macroscopically uninjured (38). Maxeiner reported nondislocated but anatomically unstable fractures of the cricoid cartilages in 10 of 191 consecutive fatal homicidal strangulation cases (39). Poquet and colleagues reported a case of hanging with cricothyroid membrane rupture diagnosed by CT scan (40). In rare cases, an arytenoid subluxation may occur after blunt external trauma to the neck, but this is reported only once in the literature. Overall, the incidence of arytenoid subluxation is relatively uncommon (41).

Victim Evaluation at Autopsy Post Resuscitation Efforts

Medical resuscitation and organ procurement procedures complicate the pathologist's ability to detect fatal homicidal neck injury. Specific findings associated with resuscitation that distort findings at autopsy include:

- Abrasions on the mouth and nasal bridge from an oxygen mask
- Intubation trauma, which can mimic strangulation injuries
- Laryngeal ulceration from pressure exerted by inflatable cuffs on intubation tubes
- Barotrauma of the lungs from mechanical ventilation
- Injuries sustained from a surgical cricothyrotomy or tracheostomy
- Needle marks and tracks of hemorrhage from jugular vein needle sticks to obtain blood or place an intravenous line (10)

Survival of the patient beyond the first day can also impede the ability to determine the extent of strangulation trauma. If resuscitation is successful, the patient may linger on mechanical ventilation for hours or days, resulting in healing of soft tissue injuries in the neck that would have been recognizable if examined earlier. In addition, toxicology is essentially meaningless in patients who survive a few days in the hospital;

therefore disproving, beyond a reasonable doubt, a defense theory that the asphyxial death was caused by overdose becomes impossible (10).

DISPOSITION OF SURVIVING STRANGULATION PATIENTS

Admit all strangulation patients with immediate presentation to the hospital for 24–36 hours (1,42). This affords several benefits (1,2):

- An observation period to monitor the victim's airway, breathing, circulation, and neurological status—important as continued neck swelling can progress up to 24–48 hours after initial assault
- An adequate period of observation to rule out occult but significant airway pathology
- An adequate time period for social services consultation for evaluation of the patient's need for social services, support, and safety planning
- An in-depth mental health evaluation, as many of these patients with a history of battering have coexistent conditions such as depression and suicidal ideation
- A period to arrange for neurosurgical and head-ears-eyes-nose-throat (HEENT) consultation as needed
- A haven of safety from their batterer, which provides time for reflection and decision-making for the patient

Another major benefit of routine hospital admission involves the community at large. Admission facilitates an in-depth evaluation of the patient at the time of admission and during the subsequent hours of observation. Much data collection and future research needs to be done in this information-scarce arena of surviving victims of strangulation (2).

Early neurosurgical and/or otolaryngologic consultation should be considered if severe neurologic and/or laryngeal injuries are suspected. In conscious patients, psychiatric consultation should be obtained if the patient is deemed severely depressed or suicidal. If the patient must be transferred and is unstable, then the airway should be secured via endotracheal intubation (1).

Should the patient decline admission, a social services consult should be obtained and care taken to explain to the patient the potential fatal consequences of possible occult underlying injuries, as well as the risk associated with strangulation as a predictor of

IPV homicide. Care must be taken to explain to the victim the numbers of cases in the literature that have documented survivors dying from delayed onset of complications (2). Should the patient still decline admission, consider a discharge noted as "against medical advice," and ask her to keep a log to monitor and document her symptoms. Give her detailed after-care instructions to return immediately if she develops any symptoms suggestive of airway or safety compromise. Thoroughly document the patient's decisional capacity, the extent of the conversation, and the care plan.

Whether or not the patient is admitted, a multi-disciplinary team approach for her care after the strangulation assault lays the ground work for an ideal "best-practice" approach to the multitude of problems she may experience in the future. In addition to primary care providers for basic needs and coordination of care, the team should include providers from mental health for posttraumatic stress disorder (PTSD) problems, neurology for sequelae of acute brain trauma, and otolaryngology to address resultant throat and neck problems.

SPECIAL CONSIDERATIONS: CHILDREN

Children often witness IPV strangulation of their parent. Strack and colleagues reported children were present in 41% of the 300 cases reported in their study. Even then, the authors felt that this figure might be low because of victim reluctance to report the presence of children or because the reporting officer failed to report their presence (6). One troubling issue regarding children witnessing parental strangulation poses the question of future behavior in the children. If a child witnesses a parent using strangulation as a form of assault, will this same child "learn" the behavior and become a strangling perpetrator when grown (5)?

Another troubling issue is that of how to best care for a child who has witnessed one parent strangling another. Is this a form of child abuse? Should it be reported to child protective services (CPS.) This issue is one that bitterly divides many in the advocacy and professional communities who support and care for IPV victims. Consider referring all children who witness IPV strangulation for further evaluation by pediatric or social services. Hospitals should establish policy regarding the care of children who witness IPV, with this policy created by a multidisciplinary committee with representation from the legal profession, hospital ethics committee, hospital administration, IPV advocacy committee, and mental health and social services professionals (5).

STRANGULATION INJURIES ARE INDICATIVE OF THE PRESENCE AND SERIOUSNESS OF INTIMATE PARTNER VIOLENCE

Clinical indicators that someone is a battered woman include delay in seeking care for an injury, injuries inconsistent with history, injuries to the face or trunk (especially genitals, breasts, or abdomen), and strangulation injuries. Furthermore, a history of strangulation is a frequent finding in cases of IPV homicides that occur some time after a strangulation assault (43). At this time, the risk of future IPV injury and homicide cannot be quantified based on current research. However there is general agreement among many in the advocacy, law enforcement, and healthcare communities who specialize in care of IPV victims that strangulation victims should be viewed as having a higher risk of IPV injury and homicide than IPV victims who have never been strangled.

AUTOEROTIC ASPHYXIATION

When evidence of strangulation exists, the question arises as to whether the strangulation was inflicted as an act of violence or self-inflicted to gain sexual pleasure or satisfaction. Clashing histories result when the victim reports that the strangulation was perpetrator-inflicted, while the perpetrator maintains that the victim engaged in asphyxiation on purpose.

Maltz notes that "autoerotic asphyxiation" is found in the *Diagnostic and Statistical Manual of Mental Health Disorders* (DSM-IV) under the diagnosis of sexual masochism, and he quotes the definition of hypoxyphilia as "involving sexual arousal by oxygen deprivation obtained by means of chest compression, noose, ligature, plastic bag, mask, or chemical (e.g., volatile nitrate)." Such practice causes disruption of blood supply to the brain, resulting in diminished oxygenation and increased carbon dioxide retention, allegedly producing sensations of light-headedness, disinhibition, exhilaration, and giddiness claimed to

reinforce masturbatory pleasure. Equipment failures and LOC during this practice sometimes results in accidental deaths (44).

It is difficult to know how common the practice is. An early 2005 computer web search for "strangulation and sex practice" using the general Google search engine returned over 16,600 sites (45). The same search done using the Google *Scholar* search engine returned only 361 websites (46). For many years, autoerotic practice was exclusively a male practice. Martz reports that autoeroticism was once thought to be a phenomenon only practiced by men; now cases of autoerotic asphyxiation, including fatalities, have been documented in women (44). Shields and colleagues have also addressed this issue (47,48).

Byard and co-workers reviewed eight fatal cases and one near-fatal case of autoerotic asphyxiation in women to increase awareness of the subtle features found in women allegedly engaging in this activity, as opposed to typical findings involved in male autoerotic behavior. The majority of women in the Byard and co-workers' review did not use unusual clothing, props, or devices to augment their activity. In addition, some of cases reported by Byard were not alone when the death occurred, further confusing the very definition of the term "autoerotic." Five were completely naked, and only one was found with elaborate clothing and extra ligatures. Six of the fatal cases had objective evidence of sexual activity, three had used neck padding to prevent chafing, and eight had failed self-rescue mechanisms. The authors contend that these findings may lead to underdiagnosis or confusion with nonaccidental death. For instance, in their nine cases, autoerotic activity was concluded in five cases, but in four cases the initial impression was homicide in two cases, attempted suicide in two cases, and accidental death during sexual activity with a partner in one case (49). In nine cases initially suspicious for autoerotic strangulation by women, two were determined to be homicide, two suicide, and one accidental during consensual activity with a partner. Shields points out the autoerotic behavior is a behavior of men, not women (48).

SUICIDAL SELF-STRANGULATION

For a number of years it has been believed that self-strangulation by methods other than hanging was not possible. Logically, this is true for manual strangulation: if a person puts her hands around her own neck and exerts pressure, then death by asphyxiation would not occur, because once consciousness is lost, so is the ability of the person to continually exert pressure on the neck. The one exception to this might occur when the victim self-stimulates the carotid body, thereby evoking a profound vagal reflex that results in asystole and death. However, while this might be theoretically true, no reports of such a death have been documented in the literature to the best of our knowledge.

If self-strangulation does occur, it would involve ligature strangulation. This is supported by the literature, which includes rare cases of suicide by ligature strangulation (50).

STRANGULATION IN PREGNANCY

Are miscarriages more common among IPV victims who have been strangled during the course of their pregnancy? And if so, are miscarriages more likely to increase in some trimesters (5)? In Strack and colleagues' study of 300 cases of strangulation, 10 victims identified themselves as being pregnant at the time of the incident, and one of these miscarried within 24 hours of the strangulation event (6).

MENTAL STATUS CHANGES FOLLOWING STRANGULATION

The medical literature, especially studies in Russia and Germany, supports the fact that early and delayed mental status changes may occur in survivors of strangulation. These changes may be secondary to the temporary brain anoxia sustained during the attack because of the development of PTSD evolving from the strangulation assault (2). Considering the profound nature of the victim's emotions, it is not surprising to learn that following a strangulation attempt, PTSD occurs almost by default (51). The manifestations of PTSD are protean, and are described in detail elsewhere in this text. Posttraumatic stress disorder is an exceedingly complex behavioral phenomenon, but the strangled victim may demonstrate concurrent effects of cerebral anoxia, as well (52). Further complicating the patient's evaluation may be the varying degrees of traumatic brain injury that occur the during the strangulation attempt, if her head were struck against a wall or floor. Add an acute or chronic

history of self-medication with alcohol or prescription or street drugs, and the assessment and subsequent treatment of the strangled victim from a pathophysiological standpoint becomes complex, indeed (53). A multidisciplinary approach, utilizing specialty services such as neurology and psychiatry, is critical in unraveling and successfully treating the strangled victim.

INTERACTING WITH THE CRIMINAL JUSTICE SYSTEM

Many clinicians who have little or no experience in interacting with law enforcement or the legal system often seek to avoid working with the legal system because their only experience with it is based on interactions (or dread of anticipated interactions) with civil malpractice cases. However, other clinicians find that involvement with law enforcement and the legal profession to secure safety and justice for DV victims can be a rewarding experience.

Victims of DV are always at risk for further assault and injury, and this is particularly true for strangulation survivors. Perpetrators who strangle once are likely to strangle again, if not their current partner then their next partner. Criminal prosecution of strangulation perpetrators may provide the time and space victims need to gain safety.

When working with law enforcement, it helps to understand that the practitioners of medicine and law have different approaches to their work. In medicine, the clinician works to provide a solution or outcome to a problem based on scientific methods to diagnose that problem and then apply the best intervention in an effort to achieve the best outcome possible. By contrast, the legal system uses an adversarial approach that advocates for or against a desired outcome. The desired outcome is determined in advance, and then all work consists of proving that outcome to be the correct or prevailing one (54).

COMMON PITFALLS IN CARING FOR STRANGULATION PATIENTS

In the authors' experience and in review of strangulation cases, there are some common pitfalls in providing care for IPV strangulation cases:

- Attempting to predict outcome based on the initial condition of the patient

- Failure to maintain cervical spine immobilization in the unstable or unconscious patient
- Failure to consider early neurosurgical and otolaryngologic consultation
- Failure to consider early psychiatric consultation or to minimally evaluate regarding possible suicidal ideology
- Failure to institute a safety plan and precautions against further assaults
- Premature discharge of patient who has been strangled within the past 24–36 hours
- Failure to inquire about a history of trauma to the neck in female patients under the age of 50 who present with signs and symptoms of a stroke or transient ischemic attack (TIA)
- Failure to provide good discharge instructions for patients who decline admission and are discharged

In addition, strangulation survivors who are IPV victims should be admitted to the hospital unless the patient appears to be stable and refuses hospital admission. The importance of hospital policy in this regard is detailed in the earlier section Disposition of Surviving Strangulation Patients.

CONCLUSION

Awareness of strangulation as a common form of IPV assault has grown this past decade. In the past few years, awareness is now growing that the long-term health consequences may be far more serious than indicated by the apparently stable appearance of survivors of an immediate attack. For instance, survivors may suffer from chronic throat or neck pain, have signs and symptoms compatible with brain damage and PTSD, plus present with a host of other physical problems mentioned in this chapter.

IMPLICATIONS FOR POLICY, PRACTICE, AND RESEARCH

Policy

- Strangulation assault should be treated as a felony offense and not a misdemeanor, given the terror experienced by the victim, the considerable risk of brain injury or fatality, and the negative long-term healthcare consequences of strangulation.

- Thorough forensic examination and documentation by trained forensic examiners should be routinely provided to strangulation victims.

Practice

- Intimate partner violence patients should be specifically asked about a history of strangulation in the past or, if presenting after acute injury, during the most recent event.
- A careful and detailed medical history and physical examination post strangulation is needed to determine baseline status and should include a detailed neurologic assessment for mild brain injury post anoxic event.
- Strangulation survivors who are IPV victims should be admitted to the hospital unless the patient appears to be stable and refuses hospital admission.

Research

- Much data collection and future research needs to be done in this information-scarce arena of surviving victims of strangulation (2).
- A multisite study of survivors of strangulation is needed to further the understanding of signs and symptoms, complications, and sequelae post strangulation.
- A clinical comparison of findings on direct and indirect laryngoscopy and CT imaging on all survivors of strangulation would be helpful to shape recommendations regarding medical management.
- Mild brain injury post strangulation may be very common and may cause neurologic impairments that may impose further risk for IPV patients.
- Study must be done of the incidence of female patients under the age of 50 who present with signs and symptoms of a stroke or TIA following strangulation assaults.

References

1. Newton K. Neck. In: Marx JA, Hockberger RS, Walls RM, eds. *Rosen's emergency medicine: Concepts and clinical practice*, 5th ed. St Louis: Mosby; 2002: 370–381.
2. McClane GE, Strack GB, Hawley DA. A review of 300 attempted strangulation cases part II: clinical evaluation of the surviving victim. *J Emerg Med.* 2001;21(3):311–315.

3. Stanley RB Jr., Hanson DG. Manual strangulation injuries of the larynx. *Arch Otolaryngol.* 1983;109:344–347.

4. Iserson KV. Strangulation: A review of ligature, manual, and postural neck compression injuries. *Ann Emerg Med.* 1984:13(3):179–185.

5. Line WS, Stanley RB, Choi JH. Strangulation: A full spectrum of blunt neck trauma. *Ann Otol Rhinol Laryngol.* 1985;94(6Part1):542–546.

6. Strack GB, McClane GE, Hawley DA. A review of 300 attempted strangulation cases part 1: criminal legal issues. *J Emerg Med.* 2001;21(3):303–309.

7. Merriam-Webster online dictionary. 2007–2008. Merriam-Webster online dictionary website. At http://www.m-w.org/cgi-bin/dictionary?book=Dictionary&va=strangulation&x=15&y=15. Accessed 1/19/2005.

8. Merriam-Webster online dictionary. 2007–2008. Merriam-Webster online dictionary website. At http://www.m-w.org/cgi-bin/dictionary?book=Dictionary&va=asphyxia&x=15&y=15. Accessed 1/19/2005.

9. DiMaio VJ, DiMaio D. *Forensic Pathology*, 2nd ed. New York: CRC Press, 2001.

10. Hawley DA, McClane GE, Strack GB. A review of 300 attempted strangulation cases part III: Injuries in fatal cases. *J Emerg Med.* 2001;21(3):317–322.

11. Gowens PA, Davenport FJ, Kerr J, et al. Survival from accidental strangulation from a scarf resulting in laryngeal rupture and carotid artery stenosis: the "Isadora Duncan syndrome." A case report and review of the literature. *Emerg Med J.* 2003;20:391–393.

12. Carson DO, Pounder DJ. Transport strangulation. (Letter to the editor.) *Forensic Sci Int.* 1996;82: 191–192.

13. Kohli A, Verma SK, Agarwal BBL. Accidental strangulation in a rickshaw: A case report. *Forensic Sci Int.* 1996;78:7–11.

14. Chou F, Conway MD. History of ocular anesthesia. *Ophthalmol Clin N Am.* 1998;11(1):1–11.

15. Crime in the United States. 2002 FBI website. At http://www.fbi.gov/ucr/cius_02/html/web/offreported/02-nmurder03.html. Accessed 2/21/2005.

16. Peelo M, Francis B, Soothill K, et al. The public construction of justice: Homicide reporting in the press. *Br J Criminol.* 2004;44:256–275.

17. DiMaio VJ. Homicidal asphyxia. *Am J Forensic Med Pathol.* 2000;21(1):1–4.

18. Campbell JC. Health consequences of intimate partner violence. *Lancet.* 2002;359:1331–1336.

19. Wilbur L, Higley M, Hatfield J, et al. Survey results of women who have been strangled while in an abusive relationship. *J Emerg Med.* 2001;21(3): 297–302.

20. Berrios DC, Grady D. Domestic violence-risk factors and outcomes. *West J Med.* 1991;155:133–135

21. Stanley RB Jr., Hanson DG. Manual strangulation injuries of the larynx. *Arch Otolaryngol.* 1983; 109:344–347.

22. Anscombe AM, Knight BH. Case report. Delayed death after pressure on the neck: Possible causal

mechanisms and implications for mode of death in manual strangulation discussed. *Forensic Sci Int.* 1996;78:193–197.

23. Kohli A, Verma SK, Agarwal BBL. Accidental strangulation in a rickshaw. *Forensic Sci Int.* 1996; 78(1):7–11.

24. O'Connor PJ, Russell JD, Moriarity DC. Anesthetic implications of laryngeal trauma. *Anesth Analgesia.* 1998;87(6):1283–1284.

25. Wu MH, Tsai YF, Lin MY, et al. Complete laryngotracheal disruption caused by blunt injury. *Ann Thoracic Surg.* 2004;77(4):1211–1215.

26. Atkins BZ, Abbate S, Fosjer SR, Vaslef SN. Current management of laryngotracheal trauma: Case-report and literature review. *J Trauma.* 2004;56(1): 185–190.

27. Goudy SL, Miller FB, Bumpous JM. Neck crepitance: Evaluation and management of suspected upper aerodigestive tract injury. *Laryngoscope.* 2002;112(5):791–795.

28. Bockholdt B, Hempelmann M, Maxeiner H. Experimental investigations of fracture of the upper thyroid horns. *Leg Med.* 2003;(5 Suppl 1): S252–255.

29. Browning ST, Whittet HB. A new and clinically symptomatic variant of thyroid cartilage anatomy. *Clin Anat.* 2000;13:294–297.

30. Malek AM, Higashida RT, Halbach NN, et al. Patient presentation, angiographic features, and treatment of strangulation-induced bilateral dissection of the cervical internal carotid artery. *J Neurosurg.* 2000;92(3):481–487.

31. Khimenko PL, Esham RH, Ahmed W. Spontaneous internal carotid artery dissection. *So Med J.* 2000;93(10):1011–1016.

32. Milligan N, Anderson M. Conjugal disharmony: A hitherto unrecognized cause of strokes. *Br Med J.* 1980;281(6237):421–422.

33. Vanezis P, Claydon SM, Chapman RC, so-Alousi LM. Internal carotid artery thrombosis following manual strangulation. *Med Sci Law.* 1993;33(1):69–71.

34. California Penal Code Section 245 and 273.5; *People v. Covino,* 100 Cal. App. 3d 660 (1980); *People v. Kinsey,* 40 Cal. App. 4th 1621 (1995) (PC273.5).

35. OES-502-Forensic Medical Report. Governor's Office of Emergency Services. Sacramento, California.

36. Khokhlov VD. The mechanisms of the formation of injuries to the hyoid bone and laryngeal and tracheal cartilages in compression of the neck. [Russian.] *Sudebno-Meditsinskaia Ekspertiza.* 1996; 39(3):13–16.

37. Delmonte C, Capelozzi VL. Morphologic determinants of asphyxia in lungs. A semiquantitative study in forensic cases. *Am J Forensic Med Pathol.* 2001;22(2):139–149.

38. Bockholdt B, Hempelmann M, Maxeiner H. Experimental investigations of fracture of the upper thyroid horns. *Leg Med.* 2003;5(Suppl 1): S252–255.

39. Maxeiner H. "Hidden" laryngeal injuries in homicidal strangulation: how to detect and interpret theses findings. *J Forensic Sci.* 1998;43(No. 4): 784–791.

40. Poquet E, Dibiane A, Jourdain C, et al. Blunt injury of the larynx by hanging. X-ray computed tomographic aspect. [French.] *J de Radiologie.* 1995;76(No. 2–3):107–109.

41. Schroeder U, Motzko M, Wittekindt C, Ecket HE. Hoarseness after laryngeal blunt trauma: A differential diagnosis between an injury to the external branch of the superior laryngeal nerve and an arytenoid subluxation. A case report and literature review. *Eur Arch Otorhinolaryngol.* 2003;260(6):304–307.

42. McLaughlin RE, Stewart A. Two cases of near asphyxiation in children, using non-releasing plastic garden ties. (Letter.) *Emerg Med J.* 2002;19:184.

43. At http://www.ojp.usdoj.gov/nij/topics/crime/violence-against-women/workshops/vawa.htm accessed on 11/21/2008 Workshop on Evaluating the Impact of Programs Under the Violence Against Women Act. 2000. Office of Justice Programs, National Institute of Justice website.

44. Maltz D. Behavioral treatment for a female engaging in autoerotic asphyxiation. *Clin Case Studies.* 2003;2(3):236–242.

45. At http://www.google.com/search?q=strangulation+and+sex+practice&ie=UTF-8&oe=UTF-8. Accessed 2/22/2005.

46. At http://scholar.google.com/scholar?q=strangulation+and+sex+practice&ie=UTF-8&oe=UTF-8&hl=en&btnG=Search. Accessed 2/22/2005.

47. Shields LBE, Hunsaker DM, Hunsaker JC. Autoerotic asphyxia, Part I. *Am J Forensic Med Pathol.* 2005;26(1):45–52.

48. Shields LBE, Hunsaker DM, Hunsaker JC, et al. Atypical autoerotic death, Part II. *Am J Forensic Med Pathol.* 2005;26(1):53–62.

49. Byard RW, Hucker SJ, Hazelwood RR. Fatal and near-fatal autoerotic asphyxial episodes in women. Characteristic features based on a review of nine cases. *Am J Forensic Med Pathol.* 1993;14(1):70–73.

50. Di Nunno N, Costantiniedes F, Conticchio G, et al. Self-strangulation: An uncommon but not unprecedented suicide method. *Am J Forensic Med Pathol.* 2002;23(3):260–263.

51. Knight JA, Taft CT. Assessing neuropsychological concomitants of trauma and PTSD. In: Wilson JP, Keane TM, eds. *Assessing psychological trauma and posttraumatic stress disorder,* 2nd ed. New York: Guilford Press, 2004.

52. Bouwer C, Stein D. Panic disorder following torture by suffocation is associated with predominantly respiratory symptoms. *Psychol Med.* 1999;29:233–236.

53. Goodman RA, Mercy JA, Rosenberg ML. Drug use and interpersonal violence. Barbiturates detected in homicide victims. *Am J Epidemiol.* 1986;124(5): 851–855.

54. Jones JW, McCullough LB, Richman BW. Ethics of serving as a plaintiff's expert medical witness. *Surgery.* 2004;136(1):100–102.

Chapter 17

Soft Tissue and Cutaneous Injury Patterns

*Daniel J. Sheridan, Katherine R. Nash,
Christine A. Poulos, Lynne Fauerbach,
and Sandra Watt*

KEY CONCEPTS

- Most injuries caused by intimate partner violence (IPV) are minor in relation to medical seriousness but are very important in the forensic care of victims of violence.
- In general, accidental injuries tend to occur in the more distal portion of extremities, whereas intentional, abusive injuries are generally more proximal.
- Abrasions can occur from assaults from dragging along rough surfaces, from fingernail scratches, and/or from being struck with an object with a rough surface.
- Health providers should identify bullet wounds but exercise extreme caution before characterizing the wounds as an "entrance" or an "exit" wound.
- A bruise is synonymous with a contusion. However, a bruise is not synonymous with ecchymosis or a hematoma.

- An incision or cutting injury is not the same as a laceration. When the skin is transected by a sharp object, it is an incision. When the skin splits or tears open from blunt or shearing force trauma, it is a laceration.
- Many injuries have embedded in their appearance a pattern suggestive of a causative object. These are called "patterned injuries."
- A "pattern of injuries" can refer to injuries in various stages of healing or a collection of injuries that appear as a pattern on the body.
- No science supports that bruises can be precisely dated by their color.
- Skin of abused patients may contain trace physical evidence on it and/or in it that needs to be collected, packaged, and labeled by the health professional prior to washing it away.

Cutaneous injuries often result from abuse and assault; however, cutaneous injuries are also, very frequently, accidentally inflicted. This chapter briefly reviews normal skin anatomy, followed by a discussion of the most frequent locations and types of injuries to the skin related to intimate partner violence (IPV).

The majority of patients victimized during IPV are women. Women who have been injured during IPV will seldom seek immediate attention, opting instead to attempt self-care. A combination of reasons have been given to the authors by battered women for not seeking *prompt* medical care of injuries from IPV. Among them are:

- Her abuser may not allow her to seek medical treatment.
- She may not want or cannot afford the costs of an emergency department visit, especially if the abuser controls the finances in the relationship.
- She has no one to help her with child care of her young children secondary to geographic and social isolation common in abuse relationships.
- Because of usually long emergency department wait times, she cannot run the risk of being away from home when her abuser returns from work.
- She may be afraid to leave older children and/ or pets home alone with her abuser without her there to protect them.

The majority of IPV injuries are relatively minor and involve soft-tissue injury to the skin and underlying tissues (1,2) However, IPV victims will seek medical care especially when their injuries do not improve on their own. Battered women are just as likely to seek medical care in primary, specialty, and emergency department settings (3).

Women in abusive relationships are more likely to seek emergency department care when an injury is relatively severe, there are multiple injuries, or when they are pressured into seeking medical care by concerned family, friends, co-workers, or the police. In addition, the health provider may discover old and/ or new cutaneous injuries (4) during routine medical visits or during an exam for another health problem (3).

REVIEW OF SKIN ANATOMY

To trained health professionals, the following discussion may seem overly simplistic. However, when testifying in court on an intimate partner abuse case, the following brief, yet simple discussion of the anatomy of the skin sets the stage for further discussions of cutaneous injuries.

The *epidermis* is the top or outer most layer of the skin, which is uniformly thin except for body surfaces that experience a lot of friction such as the soles of the feet or the palms of the hand (Figure 17–1).

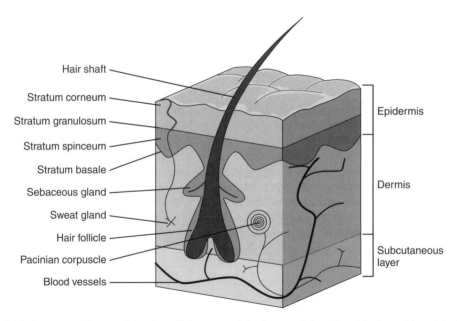

Figure 17.1 Anatomical layers of the skin. Schematic of the layers of the skin with the epidermis being the topmost outer layer, the dermis as the middle layer, and the subcutaneous (fatty) layer just above the muscle. *Drawing by Zachary C. Tai and used with his permission.*

The epidermis has no nerve endings or blood vessels. An intact epidermis prevents bacteria and viruses from entering the body through the skin (5). The epidermis becomes even thinner as a normal part of the aging process (6).

The *dermis* is often described as the middle layer of the skin. The dermis is very vascular and contains millions of nerve endings. It is very elastic (stretchable) in children and most adults, however, becomes less elastic in the elderly. When the skin becomes less stretchable, it leads to the formation of wrinkles, folds, sagging, and dryness. Another normal change related to aging is that the capillaries (microscopic thin blood vessels) become more fragile and thus more easily torn (6). Also in the dermis are sweat glands, lymph nodes, and hair follicles (roots) (5).

The deepest layer of skin is called the *subcutaneous* or fatty layer since it is composed of fat cells comprising adipose tissue. The subcutaneous layer of the skin provides insulation to cold and to heat. The subcutaneous skin layer provides a cushion of tissue that can be protective to underlying body parts (5). A normal age-related change to older adults is a decrease in the amount of subcutaneous fat (6,7). The skin in very young children, while fairly elastic, is less protective since the fibers that hold the skin together are not fully developed and will more readily tear apart if put under too much strain (8).

Below the subcutaneous layer of skin is *muscle tissue*. Trauma to the body surface can affect all layers of the skin plus the muscles and body organs underneath the skin. For example, a cut (injury made by a sharp instrument) can penetrate into the dermis (superficial cut), the subcutaneous tissue, and/or muscle (deeper cut).

LOCATIONS OF CUTANEOUS INJURIES ON THE BODY

In general, accidental injuries to the body and to the skin are more distal than proximal (4,9). Although injuries to pre-walking infants are rare, when children begin to cruise, they bruise. Commonly occurring accidental injuries to the periphery include trauma to fingers and toes, hands and feet, wrists and ankles, elbows and knees, forearms and shins, chins, foreheads, and the top of the head. In addition to injuries to bony prominences, accidental injury can include bruising to the lateral (outer) upper arms and outer thighs.

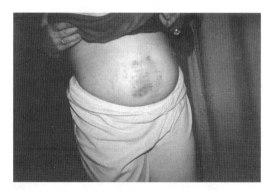

Figure 17.2 Patterned, bluish-purple punch-like contusion to the lower abdomen with circular knuckle impressions consistent with an upper-cut punch to the abdomen. (Notice the upward ecchymotic spread consistent with the patient being forced to lay supine immediately after being punched.) *Forensic photography courtesy of Dan Sheridan, RN, PhD.*

Inflicted injuries also tend to be more central in location. A review of the literature found that IPV results most frequently in injuries to the head, neck, and face (HNF) (4). Research has shown these locations are significantly associated with IPV, especially in the middle third of the face (10–12). Injuries to the upper extremities may be associated with defense injuries. Other injury locations include the chest and breast, abdomen, and the anogenital areas (Figure 17.2; Plate 10) (4,9,13). Genital injuries are very concerning, as they may be associated with greater homicide risk (14).

BLUNT FORCE INJURIES

Abrasion

An abrasion is injury to the surface of the skin caused by rubbing or scraping the skin or mucous layer (4,9,15). Abrasions can be very superficial or can involve the outermost layers of the skin. They usually begin bright red and can fade if superficial, or darken and crust when more severe (13). When the crust (scab) begins to fall off or is picked away, the newly forming skin underneath is usually lighter in color than the normal pigment of the surrounding skin.

Abrasions are common from accidental falls onto or along rough surfaces. However, abrasions can be inflicted by pushing and throwing someone onto a rough surface such as a sidewalk or asphalt road. Dragging someone along a carpeted surface can result

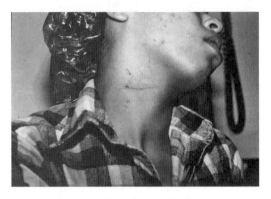

Figure 17.3 Two fingernail scratch-like abrasions to the lateral neck self inflicted in attempt to remove assailant's hands and/or inflicted by her assailant during a reported manual strangulation. *Forensic photography courtesy of Dan Sheridan, RN, PhD.*

in an abrasion, commonly called a "rug burn," even though it is not a thermal injury. Accidental and inflicted abrasions can contain trace physical evidence from the rough surface. Knowing where and the type of surface upon which the patient reportedly fell can help in the assessment of what type of trace physical evidence could and should be in the wound. The presence or absence of expected trace physical evidence can help determine if the injury is consistent or inconsistent with the presenting history.

Abrasions to the neck or chest can occur from fingernails during manual strangulation (4). The patient may have inflicted fingernail scratch abrasions to the assailant or scratched her own neck trying to pry away her assailant's hands (Figure 17.3; Plate 11). Thus, forensic examiners will scrape the undersurface of the patient's or assailant's fingernails into a clean envelope. Ligature strangulation with a rough cord-like object can result in circular or semicircular abrasions to the neck (4). Forensic examiners will swab the abrasion, before the neck is cleaned, with a saline-moistened cotton-tip applicator in case there are remnant ligature fibers.

Being punched by a person wearing a ring can result in scratch abrasions; the larger and rougher the ring, the bigger the scratch abrasion. Class rings that contain a large stone can leave a circular or semicircular abrasion in the middle of the contact bruise. If the provider has determined from the patient's history or exam that the patient has an abrasion related to a ring injury, with permission of the patient (or by statute) that information needs to be relayed to the police in

case they want to secure a suspect's ring for analysis by the crime lab. Inside the crevices of the ring may be trace evidence (skin and blood), or the ring pattern may be matched to the injury pattern.

Avulsion

An avulsion is the complete tearing away of a structure or a part (1,9,15). Although orthopedic-related avulsions to bones and ligaments occur, cutaneous-related avulsions involve the complete tearing away of a section of skin. Accidental causes of avulsions often involve getting a body part caught in a machine. Inflicted avulsions often include being struck by an object at an angle such that the force tears away a section of skin. When the skin is torn but is still partially attached, it is best described as a partial avulsion or a skin tear (1,9).

The elderly will often experience skin tears to their arms and hands. The health professional needs to obtain a thorough history to help determine if the partial avulsion to the elderly patient was caused accidentally in assisted transfer or if the skin tear was inflicted from a direct assault, the use of excessive force, or neglect by a caregiver (4,9).

Laceration

A laceration is *not* an incision or a cut. A laceration is the tearing or splitting of tissue usually from blunt or shearing force energies (1,9,13). Well-meaning health professionals erroneously use the term *laceration* to describe almost all cutaneous injuries that involve openings through the skin (1,9). Lacerations usually result in jagged, nonuniform openings through the skin with the inside edges being irregular often with visible tissue bridging. Lacerations that resemble a flap with a tag of skin still attached have already been described as partial avulsions (skin tears). Lacerations most often occur over bony surfaces and are a common accidental and inflicted injury (Figure 17.4; Plate 12) (1,9,13).

Bruise/Contusion

Blunt, compressive, and/or squeezing force injuries can result in bruising to the skin. These forces disrupt blood vessels, causing blood to extrude to surrounding tissue resulting in pain, swelling, and discoloration (Figures 17.5 and 17.6; Plates 13 and 14) (4,9,15).

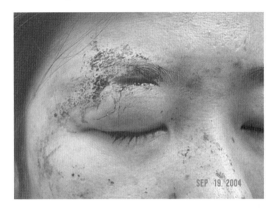

Figure 17.4 Right eyebrow laceration from blunt force trauma. *Forensic photography courtesy of Dan Sheridan, RN, PhD.*

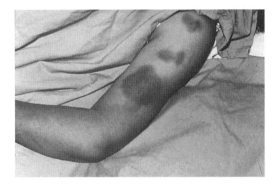

Figure 17.5 Multiple patterned contusions to the upper lateral arm consistent with history of being punched with a fist several times. *Forensic photography courtesy of Dan Sheridan, RN, PhD.*

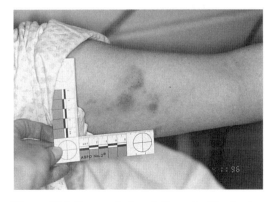

Figure 17.6 Patterned thumb/fingertip like bruises to upper arm with history of being grabbed during assault. *Forensic photography courtesy of Dan Sheridan, RN, PhD.*

The terms *bruise* and *contusion* are synonymous (1,9, 13). When the collection of blood is large and focal, the resulting injury is described as a *hematoma* (16).

Different factors can affect the amount of extravasated blood and thus the bruise's appearance. Injuries to areas with limited connective tissue support or high vascularity, such as the periorbital and genital regions, will result in greater likelihood of blood vessel leakage (17). The elderly are more easily bruised because of age-related changes that include blood vessel fragility from decreased connective tissue support (18). Bruising is more likely when there is an increase in underlying adipose tissue, which explains why women and infants tend to bruise more easily (17). If the force of impact is unable to dissipate, such as over a bony prominence, bruising is also more likely to occur subsequent to blunt force. Blunt force trauma from IPV that results in periosteal (bone) bruising can be extremely painful and take from weeks to months to heal.

The force and depth of the bruise can also affect its appearance (18). Deep bruises may take hours to days to present at the skin's surface, while superficial bruises may appear instantly (17,19). Thus, once a deep bruise becomes visible, it may appear older. Medication or disease processes that affect the body's ability to coagulate can also cause increased bruising and cutaneous bleeding (18).

Recent bruises that have discolored the skin usually have distinct outer margins and often reflect the pattern of the object that caused the trauma. Palpating a recent bruise elicits pain, and more recent bruises are often indurated (firm to touch) as compared to the adjacent nondiscolored skin (1,9,13). Cutaneous bruising from IPV is extremely common.

Ecchymosis

Ecchymosis is the leakage or oozing of blood under the skin not directly caused by blunt or squeezing force injury (1,9,15). Many health professions inaccurately call bruises/contusions ecchymoses and vice-versa. Ecchymosis is best described as the extravasation (leakage) of blood from small vessels (capillaries) from other than traumatic causes. For example, the elderly will often have a multitude of discolorations under the skin of the arms and hands that are not related to direct blunt or compression force trauma (Figure 17.7; Plate 15). A number of risk factors contribute to ecchymoses formation including

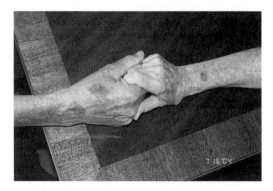

Figure 17.7 Ecchymoses, nonabuse-related lesions, to the arms and hands of an elderly couple. Tissue and blood vessel fragility common in old age can lead to bruising attributed to everyday activities. *Forensic photography courtesy of Dan Sheridan, RN, PhD.*

the use of certain medications, vitamin supplements, and the presence of abnormal serum blood values.

Ecchymotic areas under the skin are very similar in color to bruises and undergo the same color changes as bruises because the escaped blood cells are reabsorbed by the body. However, ecchymotic areas differ from bruises in that they are usually painless to palpation, nonindurated, and lack the distinct outer margins much more characteristic to bruises. The margins of ecchymotic areas are more diffuse in nature (Figure 17.8; Plate 16).

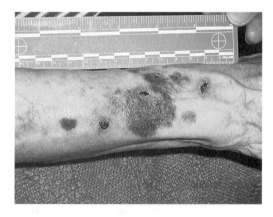

Figure 17.8 Ecchymoses with minor skin tearing (partial avulsions) to the arm. If the elderly patient is relatively active, such an injury could be nonintentional and sustained during routine activities of daily living. However, if the patient requires total care, these same injuries should prompt further assessment or an investigation for excessive force or physical abuse. *Forensic photography courtesy of Dan Sheridan, RN, PhD.*

Blunt force trauma that causes bruising may indirectly result in ecchymosis. For example, blunt force trauma to the mid face and forehead can result in bleeding under the skin that leaks downward and pools around the eyes. The discoloration to the eyes is often bilateral in nature and is unofficially called "raccoon eyes" and officially best described as *bilateral periorbital ecchymoses*. Being punched in the arm can result in a distinct oval or circular, well-marginated bruise. However, gravity may pull some of the escaped blood downward over time causing discoloration below the point of impact. This spread of escaped or leaked blood is accurately described as ecchymosis. Another example of ecchymosis related to trauma is leakage of blood under the skin from a venipuncture. The trauma was the puncture of a vessel with a needle. The blood that leaks from the punctured vein or artery to nontraumatized areas resulting in discoloration is ecchymosis.

Hematoma

A hematoma is not a synonym for a bruise. It is simply a collection of blood, which can be caused by blunt force trauma or caused by the spontaneous rupture of a weakened blood vessel (9,15). Palpable masses embedded in a large bruise are hematomas; however, a large clot in the brain from a ruptured aneurysm is also a hematoma.

SHARP FORCE INJURY

Incision

An incision, commonly called a "cut," is an injury due to a sharp object that has completely transected all layers of the skin. The skin is cut when a sharp object strikes or slides along the skin surface with enough force to divide the skin (1,9,13). When the skin is incised, the injury, in general, is longer than it is deep, as opposed to a stab wound, which is generally deeper than it is long (1,9,13). When the skin is divided by a sharp object, the inside edges of the wound are generally smooth and relatively equidistant in depth (Figure 17.9; Plate 17).

Any object that has a sharp edge can cause a cut. Innumerable sharp objects in everyday use cause cuts. Common objects used to intentionally inflict cuts include knives, razors, glass, and surgical

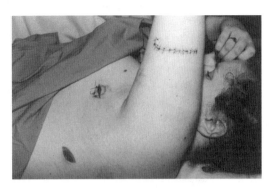

Figure 17.9 Patient stated the assailant attacked her with a knife and cut her left arm and then stabbed her in the chest. She has three sharp force injuries: one to the arm, now repaired, one to the lower chest from the assault, left open and a therapeutic incision to upper chest, now partially closed, after chest tube insertion. *Forensic photography courtesy of Dan Sheridan, RN, PhD.*

scalpel blades. If a serrated object, such as a steak knife, is used to separate the skin, the wound will have a more scalloped appearance or have multiple, nearly parallel incisions due to a sawing motion. Therapeutic incisions are performed with a scalpel in the course of providing health care.

Penetrating, Perforating, Puncture, and Stab Wounds

Puncture wounds result in a hole made by a sharp, pointed object (15,20). A stab wound is an incision (cut) made from a sharp instrument that leaves an opening deeper than it is wide (15). For example, an ice pick imbedded into an arm is best described as a puncture wound, whereas a steak knife imbedded in an arm is a stab wound.

Besant-Matthews further delineates penetrating from perforating wounds. A *penetrating wound* is an injury that enters but does not exit, "whereas a *perforating injury* passes through-and-through" (p. 191) (13). Penetrating and perforating injuries can be made by sharp and/or pointed objects, but would also include injuries from projectiles.

Chop Injuries

Being struck with heavy and sharp objects such as axes, meat cleavers, propeller blades, and machetes can result in a chop injury. A chop injury involves several mechanisms and types of resulting injury that

will produce a combination of blunt- and sharp-force injuries (13). There may evidence of both cutting and lacerating of the skin at the point of impact (16,21). Because the object has weight and mass, there may also be bruising that develops at the point of impact. If the object strikes in a sliding, glancing manner, there may also be evidence of skin abrasion.

BALLISTIC INJURIES

Most urban homicides result from firearm injury (22). From 1990–2002, two-thirds of intimate partner homicides of spouses and ex-spouses involved guns (23). In a study funded by the U.S. Centers for Disease Control and Prevention (CDC), IPV assaults were 12 times more likely to end in death if a firearm was used (24). Access to firearms is a significant predictor of domestic violence–related homicide (25). More research is needed on limiting perpetrator gun access and its correlation to decreasing intimate partner homicide (26).

A *ballistic* refers to a projectile, and *wound ballistics* is the study of how penetrating projectiles affect human tissue (27). Gunshot wounds are not always obvious, and their presence can be masked by hair, blood, and clothing. When possible, the number of holes from bullets should be counted and drawn on a body diagram. If the number is not even, a full body radiograph or computed tomography (CT/CAT) scan should be performed to evaluate any residual projectiles. Bullets can travel far from the site of penetration through soft tissue or within blood vessels.

Recognition of entrance and exit wounds has long been a controversy in trauma care across the country. Both Randall and Collins found that emergency physicians and surgeons are no more likely than chance to accurately differentiate between exit and entrance wounds, thus leading to a common recommendation to avoid attempts to differentiate between entrance and exit wounds, especially when there are multiple projectiles. Many factors influence the appearance of entrance and exit wounds (28,29). These include characteristics of the projectile, the firearm used, if the projectile passed through any objects prior to hitting the victim, the angle of impact, the type of tissue involved, the depth of penetration, whether the projectile fragmented, the projectile's shock wave, and characteristics of the resulting temporary and permanent cavities (22).

Firearms vary in power and range and include handguns, shotguns, and rifles. Handguns and rifles shoot bullets, whereas shotguns project either slugs or pellets. Projectiles can vary in size or caliber. The projectile is not the only thing shot out of a gun. With the bullet, slug, or pellets come gas, soot, gunpowder, and fire/heat. Gas can cause wound edges to rapidly expand then tear when the muzzle of the gun is held against the skin surface when fired.

Expelled dark gray to black soot will paint the surface around the bullet wound in intermediate and close range shots and can be found in the wound at contact range (13,22). Soot can easily be wiped away, so when possible, examination and photographic documentation should be done prior to cleaning the wound. However, stippling caused by hot gunpowder abrading the skin cannot be cleaned off. It will be predominantly red in color and have a punctuate abraded appearance (22). One can observe stippling at close and intermediate range fire (22). The closer the range, the more concentrated and denser the stippling will be.

Fire and heat are expelled from the end of the muzzle of a gun when it is fired. A contact gunshot can cause searing and burning around the edge of the point of contact. The imprint left can some-times be matched to the muzzle of the type of gun used. As the distance between the gun and surface is increased, heat plays less of a role in the appearance of the injury.

When medically feasible, healthcare providers need to document and collect evidence of gunshot wounds that might otherwise be lost during treatment. Gunshot wounds with soot need to be photographed, documented, and swabbed, if possible. Before going to the operating room, any injury should be docu-mented through narrative and photographs to preserve evidence of its appearance prior to it being cleansed, excised, or sutured closed. Bullets removed should be carefully packaged separately and not handled with forceps that have ridges. Any other trace evi-dence on the victim should also be collected and well documented.

BITE INJURIES

Bite marks can be an excellent source of forensic evi-dence that can easily be missed. Practitioners often minimize bite injuries. This patterned injury possesses characteristics that include an overall ovoid or round

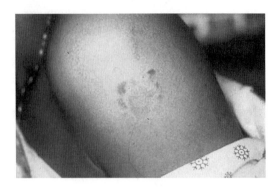

Figure 17.10 Bite injury to left upper arm. For forensic documentation, additional photos should be close up, at right angles with a right-angle ruler next to the wound. *Forensic photography courtesy of Dan Sheridan, RN, PhD.*

appearance with two U-shaped arches surrounding a bruised area. Individual tooth impressions can also be identified (Figure 17.10; Plate 18). These injuries can vary in appearance due to age of biter and victim, race of victim, number of teeth and strength of the bite, the presence of clothing, location of bite, and time elapsed since bite.

There is no way to differentiate a bite mark inflicted intentionally versus a bite mark inflicted consensually. Often combined with bite injuries are suction/compression bruises typically referred to as "hickeys." A hickey bruise can also have petechial-like hemorrhages embedded in the injury. Bites can result in transient indentations with patterned-bruising from the teeth without the breakage of skin. Bites can also result in superficial abrasions, partial or complete avulsions, or puncture wounds. Whenever there is any concern that the skin surface has been compromised or broken, prophylactic antibiotic treat-ment is prudent. The area of an identified bite mark should first be swabbed in hopes of collecting DNA from saliva deposits. Second, the injury should be photographed, if possible, with a right-angle ruler at a 90-degree angle to the skin surface (1). This process helps a forensic odontologist to identify the biter based on tooth impressions.

BURNS: THERMAL, CHEMICAL, AND FRICTION

Burns can be divided into two categories: thermal and chemical. Some sources also refer to a third category as *friction burns*, however they are more accurately called *friction abrasions* (1). Thermal burns occur due to exposure to open flames, heated implements, steam, or hot liquid or very cold surfaces. Caustic agents cause chemical burns. Thermal injuries are the most common burns seen in abusive trauma.

Burns can be further categorized by degree (30). First-degree burns injure the epidermis and exhibit erythema, whereas second-degree burns involve the epidermis and dermis layers of skin and produce blisters. Both are painful. All layers of skin (epidermis, dermis, and underlying fat tissue including nerves and blood vessels) are involved in third-degree burns. Third-degree burns are white (or charred), nonblanching due to injury of blood vessels, and nonpainful due to injury of nerve structures.

Intentional burns commonly occur in a recognized pattern (Figure 17.11; Plate 19). Cigarette burns have a recognizable round appearance and frequently occur in multiples. Occasionally, ash is still in the wound and can be collected with a moistened swab. Stocking- or glove-patterned burns, demonstrated by a clear circumferential "water-line," indicate a forced held submersion of an extremity or torso into hot liquid.

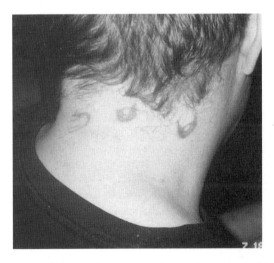

Figure 17.11 Patterned burns from a "super-heated" cigarette lighter. This patient has three, reddish-colored patterned burns to the posterior neck consistent with the shape of a disposable cigarette lighter that was "super-heated" and then pressed against the skin. (It is not known if the lighter was heated three separate times or if the lighter was heated once and pressed quickly, three times, against the skin.) *Forensic photography courtesy of Dan Sheridan, RN, PhD.*

An accidental submersion would have a splash appearance from the quick reflex of removing the extremity from exposure. A "tripod" patterned burn occurs when hands and feet are submerged, forcing the individual to keep the groin area raised to prevent further burning (31). When extremities are held against the bottom of a hot container of liquid, the skin in contact with the container will be spared, because the fluid is hotter than the surface. This creates *central sparing*.

Burns from IPV are common, especially if the assault is occurring in the kitchen. Splash burns may occur when the abuser throws hot, scalding water onto the patient from a pot cooking on the stovetop or from a cup of coffee. Glove burns will occur when the abuser forces the patient's hand into a pot on the stovetop containing hot fluid.

OTHER CUTANEOUS FINDINGS

Erythema

Erythema is an abnormal redness of the skin secondary to capillary congestion from irritation, injury, or inflammation (15,20). Erythema is a very common presentation from IPV. It can result from being slapped, punched, and/or kicked. Erythema is often a precursor to the later development of bruises. Depending on the severity of trauma, erythema could last for days or be transient. Transient erythema from minor trauma usually resolves within a relatively short period of time (minutes to hours).

Petechia(e)

Petechiae are pinpoint hemorrhages due to congestion or rupture of small capillaries. They can be attributed to vessel fragility, coagulopathies, or caused by a sudden increase in intravascular pressure. Petechiae can be diffuse or isolated and can disappear within hours or gradually clear like a bruise over days. Petechiae can result from traumatic and atraumatic causes. For example, petechiae can be caused by severe vomiting, childbirth, and other straining mechanisms that increase intraocular pressure (1). Strangulation and suffocation are common abuse-related causes of petechiae to the face and can be found all over the face and neck cephalad from the point of constriction, but are often only found in the conjunctivae and sclerae of the eyes, and over cartilage of the nose and ear (16).

Lesion

The term *lesion* is broadly used to describe a large number of abnormal changes to the skin, including wounds. However, from a forensic perspective, the primary author prefers to describe abnormal findings to the skin that are not trauma-related as lesions. Trauma to the skin that cannot be readily classified by a specific term is described as a wound.

Tenderness

Many cutaneous injuries are not visible on exam but are very tender to touch. *Tenderness*, which means sensitive or painful to touch (15,20), needs to be documented in a narrative format and by drawing the area of tenderness on a body map. In addition to drawing the area of tenderness, the provider should assess the level of pain on a 1 to 10 scale with 1 being no pain and 10 being the worst pain ever.

Traumatic Alopecia

Battered women report that their abusers often pull them or drag them by the hair. Not only is this form of abuse acutely painful, it can result in traumatic alopecia. Unless a segment of the scalp has literally been torn away in a scalping manner, traumatic alopecia can be very difficult to photograph. To document traumatic alopecia photographically, this author has carefully pulled a comb through the battered patient's hair and photographed the copious loose hairs removed by the comb. Severe traumatic alopecia can result in subgaleal hemorrhage (32).

WOUND HEALING

When cutaneous tissue is traumatized, the dynamic process of wound healing immediately begins. This process is both intracellular and extracellular. Externally, one of the first events to happen is clotting of bleeding vessels within the tissue. Medications, supplements, and abnormal hematology can prolong or prevent clotting. Obtaining a thorough history of current and recent medication and supplement use is a critical part of any trauma care. In addition, the provider may want to obtain basic hematologic and bleeding/clotting lab tests on IPV patients when multiple contusions are present, even if the injuries appear relatively minor (4).

As open injuries begin to heal, the epithelial cells at the edges of the wound begin to proliferate and granulation tissue begins to fill in the wound space. The granulation tissue forms a matrix of collagen connecting tissue that, with larger injuries, result in a visible scar (cicatrix) (33). Excessive collagen production will result in excessive scarring called a *keloid*. Keloids are more likely to form in persons with darkly pigmented skin and be located to the upper arms, back, shoulders, and chest (33).

Injuries in various stages of healing are called a *pattern of injury* (4,9,13). Intimate partner violence patients may present with a injuries in various stages of healing. If accompanied by the abuser, the couple may have rehearsed an excuse for the most recent injury, but may not have coordinated their histories to explain older injuries or scars to the skin.

BRUISE HEALING

As bruises heal, their change in color is attributed to the body's breakdown of hemoglobin from extravasated red blood cells. Initially, bruises appear red from vasodilation resulting from the inflammatory response to the trauma and leakage of any oxygenated arterial blood (18). Interstitial extravasation of deoxygenated venous blood results in a more blue or purple change in color. The inflammatory response attracts macrophages that break down the hemoglobin into biliverdin, which has a green appearance (34). During this process, some of the iron released is combined with ferritin. This results in the formation of hemosiderin, which is brown in color (34). Finally, a yellow appearance late in healing is attributed to the biliverdin being broken down into bilirubin (17).

It is common to find color charts in nursing, medical text books, and online sources that teach that the age of bruises can be relatively accurately determined by assessing the color of the bruise. However, no scientific research supports that one can accurately link the color of bruise to its age of onset. In fact, the contrary is true. In several studies, when health professionals have tried to estimate the age of bruises, they were significantly, statistically wrong.

In a study of 50 children (1 week–18 years), Baiciak and colleagues (2003) found that direct physical examination of a bruise to determine its age reliably was very difficult for physicians, despite the level of clinical training (35). They were able to make estimates between color and bruise age. Red, blue, and purple colors were more commonly seen in bruises less than 48 hours old, and yellow, brown, and green colors were most often seen in bruises older than 7 days. However, it was concluded that estimates by physicians determining bruise age within 24 hours were inaccurate and were not much better than chance alone.

Langlois and Gresham (1991) (36) conducted a study of color changes in bruises on human skin over time, using photographs of 89 subjects with an age range of 10 to 100 years. They showed photographs of bruises to physicians and found that the age of a bruise could not be determined by color changes. The colors of a bruise are dynamic, and similar colors may come and go during the time of healing. This "was assumed to be due to blood changing its position within the layers of the skin and its degradation" (36). However, the authors concluded that the appearance of a yellow coloration is highly significant, attributing it to very likely be associated with a bruise that is more than 18 hours old; but a bruise without a yellow color is not necessarily less than 18 hours old. It was also noted that little is known about what may affect bruising in children, such as differences in subcutaneous fat depth and metabolic rates (36).

A review of 50 photographs from a study by Stephenson and Bialas (1996), depicting accidental bruising in children, concluded that the sequence of color changes in determining the aging of bruises was not reliable and was much less precise than textbooks suggested (37). They discriminated that yellow coloration was not seen in photographs of injuries less of than 1 day old, but was seen in 10 out of 42 bruises more than 1 day old, and that an injury greater than 48 hours old was unlikely to be estimated as one less than 48 hours old.

Mosqueda and colleagues (7) evaluated the ability to predict the occurrence, progression, and resolution of accidental bruises in an elderly population (aged ≥65 years). The authors used a convenience sample of 101 seniors who were physically examined in their homes daily for up to 6 weeks. During the initial 2-week inspection period, 73 participants had at least one bruise occur. More specifically, 49 had one bruise, 17 had two bruises, 3 had three bruises, 3 had four bruises, and 1 had five bruises. Of all 108 observed bruises, about 90% occurred on the extremities. No bruises were observed to the neck, ears, genitalia, buttocks, or soles of the feet of the volunteer subjects. The majority of the bruises were to the arms, more specifically the lower arms (7).

The authors stated that participants who were taking medications that altered coagulation were more likely to have multiple bruises, as were participants who had functional mobility problems causing them to bump themselves or be handled by others. The authors did not report which medications taken by the subjects contributed to bruising. However, they did state that the more the subjects needed help in activities of daily living the more likely they were to have multiple bruises (7).

When the researchers discovered bruises during the daily assessments, they were visible for 4 to 41 days. The predominate color over the life of most bruises was red, with a surprising finding that yellowish discoloration occurred in 16% of the bruises on day 1 (7). The bruises took 4 to 42 days to resolve. About half resolved by day 6, with 81% of the bruises disappearing by day 11. A few bruises lingered much longer, with one bruise taking 41 days to resolve.

A commonly held and taught belief is yellowing of bruising usually occurs days after the initial trauma that caused the bruising. However, Mosqueda and colleagues (7) discovered that the yellowing of bruises in the elderly can begin within 19 to 30 hours of injury. This is consistent with Langlois and Gresham's (1991) findings from over a decade ago (36). Also consistent with earlier studies of bruising, especially in children, Mosqueda and colleagues (7) discovered the predominant color in bruises to the elderly throughout the duration of the bruise was red.

No published research to date has attempted to age bruising to women between the ages of 18 and 65 to determine if there is any accuracy in the dating of bruises on most battered women. The just-mentioned studies highlight the fact that the aging of bruises purely by looking at them is not reliable and should be avoided in written documentation and on the witness stand. Estimates of the age of a bruise can be made, especially if the approximate age of a bruise is consistent with the history of injury being given by the patient or reliable historian.

Patterned Injuries

Patterned injuries, sometimes called *geometrically patterned injuries*, are those in which the provider has reasonable certainty that the injury was caused by an unknown object, a specific object, or a specific

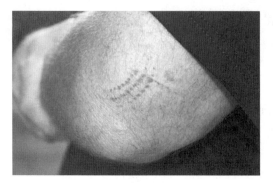

Figure 17.12 Patterned contusion (baseball seams) to elbow. Patient struck by fast, pitched ball during a sporting event. (This is an image of a nonintentional injury, but baseballs have also been thrown with intent to injure, either in a baseball game or during an intimate partner physical assault.) *Forensic photography courtesy of Dan Sheridan, RN, PhD.*

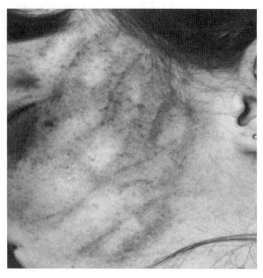

Figure 17.14 Bruising to the face with parallel raised welts and central clearing consistent with the strike of an open hand. The outline of the fingers, including the flexor creases is clearly evident. *Forensic photography courtesy of Dan Sheridan, RN, PhD.*

mechanism. For example, being struck with a baseball may leave seam (stitching) marks to the skin (Figure 17.12; Plate 20). Being punched when the assailant is wearing a ring may result in a semicircular abrasion or laceration (Figure 17.13; Plate 21). Being forcefully slapped may result in a classic pattern imprint to the skin that begins with distinct generalized erythema but then develop into parallel linear bruises outlining the outer edges of the fingers (Figure 17.14; Plate 22). Being struck with a solid object can result in a bruise with central clearing, in which the blood is displaced laterally around the area where the solid object made contact (Figure 17.15; Plate 23) (38). Being struck with a looped cord can result in patterned looped bruises or erythema (Figure 17.16; Plate 24). Abrasions can also be patterned to match a zipper against the skin when it is compressed or dragged across the skin surface (Figure 17.17; Plate 25).

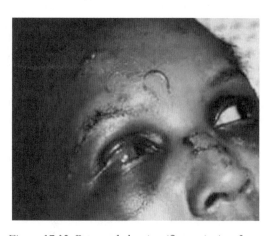

Figure 17.13 Patterned abrasion (finger ring) to forehead. Punch injury with patterned, ring-shaped abrasion to mid forehead. Other injuries to face include bilateral periorbital ecchymoses. *Forensic photography courtesy of Dan Sheridan, RN, PhD.*

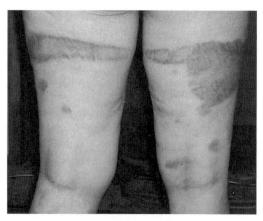

Figure 17.15 Horizontal patterned bruise with central clearing that extends across both legs. This injury pattern is consistent with being struck with a solid object, in this case a cane. There are other bruises in various stages of healing. *Forensic photography courtesy of Dan Sheridan, RN, PhD.*

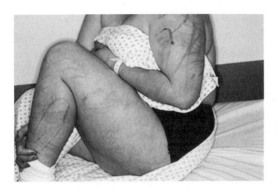

Figure 17.16 Patterned bruising, "loop-cord" injury. Multiple reddish-colored, looped, cord-like bruises in a pattern consistent with patient's history of laying on her right side, in a curled defensive posture while being whipped with a looped telephone cord. *Forensic photography courtesy of Dan Sheridan, RN, PhD.*

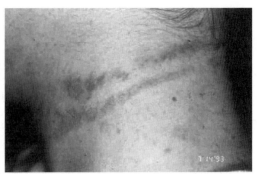

Figure 17.18 Patterned abrasion (ligature marks) to neck. Two circumferential ligature marks to the neck, the lower one newer than the upper one, secondary to being brighter red and having more intact margins. *Forensic photography courtesy of Dan Sheridan, RN, PhD.*

STRANGULATION

Strangulation is a common abuse in domestic violence, usually occurring later in an abusive relationship (39). There are three types of strangulation: ligature, manual, and mechanical. Common ligatures include ropes, stockings, belts, electrical cords, and clothing. Ligature strangulation can leave circumferential linear markings or abrasions on the neck, or the ligature mark may be confined to just one part of the neck where the most force was applied (40) (Figure 17.18; Plate 26). Ligature marks can sometimes be matched to the object that caused them. Manual

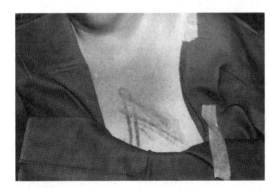

Figure 17.17 Parallel "train track" abrasions are consistent with a zipper abrading the skin. Patient said she was wearing a zippered heavy cotton pull-over shirt and her boyfriend grabbed her by the front of the shirt and shoved her against the wall, forcing the zipper up and then down against the skin. *Forensic photography courtesy of Dan Sheridan, RN, PhD.*

strangulation involves "choking" the victim either by using hands, a head lock "choke-hold," or a leg scissors hold. This type of strangulation sometimes leaves very little external findings (16). Manual strangulation also includes applying direct pressure to the neck with the elbow, knee, or foot.

With ligature and manual strangulation, the victim may fight to remove the hands or rope hurting them. Fingernail scratches on the neck may be seen (4). Petechiae, subconjunctival hemorrhages, and face and tongue swelling can also be present post strangulation. Other signs, symptoms, and sequelae of strangulation are discussed in Chapter 16.

Mechanical strangulation is usually accidental in nature and is rarely seen in intentional, interpersonal violence. Mechanical strangulation occurs when a person's head and neck get wedged in tight places such as between bed guard rails, staircase rails, or furniture. A subtype of strangulation is applying pressure to the chest, thus preventing it from expanding while also applying pressure to the neck. *Burking* is a type of mechanical strangulation that involves someone sitting on the chest of another, eventually suffocating them (16).

DEFENSIVE INJURIES

Obtaining a thorough history is important in helping to determine if injuries are accidental in nature or intentional. A lacrosse player may have numerous bruises to the forearms in various stages of healing from being

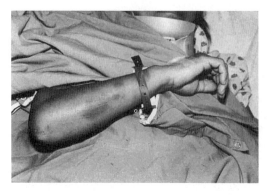

Figure 17.19 Mid forearm bruises consistent with de-fensive posturing of holding arm up to protect face and anterior neck/chest. *Forensic photography courtesy of Dan Sheridan, RN, PhD.*

struck and "checked" by a lacrosse stick. However, bruises to the forearms of a young woman, especially to the ulnar surface, may be suggestive of defensive injuries from raising her arms to block punches and/ or kicks from an abusive partner (Figure 17.19; Plate 27). Victims may defend themselves by covering their faces with their hands (so hands get bruised and swollen), by curling into a protective fetal position (so injuries appear on the side or back of the body), or by punching, scratching, or biting their assailant (Figure 17.20; Plate 28).

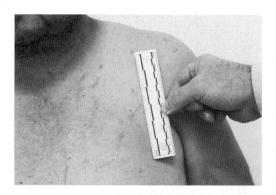

Figure 17.20 Suspect exam reveals linear abrasions to chest. Long, linear, fan-patterned abrasions are consis-tent with claw marks that could be sustained in a fight or as a victim struggles to defend or escape. *Forensic photos courtesy of the Office of the District Attorney, Placer County, CA.*

THE SKIN AS A REPOSITORY OF OTHER EVIDENCE

In addition to injuries to the skin from IPV, the skin often contains many types of trace physical evidence. Historically, health providers were never trained nor would they consider saving miscellaneous debris imbedded on the skin or in the injury. The dirt, leaves, sand, spittle, blood, or fabric fibers washed away and destroyed by well-meaning health professionals may make the difference between a successful prosecution of the crime of domestic violence or not. Unless abso-lutely contraindicated by the acute medical needs of a patient, medical providers should take a minute or two to scrape, swab, and collect any trace evidence on the patient's skin. Most types of trace physical evidence on the skin of IPV patients can be swabbed or brushed into specimen containers, sealed with tape, and labeled with a patient identification label. Areas of the body that have been licked by a reported assailant can be swabbed with a moistened cotton-tip applicator moist-ened with sterile water and then swabbed a second time with a dry swab. The swabs can be placed, when dried, in a clean envelope, sealed with tape, and labeled.

Clothing removed during treatment should be individually packaged in paper bags, sealed with tape, and labeled with a patient identification tag. Paper is preferred over plastic since any moisture in the cloth-ing will evaporate from a paper bag. Moist clothing in a plastic bag is more prone to destruction from mold and bacterial growth.

CONCLUSION

In this chapter, a brief overview of the structures of the skin was presented. Definitions of the most common injuries to the skin were provided, highlighting a few medical forensic terms that are frequently misused by health providers. Intimate partner violence patients, especially women in abusive relationships, may not seek medical attention for many cutaneous injuries, opting instead to self-care. Health providers need to screen for IPV in all patients, even those presenting for routine medical care or other ailments. Cutane-ous injuries need to be fairly documented in written progress notes, by the use of body maps and by photo-graphs. The skin may contain important trace physical evidence on it and in it, and health facilities must have evidence collection and preservation policies in place.

IMPLICATIONS FOR POLICY, PRACTICE, AND RESEARCH

Policy

- Forensic care is a component of health care of victims of violence and abuse, and therefore health systems and criminal justice professionals should collaborate to create standardized procedures for the examination, documentation, and collection of physical evidence for victims of IPV.
- Standardized training should be developed and provided as a means of establishing and maintaining quality of medical forensic skills.
- Forensic care should be provided without cost to the victim, perhaps through victim of crime resources.

Practice

- All patients with cutaneous injuries without an absolutely known cause need to be assessed for IPV.
- Patients who present with delays in treatment for their cutaneous injuries need to be assessed for IPV.
- Patients with bruises in various stages of healing, especially in the absence of reasonable histories of injury, need to be assessed for IPV.
- Patients whose cutaneous injuries are not consistent with the history being provided need to be assessed for IPV.
- Health providers need to be more thorough in their written descriptions of cutaneous injuries in medical records.
- Health providers should utilize body maps to draw in areas of visible cutaneous injury and to mark areas of nonvisible tenderness.
- Health providers need to better utilize medical photographic documentation of cutaneous injuries before the injuries are cleaned, after the injuries are cleaned, and after the injuries are treated. Serial photography should be made available to IPV patients in healthcare settings since a cutaneous injury inflicted today might be more visible and show more distinct patterns tomorrow.

Research

- Little is known about the types, locations, and healing process of IPV patients who are injured but do not seek traditional healthcare institutional services. While studying routine bruising in the elderly, Mosqueda and colleagues (2005) were able to do daily assessments of the elderly in their homes. Being able to do daily assessments of a possibly abused woman in her home by a trained research associate is not practical and not safe for all parties. However, abused women with minor injuries who enter shelter settings shortly after an abusive episode could be assessed on a daily basis, to better understand cutaneous injuries.
- Further research is needed to study nonabusive cutaneous injuries to women in general, especially in regards to bruising and tissue healing. Most of the published research on bruising has focused on children and/or the elderly. Much less is known about bruising to the largest population of IPV patients—women. Although a growing body of literature looks at the effects of medications on bleeding and bruising, more research is needed on the role of supplements and vitamins and their role in bleeding and bruising.

References

1. Sheridan D. Treating survivors of intimate partner abuse: Forensic identification and documentation. In: Olshaker J, Jackson M, Smock W, eds. *Forensic emergency medicine.* Philadelphia: Lippincott, Williams & Wilkins; 2007:202–222.
2. Tjaden P, Thoennes N. *Full report of the prevalence, incidence and consequences of violence against women: Findings from the national violence against women survey.* Washington DC: National Institute of Justice, 2000.
3. Plichta S. Intimate partner violence and physical health consequences: Policy and practice implications. *J Interpers Violence.* 2004;19(11):1296–1323.
4. Sheridan D, Nash K. Acute injury patterns of intimate partner violence. *Trauma Violence Abuse.* 2007;8(3):281–289.
5. Jarvis C. *Skin, hair and nails: Physical examination and health assessment.* Philadelphia: Saunders, 2004.
6. Webster G. Common skin disorders in the elderly. *Clin Cornerstone.* 2001;4:9–44.
7. Mosqueda L, Burnight K, Liao S. The life cycle of bruises in older adults. *J Am Geriatr Soc.* 2005;53(8):1339–1343.
8. Edward C, Marks R. Evaluation of biomechanical properties of human skin. *Clin Dermatol.* 1995;13:375–380.

9. Sheridan D. Forensic identification and documentation of patients experiencing intimate partner violence. *Clin Fam Pract.* 2003;5(1):113–143.

10. Le B, Dierks E, Ueeck-Homer L, Potter B. Maxillofacial injuries associated with domestic violence. *J Oral Maxillofacial Surg.* 2001;59: 1277–1283.

11. Muelleman R, Lenaghan P, Pakiese R. Battered women: Injury locations and types. *Ann Emerg Med.* 1996;28(5):486–492.

12. Ochs H, Neuenschwander M, Dodson T. Are head, neck and facial injuries markers for domestic violence? *J Am Dent Assoc.* 1995;127:757–761.

13. Besant-Matthews P. Blunt and sharp injuries. In: Lynch V, Duval J, eds. *Forensic nursing.* St. Louis: Elsevier Mosby; 2006:189–200.

14. Wadman M, Muelleman R. Domestic violence homicides: ED use before victimization. *Am J Emerg Med.* 1999;17(7):689–691.

15. Crowell NA BA. *Understanding violence against women.* Washington DC: National Academy Press, 1996.

16. DiMaio V, DiMaio D. *Forensic pathology,* 2nd ed. Boca Raton, FL: CRC Press, 2001.

17. Venezis P. Bruising: Concepts of ageing and interpretation. In: Rutty G, ed. *Essentails of autopsy practice.* Vol. 1. London: Springer; 2001:221–240.

18. Nash K, Sheridan D. Can one accurately date a bruise? State of the science. *J Forensic Nurs.* 2009;5(1):31–37.

19. Randeberg L, Winnem A, Langlois N, Larsen E. Skin changes following minor trauma. *Lasers Surg Med.* 2007;39:403–413.

20. Venes D, Thomas C. *Taber's cyclopedic medical dictionary.* Philadelphia: FA Davis, 2001.

21. Lew E, Matshes E. Sharp force injuries. In: Dolinak D, Matshes E, Lew E, eds. *Forensic pathology: Principles and practice.* Burlington, MA: Elsevier; 2005:143–162.

22. Lew E, Dolmak D, Matshes E. Firearm injuries. In: Dolinak D, Matshes E, Lew F, eds. *Forensic pathology: Principles and practice.* Burlington, MA: Elsevier; 2005:163–200.

23. Justice Bo. *Homicide trends in the US: Intimate homicide.* Washington DC: Department of Justice; 2006.

24. Saltzman L, Mercy J, O'Carroll P, et al. Weapon involvement and injury outcome in family and intimate assaults. *JAMA.* 1992;267:3043–3047.

25. Koziol-McLain J, Webster D, McFarlane J, et al. Risk factors for femicide-suicide in abusive relationships: Results from a multi-site case control study. *Violence Vict.* 2006;21:3–21.

26. Garcia L, Soria C, Hurwitz E. Homicides and intimate partner violence: A literature review. *Trauma Violence Abuse.* 2007;8:370–383.

27. Spitz W. *Medicolegal investigation of death,* 3rd ed. Springfield, IL: Charles C Thomas, 1976.

28. Randall T. Clinician's forensic interpretations of fatal gunshot wounds often miss the mark. *JAMA.* 1993;269(16):2058–2061.

29. Collins K, Lantz P. Interpretations of fatal, multiple, and exiting gunshot wounds by trauma specialists. *J Forensic Sci.* 1994;39(1):94–99.

30. Clark S, Ernst M, Haglund W, Jentsen J. *Medicolegal death investigator.* Big Rapids, MI: Occupational Research and Assessment, Inc., 1996.

31. LaSala K, Lynch V. Child abuse and neglect. In: Lynch V, Duval J, eds. *Forensic nursing.* St. Louis, MO: Elsevier Mosby, 2005.

32. Dolinak D, Matshes E. Forensic neuropathology. In: Dolinak D, Matshes E, Lew E, eds. Burlington, MA: Elsevier; 2005:423–465.

33. Jenny C. Cutaneous manifestations of child abuse. In: Reese R, Ludwig S, eds. *Child abuse: Medical diagnosis and management.* Philadelphia: Lippincott, Williams & Wilkins; 2001:23–45.

34. Hughes V, Ellis P, Burt T, Langlois N. The practical application of reflectance spectrophotometry for the demonstration of haemoglobin and its degradation in bruises. *J Clin Pathol.* 2003;57:355–359.

35. Bariciak E, Plint A, Gaboury I, Bennett S. Dating of bruises in children: An assessment of physician accuracy. *Pediatrics.* 2003;112(4):804–807.

36. Langlois N, Gresham G. The aging of bruises: A review and study of the colour changes with time. *Forensic Sci Int.* 1991;50:227–238.

37. Stephenson T, Bialas Y. Estimation of the age of bruising. *Arch Dis Child.* 1996;74:53–55.

38. Smock W. Forensic emergency medicine. In: Olshaker J, Jackson M, Smock W, eds. *Forensic emergency medicine.* Philadelphia: Lippincott, Williams & Wilkins; 2001:63–83.

39. Wilbur L, Higley M, Hatfield J, et al. Survey results of women who have been strangled while in an abusive relationship. *J Emerg Med.* 2001;21(3): 297–302.

40. Sheridan D, Fernandez L, Pelt DV, et al. Intimate partner violence and sexual assault. In: Schuiling K, Likis F, eds. *Women's gynecologic health.* Boston: Jones & Bartlett Publishers; 2006:293–320.

Chapter 18

Intimate Partner Violence and Pregnancy

Peggy E. Goodman

KEY CONCEPTS

- Intimate partner violence (IPV) is as prevalent during pregnancy as other commonly screened-for complications of pregnancy such as gestational diabetes and preeclampsia.
- Lack of choice in reproductive health matters within an abusive relationship because it results in an increased prevalence of sexually transmitted infections (STIs), human immunodeficiency virus (HIV)/acquired immunodeficiency syndrome (AIDS), and unwanted pregnancies.
- Diagnosis of pregnancy may be an incidental finding during evaluation for other medical problems, and may be associated with delayed prenatal care and poorer antenatal outcomes.
- The postpartum period is often as dangerous, if not more so, than the preconception and pregnancy periods for IPV relationships.
- Femicide is a leading cause of maternal death.

Intimate partner violence (IPV) affects the preconception period through the postpartum period. It is a contributory factor in high-risk sexual behavior, infection with sexually transmitted infections (STIs) and human immunodeficiency virus (HIV), multiple pregnancies, and pregnancy loss. Pregnancy is a particularly complex event in the context of IPV. In addition to the numerous anatomic, physiologic, and psychologic changes regarding the relationship of the woman and the developing fetus, the additional psychosocial factors occur between the woman and her abuser. When considering IPV during pregnancy, it is important to remember that both the mother and the fetus are at risk. On account of the pregnancy, an increased number of interactions between the healthcare provider and abused woman may occur, compared to the nonpregnant state. This results in an increased number of opportunities for intervention.

PREVALENCE

The prevalence of IPV during pregnancy is difficult to estimate, given the different types (emotional, physical, and sexual) of abuse and the types of data collected. The estimated prevalence is 3.9%–8.3% of pregnant women, with a range of physical IPV from 0.9% to over 30% (1). This makes IPV as common as gestational diabetes (1.4%–6.1%) (2) and preeclampsia (2%–7%) (3), two conditions routinely screened for during pregnancy. Even this is likely to be an underestimate, since victims of abuse may have greater difficulty accessing medical and law enforcement services or are less willing to disclose their abuse because of stigma or the increased risk of personal harm.

Although no typical victim of abuse exists, many studies, including population-based analyses of IPV events requiring police involvement (4), analysis of maternal demographics at time of delivery (5), and face-to-face interviews with patients during prenatal screening (6,7) have all shown characteristics that increase the likelihood of abuse during pregnancy (Table 18.1). It is inconclusive whether race is a factor; one study (8) found a higher prevalence of abuse in White females, although other studies show a greater difference based more on socioeconomic status than

Table 18.1. Characteristics that Increase the Likelihood of Abuse of Abuse During Pregnancy

- Age under 20 years old
- Fewer than 12 years of education
- Fewer economic resources
- Use of alcohol, tobacco, or other drugs (ATOD)
- Prior sexually transmitted infections
- Unmarried status
- Current or prior unintended pregnancy and/or termination
- Interpregnancy duration of less than 24 months
- History of suicide attempts, depression, or other psychiatric illness

From Lipsky S, Holt VL, Easterling TR, Critchlow CW. Impact of police-reported intimate partner violence during pregnancy on birth outcomes. *Obstet Gynecol.* 2003;102(3):557–564; Janseen PA, Holt VL, Sugg NK, et al. Intimate partner violence and adverse pregnancy outcomes: a population-based study. *Am J Obstet Gynecol.* 2003;188(5):1341–1347; Hillard PJ. Physical abuse in pregnancy. *Obstet Gynecol.* 1985;66(2):185–190; and Bohn DK, Tebben JG, Campbell JC. Influences of income, education, age, and ethnicity on physical abuse before and during pregnancy. *J Obstet Gynecol Neonatal Nurs.* 2004;33(5):561–571.

on race (9). It is important to note that most of these characteristics also pertain to both pregnant and nonpregnant abused females, and many of the characteristics, such as substance abuse, depression, and STIs, are recognized as consequences, rather than causes of prior or ongoing abuse.

Numerous studies have looked at patterns of abuse prior to, during, and after pregnancy, although the majority of these studies provided a "snapshot," rather than longitudinal analysis, of the problem. Abuse in a relationship usually precedes the pregnancy, with 23%–28% of women reporting physical or sexual abuse in the year prior to their first prenatal visit (10,11), and 13.9% reporting their first incident of abuse during the current pregnancy (12). These studies conclude that physical abuse increases in 63.9% of the pregnancies, remains the same in 20%–30%, and decreases in approximately 5% (12–14).

The concept of reproductive choice includes a number of variables: consent, timing, type of intercourse or other sexual activity, pregnancy prophylaxis, disease prophylaxis, and pregnancy retention. All of these can be severely restricted in an abusive relationship (15). Studies show a 29%–78% prevalence of unplanned pregnancy (16,17); one study shows that only 40% of the women with unintended pregnancies were allowed by their partner to use some form of contraception (18). In cases of unintended pregnancy, women have 2.5 times the risk of experiencing physical abuse compared with those whose pregnancies are intended (16). In a study involving a population with good access to medical care, 29% of these women had unintended pregnancies, and women who reported that their partner did not want the pregnancy were 7.4 times more likely to consider the pregnancy as unintended than women whose partner did want the pregnancy (18).

Similarly, the STI and HIV status of the abusive partner may be unknown, with no opportunity for preventive action or protective measures to be incorporated. Condoms are less likely to be used by abusers and not insisted on by abused partners due to anticipated negative and potentially violent repercussions (19–21). These diseases can also affect the development and subsequent health of the fetus.

When pregnancy occurs, many variables affect whether a woman conceals or discloses the pregnancy. These include perceived preference of the partner, belief that a child will help "bring the couple together," presence and degree of current abuse, circumstances of conception (e.g., date or marital rape), the timing of the pregnancy, and pessimism (doesn't want to bring child into abusive relationship).

Several studies (13,22,23) note that the prevalence of abuse that occurs during pregnancy is two to three times greater in frequency or severity, particularly in the first trimester of an unintended pregnancy (24). Proposed explanations include jealousy or anger toward the fetus, who receives more attention than the adult partner; perception that the pregnancy interferes with the woman's role as caretaker for her partner; loss of control for the partner (unless the partner later "regains control" by causing a miscarriage or otherwise forcing termination of the pregnancy); increased substance abuse by the partner; stress of becoming a parent; and "routine" escalation of violence within the abusive relationship (24).

The increased stress in the relationship and resentment by the mother toward the fetus, particularly in cases of unintended pregnancy or rape, can lead to rejection of the child, with failure of normal parent–child bonding and long-term psychologic consequences.

In women seeking an abortion, 39.5% self-report their primary reason for pregnancy termination as "abuse" (25). Overall, the most common reason given for pregnancy termination is "relationship issues." Another study reports that 16%–19% of IPV victims with rape-related pregnancies electively terminate the pregnancy (26). A study by Campbell found that abused women are significantly less likely to inform their partner of the pregnancy or involve the partner in the decision to abort than are women who are nonabused; single women and Black women are more likely to continue their pregnancies despite their partners' preferences (22).

CLINICAL PRESENTATIONS OF INTIMATE PARTNER VIOLENCE IN PREGNANCY

Clinical presentation of the abused pregnant woman can vary greatly. Her first presentation may occur during a healthcare visit for an illness or injury seemingly unrelated to either abuse or pregnancy (Table 18.2) (27). Pregnant patients also present to healthcare services when they develop acute abdominal pain or vaginal bleeding, which can be spontaneous or caused by trauma.

It is well established that victims of IPV often show manifestations of chronic stress and are generally

---

Table 18.2: Effects of Intimate Partner Violence on Pregnancy

Prenatal

- Increased incidence of sexually transmitted infections, including HIV
- Increased number of unplanned pregnancies
- Late recognition of pregnancy
- Late entry into healthcare system
- Continued high-risk behaviors (e.g., alcohol, tobacco, other drug use)
- Poor physical and mental health
- Increased incidence of miscarriage
- Increased risks of trauma to mother and fetus

Peripartum

- Premature labor
- Premature rupture of membranes
- Placental abruption
- Acute maternal distress (e.g., poorly controlled chronic disease, femicide)
- Fetal distress

Birth

- Intrauterine growth retardation/low birth weight (IUGR/LBW)
- Premature birth
- Alcohol, tobacco and other drug (ATOD) withdrawal syndromes

---

perceived to be in poorer health (28–30). They appear to have a higher prevalence of neuropsychiatric illnesses such as anxiety disorders, sleep disorders, substance abuse, chronic pain syndromes, depression, chronic fatigue, and posttraumatic stress disorder (PTSD). Other frequent clinical presentations include gastrointestinal symptoms such as anorexia, eating disorders, ulcers, chronic abdominal pain, or functional bowel disease; cardiac symptoms such as hypertension, chest pain, palpitations, and hyperventilation; and gynecologic problems such as STIs, HIV infection, vaginal bleeding, vaginal infections, fibroids, decreased libido, genital irritation, dyspareunia, chronic pelvic pain, urinary tract infections (UTI), and infertility (31–35).

A patient may not know she is pregnant, or may know but choose not to disclose her pregnancy, or the pregnancy may be diagnosed as an incidental finding during evaluation for other conditions. She may also not disclose a history of abuse, even when asked directly, due to reasons such as embarrassment, confidentiality concerns, fear of partner retaliation, or belief that the provider will not be able to help (36–38). As a result, these two factors, occurrence of abuse and pregnancy determination, are among the most important areas of assessment. These alert the examiner that there are two victims to be evaluated and thus facilitates appropriate assessment, treatment, intervention, and referral.

Teenage Pregnancy

Young age at time of first sexual activity is among the recognized risk factors for IPV. Adolescents are more likely to engage in high-risk behaviors such as unprotected sexual intercourse, with higher rates of pregnancy and sexually transmitted infections, including HIV/AIDS (39). Peer pressure and parental influences greatly affect the decision to have early intercourse (40).

A partner more than 3 years older, multiple partners, and poor support systems are major risk factors contributing to early pregnancy and increased incidence of IPV (41). Financial dependence on a partner and lack of parental support can facilitate isolation from positive support systems that would be protective against IPV. Although access to health care is often more available to minors, they may be less aware of and able to seek out these resources, with an even higher incidence of poor fetal outcome (42).

Delayed Prenatal Care

Intimate partner violence during pregnancy often results in late entry into prenatal care, which is associated with an increased risk of poor fetal outcome. Abused women were 1.8 times more likely to delay prenatal care compared to women who were not abused, and were twice as likely to begin prenatal care in their third trimester (26). Two to three times as many low-birth-weight infants are born to abused women than to nonabused women (43–45). In cases of alcohol or substance abuse, approximately two-thirds of the abused pregnant women decreased or stopped their use when they found out they were pregnant, so delayed diagnosis of pregnancy can have significant ramifications to fetal health (46).

Preterm Labor

Preterm labor is a continuing challenge, occurring in approximately 12.5% of all pregnancies (47).

Although preterm labor in otherwise uncomplicated pregnancies in nonabused females can often be delayed with rest and tocolytic agents, the multifactorial risks related to IPV (including lack of adequate prenatal care, comorbid medical conditions, substance abuse, and repeated trauma) contribute to a higher incidence of preterm delivery (14%–16%) than in nonabused females (48,49).

The most likely cause of preterm labor (premature contractions with cervical thinning or dilation) in a trauma patient is placental abruption (separation of the placenta from the wall of the uterus), which usually occurs after 16 weeks gestation when the inelastic placenta is firmly adherent to the thinning uterine wall. Blunt trauma can result in shearing forces that cause a partial or full separation of the placenta, with varying degrees of subchorionic hemorrhage. Signs of placental abruption, including spontaneous rupture of membranes, vaginal bleeding, and uterine tenderness may not occur after trauma, and their presence or absence is not a reliable indicator of adverse fetal outcome. Post-traumatic placental abruption has a 67%–75% rate of fetal mortality (50).

Low Birth Weight

There appears to be a positive association between IPV and low birth weight, miscarriage, and preterm birth (delivery prior to 37 weeks gestation). Rates of low birth weight among IPV victims are 1.5 to 2.5 times higher than among non-victims, and rates of preterm birth range from 2.5 to 4 times higher in three studies (49,51,52), although two studies report no association of abuse with adverse pregnancy outcome (53,54). Some of these studies did not distinguish between verbal and physical abuse, some had small study samples, and some used mail or telephone surveys rather than face-to-face interviews (5,28,55). When the IPV warranted law enforcement intervention, women reporting any violence were more than 1.5 times as likely to have a low-birth-weight infant or preterm birth than women who did not report violence during their pregnancy (5).

Miscarriage and Pregnancy Loss

Intimate partner violence is associated with a threefold increased risk of pregnancy loss, with more than half of these (58%) occurring prior to 37 weeks gestation (4). The effects of chronic stress on pregnancy are being studied, although most data are retrospective or observational rather than prospective, randomized, and blinded, because of potential risks to the fetus. One area of interest is the relationship between elevated levels of corticotropin releasing hormone (CRH) and risks of miscarriage or preterm labor. Thus far, the results have been contradictory and inconclusive (56,57). One study noted that women with high levels of chronic stress, as measured by the Prenatal Social Environment Inventory (PSEI), were more likely to use cigarettes and marijuana during pregnancy, but did not have a higher risk of spontaneous abortion. However, they did not find a relationship between acute stress, measured by the Index of Spouse Abuse, and health behavior (57). In another study, women with a spontaneous miscarriage had a slightly earlier gestational age and lower levels of estradiol and progesterone compared with the control group, but exposure to violence did not appear to influence the risk of spontaneous abortion (54).

Postpartum

The postpartum period is a particularly dangerous time for the mother, frequently with an increase in significant IPV during the first month postpartum (11,24,58). Added to the abusive relationship are the additional stressors of parenting. These include attention to the increased needs of the newborn, with relative inattention to the partner; lack of "control" over the newborn's eating, sleeping, and elimination patterns; increased financial obligations; and concerns about parenting abilities (24).

If the mother had a preterm or complicated delivery, or delivered an ill or addicted infant, the additional health problems may increase the volatility of the relationship. It has also been proposed, although not proven, that a stressed mother might have higher levels of circulating serum catecholamines, resulting in a more irritable, "jittery" infant (59,60). Bonding issues may also occur, based on ambivalence toward the infant by one or both of the parents related to the intendedness of the pregnancy.

Postpartum Depression

Postpartum depression (PPD) is a problem affecting mothers in the 12 months after giving birth. Depending on the criteria used for diagnosis, it ranges from 13% using the *Diagnostic and Statistical Manual of Mental Disorders* (DSM-IV) criteria of clinically diagnosed depression, to as much as 30% of new mothers with subclinical symptoms ranging from mild malaise, a sense of being overwhelmed, and the "blues," to severe depression and despair resulting in suicidal and/or homicidal ideation (61). Based on an analysis of Pregnancy Risk Assessment Monitoring System (PRAMS) data, Gross demonstrated a 1.6 times likelihood of PPD if physical abuse had occurred during pregnancy (62).

The main theories about the etiology of PPD include hormonal shifts postpartum and parental stresses, including health, financial, and relational stresses with the partner. Although it has not been well-studied specifically in the context of IPV, the lack of partner and other family support, negative perceptions about the pregnancy and pain of delivery, and the increased stress of the new infant in the home (financial stress, lack of sleep, crying and other distractions, and diversion of attention away from the partner), have been proposed as resulting in a posttraumatic stress-like disorder (51,63,64) with an increased incidence of PPD (65).

Substance Abuse

Substance abuse plays a significant role in poor birth outcome, including birth defects, intrauterine growth retardation (IUGR), placental abruption, miscarriage, preterm labor, and intrauterine fetal demise (66–70). In the context of IPV, chronic stress and "self-medication" may contribute to the increase or continuation of substance abuse (5). Women who suffer physical and sexual abuse are more likely to abuse substances both prior to and during pregnancy than women who are emotionally abused, and both groups have a higher prevalence of substance abuse than nonabused women (46,71,72). Abused pregnant women have more severe alcohol and psychiatric problems than do nonabused women, and the partners of abused women are almost twice as likely to abuse alcohol and/or illicit drugs than are partners of nonabused women (50% versus 28.6%) (73,74). Only 5%–10% of pregnant substance abusers receive professional help for their drug abuse problems. Many reasons for this are given, including lack of insurance, transportation, child care; risk of job or housing loss; lack of family or other social support; lengthy waiting lists; type and severity of addiction; and race, marital status, and IPV history (73,75).

Abdominal Trauma

Blunt and penetrating injuries of the abdomen are among the most common causes of fetal and maternal morbidity and mortality when trauma occurs during pregnancy. Blunt injuries to the abdomen are more common than penetrating injuries, and can be caused directly by a blow such as a punch or kick, or indirectly, as by being pushed down stairs or into a wall. Although blunt injuries are much more common, penetrating injuries are more likely to be fatal. Both types of injuries have direct effects (e.g., fracture, organ disruption, hemorrhage) as well as indirect effects (hypoxemia, vasoconstriction, hypotension, anemia), which can result in significant disability or death (76,77).

Trauma affects 6%–7% of pregnancies and is a leading cause of maternal death. Rates of fetal mortality after maternal blunt trauma range from 3.4% to 38%, mostly due to placental abruption, maternal shock, and maternal death with resulting fetal hypoxia. Trauma to the fetus from blunt trauma in the first trimester is not due to direct injury, since the fetus is small, cushioned by amniotic fluid, and the uterus is shielded by the pelvis. Maternal hemorrhage, hypotension, and hypoxemia result in decreased perfusion of all tissues, including the fetus. In the second and third trimesters, the uterus is exposed above the pelvic brim, is thinner and less muscular, and there is relatively less amniotic fluid to cushion the enlarging fetus, resulting in a higher incidence of direct fetal injury. Fetal loss can occur even when minimal injury has occurred to the mother (78).

FEMICIDE

Femicide, or the killing of women and girls, is a leading cause of maternal death, and accounts for 36%–63% of trauma deaths during pregnancy (79,80) or 1.7 maternal deaths per 100,000 live births (81). In 67%–80% of these cases, there was evidence of physical abuse by the current or former partner prior to the femicide (23), and 41%–43% had used healthcare agencies within the 2 years preceding their femicide (82,83). Guns were used in approximately 80% of the completed femicides (84). Access to a gun is associated not only with a higher risk of death, but also with higher levels of all types of abuse.

Strangulation, or manual asphyxiation, is now being acknowledged as an underrecognized, potentially lethal form of physical injury. The proposed mechanisms, depending on degree and duration of strangulation, are occlusion of venous return from the brain, causing increased intracerebral pressure; cerebral ischemia from subsequent arterial occlusion; other neurovascular compromise from surrounding soft tissue edema; and potentially, airway occlusion, although tracheal cartilages make this a much less likely etiology than initially believed. Initially, 67% have no symptoms, although hoarseness and dysphagia may occur as edema develops. Within the first 24 hours, 42% have no visible injury and another 40% may have only minor-appearing abrasions or contusions. This lack of significant initial signs and symptoms has led to concerns about the victim's credibility when reporting symptoms related to attempted strangulation, although it is hoped that greater awareness will lead to improved identification and intervention when these events occur (85,86,87).

Extensive research clearly shows that murder of a female by her partner is four to times more likely than the murder of a male by his partner (84). Other forms of violent death of pregnant women are underresearched and poorly understood (88). Although homicide rates in the United States have decreased over the past 5 years, the rate of femicide has not decreased proportionately. The Danger Assessment (DA) tool (89) provides a highly accurate assessment of the risk of lethal assault based on the factors in a victim's environment.

INTIMATE PARTNER VIOLENCE INTERVENTIONS FOR THE PREGNANT PATIENT

Most healthcare providers believe that routine inquiry should be the initial intervention to identify IPV among pregnant patients (27). Since pregnancy may be the primary opportunity for a healthy female to interact with healthcare providers and the healthcare system, it provides an opportunity to discuss with a patient her home situation, safety issues, and options.

The American College of Obstetrics & Gynecology (ACOG) recommends routine assessment, at least annually during routine gynecologic visits in the nonpregnant patient, as well as during family planning and preconception visits. If the patient is pregnant, they recommend assessment at least once during each trimester and at the postpartum visit (90).

Despite these recommendations, many obstetricians and other primary care providers have very low rates of asking about and detection of IPV. The ACOG found that only 27% of its members routinely asked new patients about IPV, compared to 95% who screened for tobacco use, 93% who screened for alcohol use, 80% who inquired about diet and exercise, and 73% who asked about seatbelt use. They also found that 68% –72% of ACOG members asked patients about IPV only when they suspected abuse, and only 5% asked about IPV during a postpartum visit (91).

An increasing number of "face-to-face" programs provide intervention at various locations, through a variety of providers. Settings include health clinics, domestic violence programs, social service programs, and childbirth classes.

The Domestic Violence Survivor Assessment (DVSA) tool (92) has shown that individual psychotherapeutic counseling of IPV survivors is one of the more effective interventions to help survivors progress toward a nonviolent life. Generally lasting for less than 6 months, it was more effective in this study than group counseling or referral of services. Although not specifically addressing pregnancy as an issue, the individual approach allows concurrent issues such as pregnancy, substance abuse, or mental health to be addressed more effectively than in a group situation.

Studies looking at barriers to routine inquiry continue to find physicians uncomfortable with asking about abuse, and uncertainty regarding available resources and reporting requirements. Specific screening tools and action items are more readily accepted and integrated into practice by healthcare providers than general guidelines (93). The Health in Pregnancy (HIP) computer program (94) is among the screening tools used to identify patients at risk and cue the healthcare provider to discuss IPV with patients during prenatal visits. The incidence of IPV discussion in this study increased from 23.5% to 85% with cueing, although a small sample size was used (94). Other instruments that evaluate lethality (89) and assist clients with the development of safety plans suggest that safety-promoting behaviors are enhanced through periodic telephone follow-up. These studies are carefully designed to ensure that the follow-up contact does not endanger the client (95).

IMPLICATIONS FOR POLICY, PRACTICE, AND RESEARCH

Policy

- Maternal health policy and programs should include programs promoting healthy relationships and resources to improve client lifestyle, safety, nutrition, education, access to health care, and financial independence, as these are all related to maternal health outcomes.
- Maternal mortality review by public health departments should include review of pregnancy-associated deaths by injury, homicide, and suicide for further means of preventing maternal mortality. These could be coordinated with state IPV fatality review teams.
- Policies should be developed to increase and improve the quality and availability of healthcare and social service resources for victims of IPV and their children.

Practice

- Preconception care should specifically assess for prior or current violence victimization and should provide education and counseling regarding healthy relationships.
- Clinicians should routinely assess patients of child-bearing age for emotional, sexual, and physical abuse. They should also provide information to their patients about options to practice "safe-sex," with information about pregnancy and STI prophylaxis. They should also be aware of local resources, so that they may advise and appropriately refer patients with signs or symptoms suggestive of IPV.
- Healthcare practitioners should inquire about patient safety, including exposure to violence, at each trimester visit and the postpartum visit, because research indicates that higher rates of disclosure occur when the assessment is done multiple times during the prenatal care period.
- Clinicians should routinely screen for high-risk lifestyle behaviors, such as unprotected sexual intercourse, and alcohol, tobacco, and substance abuse as these too are all associated with higher risk for IPV.

Research

- The multifactorial nature of pregnancy risks makes it difficult to determine the precise role IPV plays in poor birth outcomes. Since IPV is recognized to increase high-risk behavior such as substance abuse and impair access to health care, factors such as these should be addressed as vigorously as possible to allow further evaluation of neuroendocrine and other physiologic responses to IPV.
- Population-based samples with ethnic and socioeconomic diversity should be attempted to maximize the representation of society as a whole. Many current studies are site-based, representing a more limited demographic group.
- Larger, population-based samples should improve analysis of outcomes, with an improved ability to discover more subtle outcomes beyond the statistical power of current studies.
- Restrictions on research in pregnant women make it difficult to study the effects of IPV on pregnant women and the developing fetus, but without this research it is difficult to develop evidence-based policies and best practices for care of the pregnant IPV victim.

References

1. Bailey BA, Daugherty RA. Intimate partner violence during pregnancy: Incidence and associated health behaviors in a rural population. *Matern Child Health J.* 2007;11(5):495–503.
2. Jovanovic L, Pettitt DJ. Gestational diabetes mellitus. *JAMA.* 2001;286(20):2516–2518.
3. Sibai B, Dekker G, Kupferminc M. Pre-eclampsia. *Lancet.* 2005;365(9461):785–799.
4. Lipsky S, Holt VL, Easterling TR, Critchlow CW. Impact of police-reported intimate partner violence during pregnancy on birth outcomes. *Obstet Gynecol.* 2003;102(3):557–564.
5. Janssen PA, Holt VL, Sugg NK, et al. Intimate partner violence and adverse pregnancy outcomes: a population-based study. *Am J Obstet Gynecol.* 2003;188(5):1341–1347.
6. Jesse DE, Walcott-McQuigg J, et al. Risks and protective factors associated with symptoms of depression in low-income African American and Caucasian women during pregnancy. *J Midwif Women Health.* 2005;50(5):405–410.
7. Hillard PJ. Physical abuse in pregnancy. *Obstet Gynecol.* 1985;66(2):185–190.
8. McFarlane J, Parker B, Soeken K, Bullock L. Assessing for abuse during pregnancy. Severity and frequency of injuries and associated entry into prenatal care. *JAMA.* 1992;267(23):3176–3178.
9. Bohn DK, Tebben JG, Campbell JC. Influences of income, education, age, and ethnicity on physical abuse before and during pregnancy. *J Obstet Gynecol Neonatal Nurs.* 2004;33(5):561–571.
10. Jasinski JL. Pregnancy and domestic violence: a review of the literature. *Trauma Violence Abuse.* 2004;5(1):47–64.
11. Martin SL, Mackie L, Kupper LL, et al. Physical abuse of women before, during, and after pregnancy. *JAMA.* 2001;285(12):1581–1584.
12. Stewart DE, Cecutti A. Physical abuse in pregnancy. *Can Med Assoc J.* 1993;149(9):1257–1263.
13. Jasinski JL, Kantor GK. Pregnancy, stress and wife assault: Ethnic differences in prevalence, severity, and onset in a national sample. *Violence Vict.* 2001;16(3):219–232.
14. Koenig LJ, Whitaker DJ, Royce RA, et al. Physical and sexual violence during pregnancy and after delivery: A prospective multistate study of women with or at risk for HIV infection. *Am J Pub Health.* 2006;96(6):1052–1059.
15. Pallitto CC, Campbell JC, O'Campo P. Is intimate partner violence associated with unintended pregnancy? A review of the literature. *Trauma Violence Abuse.* 2005;6(3):217–235.
16. Goodwin MM, Gazmararian JA, Johnson CH, et al. Pregnancy intendedness and physical abuse around the time of pregnancy: Findings from the pregnancy risk assessment monitoring system, 1996–1997. PRAMS Working Group. Pregnancy Risk Assessment Monitoring System. *Matern Child Health J.* 2000;4(2):85–92.
17. Petersen R, Gazmararian JA, Anderson Clark K, Green DC. How contraceptive use patterns differ by pregnancy intention: Implications for counseling. *Womens Health Issues.* 2001;11(5):427–435.
18. Green DC, Gazmararian JA, Mahoney LD, Davis NA. Unintended pregnancy in a commercially insured population. *Matern Child Health J.* 2002;6(3):181–187.
19. Wingood GM, DiClemente RJ. The effects of an abusive primary partner on the condom use and sexual negotiation practices of African-American women. *Am J Pub Health.* 1997;87(6):1016–1018.
20. Hamburger ME, Moore J, Koenig LJ, et al. HIV Epidemiology Research Study Group. Persistence of inconsistent condom use: relation to abuse history and HIV serostatus. *AIDS Behav.* 2004;8(3):333–344.
21. Johnson PJ, Hellerstedt WL. Current or past physical or sexual abuse as a risk marker for sexually transmitted disease in pregnant women. *Perspect Sex Reprod Health.* 2002;34(2):62–67.
22. Campbell JC, Pugh LC, Campbell D, Visscher M. The influence of abuse on pregnancy intention. *Women's Health Issues.* 1995;5(4):214–223.
23. Campbell JC, Webster D, Koziol-McLain J, et al. Risk factors for femicide in abusive relationships: Results from multisite case control study. *Am J Pub Health.* 2003;93(7):1089–1097.

24. Macy RJ, Martin SL, Kupper LL, et al. Partner violence among women before, during, and after pregnancy: Multiple opportunities for intervention. *Women's Health Issues.* 2007;17(5):290–299.

25. Glander SS, Moore ML, Michielutte R, Parsons LH. The prevalence of domestic violence among women seeking abortion. *Obstet Gynecol.* 1998;91(6):1002–1006.

26. McFarlane J, Malecha A, Watson K, et al. Intimate partner sexual assault against women: frequency, health consequences, and treatment outcomes. *Obstet Gynecol.* 2005;105(1):99–108.

27. Shadigian EM, Bauer ST. Screening for partner violence during pregnancy. *Int J Gynaecol Obstet.* 2004;84(3):273–280.

28. Coker AL, Sanderson M, Dong B. Partner violence during pregnancy and risk of adverse pregnancy outcomes. *Paediatr Perinatal Epidemiol.* 2004;18(4):260–269.

29. Loxton D, Schofield M, Hussain R, Mishra G. History of domestic violence and physical health in midlife. *Violence Against Women.* 2006;12(8):715–731.

30. Centers for Disease Control and Prevention (CDC). Adverse health conditions and health risk behaviors associated with intimate partner violence—United States, 2005. *MMWR.* 2008;57(5):113–117.

31. Campbell JC. Health consequences of intimate partner violence. *Lancet.* 2002;359(9314):1331–1336.

32. Sutherland C, Bybee D, Sullivan C. The long-term effects of battering on women's health. *Womens Health.* 1998;4(1):41–70.

33. Muelleman RL, Lenaghan PA, Pakieser RA. Nonbattering presentations to the emergency department of women in physically abusive relationships. *Am J Emerg Med.* 1998;16(2):128–131.

34. Abbott J. Injuries and illnesses of domestic violence. *Ann Emerg Med.* 1997;29(6):781–785.

35. John R, Johnson JK, Kukreja S, et al. Domestic violence: prevalence and association with gynaecological symptoms. *BJOG.* 2004;111(10):1128–1132.

36. Bacchus L, Mezey G, Bewley S. Experiences of seeking help from health professionals in a sample of women who experienced domestic violence. *Health Social Care Comm.* 2003;11(1):10–18.

37. Lutenbacher M, Cohen A, Mitzel J. Do we really help? Perspectives of abused women. *Pub Health Nurs.* 2003;20(1):56–64.

38. Fugate M, Landis L, Riordan K, et al. Barriers to domestic violence help seeking: Implications for intervention. *Violence Against Women.* 2005;11(3):290–310.

39. Sandfort TGM, Orr M, Hirsch JS, Santelli J. Long-term health correlates of timing of sexual debut: results from a national US study. *Am J Pub Health.* 2008;98(1):155–161.

40. Hillis SD, Anda RF, Dube SR, et al. The association between adverse childhood experiences and adolescent pregnancy, long-term psychosocial consequences, and fetal death. *Pediatrics.* 2004;113(2):320–327.

41. Monasterio E, Hwang LY, Shafer MA. Adolescent sexual health. *Curr Prob Pediatr Adolesc Health Care.* 2007;37(8):302–325.

42. Chen XK, Wen SW, Fleming N, et al. Teenage pregnancy and adverse birth outcomes: A large population based retrospective cohort study. *Int J Epidemiol.* 2007;36(2):368–373.

43. Yost NP, Bloom SL, McIntire DD, Leveno KJ. A prospective observational study of domestic violence during pregnancy. *Obstet Gynecol.* 2005;106(1):61–65.

44. Dietz PM, Gazmararian JA, Goodwin MM, et al. Delayed entry into prenatal care: Effect of physical violence. *Obstet Gynecol.* 1997;90(2):221–224.

45. McFarlane J, Parker B, Soeken K. Abuse during pregnancy: Associations with maternal health and infant birth weight. *Nurs Res.* 1996;45(1):37–42.

46. Martin SL, Beaumont JL, Kupper LL. Substance use before and during pregnancy: Links to intimate partner violence. *Am J Drug Alcohol Abuse.* 2003;29(3):599–617.

47. Martin JA, Hamilton BE, Sutton PD, et al. Births: Final data for 2004. *Natl Vital Stat Rep.* 2006;55(1):1–101.

48. Cokkinides VE, Coker AL, Sanderson M, et al. Physical violence during pregnancy: Maternal complications and birth outcomes. *Obstet Gynecol.* 1999;93 (5 Pt 1):661–666.

49. El Kady D, Gilbert WM, Xing G, Smith LH. Maternal and neonatal outcomes of assaults during pregnancy. *Obstet Gynecol.* 2005;105(2):357–363.

50. Shah KH, Simons RK, Holbrook T, et al. Trauma in pregnancy: Maternal and fetal outcomes. *J Trauma-Inj Infect Crit Care.* 1998;45(1):83–86.

51. Rosen D, Seng JS, Tolman RM, Mallinger G. Intimate partner violence, depression, and posttraumatic stress disorder as additional predictors of low birth weight infants among low-income mothers. *J Interpers Violence.* 2007;22(10):1305–1314.

52. Boy A, Salihu HM. Intimate partner violence and birth outcomes: A systematic review. *Int J Fertil Womens Med.* 2004;49(4):159–164.

53. Jagoe J, Magann EF, Chauhan SP, Morrison JC. The effects of physical abuse on pregnancy outcomes in a low-risk obstetric population. *Am J Obstet Gynecol.* 2000;182(5):1067–1069.

54. Nelson DB, Grisso JA, Joffe MM, et al. Violence does not influence early pregnancy loss. *Fertil Steril.* 2003;80(5):1205–1211.

55. Neggers Y, Goldenberg R, Cliver S, Hauth J. Effects of domestic violence on preterm birth and low birth weight. *Acta Obstet Gynecol Scand.* 2004;83(5):455–460.

56. Boyles SH, Ness RB, Grisso JA, et al. Life event stress and the association with spontaneous abortion in gravid women at an urban emergency department. *Health Psychol.* 2000;19(6):510–514.

57. Nelson DB, Grisso JA, Joffe MM, et al. Does stress influence early pregnancy loss? *Ann Epidemiol.* 2003;13(4):223–229.

58. Hedin LW. Postpartum, also a risk period for domestic violence. *Eur J Obstet Gynecol Reprod Biol.* 2000;89(1):41–45.

59. Phillips DI. Programming of the stress response: a fundamental mechanism underlying the long-term effects of the fetal environment? *J Intern Med.* 2007;261(5):453–460.

60. Field T, Diego M, Hernandez-Reif M, et al. Prenatal maternal biochemistry predicts neonatal biochemistry. *Int J Neurosci.* 2004;114(8):933–945.

61. Records K, Rice MJ. A comparative study of postpartum depression in abused and non-abused women. *Arch Psychiatr Nurs.* 2005;19(6):281–290.

62. Gross KH, Wells CS, Radigan-Garcia A, Dietz PM. Correlates of self-reports of being very depressed in the months after delivery: Results from the Pregnancy Risk Assessment Monitoring System. *Maternal Child Health J.* 2002;6(4):247–253.

63. Mezey G, Bacchus L, Bewley S, White S. Domestic violence, lifetime trauma and psychological health of childbearing women. *BJOG.* 2005;112(2): 197–204.

64. Cigoli V, Gilli G, Saita E. Relational factors in psychopathological responses to childbirth. *J Psychosomat Obstet Gynecol.* 2006;27(2):91–97.

65. Kendall-Tackett KA. Violence against women and the perinatal period: The impact of lifetime violence and abuse on pregnancy, postpartum, and breastfeeding. *Trauma Violence Abuse.* 2007;8(3): 344–353.

66. Centers for Disease Control and Prevention (CDC). Alcohol consumption among women who are pregnant or who might become pregnant—United States, 2002. *MMWR.* 2004;53(50):1178–1181

67. Fajemirokun-Odudeyi O, Lindow SW. Obstetric implications of cocaine use in pregnancy: a literature review. *Eur J Obstet Gynecol Reprod Biol.* 2004;112(1):2–8.

68. Park B, McPartland JM, Glass M. Cannabis, cannabinoids and reproduction. *Prostaglandins Leukotrienes & Essential Fatty Acids.* 2004;70(2):189–197.

69. Higgins S. Smoking in pregnancy. *Curr Opin Obstet Gynecol.* 2002;14(2):145–151.

70. Greenfield SF, Manwani SG, Nargiso JE. Epidemiology of substance use disorders in women. *Obstet Gynecol Clin N Am.* 2003;30(3):413–446.

71. Haller DL, Miles DR. Victimization and perpetration among perinatal substance abusers. *J Interpers Violence.* 2003;18(7):760–780.

72. Ahluwalia IB, Mack KA, Mokdad A. Mental and physical distress and high-risk behaviors among reproductive-age women. *Obstet Gynecol.* 2004; 104(3):477–483.

73. Haller DL, Miles DR, Dawson KS. Factors influencing treatment enrollment by pregnant substance abusers. *Am J Drug Alcohol Abuse.* 2003;29(1): 117–131.

74. Tuten M, Jones HE, Tran G, Svikis DS. Partner violence impacts the psychosocial and psychiatric status of pregnant, drug-dependent women. *Addictive Behav.* 2004;29(5):1029–1034.

75. Martin SL, Kilgallen B, Dee DL, et al. Women in a prenatal care/substance abuse treatment program: links between domestic violence and mental health. *Matern Child Health J.* 1998;2(2):85–94.

76. Shah AJ, Kilcline BA. Trauma in pregnancy. *Emerg Med Clin N Am.* 2003;21(3):615–629.

77. Grossman NB. Blunt trauma in pregnancy. *Am Fam Physician.* 2004;70(7):1303–1310.

78. Tsuei BJ. Assessment of the pregnant trauma patient. *Injury.* 2006;37(5):367–373.

79. Dannenberg AL, Carter DM, Lawson HW, et al. Homicide and other injuries as causes of maternal death in New York City, 1987 through 1991. *Am J Obstet Gynecol.* 1995;172(5):1557–1564.

80. Fildes J, Reed L, Jones N, et al. Trauma: The leading cause of maternal death. *J Trauma-Injury Infect Crit Care.* 1992;32(5):643–645.

81. Chang J, Berg CJ, Saltzman LE, Herndon J. Homicide: A leading cause of injury deaths among pregnant and postpartum women in the United States, 1991–1999. *Am J Pub Health.* 2005;95:471–477.

82. Sharps PW, Koziol-McLain J, Campbell J, et al. Health care providers' missed opportunities for preventing femicide. *Prevent Med.* 2001;33(5): 373–380.

83. Wadman MC, Muelleman RL. Domestic violence homicides: Emergency department use before victimization. *Am J Emerg Med.* 1999;17(7):689–691.

84. Campbell JC, Glass N, Sharps PW, et al. Intimate partner homicide: Review and implications of research and policy. *Trauma Violence Abuse.* 2007;8(3):246–269.

85. Hawley DA, McClane GE, Strack GB. A review of 300 attempted strangulation cases. Part III: Injuries in fatal cases. *J Emerg Med.* 2001;21(3):317–322.

86. McClane GE, Strack GB, Hawley D. A review of 300 attempted strangulation cases. Part II: Clinical evaluation of the surviving victim. *J Emerg Med.* 2001;21(3):311–315.

87. Strack GB, McClane GE, Hawley D. A review of 300 attempted strangulation cases. Part I: Criminal legal issues. *J Emerg Med.* 2001;21(3):303–309.

88. Martin SL, Macy RJ, Sullivan K, Magee ML. Pregnancy-associated violent deaths: The role of intimate partner violence. *Trauma Violence Abuse.* 2007;8(2):135–148.

89. Campbell JC. Danger Assessment. At http://danger-assessment.org. Accessed 11/4/08.

90. American College of Obstetricians and Gynecologists Committee on Health Care for Undeserved Women. ACOG Committee Opinion No. 343: Psychosocial risk factors: Perinatal screening and intervention. *Obstet Gynecol.* 2006;108(2):469–477.

91. Horan DL, Chapin J, Klein L, et al. Domestic violence screening practices of obstetrician-gynecologists. *Obstet Gynecol.* 1998;92(5):785–789

92. Dienemann J, Glass N, Hanson G, Lunsford K. The Domestic Violence Survivor Assessment (DVSA): A tool for individual counseling with women experiencing intimate partner violence. *Issues Mental Health Nurs.* 2007;28(8):913–925.

93. Taylor P, Zaichkin J, Pilkey D, et al. Prenatal screenin g for substance use and violence: Findings from physician focus groups. *Matern Child Health J.* 2007;11(3):241–247.

94. Calderon SH, Gilbert P, Jackson R, et al. Cueing prenatal providers effects on discussions of intimate partner violence. *Am J Prevent Med.* 2008;34(2): 134–137.

95. McFarlane J, Malecha A, Gist J, et al. Increasing the safety-promoting behaviors of abused women. *Am J Nurs.* 2004;104(3):40–50.

Chapter 19

Intimate Partner Sexual Abuse

Carolyn Sachs and Linda J. Gomberg

KEY CONCEPTS

- Most perpetrators of sexual assault are not strangers but are well known to their victims.
- Approximately 8%–14% of women suffer sexual abuse from an intimate partner or former intimate partner during their lifetimes.
- Intimate partner sexual abuse (IPSA) includes sexual assault/battery, rape, sexual contact without consent, coercion, intimidation, and acquiescence.
- Traditional societal biases continue to blame victims of intimate partner sexual abuse to a greater extent than victims of sexual assault by a stranger.
- Intimate partner sexual abuse is associated with harmful psychological and physical sequela at least as severe as sexual assault by other perpetrators.
- Federal and state laws enacted over the last several decades make spousal rape a crime throughout the United States, although the details of and exemption from such laws vary by state.
- Support and services must be available to specifically address the health consequences of women who suffer from IPSA.

DEFINITIONS OF SEXUAL ABUSE IN RELATIONSHIPS WITH INTIMATE PARTNER VIOLENCE

Although many people use the term *sexual assault* synonymously with rape, sexual assault more accurately refers to any sexual contact of a person by another without appropriate legal consent (1). Physical force may be used to overcome the victim's lack of consent, but contrary to popular opinion, lack of voluntary consent for sexual contact by intimidation or threats is tantamount to no consent (2). "The commonly shared societal (mis)perception of rape is that it involves some kind of physical force. A woman walking through a deserted parking lot as a strange man grabs her by the throat . . . is the typical image that comes to mind" (3). However, most perpetrators of sexual assault are not strangers, but are well known to the victims (4–6). The literature is somewhat inconsistent in defining and distinguishing strangers, acquaintances, and intimate partners, with at least one article distinguishing first date acquaintances from longer-term relationships and others defining only current partners as intimates; further, in order to be considered intimates those partners must be in a "committed" relationship (7–9). For purposes herein, however, intimate partner sexual abuse (IPSA) will be said to occur when a current or former intimate partner or spouse uses physical force to compel the other to engage in a sexual act; attempts or completes the sex act with one who is unable to understand the nature of the act, decline participation, or communicate unwillingness because of illness, disability, the influence of alcohol or other drugs, or because of remote or proximal coercion, intimidation, pressure, or acquiescence; or when there is abusive sexual contact (10,11).

State laws vary slightly in their descriptions of the exact acts that define abusive sexual contact, which populations are legally unable to give consent, and specific definitions of consent; even the definition of rape may take on nuances of differing degrees of abusive sexual contact depending upon legal, medical, and author perspective (11,12). However, a generally accepted legal definition of consent is recognized as the "voluntary agreement or acquiescence by a person of age or with requisite mental capacity who is not under duress or coercion and who has knowledge or understanding" and has reached the age of majority (Merriam-Webster, 1996; 12). The key word here is "voluntary," and it is now understood within the legal and healthcare systems that any unwanted sexual contact is abusive and damaging (12).

Although societal views may minimize the seriousness of IPSA, review of the available literature finds IPSA to be every bit as physically brutal and psychologically devastating as stranger sexual assault, and more so than sexual assault by acquaintances who are not intimate partners (9,10,13).

LEGAL AND SOCIAL BIASES SURROUNDING INTIMATE PARTNER SEXUAL ABUSE

Old British legal doctrine first espoused by then Chief Justice Matthew Hale (1736) condoned what today is considered spousal rape with the following statement: "The husband cannot be guilty of a rape committed by himself upon his lawful wife, for by their mutual matrimonial consent and contract the wife hath given up herself in this kind unto her husband, which she cannot retract" (13). Blackstone expanded on this concept by writing about a "marital unity" wherein the woman lost her identity as an individual upon marriage, being subsumed into a legal unit controlled by her husband (13). This finding, now termed the "marital rape exemption" has a history in the United States legal system since at least 1857, when the Massachusetts *Commonwealth v. Fogarty* decision implied, in part that "once married, a woman does not have the right to refuse sex with her husband" (12,13). The marital rape exemption guided legal practice in the United States for over a century, so that, prior to the late 1970s, not a single state recognized marital rape as a crime (12). To be raped, a woman must be able to withhold consent; since a married woman could not revoke the consent granted upon marriage, rape could not be legally charged.

Marital rape surfaced as a legal and media issue in 1978 when an Oregon man became the first person prosecuted in a criminal trial for raping his wife (14). During that time, Laura X, an advocate for IPSA survivors, founded the National Clearinghouse on Marital and Date Rape (15). She subsequently worked to help several states enact laws that criminalized spousal rape. According to the National Clearinghouse on Marital and Date Rape, "as of July 1993, marital rape was a crime in all 50 states in at least one section of the sexual offense codes, usually regarding force." However, as mentioned earlier, even though lack of consent is an element of rape in all definitions, the various states do define rape differently, and in 33 states there are still some exemptions given to husbands and common-law partners from sexual assault prosecution. In these states, if a woman is unable to consent under the law (due to altered mental status or mental or physical impairment, etc.), a spouse or cohabitant may be exempt from prosecution (16). The existence of a variety of intimate partner exemptions in these 33 states supports long-standing societal and legal biases that consider IPSA less serious than sexual assaults by other perpetrators. It also harkens back to the 17th century notion that wives are the property of their husbands, who cannot commit a crime against their own property (16).

That the general public still views IPSA to be a lesser crime than sexual assault by perpetrators who do not have an intimate relationship with the victim is supported by substantial evidence. Kirkwood queried a convenience sample of undergraduate students at the University of Maryland concerning their opinions about the seriousness of rape. The criterion used was the relationship between the perpetrator and victim. A subset of students (27%) felt that perpetrator's relationship with the victim made a difference in rape severity; this subset ranked stranger rape a 3.9 and spousal rape a .55 on a crime severity scale of 1 to 4, with 4 having the highest severity. Approximately 30% of male subjects and 20% of female subjects felt that nonconsensual intercourse between spouses was not rape (14). Frese, Moya, and Megias surveyed 182 undergraduate psychology students and asked them to rate perceived severity of rape based on Rape Myth Acceptance theories and perpetrator relationship (17). Even these educated undergraduate students judged stranger rape as more traumatic than rape by an intimate partner, and responded they would be less likely to advise intimate partner rape victims to report the crime to police than victims of stranger or acquaintance rape. Bennice and Resick eloquently summarized this concept with the following statement: "As the victim–offender relationship becomes more intimate, the likelihood that the incident is defined as rape decreases, attribution of blame to the victim increases, and the level of perceived harm decreases" (18).

CURRENT SEXUAL ASSAULT LAWS AND PROSECUTIONS

The explanation of current sexual assault legislation in the United States is complicated by the fact that the country operates under 50 different state legislatures with constantly changing laws, multiple court systems, federal criminal codes, and/or court decisions that may reinterpret, contradict, and/or overlap each other. Further, although prosecution of sexual criminal offenses is most commonly within the state jurisdiction, in specific instances, the federal courts may prosecute. For this purpose, Title 18 of the United States Codes, commonly referred to as the Federal Criminal Code and entitled Crimes and Criminal Procedure, defines aggravated sexual abuse as "sexual abuse by force or threat of force, or sexual abuse by

other means" (Chapter 109A, §2241) (11). Sexual abuse by force or threat of force is aggravated "when a person knowingly causes another person to engage in a sexual act, or attempts to do so, by using force against that person, or by threatening or placing that person in fear that that person will be subjected to death, serious bodily injury, or kidnapping" (§2241) (11). Aggravated sexual abuse by other means occurs "when a person knowingly renders another person unconscious and thereby engages in a sexual act with that other person; or administers to another person by force or threat of force without the knowledge or permission of that person, a drug, intoxicant, or similar substance and thereby (a) substantially impairs the ability of that person to appraise or control conduct and (b) engages in a sexual act with that person" (§2241) (11). State laws and state resources can be found in the National State Coalition List (19).

Successful adjudication of sexual assault crimes has been shown to correlate with young victim age, use of a weapon, and findings of bodily and/or anogenital trauma (20,21). Despite a legal history of minimizing IPSA in the United States, increased prosecution rates for IPSA have recently been noted. One Washington state emergency department–based study of reported sexual assaults in 888 women found that perpetrators of IPSA were three times as likely to be prosecuted as perpetrators of stranger or acquaintance sexual assaults (22). Eighteen years earlier in a Midwestern state, a similar emergency department–based study found the opposite result, with IPSA perpetrators being prosecuted less often than others (23). However, it is likely that a greater percentage of IPSA victims fail to report the assault than do victims assaulted by perpetrators of acquaintance or stranger sexual assault. This likelihood is supported by data from the government-sponsored National Crime Victimization Survey (NCVS), a survey of approximately 77,000 households. This survey found that almost six times as many women victimized by intimates (18%) as those victimized by strangers (3%) said that they did not report their violent victimization to police because they feared perpetrator retaliation (4). One could conjecture that the increased prosecution rate for IPSA found in Wiley's more recent study reflects a selection bias, with the women who were victims of IPSA and presented to the emergency department probably having more severe injuries and therefore being more likely to report the assault (22).

INCIDENCE AND PREVALENCE OF SEXUAL ASSAULT AND INTIMATE PARTNER SEXUAL ABUSE

Quantification of the true incidence of sexual assault in the United States remains problematic due to differing survey methodology, disparate definitions of which acts constitute sexual assault and/or rape, and low disclosure rates by victims for reasons ranging from shame and stigma to fear of revictimization (24). If one examines national incidence data of sexual assaults using reports to law enforcement, the number will grossly underestimate the true incidence of sexual assault, as less than one in five victims report the crime to police (25). The Federal Bureau of Investigation (FBI) compiles such data annually and publishes the data in the Uniform Crime Reports (UCR). According to the UCR, in 2006, law enforcement received reports of "forcible rape" from 92,455 females victims. *Forcible rape*, as defined in the Uniform Crime Reporting Program, "is the carnal knowledge of a female forcibly and against her will. Assaults and attempts to commit rape by force or threat of force are also included." In these 92,455 cases, 24,535 arrests were made, and 40.9% of the cases were cleared by either arrest or other circumstances such as the victim refusing to cooperate with the prosecution (26).

To better obtain the true estimate of sexual assault in the United States, other investigators have performed population-based survey studies. One frequently referenced population-based estimate comes from the National Crime Victimization Survey (NCVS). This random-digit dial telephone survey collects data yearly on nonfatal violent crimes against males and females 12 years of age and older (4). According to this survey data, 261,950 sexual assaults occurred in 2000, and 169,340 occurred in 2003. This study found that 17% of all disclosed sexual assaults were perpetrated by an intimate or formerly intimate partner. The NCVS queries subjects about all sexual assaults, not just rape, but uses only two questions to ask about the events and reduces most events occurring in the prior 6 months to a single reported event. The survey also uses the term "rape" when asking about forced sex, and requires subjects to identify themselves as "rape victims." Because of its methodology, the NCVS is considered by many experts to provide an underestimate of the true incidence of rape and sexual assault in the nation (27).

Another source of information on the national incidence and lifetime prevalence of sexual assault in the United States comes from the National Violence Against Women Survey (NVAWS) a national survey that was conducted from November 1995 to May 1996. This random-digit dial telephone survey of adults, 18 to 65 years of age, queries subjects only about forcible rape, with rape being defined as nonconsensual penetration or attempted penetration of the mouth, anus, or vagina, and then has five follow-up questions to gather information on the events. Using this definition of rape, the NVAWS found 18% of U.S. women and 3% of U.S. men experienced attempted or completed rape at some time in their adult life. Additionally, 7.7% of women experienced intimate partner violence (IPV) rape during their lives, with 0.2% experiencing it in the last 12 months. The calculated 1-year incidence of rape (with average 2.9 rapes per woman who reported any rape that year) from this survey is 876,100 women per year and 111,300 men per year (27). This is a much higher number than that extrapolated from data in the NCVS. Importantly, the NCVS includes victims ages 12 years and older, while NVAWS includes 18 years and older. However, the NCVS definition is more liberal and includes other sexual acts besides rape. The NVAWS uses five questions, while the NCVS only uses two questions to determine the occurrence of rape. As stated before, the NCVS counts many events that occurred in last 6 months as one event, versus the NVAWS, in which all events are recorded separately. These disparate estimates of the yearly incidence of sexual assault from two well-designed national telephone surveys underscore the fact that, despite well-planned research, the true national incidence of sexual assault remains unclear (27,28).

The National Woman's Study (NWS) is a third methodologically sound, population-based sample of women 18 years and older that sought to define, among other elements, the lifetime prevalence of sexual assault and/or rape. In its first wave, which included 4,009 women, this telephone survey study found 15.1% of women reported experiencing a completed rape (29). The NWS used questions that avoid mandating that subjects identify themselves as rape victims, but rather questioned subjects about specific acts. The questions are believed to be more likely to elicit a true response from subjects than are other national population-based studies (27).

Multiple studies of college students reveal a striking risk for sexual assault during those years. Gross' convenience sample of 903 female undergraduate students at the University of Mississippi reported a 27% incidence of unwanted sexual contact and an almost 19% incidence of forced penetration (anal, oral, or vaginal) since college matriculation. Seven percent reported that intercourse without consent was related to drug or alcohol intoxication (30). The 1995 National College Health Risk Behavior Survey found that 20% of students who responded to this mailed survey reported that they had experienced rape in their lifetimes (31). Banyard queried 416 college students in New Hampshire and found that 6% had unwanted intercourse over the previous 6 months. In 50% of those cases, the perpetrator was a partner or former partner (32).

Studies in clinical populations have found an even higher prevalence of sexual assault and also a higher prevalence of IPSA than the just-mentioned population-based samples. Coker's 1997–1998 cross-sectional study of 1,443 women patients ages 18–65 in a family practice setting in Columbia, South Carolina found a lifetime prevalence of IPSA of 23.1%, with 7.7% reporting IPSA in their current relationship. She used three questions from the Index of Spousal Abuse (ISA) to define IPSA: partner hurts you badly during sex, partner physically forces you to have sex, and partner injured your breasts or genitals (33). Feldhaus' survey in Denver of 360 female emergency department patients with current partners found a 39% lifetime prevalence of sexual assault. In 18% of those sexual assaults, the perpetrator was an intimate or formerly intimate partner (34). Another emergency department–based study of women aged 15 years and older presenting for a sexual assault exam found that 12% of 744 victims examined were assaulted by an intimate partner (35). Similarly, Jones found that 21% of the 849 consecutive female sexual assault victims seen at their comprehensive center reported their partner or former partner as the perpetrator (6).

Although rates of sexual assault vary depending on the definition and survey methodology, it is clear from these population-based and clinical studies that at least one in five women suffer abusive sexual acts at some point in their adult lives. Many studies fail to carefully define perpetrators; hence most underestimate the number of sexual assaults perpetrated by a partner or former partner. However, based on the available evidence, it can be seen from the studies surveyed that the percentage of reported sexual assaults perpetrated by a current or former partner is likely to be around 20%.

INTIMATE PARTNER SEXUAL ABUSE WITHIN THE BROADER SCOPE OF SEXUAL ASSAULT AND INTIMATE PARTNER VIOLENCE

Sexual abuse by a partner or former partner remains an under-researched subject, with less than its appropriate representation in the medical and sociologic literature based on the sheer number of events and persons whose lives are marked by such an event. Conversely, the literature is filled with research and analysis of physical and emotional IPV and sexual assault (16). Consequently, most of the available literature examining IPSA does so in the context of how these victims differ from sexual assaults by other perpetrators or how they differ from IPV victims whose perpetrators do not assault them sexually.

Intimate Partner Sexual Abuse Compared to Sexual Assault by a Nonintimate Partner

Data from NVAWS demonstrated that female rape victims reported physical injury 31.5% of the time. However, for the subset of rape victims abused by an intimate partner 36.2% suffered injury and 31% required medical treatment. Logistic regression analysis of that same data, controlling for other variables that increase injury, continued to show that women raped by a partner or former partner were more likely to suffer injury than those raped by an acquaintance with statistical significance (5). Mahoney investigated the impact of victim–offender relationship using NCVS data and determined that a rape victim whose perpetrator was a spouse was more likely to experience repeated rape than a victim who was assaulted by an acquaintance or stranger. In this data set, IPV rape victims were less likely than acquaintance and stranger rape victims to seek help from medical, legal, and social services (36). However, as Mahoney noted, the NCVS data defined married persons as current and former spouses, acquaintances as known assailants, and strangers as unknown or only known by sight. Therefore, the entire category of "boyfriend" became "problematic" for accurate intimate partner reporting (p. 1014). An acquaintance perpetrator could have been anyone from live-in boyfriend to a first date.

Studies in clinical settings have produced similar results. Overall, approximately one-third to one-half of the victims seeking medical examinations for sexual assault reveal genital and/or bodily injuries (37–40). Sugar's clinical report of 744 victims demonstrated that assaults by either strangers or by intimate partners resulted in more than twice the incidence of general body trauma than those by friends or acquaintances (35). Stermac's sample of sexual assault victims seeking forensic examination also demonstrated that spouses/ex-spouses and boyfriends were more likely to use violent force than acquaintances (41). Logan and colleagues reviewed data that showed IPSA victims received fewer genital but more soft-tissue and external injuries than the other groups, in addition to more violent external injuries (9). In their own study, they found that nongenital injuries suffered as a result of IPSA were "even greater than nongenital injuries sustained from strangers" (p. 1072). They used, as their measure of violence, the medical results from records of forensic exams of women who presented to hospital emergency departments. A limitation of their study is that it includes only patients reporting at one hospital, and the study continued over a period of 4 years, thereby gathering somewhat diverse data.

In summary, these studies reveal that sexual abuse perpetrated by partners/ex-partners is at least as violent, if not more so, than sexual assaults perpetrated by strangers or acquaintances. Other studies also seem to indicate that women who experience IPSA also experience increased incidences of sexually transmitted infections (STI) and other infections (42).

Intimate Partner Violence with Sexual Abuse Compared to Intimate Partner Violence Without Sexual Abuse

The trend toward increased severity of abuse can also be found in the subset of IPV victims whose perpetrators use sexual violence, as compared to IPV victims who do not disclose sexual violence. Campbell's 1999 investigation of a convenience sample of 159 IPV victims recruited through the newspaper found that 46% of these victims also reported IPSA by the physically abusive partner. Intimate partner violence victims who were also sexually abused by their partners reported more negative health symptoms, gynecologic symptoms, and risk factors for becoming an IPV homicide victim. There was also a direct correlation in the numbers of sexually abusive events with the severity of symptoms of depression (43). Coker's study of family practice patients found that IPV relationships that also involved sexual abuse were much more violent

than IPV relationships with physical violence alone (33). McFarlane's analysis of IPV victims from the Houston District Attorney's office found that perpetrators of IPSA were more likely than other perpetrators to threaten to harm the children (44). These studies underscore the concern that IPV perpetrators who also use sexual violence against their victims comprise a more violent and dangerous subset of abusers.

HEALTH IMPACT OF INTIMATE PARTNER SEXUAL ABUSE

Physical Health

Multiple studies in various clinical arenas have demonstrated the associations between IPSA and risky sexual practices. In one emergency department–based sample, abused women were almost five times more likely than nonabused women to have had an STI, and four times more likely to engage in high-risk sexual relations (45). The authors suggest the need for the development of HIV risk-reduction strategies that address the needs of women in IPV relationships. Another retrospective case control study found that women experiencing IPV had STIs at rates three times greater than the general population (46). Wingood's survey of 165 young African-American women in San Francisco found those in IPV relationships were less likely than others to use condoms and were much more likely to experience abuse when they discussed condom use with their partners (47). Wingood later studied the risks of STIs related to IPSA (48). In this shelter-based study of 203 IPV victims, the 43% who suffered rape by their partners were also more likely to have an STI. Further, it should also be noted that unprotected sex translates to higher rates of unwanted pregnancy (49). Both sexual assault and IPV treatment and prevention programs must address STI and HIV concerns; conversely, HIV and STI treatment providers must also address IPV prevention, detection, and treatment strategies. Bourassa and Berube found that a disproportionate number of women desirous of elective abortions had suffered IPV, and these researchers concluded that the number was sufficient to justify assessment for IPV during preabortion visits (49).

In 2000, although not specifically addressing IPSA, Gielen and colleagues reported that in a sample of 237 HIV-positive women, 27% had experienced sexual abuse of some sort. The majority (62%) had experienced violence in their history. From these and other studies the authors inferred "high rates of historical violence" that underscored a "need for . . . intervention for domestic violence in all settings that provide health care to women living with HIV" (50). More specifically, Coker concluded after recruiting 1,152 women who reported experiencing psychological (23%), physical, and/or sexual (77%) IPV that the experience may increase the risk of cervical neoplasia (46). Of the women studied, 234 had been diagnosed with cervical dysplasia; 14 actually had cervical cancer. They further noted that their findings were consistent with the findings of several other studies that "reported associations between IPV and STIs, pelvic inflammatory disease, chronic pelvic pain, and bladder, kidney, or other urinary tract infections."

Mental Health

The psychological sequelae of sexual assault have been well described in the literature (51). Victims often develop post-rape symptomatology marked by numbed responsiveness to the external world, sleep disturbances, guilt feelings, memory impairment, activity avoidance, and other manifestations that together are termed *rape trauma syndrome* (RTS). Rape trauma syndrome is a pattern of symptoms, similar to PTSD, first described by Burgess and Holstrom in 1974, after performing a qualitative observational study of rape victims who presented to Boston City Hospital (52). Rape victims are more likely than victims of other crimes to suffer from PTSD and mood disorders as a result of the event (53). Recent research has also demonstrated an increase in suicidality associated with sexual assault. In Tiet's study of more than 34,000 veterans at substance abuse or mental health clinics, those veterans who experienced sexual assault within the prior month had an increased risk of a suicide attempt of almost fivefold those veterans without sexual assault (54). Similarly, the 1995 National College Health Risk Behavior Survey demonstrated that students who suffered a sexual assault were more likely to express suicidality, smoke, and risk drinking while driving than students who lacked such a history (31).

Psychological trauma suffered by IPSA victims often equals or exceeds that found in other types of sexual assault (55). This trauma often begins in adolescence. One study of 81,247 Minnesota high school students found a prevalence of date rape of 4.4% in girls and 3.5% in boys. Those who suffered date rape

were more likely to develop eating disorders and express suicidality (56). Weaver also showed an association of IPSA with suicidality (57). One multicenter population-based survey of 6,024 subjects found that spousal assaults (in addition to repeated assaults, physically threatening assaults, and those resulting in intercourse or sexual disturbances) were most strongly related to subsequent impaired functioning (58). Analysis of data from the NVAWS found that those who suffer injury during sexual assault (such as the case in IPSA) are more likely to suffer resultant PTSD, even when controlling for other factors that cause PTSD (8,29). McFarlane also examined this aspect of IPSA in her study of 148 women IPV victims who presented to the family violence unit of the District Attorney's office in Houston, Texas (44). Among these women, 68% reported IPSA defined as oral, anal, or vaginal intercourse against the victim's will or involving the use of an object on the victim in a sexual way. The victims who suffered IPSA were more likely than other victims to express suicidality and abuse drugs or alcohol. In her study of 62 women suffering from IPV, Bennice also found that sexual violence within the relationship led to greater mental health distress in the form of increased PTSD symptoms (13). Cole examined the physical and mental health consequences of IPSA in a sample of women victims of IPV seeking restraining orders against male perpetrators (59). Multivariate analysis showed that women with sexual victimization within the IPV relationship had significantly more mental health problems than women who lacked a sexual component of IPV. Campbell's sample of 159 IPV victims demonstrated that victims who were also sexually abused by their partner reported more negative health symptoms and increasing numbers of episodes of sexual abuse correlated with increased depression (43). In one series, over one-half of the women sexually abused by spouses or other family members reported three or more rapes by the same perpetrator (6). Hence, among women who suffer physical abuse by a partner, those who also experience IPSA are clearly at increased risk for depression, suicidality, substance abuse, and PTSD (13,43,44).

INTERVENTION FOR VICTIMS OF INTIMATE PARTNER SEXUAL ABUSE

Although IPSA is at least as physically brutal and more likely to lead to mental health sequela as other sexual assaults, IPSA victims are less likely to receive help after the attack. Data from the NVAWS shows that 35% of rape victims receive medical care for injuries suffered from the assault. In this population-based study, IPSA victims were less likely to receive medical treatment after the assault, with only 31% doing so (16). One clinical sample based in an emergency department found a similar trend. Those who reported IPSA were much less likely to report the event or obtain services than were those assaulted by a stranger. Victims of IPSA were significantly less likely to report the assault to police (18% versus 79%), to receive medical care (29% versus 70%), or to contacted a social service agency (24% versus 30%) (34). After IPSA victims do make the decision to get help, they may be more likely to follow through with care. Stermac's cross-sectional study of 547 women presenting for a sexual assault examination reported that the victims who were assaulted by intimates were more likely to present with a shorter postcoital interval and more likely to complete a forensic exam than were those assaulted by other categories of perpetrators (41). Sexual assault by an intimate partner is likely to be repeated over and over again, with the majority of events never disclosed to anyone. It may take days, weeks, months, or even years for victims to view nonconsensual intercourse as rape (60). It appears that there may be a certain threshold of violence or serious threats that leads a victim to eventually break the silence. Once this threshold is reached and they seek help, victims may be more intent on completing the process.

IMPLICATIONS FOR POLICY, PRACTICE, AND RESEARCH

Policy

- Some state laws must be amended to make charges filed against perpetrators of IPSA crimes as severe as other sexual assault charges.
- Governmental and private agencies that supply funding to IPV support services must ensure that advocates and peer counselors receive adequate training in IPSA.
- Governmental and private agencies that supply funding to sexual assault support services must ensure that advocates and peer counselors receive adequate training in IPSA.

- Intimate partner violence advocacy organizations must work with the media and criminal justice professionals to dispel myths and biases surrounding IPSA and spousal rape.
- Educators of middle and high school students must specifically include course work on healthy relationships and the topic of voluntary consent for sexual relationships for both male and female adolescents.

Practice

- Sexual assault response teams must be trained to address the complexities and different needs of victims of IPSA, including the recognition and documentation of various forms of sexual abuse often experienced by victims of IPSA.
- Sexual assault forensic documentation forms should be modified to include space to record additional history of assaultive behavior often experienced by victims of IPSA.
- Sexual abuse by a partner or former partner should trigger an immediate referral to an advocate skilled in IPV counseling, if this not provided by the sexual assault advocate.
- Clinicians need to be aware of legal obligations to contact legal authorities, who may provide an emergency protective order (EPO), with specific regard to IPV crimes, including IPSA.
- Clinicians should routinely inquire about a history of past or present sexual abuse in all patients and be prepared to assist patient's medical and psychosocial needs.

Research

- Explore the efficacy of sexual assault prevention programs that target youth by designing long-term outcome population-based studies.
- Investigators should partner with state marriage licensing boards to perform a randomized controlled trial of spousal rape prevention. For instance, the board could provide information about spousal rape and appropriate consent to a random sample of couples seeking marriage licenses and determine the incidence of subsequent spousal rape in the intervention group versus an uninformed control group over time.
- Evaluate the efficacy of various cognitive, psychological, pharmacologic, and behavioral

treatments for the mental health consequences suffered by victims of IPSA.

- Evaluate the effectiveness of early intervention to prevent the onset of PTSD in IPSA victims.

References

1. Groth S. *Evaluation and management of the sexually assaulted or sexually abused patient.* Dallas, Texas: American College of Emergency Physicians, 1999.
2. *Merriam-Webster's Dictionary of Law.* Merriam-Webster, Inc., 1996.
3. Basile K. Rape by acquiescence: The ways in which women "give in" to unwanted sex with their husbands. *Violence Against Women.* 1999;5(9): 1036–1058.
4. Rennison CM. Bureau of Justice Statistics; National Crime Victimization Survey; Criminal Victimization. *Violence Against Women.* 2000;5:1036–1058.
5. Tjaden P, Thoennes N. *Full report of the prevalence, incidence, and consequences of violence against women: Findings from the National Violence Against Women Survey.* National Institute of Justice Centers for Disease Control and Prevention (NIJCDC), 2000.
6. Jones J, Wynn B, Kroeze B, et al. Comparison of sexual assault by strangers versus known assailants in a community-based population. *Am J Emerg Med.* 2004;22(6):454–459.
7. Shackelford T, Goetz A. Men's sexual coercion in intimate relationships: Development and initial validation of the sexual coercion in intimate relationships scale. *Violence Victims.* 2004;19(5):541–556.
8. Temple J, Weston R, Rodriguez B, Marshall L. Differing effects of partner and non-partner sexual assault on women's mental health. *Violence Against Women.* 2007;13:285–297.
9. Logan T, Cole J, Capillo A. Differential characteristics of intimate partner, acquaintance and stranger rape survivors examined by a sexual assault nurse examiner (SANE). *J Interpersonal Violence.* 2007;22:1066–1076.
10. Basile K, Arias D, Desai S, Thompson M. The differential association of intimate partner physical, sexual, psychological and stalking violence and posttraumatic stress symptoms in a nationally representative sample of women. *J Traumatic Stress.* 2004;17(5):413–421.
11. Crimes and Criminal Procedure, 18 US Court, §2241–2246 (2005).
12. Bergen R. Marital rape. *Applied research forum: National electronic network on violence against women,* 1999. At http://www.vaw.umn.edu/vawnet/. Accessed 9/27/2007.
13. Bennice J, Resick P. Marital rape: history, research, and practice. *Trauma Violence Abuse.* 2003;4(3): 228–246.
14. Kirkwood MK, Cecil DK. Marital rape: A student assessment of rape laws and the marital exemption. *Violence Against Women.* 2001 2001;7(11): 1234–1253.
15. X L. Accomplishing the impossible: An advocate's notes from the successful campaign to make marital and date rape a crime in all 50 US states and other countries. *Violence Against Women.* 1999;5(9):1064–1081.
16. Bergen R. Studying wife rape: Reflections on the past, present, and future. *Violence Against Women.* 2004;10(12):1407–1416.
17. Frese B, Moya M, Megius J. Social perception of rape: How rape myth acceptance modulates the influence of situational factors. *J Interpersonal Violence.* 2004;19(2):143–161.
18. Bennice J, Resick P, Mechanic M, Astin M. The relative effects of intimate partner physical and sexual violence on post-traumatic stress disorder symptomatology. *Violence Victims.* 2003;18(1):87–94.
19. State Coalition List. 2005. At http://www.ncadv.org/resources/StateCoalitionList_73.html. Accessed 11/1/2008.
20. Rambow B, Adkinson C, Frost T, Peterson G. Female sexual assault: Medical and legal implications. *Ann Emerg Med.* 1992;21(6):727–731.
21. McGregor M, DuMont J, Myhr T. Sexual assault forensic medical examination: Is evidence related to successful prosecution? *Ann Emerg Med.* 2002;39(6):639–647.
22. Wiley J, Sugar N, Fine D, Eckert L. Legal outcomes of sexual assault. *Am J Obstet Gynecol.* 2003;188(6):1638–1641.
23. Tintinalli JE, Hoelzer M. Clinical findings and legal resolution in sexual assault. *Ann Emerg Med.* 1985;14(5):447–453.
24. Fanlick P. Victim responses to sexual assault: Counterintuitive or simply adaptive? At http://www.ndaa.org. Accessed 09/02/2007.
25. Resnick H, Acierno R, Holmes M, et al. Predictors of post-rape medical care in a national sample of women. *Am J Prevent Med.* 2000;19(4): 214–219.
26. Federal Bureau of Investigation. *Uniform Crime Report: Crime in the United States* (2006). Washington DC: Department of Justice, Federal Bureau of Investigation, 2007.
27. Kilpatrick D, Ruggerio K. Making sense of rape in America: Where do the numbers come from and what do they mean? *J Interpersonal Violence.* 2004;19:1204–1234.
28. Tjaden P, Thoennes N. Full report of the prevalence, incidence and consequences of violence against women: Findings from the national violence against women survey. Washington DC: *National Institute of Justice,* 2000.
29. Acierno R, Resnick H, Kilpatrick D, et al. Risk factors for rape, physical assault, and posttraumatic stress disorder in women: Examination of

differential multivariate relationships. *J Anxiety Disorders*. 1999;13(3):541–563.

30. Gross A, Winslett A, Roberts M, Gohm C. An examination of sexual violence against college women. *Violence Against Women*. 2006;12(18):288–300.

31. Brener N, McMahon P, Warren C, Douglas C. Forced sexual intercourse and associated health-risk behaviors among female college students in the United States. *J Consult Clin Psychol*. 1999;67(2):252–259.

32. Banyard V, Plante E, Cohn C, et al. Revisiting unwanted sexual experiences on campus: A 12-year follow-up. *Violence Against Women*. 2005;11(4):426–446.

33. Coker A, Smith P, McKeown R, King M. Frequency and correlates of intimate partner violence by type: Physical, sexual, and psychological battering. *Am J Pub Health*. 2000;90:533–539.

34. Feldhaus K, Houry D, Kaminsky R. Lifetime sexual assault prevalence rates and reporting practices in an emergency department population. *Ann Emerg Med*. 2000;36(1):23–27.

35. Sugar N, Fine D, Eckert L. Physical injury after sexual assault: Findings of a large case series. *Am J Obstet Gynecol*. 2004;190(1):71–76.

36. Mahoney P. High rape chronicity and low rates of help-seeking among wife rape survivors in a non-clinical sample. *Violence Against Women*. 1999;5(9):993–1013.

37. Gray-Eurom K, Seaberg D, Wears R. The prosecution of sexual assault cases: Correlation with forensic evidence. *Ann Emerg Med*. 2002;39(1):39–46.

38. Lauber A, Souma M. Use of toluidine blue for documentation of traumatic intercourse. *Obstet Gynecol*. 1982;60(5):644–648.

39. Grossin C. Analysis of 418 cases of sexual assault. *Forensic Sci Intern*. 2003;131(2–3):125–130.

40. Riggs N, Houry D, Long G, et al. Analysis of 1.076 cases of sexual assault. *Ann Emerg Med*. 2000;35(4):358–362.

41. Stermac L, Del Bove G, Addison M. Violence, injury, and presentation patterns in spousal sexual assaults. *Violence Against Women*. 2001;7(11):1218–1233.

42. Gielen AC, O'Campo PJ, Campbell JC, et al. Women's opinions about domestic violence screening and mandatory reporting. *Am J Prevent Med*. 2000;19(4):279–285.

43. Campbell J, Soeken K. Forced sex and intimate partner violence: Effects on women's risk and women's health. *Violence Against Women*. 1999;5(9):1017–1035.

44. McFarlane J, Malecha A. Intimate partner sexual assault against women and associated victim substance use, suicidality and risk factors for femicide. *Issues Mental Health Nurs*. 2005;26(9):953–967.

45. El-Bassel N, Gilbert L, Krishnan S, et al. Partner violence and sexual HIV-risk behaviors among women in an inner-city emergency department. *Violence Victims*. Winter 1998;13(4):377–393.

46. Coker A, Sanderson M, Fadden M, Pirisi L. Frequency and correlates of intimate partner violence by type: Physical, sexual and psychological battering. *Am J Pub Health*. 2000;90(4):553–559.

47. Wingood G, DiClemente R. The effects of an abusive primary partner on the condom use and sexual negotiation practices of African-American women. *Am J Pub Health*. 1997;87(6):1016–1018.

48. Wingood G, DiClemente R, Raj A. Identifying the prevalence and correlates of STDs among women residing in rural domestic violence shelters. *Women's Health*. 2000;30(4):15–26.

49. Bourassa D, Berube J. The prevalence of intimate partner violence among women and teenagers seeking abortion compared with those continuing pregnancy. *J Obstet Gynaecol Can*. 2007;29(5).

50. Gielen A, Fogarty L, O'Campo P, et al. Women living with HIV: Disclosure, violence, and social support. *J Urban Health: Bull NY Acad Med*. 2000;77(3):480–491.

51. Winfield I, George L, Swartz M. Sexual assault and psychiatric disorders among a community sample of women. *Am J Psychiatry*. 1990;147(3):335–341.

52. Burgess A, Holmstrom L. Rape trauma syndrome. *Am J Psychiatry*. 1974;131(9):981–986.

53. Faravelli C, Giugni A, Salnatori S, Ricca V. Psychopathology after rape. *Am J Psychiatry*. 2004;161(8):1483–1485.

54. Tiet Q, Finney J, Moos R. Recent sexual abuse, physical abuse, and suicide attempts among male veterans seeking psychiatric treatment. *Psychiatric Serv*. 2006;57(1):107–113.

55. Koss M, Gidycz C, Wisniewski N. The scope of rape: Incidence and prevalence of sexual aggression and victimization in a national sample of higher education students. *J Consult Clin Psychol*. 1987;55(2):162–170.

56. Ackard D, Neumark-Sztainer D. Date violence and date rape among adolescents: Associations with disordered eating behaviors and psychological health. *Child Abuse Neglect*. 2002;26(5):455–473.

57. Weaver T, Allen J, Hopper E, et al. Mediators of suicidal ideation within a sheltered sample of raped and battered women. *Health Care Women Intern*. 2007;28(5):478–489.

58. Golding J. Sexual assault history and limitations in physical functioning in two general population samples. *Res Nurs Health*. 1996;19(1):33–44.

59. Cole J, Logan T, Shannon L. Intimate sexual victimization among women with protective orders: Types and associations of physical and mental health problems. *Violence Vict*. 2005;20(6):695–715.

60. Harned M. Understanding women's labeling of unwanted sexual experiences with dating partners: A qualitative analysis. *Violence Against Women*. 2005;11(3):374–413.

Chapter 20

A Public Health Approach to Intimate Partner Violence

Meghan E. Howe and Elaine J. Alpert

KEY CONCEPTS

- Public health is a multidisciplinary, collaborative, science-based, and advocacy-oriented approach to the health of populations.
- Intimate partner violence (IPV) impacts the mental and physical well-being of many individuals, which in turn impacts the health, safety, and economy of communities. Therefore, it is a public health problem.
- The public health approach involves four steps: surveillance, risk factor identification, intervention, and dissemination of effective interventions.
- An effective public health response to IPV occurs on three levels: a primary approach to prevent IPV, a secondary approach to minimize the chronic impact of IPV, and a tertiary approach to respond to critical cases.
- To understand if an intervention program works and why, formative, process, and outcome evaluation must be incorporated into an intervention from the development stages.
- The social-ecological model is useful for mapping the multiple influences on IPV, and the Spectrum of Prevention is a useful framework for planning comprehensive interventions.
- Most healthcare and public health professionals will be exposed to IPV in their careers, and thus need to develop core competencies for addressing the issue.

Although we must be ready to provide care for . . . victims of violence, it is critical that we also find ways to prevent injuries, disabilities, and deaths from violence from occurring in the first place, or from recurring. The public health approach looks for ways to interrupt the cycle of violence and stop a pattern that often begins in infancy and childhood and carries over into adulthood . . . The public health approach with its emphasis on prevention complements the work done

in [other] areas . . . The public health approach
also stresses the importance of bridging not only
different disciplines, but also different parts of
government, the private and public sectors, practi-
tioners and researchers, racial and ethnic groups,
and conservative and liberal ideas. Effective solu-
tions will also bridge the gap between those who
want to study the problem to find out what works
before taking action and those who sense the
urgency to do something now (1).

Linda Saltzman, Ph.D. and
Denise Johnson, MS (1996)

An understanding of public health as a discipline, and
of the public health approach to understanding and
addressing complex health and social welfare issues,
is critical to the development, implementation, and
dissemination of successful intervention and prevention strategies. The multidisciplinary nature of
public health is ideally suited to a prevention-focused
response to intimate partner violence (IPV). This
chapter will provide an overview of the discipline
of public health and will introduce a public health
perspective into our examination of IPV.

Public health addresses complex endemic, epidemic, and pandemic problems from a science-based,
multidisciplinary vantage point. The work of public
health is accomplished by organizing and coordinating the efforts of diverse disciplines, such as healthcare, public safety, and community advocacy. The
public health approach provides an effective framework for developing a prevention-focused, coordinated
response to IPV. Viewing IPV as a public health problem is not an attempt to preempt work being done in
other fields; rather, it is an effort to organize the work
being done and address complex problems in a manner that is systematic, pragmatic, and sustainable.

DEFINING AND UNDERSTANDING
PUBLIC HEALTH

Public health, broadly speaking, refers to the health of
communities or populations, as opposed to the health
of individuals. Public health addresses the big picture,
looking at the health of populations overall, bringing
together diverse viewpoints, and making informed
recommendations on addressing problems. The field
of public health maintains a broad definition, so that
it is able to address the full range of factors that affect
quality of life for individuals and communities.

According to the American Public Health Association, the mission of public health is to "promote physical and mental health and prevent disease, injury, and
disability. . . . Both distinct from and encompassing
clinical services, public health's role is to assure the
conditions necessary for people to live healthy lives,
through community-wide prevention and protection
programs." Alpert and colleagues define public health
as "a prevention-focused, multidisciplinary, collaborative, culturally sensitive, science-based discipline that
is focused on the health of populations and on the
social, emotional, and physical well-being of communities" (2).

Science-based advocacy using the public health
approach can be a powerful tool for health, safety,
and lasting social change. It is for these reasons that
the knowledge and expertise gained through the lens
of public health can be key to the intervention and
prevention of IPV. Anything that stands in the way of
the well-being of an individual or a community can be
considered a public health problem. Although some
may consider this definition to be too broad, most
public health practitioners would argue that narrower
distinctions would be artificial. The well-being of individuals and communities is dependent on a variety of
interdependent factors, including everything from
genetic predisposition to disease to the unemployment rate. Decades of research, as well as common
sense, tells us that the physical and mental health of
individuals is dependent on biological, environmental, and social factors, and a response that does not
consider all three would be incomplete, at best. The
field of public health considers the entire interwoven
web of determinants in order to meet a mandate of
improving the public's health.

Characteristics of Public Health

Five characteristics of public health, taken together,
distinguish the field from clinical healthcare disciplines (3,4).

Public Health Is Multidisciplinary

Public health is a discrete discipline in and of itself.
That said, the aggregate expertise of scholars and
practitioners from a multiplicity of perspectives
comprise an expanding body of knowledge on public health issues, and thus help create a dynamic
coordinated public health response that may be

geographically and culturally tailored. The fields of health care, law enforcement, education, human services, and many others need to contribute their own expertise both individually and in combination to address the multiple and interrelated complexities of IPV.

Public Health is Collaborative

The various disciplines contributing to the public health response to IPV, or to any other public health problem, must cooperate, communicate, and collaborate in order to affect a lasting and beneficial response. A key role of the public health practitioner is to assemble diverse stakeholders, particularly those who would not naturally work together, and encourage respectful sharing of information and the development of a science-based, culturally competent, coordinated response. In addition to a spectrum of more traditional professional fields, nontraditional service providers; patients or clients; and members of the community need to be involved in the public health response to IPV.

Public Health Is Science-Based

Public health uses science to identify, describe, and solve complex health and social welfare problems. Public health incorporates theoretical and applied research into the development and implementation of programs, and then evaluates their effectiveness so that resources can be focused on initiatives that work. Rigorous research and careful evaluation are key to sound public health practice. These tasks take time, money, effort, and creativity, and can be quite challenging, particularly when fast, simple answers are sought in the wake of tragedy or in response to fear or threat. A science- or evidence-based approach ensures that implemented programs have an optimal chance of being lasting and efficacious.

Public Health Is Advocacy-Oriented

Public health practitioners translate new knowledge into action in order to inform policy and funding decisions, advocate for program implementation, and guide further work in the field. Many public health practitioners are passionate about their work and do not shy away from taking a strong, proactive advocacy stance, which is informed by science.

Public Health Is Population-Focused

Clinically focused health and human service professions are, by definition, oriented toward the care of individuals, not populations. Public health takes a broader, population-oriented view, focusing on the community as a whole (or at times segments of a community), and the range of risk and resilience in individuals in their roles as members of a culture, community, or society. Whereas acute clinical strategies may yield substantial, and at times life-saving benefit for individuals, the community at-large may not see a benefit. Conversely, population strategies that yield maximum benefit for a community may yield little or no benefit for a given individual. The small percentage of the population that is at very high risk often does not benefit directly from population-based prevention and intervention. However, a substantial percentage of those who are at low to medium risk may derive a great deal of benefit. We can see that the interests and needs of individuals and those of the community may conflict, particularly in fiscally constrained times. This conflict is known as the "prevention paradox" (5). One of the tasks of public health, therefore, is to try to strike a balance between individual and community needs, and to advocate for judicious and balanced allocation of resources geared to both intervention and prevention.

THE PUBLIC HEALTH APPROACH

An issue becomes a public health problem when it is transformed from the realm of the *given* to that of the *unacceptable*. To apply the public health approach to the intervention and prevention of IPV, we must focus attention and resources on naming the problem itself, understanding its epidemiology, identifying risk factors, developing and evaluating prevention-focused programs, and disseminating programs that are shown to be effective, or that at least have promise in defined populations. A science-based understanding of the perspectives of stakeholders, particularly those of vulnerable populations such as survivors, children, and community residents, is key to an effective public health response to IPV. Understanding attributes such as safety, autonomy, and resilience; and addressing in a culturally sensitive manner issues such as housing, employment, and literacy are essential components of the public health response to IPV (6,7).

The "public health approach" involves four basic steps: (1) surveillance, (2) risk factor identification, (3) intervention, and (4) dissemination (8).

Surveillance: Identify, Define, and Describe the Problem

As aptly put by Saltzman and Johnson, (1), the key question that is asked in this stage is, "What is the problem and how big is it?" When public health practitioners are faced with a new problem, they attempt to gather as much information as they can about its scope, magnitude, and impact, and they put the problem into a context of what is known about the problem itself or similar issues. It is the job of public health to "connect the dots," by naming an issue as a problem, describing who is being affected and how, and elucidating commonalities among different cases. In the case of IPV, early, groundbreaking work by Stark and Flitcraft (9); Martin (10); Straus, Gelles, and Steinmetz (11); Burgess (12); and others helped to define and describe the problem by identifying recurring patterns of signs and symptoms, thus giving a name and a sense of urgency to a previously silent epidemic.

Risk Factor Identification: Delineate Risk Factors

Public health is prevention-focused, so in addition to treating those affected by health issues, the field attempts to discern which categories of people are most at risk and in need of early interventions or other services. The main question at this step is, "What is the cause of the problem?" Addressing this phase of inquiry is often the purview of epidemiologists working in partnership with others. The second step attempts to find differences between those who are impacted by a health issue and those who are not, and then confirm a relationship between risk and outcome through experiment or observation.

Intervention: Develop, Implement, and Evaluate Interventions

The main question at this step is, "What works to prevent the problem, and how do we know that it works?" Once an issue has been described and risk factors are known, interventions are developed to address the issue itself and its risk factors. Once an intervention has been implemented, it must be evaluated to determine its effectiveness in addressing the problem. Types of public health interventions and methods of evaluation are discussed in more detail later.

Dissemination: Promote and Replicate Promising Programs

The question asked at this step is, "How can we employ effective models on a larger scale?" To promote science-based programming, public health encourages the replication of programs that are evaluated and show promise. Researchers and practitioners share information by publishing and disseminating details of program implementation and evaluation, by forming collaborations to replicate programs, and by communicating formally and informally with colleagues. Public health tries to avoid "reinventing the wheel." Promising programs are often distributed widely, modified for use with different populations, and then evaluated again.

EXAMPLE OF PUBLIC HEALTH APPROACH TO INTIMATE PARTNER VIOLENCE

The hypothetical example (Sidebar 20.1) illustrates the four steps of the public health approach more clearly with respect to IPV.

The emergency department staff in a local hospital notice that some women present on multiple occasions with broken bones, contusions, burns and other injuries, and that the explanations given for these traumatic events are not consistent with the observed injury patterns. Each time, the emergency department staff treats the injuries; however, one day, a physician and a nurse raise the question that the injuries may not be accidental but intentionally inflicted. They worry that the injuries may be just the tip of the iceberg in terms of the patient's health and safety needs. They hypothesize that if they can stop the injury from occurring in the first place, or stop it from occurring again, the patient's overall health might improve and precious healthcare resources could be recovered.

Sidebar 20.1 Case Study.

Step 1: Identify, Define, and Describe the Problem

The emergency department staff will ask, what is happening here? Are we seeing a pattern or trend, or are we "just" a busy emergency department with many patients of all kinds? What are the characteristics of these cases, and how do they compare to our understanding of how IPV presents in emergency settings? What is the scope and magnitude of the problem? The physicians decide to discuss the issue with hospital-based psychologists and social workers, local epidemiologists from the state public health department, and advocates from the local domestic violence agency.

The staff determines that the physical injuries they are seeing are consistent with signs of abuse, and an informal chart review of visits over the past 12 months shows that 20% of emergency department visits for women fit this pattern. Further, these patients seem to have a higher than usual frequency of visits to the emergency department for nontrauma causes, including alcohol and other drug intoxication, suicide attempts, headaches, back pain, and other medical and psychiatric ailments. Considering the prevalence of IPV as reported in the literature and the hospital's catchment area, the staff estimates that 22 per 1,000 women may be affected by abuse requiring medical attention in a given year. They identify IPV as a health problem in their community, and also acknowledge that routine inquiry for abuse has not been undertaken in the emergency department. They proceed to move to the next step in respect to female patients, and agree to conduct further inquiry into the possibility of victimization of males, both in heterosexual and same-sex relationships. They agree to seek a better understanding of risk factors in the patients they see, and to develop a questionnaire for use in the emergency department.

Step 2: Delineate Risk Factors

Now that IPV has been identified as an important problem in their patient population, the emergency department staff and their colleagues want to identify cases of IPV more efficiently, and to prevent new, recurrent, or more severe cases in their patient population. They also suspect that they have not been seeing every case of IPV occurring in the community served by the emergency department. Some women have never come to the emergency department, some came only once, some come repeatedly. There also may be males who are victims and have been neither identified nor helped. They know that they need to better address the needs of those women who had come to the emergency department in the past, but they also want to prevent new cases and reach women, and men, who may be abused but have not sought care in the emergency department. Therefore, they have to determine what the risk factors for abuse are in their patient population. They review the literature on IPV and meet with community-based experts to learn what risk factors are known, and they compare their new knowledge with the data they accrued in the first step. In their community, they find one pattern that was previously unrecognized. Women who are unemployed or new to the country seem more likely to be abused. The group decides to focus on unemployed, immigrant women, who make up the majority of the cases they have seen in the last 12 months.

Step 3: Develop, Implement, and Evaluate Interventions

The emergency department staff already refers confirmed cases to the local IPV agency, but they want to identify and refer more patients, and also implement a prevention program. They partner with the local IPV agency and brainstorm about how the problem they have identified can be addressed with the resources available to them. Why are unemployed immigrant women more likely to be abused? Perhaps their home environments are more strained because of lack of income. Maybe they are isolated in their homes because of physical restraint, language or cultural barriers, or lack of familiarity with American laws and customs. Maybe they are unable to support themselves and their children independently, and therefore remain in abusive relationships to assure food and shelter. Perhaps some are undocumented and fear deportation if they identify themselves to "authorities" by seeking help. The planning group reviews dozens of ideas, and they focus on the isolation and economic dependence that these women may be experiencing. They review the literature, and identify a domestic violence program that focuses on job skills as a means of helping women achieve safety and independence through economic self-sufficiency.

The IPV agency secures funding to develop and pilot a job-skills program, which it implements in partnership with the emergency department over a

2-year period. Women who present to the emergency department with injuries or illnesses suspicious for IPV, plus all women identified by the newly developed screening tool, are invited to participate in the program. The emergency department, in partnership with the IPV agency, incorporates an evaluation component into the program that measures the number of women who are identified as IPV survivors in the emergency department, and also tracks referrals to the job skills program, attendance, job placement, job retention, and subsequent visits to the emergency department. The new IPV and emergency department partners also work with the local court to track requests for orders of protection over time. At the end of the program, the evaluation shows that the program is both known and well received in the community, and that the number of women enrolling in and completing the job skills program has increased. They also demonstrate that the number of women presenting to the emergency department with minor injuries has decreased, and that the number of requests for orders of protection has increased. However, the evaluation also showed the number of women presenting to the emergency department with severe injuries did not decrease, and that those experiencing severe violence were less likely to participate in the job skills program.

Step 4: Disseminate Promising Programs

The emergency department staff and the IPV agency publish their findings, and the results are seen by nurses in another community who have made similar observations about women presenting with injury. The nurses consult with the emergency department/IPV partners to help them implement a similar program in their community. However, they modify the program to add a hotline component for women who cannot leave their homes to attend the job training program in an attempt to reach out to those experiencing severe abuse. They also develop a revised evaluation tool to track their success, and the process begins again.

The public health approach requires "thinking outside the box" and open-minded collaboration, and does not need to be done exclusively by "public health officials." The public health approach provides guidance for addressing virtually any problem related to health and safety, and leaves room for flexibility and creativity while encouraging action that is science-based and geared to prevention and advocacy.

THE EVOLUTION OF PREVENTION

Once a new public health problem is identified, society's response follows a predictable evolutionary trajectory. Key to understanding the evolution of society's response to IPV are the concepts of primary, secondary, and tertiary prevention (13). Each prevention strategy has a different goal and therefore different approach. We will begin by looking at the response to the most severe and immediate need, the tertiary response.

The tertiary response, also called *tertiary prevention*, is an immediate response to crisis, designed to prevent a severe outcome. Medical personnel, police, and other first responders provide tertiary prevention services on a daily basis. Tertiary prevention responses to IPV include crisis hotline services, emergency shelter admissions, law enforcement responses to calls for assistance, and assistance with applications for emergency orders of protection.

Tertiary prevention is the most immediate response to an urgent or newly conceptualized health need, and it is often the logical initial response to an emerging public health problem. Pioneers in IPV work concerned themselves first with the immediate safety needs of victims, such as emergency police action, care in an emergency department, or refuge in a shelter. Such services, often life-saving, are provided to a small number of individuals at substantial cost, yet funders can nonetheless be assured that those receiving services are truly in need of them. Although effective in reaching individuals in dire need, the tertiary response is, by necessity, reactive and is not designed to prevent a problem from occurring in the first place. To further safeguard the public's health, more proactive responses must be used.

Secondary prevention services, often developed and implemented later in society's awareness of a new public health problem, are provided as a means of detecting an otherwise unapparent problem early in its course, so as to prevent later or more severe complications. Secondary prevention strategies also can be provided to individuals who previously faced a crisis situation and are now trying to manage its chronic manifestations, thus avoiding more serious complications in the future. Inquiring about IPV in the healthcare setting is essential to secondary prevention, as routine inquiry (called "screening" by some) aids in case finding and early disclosure, and helps direct patients to supportive services before an existing, yet nonemergent abusive situation deteriorates. Alternatively, an individual who has disclosed abuse may decide to join a support group, thereby reducing her sense of isolation and disempowerment, and learning safety and self-esteem strategies to negotiate the future. Both are examples of secondary prevention at work. Secondary interventions may include routine inquiry for "subclinical" abuse that may exist in a state prior to being clinically obvious to the practitioner, and providing clinical services for survivors and their children in order to maintain or improve their health and safety. Identification through routine inquiry and early intervention services incur lower costs per case than tertiary services, but may need to be provided over a longer period of time and to a larger segment of the population, including to some who may never need them (i.e., those who may be asked about abuse but are not victims). Since providers cannot see into the future, they cannot know who might benefit from secondary prevention, thus a wider population net must be cast for secondary prevention programs to work. It bears notice that routine inquiry regarding IPV, even when negative, is almost universally remembered and appreciated by patients. The simple act of inquiring serves as a useful tool for patient education and awareness about IPV, and becomes a valuable intervention that changes the social norm.

Secondary prevention can be essential in improving the outlook for those whose IPV is disclosed as a result of being asked, or in improving the quality of life and preventing further adverse outcomes for someone who has survived a crisis. However, secondary prevention strategies do not prevent a given problem from occurring in the first place. To fulfill the public health goal of population-based prevention, we must look to the final and most challenging level of response, primary prevention.

Primary prevention has the potential to make the most significant impact on a population and to promote lasting social change by preventing a health problem from occurring entirely. Although primary prevention efforts tend to be long-range in scope, they are of value to society because they reduce the need for more resource-intensive secondary and tertiary prevention services. It takes a long time, however, to see the effects of primary prevention, and it is not easy to measure that which *doesn't happen*. It is also difficult to obtain funding for primary prevention efforts, precisely because of the long timeline involved and the lack of prompt political payoff for those whose job

it is to allocate funds. Despite this, effective primary prevention is generally considered the ultimate goal of public health.

The aim of primary prevention in IPV is to change social norms about what kind of behavior is normative, acceptable, or desirable in a relationship. Examples of primary prevention initiatives include social norms-oriented violence prevention education programs in schools and programs that focus on changing social norms about men's involvement as partners and allies in the prevention of IPV. Primary prevention programs cost little per person, but they must be provided to a significant percentage of the population and for a very long time in order to be effective. Some may view primary prevention as an unnecessary expense, lacking in tangible benefit, which takes resources away from those "most in need." However, this is the only strategy that has the potential to change social attitudes regarding violence, and truly prevent victimization from occurring. Primary prevention, if executed in a well-thought-out manner, can be very powerful. For this reason, public health practitioners argue that it is worthwhile to devote resources directed toward primary prevention as soon as is feasible, so the entire population can benefit and ultimately reduce the need for crisis-related and survivor services. That being said, it is unrealistic to assume that primary prevention is the answer to all public health issues. A comprehensive public health response incorporates integrated interventions at all three levels.

Although primary prevention is the ultimate goal, programs focused on this strategy are difficult to implement and prove successful, and difficult to fund. As a science-based discipline, public health practitioners judge their success on the measurable outcomes of their programs. In addition, stakeholders in the process, including the government, members of the public, and funders, expect a tangible benefit from public health programs in order to justify the continued use of resources. When tertiary and secondary prevention efforts are successful, that tangible benefit is usually very clear. Because it is nearly impossible to measure that which has not occurred, when a primary prevention campaign is successful in preventing a negative outcome, there often is uncertainty as to whether the campaign was truly successful, or whether there was nothing to prevent in the first place and resources were wasted. This dilemma is exacerbated with IPV because the problem is so vastly underreported. Because of variations in definition and reporting, and multiple challenges to disclosure, it is difficult to "measure" IPV. Thus, determining trends over time and gauging the success of interventions are daunting, yet by no means impossible, tasks. To achieve the public health goal of science-based prevention, well-conceived and executed evaluation strategies should be incorporated into program design and implementation. The next section provides a summary of evaluation methods used in public health.

EVALUATION AS A CRITICAL FUNCTION OF PUBLIC HEALTH

Evaluation is often thought of as a post-hoc activity that takes place at the end of a program to see if it worked. Although outcome evaluation is a necessary component of program assessment, it is only one part of what is needed to assess the value of programs and services. Evaluation clearly serves the function of assessing outcomes; in other words, determining whether a program did what it's supposed to do. However, evaluation serves several other functions as well, and the evaluation process needs to begin even before the intervention commences.

There are three major types, or levels, of evaluation: formative, process, and summative or outcome.

Table 20.1 lists each category of evaluation, its main purpose, and examples of evaluation activities.

The first type of evaluation, formative evaluation, informs an intervention before it begins. Formative evaluation ensures that the proposed program truly meets the needs of the target population, and that the program staff are asking the right questions and placing emphasis on appropriate components of the planned program (14). Through the use of one-on-one interviews or surveys with stakeholders, focus groups, and public forums, formative evaluation helps the practitioner learn more about the intended audience and its needs and preferences for emerging content. This process helps the designer, during the early development stages, increase the likelihood that the final product will achieve its stated goals (15). For example,

> Funding is secured to adapt an IPV poster campaign, originally designed for an English-speaking audience, for use with Latina immigrants in a community. The desired outcome of the program is to increase calls to the local hotline, which has just added Spanish-speaking staff.

Formative evaluation, undertaken at the earliest stages of a planned intervention, may reveal that in addition to the obvious need to translate the words on

Table 20.1 Program Evaluation Summary

Category	Purpose/Question	Examples
Formative	Does the program make sense?	• Focus group with target population • One-to-one interviews with prospective participants • One-to-one interviews with key informants and opinion leaders • Public forums
Process	Is the program being implemented as intended?	• Inspections of participant attendance records • Audits of log books and other program materials • Direct observation of program in process • Participant "satisfaction" surveys • Interviews with program staff
Outcome/summative	Is the program effective?	• Post-test (immediate and follow-up) • Measurements of morbidity and mortality over time

the informational poster into Spanish, messages and images on the posters do not reflect the cultural values and priorities for the targeted community members. As a result of the formative evaluation, alterations in the tone and format of the poster will be made, so as to reach the target population more effectively. Without conducting a formative evaluation, the poster campaign would likely be ineffective, and might possibly even alienate the population intended to benefit from the program.

Formative evaluation should be conducted whenever a new program is about to be implemented or when an existing program is being modified for a new use or population. Although formative evaluation is critical to the success of most programs, it is often overlooked because of the misperception that evaluation happens after a program is concluded. A plan for formative evaluation, therefore, is best incorporated into the design stage of any new or revised program.

The second form of evaluation, also frequently overlooked, is *process evaluation*: the measure of how well a program is being implemented (16). Process evaluation helps determine if a program is being conducted as intended, and how well the program components are understood and received by participants. Process evaluation allows program staff to make needed revisions while the program is running (15). Process evaluation measures may include inspecting participant attendance or compliance records, engaging in direct observation of program implementation, administering participant satisfaction questionnaires, reviewing log books that record critical implementation events, conducting media analyses for news events that might affect program implementation or outcomes, and conducting direct interviews with program staff.

A process evaluation of the Spanish poster initiative may include tracking the number and locations of posters distributed throughout the community; surveying Latina community members to learn if they recall seeing the posters, if they can recall the content, and what they liked or did not like about the posters; and asking Spanish-speaking callers to the hotline how they found out about the hotline and why they decided to make the call. These data indicate whether the program was implemented as intended and how well it was received by the target audience. The data can then be used to inform changes in implementation, such as moving posters to different locations, or to inform the outcome evaluation.

The process evaluation can also include project management information, such as the extent to which the project adhered to its projected budget and timeline. These data are helpful in analyzing how efficiently resources were used. For example, the initial project plan may have allocated $5,000 and two staff members and planned to reach 5,000 people over a 3-month period. If the project actually spent $7,000 and used three staff people to reach 5,000 people, the project was not implemented as intended, even though it reached its target goals. Process data can help the staff articulate "lessons learned" regarding how to make the program more efficient in the future, or can serve as a warning to other providers that the cost of using this program model is higher than originally anticipated.

Outcome, or *summative evaluation* is the most well-known of the evaluation trio, and asks the question, "Is/was the program effective?" (17). To measure outcomes, a number of factors must be in place:

- The desired outcomes of the program must be clearly stated.
- An indicator, or proxy measure, for the outcome must be identified.
- A system must be in place to collect data related to the proxy measure, and the data must be collected consistently.

Continuing with the previous example:

> There are 10,000 Latina women in the community. The project staff projected that half of them (5,000) would see the posters, that 20% of those who saw the posters (1,000) would be living with IPV, and that 10% of those people (100) would actually call the hotline. They devised a brief three-question survey of all hotline callers to find out how they became aware of the hotline and its services. The hotline staff was instructed to track the number of hotline calls they answered, how many callers were surveyed, and to record the answers to the three questions.
>
> At the conclusion of the 3 months, the results are reviewed and the staff determines that:

- 357 calls were received from Spanish-speaking callers.
- 249 (70%) of these callers were surveyed.
- 25 (10%) of the callers surveyed cited the posters as the reason they called.

The data suggest that the program did not meet its target outcome of 100 calls attributable to the poster program. Although disappointing, it is premature to call this program a failure. Staff members reported that they chose not to survey 107 callers whom they determined to be extremely fearful or agitated, as they needed to focus entirely on safety and crisis issues. This group, clearly different from the "nonagitated" callers, might have been more likely to have seen the poster and been motivated to act by its appearance and content. Alternatively, many members of this group may be isolated in their homes and unable to view the posters. They might have learned there was a Spanish-speaking hotline by watching the news. The outcome results prompted program staff to conduct focus groups in the community to gain an additional measure of how well the program was received. Although the focus groups would also exclude the potential population of victims isolated in their homes, it would provide an alternate measure of community response to the campaign.

Too often, evaluation is an afterthought in the implementation process. A program is instituted, and the stakeholders and funders ask for evidence to see if it has been effective. Evaluation after the fact is usually unsuccessful for several reasons. First, if the program is not designed with evaluation in mind, then the information needed to conduct a successful evaluation may not be available. For example, a post-test to measure knowledge gained through an education program is only useful if a pre-test was completed at baseline. Second, if an after-the-fact evaluation shows that a program is unsuccessful, there may be no way to know why. The program may have shown no effect because of a faulty theoretical basis or because the program was implemented incorrectly. A process evaluation, if conducted throughout the implementation phase of a program and in synergy with an outcome evaluation, could provide that information.

Any program that has been implemented widely has consumed resources and can appear to take on a life of its own. Late in a process, particularly if either formative and process evaluation measures were omitted or poorly conducted, it can be difficult to go back to the drawing board. Thus, if an outcome evaluation shows no beneficial effect, the program may either be abandoned or continued without modification (even if faulty) because it would be too resource-intensive to make changes so late in the process. Even if the results of the process evaluation are incorporated, it might be expensive, inefficient, and perhaps even counterproductive to attempt major changes at a late stage in any process. Effective, prospectively thought-out evaluation strategies enable researchers and practitioners to design, conduct, and disseminate interventions most effectively.

The previous sections provided a basic overview of public health and the public health response. Examples of how IPV can be viewed in this model have been incorporated. The next section examines how public health frameworks can be applied to the field of IPV.

THE SOCIAL-ECOLOGICAL MODEL

Because public health issues are so complex and multifaceted, interventions developed to address them must consider the multiple levels of influence at work. The social-ecological model is used most often. Originally described by McLeroy, Bibeau, Steckler, and Glanz (18) as a model to show various levels of influence on behavior, it is also applied to public health issues as a way to categorize contributing factors (19,20). The model considers five levels of reciprocal influence on individual behavior:

- *Intrapersonal.* The effect that one's own knowledge, attitudes, and beliefs can have on one's behavior
- *Interpersonal.* The impact of another person or group of people, including the advice or actions of a peer, or one's sense of others' expectations
- *Institutional.* The impact of an organization's policies, procedures, or environment on individual behavior
- *Community.* The influence of social norms and formal or informal limitations or expectations on an individual
- *Public policy.* The impact of laws and governmental policies and procedures on individual behavior

The individual is influenced at each of these levels and also has the potential to exert influence at each level.

The intrapersonal level is often referred to as "self-talk." A survivor of IPV who is considering leaving her abuser will reflect on many things before changing her behavior and taking action. She may be influenced by her existing knowledge about IPV and the resources that are available to her, or she may question her self-efficacy in being able to leave successfully. She may also explore her beliefs about relationships, independence, law enforcement, and a myriad of other considerations. Her knowledge, attitudes, and beliefs on each subject, in addition to the relative priority that she gives to each, will influence her course of action.

The interpersonal level describes the influence individuals and groups have on each other. This level has considerable meaning in the context of IPV, in which interpersonal influence is being coerced and manipulated. Abused individuals may choose not to disclose their victimization to anyone because their love and fear of the abusive individual is the dominating force in their life, and it controls their behavior on a mental, emotional, or physical level. Interaction with a caring, trusted adult can help to build another, more positively focused relationship that leads the survivor to disclose the abuse and seek help. Conversely, being rejected, not believed, or treated callously while trying to disclose could cause the survivor to withdraw further.

At the institutional level, behavior may be influenced both directly and indirectly. For example, a worksite may have a published policy regarding IPV that creates a climate of zero tolerance for abuse. Such a worksite may have an employee assistance program that provides counseling to a victim of IPV and directly influences her decision to leave a relationship. On the other hand, even worksites that have no services related directly to IPV may offer flexible personal days that could make it easier for a survivor to attend a hearing regarding child custody or to obtain an order of protection.

The community level exerts influence primarily through promulgating and supporting social norms. Cultural attitudes about gender roles in a community influence definitions of IPV, as well as what is considered a crime. Religious beliefs about marriage and divorce may impact a victim's decision about leaving a relationship.

The public policy level is the farthest removed from the individual, but can have a great deal of influence because it represents legal and policy/regulatory authority. Influence at this level depends not only on the specific policies that are promulgated, but also on the extent to which they are enforced. Funds allocated to teen dating violence prevention programs can be useful if they fund effective, evaluated programs. Strict laws against IPV are only helpful if

law enforcement responds to calls and the legal system supports the safety and financial independence of survivors.

Using the social-ecological model, practitioners can map a range of influences on the behaviors of abusers, survivors, families, communities, and society. The model offers a rational process to understand complex interrelationships and better informs a prevention-focused understanding of the problem. An understanding of the social-ecological model allows one to create cohesive strategies that can be used to craft effective interventions. One excellent model for operationalizing interventions for IPV is Cohen and Swift's (21) Spectrum of Prevention, developed by the Contra Costa County Prevention Program for use in injury prevention programs. The Spectrum of Prevention uses a social-ecological framework, and goes further in that it specifies the realms in which action should be taken. The Spectrum is summarized below.

- *Strengthen individual knowledge and skills.* As a foundation of most behavior change programs, many individuals need relevant, personalized information and the opportunity to ask questions.
- *Promote community education.* In an effort to reach a wide swath of the population, community education campaigns provide information through community-focused initiatives.
- *Educate providers.* Direct-care providers have the most access to individuals who are victims of or at risk for IPV, and need to be educated about the issue itself, who is at risk, and what services are available.
- *Foster coalitions and networks.* To facilitate this collaboration, stakeholders should be brought together in formal and informal networks to encourage productive working relationships.
- *Change organizational practices.* Since institutional policies shape behavior by encouraging or discouraging certain practices, facilitating change within an organization can have an impact on the behavior of individuals affiliated with an organization, as well as on the community.
- *Influence policy and legislation.* Federal, state, and local governments have widespread influence on a community and its inhabitants by setting social norms and controlling public spending. To implement a community-based intervention, policy and legislation must support the provision of resources to support these efforts.

The Spectrum of Prevention and its six components provide a framework for taking integrated action against IPV on a community level. The Spectrum reiterates the need for a comprehensive, prevention-focused public health response. No matter how many individuals or organizations commit to acting at one level of the spectrum, an effective response is not possible unless a coordinated response is mounted at all levels.

CONCLUSION

The public health approach has advanced our understanding of IPV and our capacity to develop, implement, and disseminate successful intervention and prevention strategies. An understanding of the public health approach to IPV intervention and prevention is crucial for both students and practitioners of public health who wish to participate actively in a coordinated community response to this problem. We have certainly come a long way in a relatively short time, but we still have far to go to achieve true prevention. We owe it to our patients and clients, and indeed, to our entire society, to work together to address, and ultimately prevent, this significant threat to the public's health.

IMPLICATIONS FOR POLICY, PRACTICE, AND RESEARCH

Policy

- A coordinated community response is required at multiple levels of the social structure in order to effectively address IPV. Legislation, regulations, and funding allocations must reflect a commitment to a multifaceted response.
- A critical mass of public health professionals and other stakeholders must be willing, ready, and able to respond to the issue of IPV. Professional education and development programs must institutionalize IPV education to raise awareness and create a body of competent professionals.

Practice

- Interventions must be implemented at all levels of the Spectrum of Prevention to create an effective, sustainable response to IPV.

Practitioners with varying interests, abilities, and resources must collaborate to mount this coordinated effort.
- Resources are wasted when practitioners are constantly reinventing the wheel. Effective, science-based practices need to be widely disseminated and replicated in order to maximize the benefit of best practices.

Research

- Focus must return to conducting surveillance research using sound methodology and standardized definitions.
- Practice must be informed by rigorous evaluation research. Well-designed and executed evaluation is the only way to understand which IPV intervention programs are effective, and to ensure that precious resources are allocated in the most beneficial way.

References

1. Saltzman L, Johnson D. CDC's family and intimate violence prevention team: Basing programs on science. *J Amer Women's Med Assoc.* 1996;51(3):83–86.
2. Alpert EJ, Shannon D, Velonis A, et al. Family violence and public health education: A call to action. *Violence Against Women.* 2002; 8(6):746–778.
3. Mercy JA, Rosenberg ML, Powell KE . Public health policy for preventing violence. *Health Affairs* 1993;12:7–29.
4. World Health Organization. *World Report on Violence and Health.* Geneva, Switzerland: World Health Organization, 2002.
5. Rose G. Strategy of Prevention: Lessons from cardiovascular disease. *Br Med J.* 1981;282:1847–1851.
6. Sullivan CS, Basta J, Tan C, Davidson WS. After the crisis: A needs assessment of women leaving a domestic violence shelter. *Violence Vict.* 1992;7(3):167–275.
7. Sullivan CM, Davidson WS. The provision of advocacy services to women leaving abusive partners: The examination of short-term effects. *Am J Comm Psychol.* 1991;19(6):953–960.
8. Graffunder CM, Noonan RK, Cox P, Wheaton J. Through a public health lens: Preventing violence against women: An update from the US Centers for Disease Control and Prevention. *J Women Health.* 2004; 13(1): 5–15.
9. Stark E, Flitcraft A. Wife abuse in the medical setting: An introduction for health personnel. *Domestic Violence Monograph Series, No. 7.* Rockville, MD: National Clearinghouse on Child Abuse and Neglect, U.S. Department of Health and Human Services, 1981.

10. Martin D. *Battered wives*. San Francisco, CA: Volcano Press, 1976.

11. Straus M, Gelles RJ, Steinmetz SK. *Behind closed doors: Violence in the American family*. Garden City, NY: Anchor Press/Doubleday; 1980.

12. Burgess AW, Holmstrom LL. Rape trauma syndrome. *Amer J Psychiatry*. 1974;131:413–418.

13. Wolfe DA, Jaffe, PG. Emerging strategies in the prevention of domestic partner violence. *Future Child*. 1999; 9(3):133–144.

14. Centers for Disease Control and Prevention. *Demonstrating your program's worth: A primer on evaluation for programs to prevent unintentional injury*. Atlanta, GA: Centers for Disease Control, 2000; 27–42.

15. Flagg BN. *Formative evaluation for educational technologies*. Mahwah, NJ: Lawrence Erlbaum Associates, 1989.

16. Grembowski D. *The practice of health program evaluation*. Thousand Oaks, CA: Sage Publications, 2001.

17. Scheirer MA. Designing and using process evaluation. In Wolely JS, Hatry HP, Newcomer KE, eds., *Handbook of practical program evaluation*. San Francisco: Jossey Bass;1994:40–68.

18. McLeroy KR, Bibeau D, Steckler A, Glanz K. An ecological perspective on health promotion programs. *Health Educ Q*. 1988; 15:351–377.

19. Stoklos D. Translating social ecological theory into guidelines for community health promotion. *Am J Health Promot*. 1996; 10(4), 282–298.

20. Glanz K, Rimer B. *Theory at a glance: A guide for health promotion practice*. Washington, DC: National Institutes of Health;1997:15–16.

21. Cohen L, Swift S. The spectrum of prevention: Developing a comprehensive approach to injury prevention. *Injury Prevent*. 1999; 5:203–207.

Chapter 21

Primary Prevention of Intimate Partner Violence: Toward a Developmental, Social-Ecological Model

Daniel J. Whitaker, Diane M. Hall, and Ann L. Coker

KEY CONCEPTS

- Primary prevention of intimate partner violence (IPV) has traditionally focused on school-based interventions for middle and high schools students.
- Two programs have been found to prevent IPV: the Safe Dates program, and the Youth Relationship Project.
- Conceptual models for the primary prevention of IPV should be expanded to be more developmentally and ecologically focused.
- A developmental perspective seeks to understand the early precursors of IPV. Such a perspective would seek to understanding the trajectories of partner violence and related behaviors, and would understand risk and protective factors as being developmentally specific.
- An ecological perspective would focus on a range of risk and protective factors at various levels of influence (individual, family, dyad, group, and societal level) and on how those levels interact to produce IPV.
- Current developmental studies implicate individual, peer, and family factors as being important longitudinal predictors of IPV perpetration.
- Several issues are critical to deal with in terms of bringing a developmental, ecological perspective to the study of IPV. Those include understanding trajectories of partner violence, understanding different types of perpetrators and perpetration behaviors, and understanding the role of sex and gender in the development of IPV.

The goal of this chapter is to provide an overview of primary prevention efforts for intimate partner violence (IPV). To do that, we first define primary prevention and discuss approaches to primary prevention as well as challenges to thinking about and conducting primary prevention of IPV. We then review current primary prevention efforts for IPV to describe the types of approaches that have been tested in the field and the results of those findings. Based on the limited data regarding primary prevention efforts, we suggest a broad expansion is needed in how primary prevention of IPV is conceptualized and implemented. Specifically, we suggest that a more developmental and ecological approach is needed, one that considers how IPV develops and one that considers how the various spheres of influence operate to produce (or prevent) IPV. To support this, we present the most recent data on developmental studies of individuals who perpetrate IPV. We conclude by discussing ways in which various sectors, including families, schools, communities, and the medical community, can work to prevent IPV.

PUBLIC HEALTH APPROACH TO PRIMARY PREVENTION

Primary prevention refers to prevention efforts that seek to "prevent the onset of a targeted condition," (1), or in other words, to prevent a problem before it begins. In the field of IPV, primary prevention is aimed at preventing an *initial* occurrence of IPV perpetration. Secondary prevention is aimed at intervening with known perpetrators or victims to prevent the *recurrence* of IPV perpetration. Tertiary prevention generally involves working with identified victims to prevent the negative health impacts of IPV. Primary prevention can be targeted toward a *universal* population, meaning all individuals without consideration of risk factors, or a *selected* population, meaning targeting a population that is at increased risk of experiencing IPV, but has not yet done so. The primary/secondary distinction refers to the "timing" of prevention efforts, whereas the universal/selected distinction refers to the risk level of the targeted population. Although the two can be related, they also are distinct. For example, a universal intervention strategy (e.g., media campaign) can be targeted at individuals who have not yet perpetrated IPV and those who have, and thus is both primary and secondary prevention.

Standard definitions of IPV include acts of physical aggression (such as pushing, hitting, slapping, and kicking), sexual aggression, threats of physical or sexual aggression, and psychological/emotional abuse,

which is considered IPV only when there has been prior physical, sexual, or threats of physical or sexual violence (2). Given these definitions, the boundaries between primary and secondary prevention efforts have a substantial gray area, and conducting strict primary prevention (i.e., without secondary prevention) can be difficult. Because acts of IPV vary in intensity, it is sometimes unclear when physical aggression begins (e.g., would an individual who has pushed a partner out of the way to leave an argument be considered a perpetrator and thus not "eligible" for primary prevention?). Also, IPV may be recurrent, or it may be an isolated incident that does not recur (3). Finally, some evidence suggests that, among younger individuals, IPV perpetration tends to cease when they move to a new relationship (4,5). This suggests that IPV may be defined as a relationship-specific phenomenon, at least for younger populations. Finally, the very nature of what constitutes an "intimate partner" can be unclear, particularly among teenagers.

In practice, most IPV prevention programs have included both primary and secondary prevention efforts. For example, most interventions delivered in middle or high schools are universal (i.e., they include teens who have and have not perpetrated IPV), thus acting as both primary and secondary prevention. This is not necessarily problematic, because it is not clear whether primary and secondary prevention efforts at preventing adolescent IPV perpetration *should* be different (i.e., will the intervention need to differ if violence has already occurred?). It also is not clear whether preventive interventions must be different for universal versus selected populations (i.e., will the intervention be appropriate for everyone, or will it need to vary based on type of risk?). In part, this will depend on the type of factor that is used to identify the selected population. For example, the attachment histories and emotional regulation of children who have been the victims of child maltreatment or who have witnessed IPV in the home have been hypothesized to affect their behavior in adult intimate relationships (6); thus, an intervention that addresses those factors may be particularly relevant to such a targeted population. In contrast, teens from disadvantaged backgrounds may be targeted because socioeconomic status (SES) is a strong risk factor for IPV involvement (7), but low SES may not be a target of the intervention.

CURRENT PRIMARY PREVENTION
EFFORTS

Most current primary prevention efforts consist of school-based teen dating violence programs; we argue below that these are just one of many strategies the field will need for effective primary prevention of IPV. Several reviews of the dating violence literature discuss those programs (8,9), including a recent systematic review published in 2006 (10) that summarized evaluated programs published since 1990. Here, we briefly discuss the state of the evaluated primary prevention literature to date.

Whitaker and colleagues (10) conducted a systematic review of primary prevention studies targeting the perpetration of IPV that were published between 1990 and April 2003. Search strategies revealed 15 papers evaluating 11 different programs. All but one were school-based programs delivered to either middle or high school students, and delivered to universally selected populations, that is, not targeted to kids at high risk for IPV (11). All included both boys and girls together as part of the intervention (in contrast to interventions in adult IPV, where it is most common to have gender-specific groups). Although descriptions of the actual interventions were limited (likely due to journals' space limitations), there appeared to be little variability in the approaches taken by the various programs. Most programs were based on some combination of feminist theory and/or social learning theory. Specifically with regard to feminist theory, programs focused on gender roles, knowledge about why dating violence occurs, attitudes, power, and control. With regard to social learning theory, programs tended to focus on changing attitudes and cognitions. Only a few mentioned attempting to deliver skill-based components through role plays or other techniques that actively engaged participants. Only two included noncurriculum based activities. Foshee's Safe Dates included a 10-session curriculum, a poster contest, a theater production, community-based activities, and training for local community-based providers. Wolfe's Youth Relationship Project (YRP) included an 18-session curriculum, community action planning, and the development of a fund-raising or community awareness project. In general, the programs were short in duration. About half the programs were less than 5 hours in duration. The Youth Relationship Project was the longest, with 36 hours of curriculum (plus the community-based activities).

Overall, the research methods employed were relatively weak. Although six of the 11 studies used randomized designs, the overall study quality reported by Whitaker and colleagues was low. Six of 11 studies did not report fidelity to the intervention, and three others used self-report measures of fidelity. Five did not report attrition rates, and three others had attrition rates as high as 40%. Follow-up periods for assessments were generally too short, with only two extending beyond 6 months. All studies included knowledge and attitudes as outcomes, but only four of the 11 studies measured perpetration behavior as an outcome. Most studies (nine of 11) found some positive outcome with regard to knowledge, attitude, or behavior, and of the four studies examining behavioral outcomes, two (Safe Dates and YRP) found positive outcomes for behavior (i.e., reductions in the use of dating aggression).

Although the overall body of dating violence studies was weak, two notable exceptions reported very promising results. The Safe Dates program was a highly rigorous study conducted in 14 middle and high schools in rural North Carolina. As already mentioned, the intervention included both a curriculum- and several noncurriculum-based activities. The study used a strong design, including randomization of schools to intervention and control conditions, fidelity observations, good retention of participants, and several follow-up assessments, the last of which was 4 years after the intervention. The results at 4 years showed that students receiving Safe Dates compared to control students reported less psychological, physical (moderate severity only), and sexual dating violence perpetration, as well as less physical dating violence victimization, again moderate severity only (12). Safe Dates was equally effective for boys and girls, and showed positive effects both for teens who had not perpetrated dating violence at baseline and those who had perpetrated dating violence relative to control students. Mediational analyses found that the primary mediators of behavior change were beliefs about gender norms, dating violence norms, and awareness of community services (13).

The Youth Relationships Project (11) was conducted with 158 adolescents aged 14–16 whose parents were involved with child protective services. The curriculum was a series of 18 two-hour sessions with the goal of promoting healthy, nonviolent relationships and preventing abusive ones. The program was designed to improve decision making and to help youth learn nonviolent means of communication.

The YRP utilized a strong research design, randomly assigning teens to the intervention or a wait-list control group. As with Safe Dates, intervention fidelity was carefully monitored, study attrition was low, behavioral outcomes (and mediators) were measured, and there was a lengthy follow-up period of 18 months. Findings of the YRP indicate that, at the 18-month assessment point, girls and boys in the intervention group were 3.2 and 1.9 times less likely as control girls and boys to perpetrate physical IPV. One puzzling finding regarding the YRP was that, although behavioral changes were found for both perpetration and victimization, five constructs targeted in the intervention hypothesized to mediate behavior change (e.g., conflict resolution, communication) did not show any impact from the intervention. Thus, why the YRP affected behavior is unclear.

Since the publication of Whitaker and colleagues' review, a few other trials of dating violence prevention programs have been conducted. Jaycox and colleagues (14) conducted a randomized trial of the Ending the Violence curriculum, a three-session legal-based intervention that focuses on the basics of IPV, laws regarding IPV, and legal processes and safety planning. The randomized trial included over 2,000 9th grade Latinos in Los Angeles. Findings indicate that the program resulted in changes in knowledge and help-seeking measures (particularly with regard to using lawyers), but no program effects were found on behaviors at the 6-month assessment point.

In a yet-to-be-published study, Campbell and colleagues conducted a multifaceted dating violence program in inner-city middle schools that included a four-session curriculum, several arts-based components (e.g., theater, web design), discussion groups, and teacher training. Two schools received the intervention, and two similar schools were used as controls. The evaluation results showed a reduction in IPV perpetration and victimization relative to the comparison schools, but the study had methodological problems common to research conducted in inner-city schools, including a relatively weak design, low participation rates, and the use of successive samples, rather than a longitudinal sample, for baseline and post-test (i.e., the same students did not necessarily participate in the baseline and post-test).

A third study conducted in the Cleveland area (15) evaluated two interventions against a control in a randomized trial: an interaction-based curriculum focusing on healthy relationships, and a law-based curriculum focusing on laws, definitions, and penalties. Both interventions were five 40-minute sessions and were delivered to 6th and 7th graders. Several outcomes were measured, including violent perpetration and victimization toward peers, dating partners, and dating "interests"; sexual harassment perpetration and victimization; intentions; and bystander behaviors. Assessments were conducted post-intervention and at 6 months following the intervention. Few intervention effects were found at post-test, and some conflicting findings were reported at 6 months, with healthy relationship curriculum students reporting less victimization from peers and dating interests, but more perpetration of aggression toward dating partners.

In addition to school-based interventions, the other major form of IPV primary prevention efforts is that of media campaigns. Media campaigns can take various forms including posters, television and radio spots, public service announcements, and the like. Media campaigns often have many goals: to increase awareness of IPV, to change attitudes and norms about IPV, to increase public support for IPV prevention and intervention, or to reduce the incidence and prevalence of IPV. Media campaigns can be targeted broadly to an entire population, or can target specific subgroups of individuals. Several media campaigns have been initiated (e.g., The Family Violence Prevention Fund's There's No Excuse for Domestic Violence and Coaching Boys Into Men), but to date there are no evaluation data indicating such media campaigns are effective at changing behavior. It remains to be seen whether media-based approaches, such as Coaching Boys Into Men, can effectively change behavior by itself or augment the effects of curriculum-based efforts such as Safe Dates. Many have suggested that media campaigns should be used in conjunction with more comprehensive program or policy changes to change behavior (16).

In sum, primary prevention efforts for IPV have consisted primarily of school-based dating violence curriculum and to a lesser extent media-based approaches. School-based approaches to dating violence prevention are surely an important component of a societal effort to prevent IPV. We argue, however, that an expansion of primary prevention efforts for IPV is needed, one that is ecological, in that it takes into account multiple spheres of influence, and developmental, in that it considers the developmental precursors of IPV. Schools are but one important way in which to reach youth, and school-based curricula target primarily individual-level factors (e.g., knowledge, attitudes, and skills).

WHY A DEVELOPMENTAL, SOCIAL-ECOLOGICAL MODEL OF INTIMATE PARTNER VIOLENCE?

We propose that prevention efforts for IPV should become more *developmental* and *social-ecological*. A developmental perspective suggests that we must understand IPV and its prevention in the context of child and adolescent development. That is, to properly prevent IPV, we must seek to understand how intimate relationships develop, how relationship violence *and* nonviolence develops, what skills are needed to develop nonviolent relationships (and/or what skills are absent in violent ones), and most importantly, how and when those skills may develop. The "how" and "when" speak to the importance of understanding developmentally specific risk and protective factors. That is, key influences may be at work at certain developmental time points that are relatively less important at other developmental time points (e.g., an experience at age 5 may lead to a very different outcome than the same event experienced at age 12).

The social-ecological perspective (17) on the prevention of IPV suggests that a broad range of factors may influence IPV perpetration. For example, under Jessor and Jessor's (18) framework, risk and protective factors at various levels of influence—individual, family, peer, social, cultural—contribute to risk behavior (including IPV), and interventions that address multiple levels may be needed. The combining of a developmental and social-ecological approach suggests that we must examine if and how the specific risk and protective factors at the various levels of the social-ecology may change over time with development. For example, in early childhood, family factors may be particularly important; as children reach adolescence, however, the relative influence of peers and media may increase. Thus, it is important to understand the influence of risk and protective factors in the context of development.

Why is a developmental and social-ecological framework important? As we discussed earlier, the majority of primary prevention efforts for IPV have been conducted in a single context (schools) and have targeted mainly individual-level factors such

as knowledge and attitudes. Most broad theories of IPV suggest a range of factors that may lead to IPV (19–22). Although theories of IPV are often discussed as either "feminist" or "family conflict" theories, most theories within each category propose a number of factors that span the levels of the social ecology. For example, Riggs and O'Leary's (21) model includes individual, family, and social environmental factors. Likewise, Heise's (22) model, which is rooted in the notion of gender inequities, discusses factors at individual, family, relationship, and social levels as important in determining IPV perpetration. Although such models are clearly ecological, there has been less attention given to developmental aspects, and very little longitudinal data that have provided a strong test of these models. Developmental studies are needed to examine risk and protective factors at various levels of the social-ecological model, and to examine the processes by which IPV perpetration develops. Such studies would go a long way toward informing primary prevention efforts.

We believe taking such a developmental and social-ecological perspective on IPV prevention will have two major implications for primary prevention: prevention would begin much earlier than adolescence and would seek to understand processes involved in the development of IPV perpetration and non-perpetration; and prevention efforts would consider and be conducted in a range of venues that tap social-ecological influence points. Fortunately, many lessons can be borrowed from existing prevention efforts for other teen risk behaviors (e.g., youth violence, delinquency, substance use), where such a developmental social-ecological framework has been applied with encouraging results. We briefly review how progress has been made in the field of youth violence prevention to illustrate what is possible, and then discuss the two implications of the developmental, social-ecological model in some detail.

Progress in Youth Violence

Efforts to prevent youth violence have changed greatly over the past three decades. The proliferation of prevention programs for youth violence began in the 1970s. Early youth violence prevention programs tended focus on single risk factors at the individual level (23). The limited success of early approaches prompted some to call into question whether youth violence was at all preventable. Today, however, state-of-the-art youth violence prevention studies may address multiple risk factors simultaneously, intervene in multiple contexts, and offer universal and selective intervention strategies (e.g., 24,25–27). Several bodies of etiological research have converged and facilitated this transition. Those include rigorous longitudinal studies examining the trajectories of youth violence along with specific risk and protective factors; studies of the micro-level interactive processes that reinforce aggressive behavior; and studies showing the impact of programs that promote positive social, emotional, and behavioral skills across a variety of contexts for the prevention of problem behaviors (28). In addition, several studies have examined how larger community and societal factors, such as social cohesion (29), poverty (30), and media (31,32) influence youth violence. This area of research is new but promising. One study found that deconcentrating areas of poverty reduced adolescent violent behavior, although we need a better understanding of the mechanisms involved (33).

Studies examining the trajectories of youth violence showed that at least two different trajectories for youth violence exist: early- and late-onset (34–36). Early-onset violence is characterized by problem behavior that begins early in childhood, and, for some children, escalates as they grow older (37); late-onset violence typically first occurs in adolescence and is associated with fewer problems in childhood (34,35,38). A majority of violent youth follow the late-onset trajectory (39), but those who follow the early-onset trajectory commit more persistent and serious violence (38,40,41). This work suggested the prevention of serious violence must begin prior to adolescence and should be based on early behavioral markers for later serious aggression (42–44). In the field of IPV, similar typologies have been proposed (discussed later), but no studies examine the development of "types" of perpetrators or perpetration.

Other research showed that there are different risk factors for youth violence by developmental stage. Lipsey and Derzon's (45) meta-analysis summarized predictors of later youth violence for younger (ages 6–11) and older children (ages 12–14). For younger children, the strongest modifiable predictors of later violence were nonserious delinquency, substance use, low SES, and antisocial parents. For older children, the strongest modifiable predictors for violence were a lack of strong social ties, antisocial peers, and poor school attitude and performance. Findings such as these suggest that preventive interventions that target

younger versus older children may utilize different strategies and have different types of focus.

Research on the development of youth violence has also focused on the specific social processes that can lead to violent behavior. For example, Patterson and colleagues (46,47) have studied the "microsocial exchanges" in home environments of aggressive children and documented how negative reinforcement within families of aggressive children contributes to the escalation of aggressive behavior. These findings were used to develop parent-training methods to interrupt the cycles of negative reinforcement and curtail aggressive behavior and have since been incorporated into large-scale community interventions (48). In the case of IPV prevention, some studies have shown differences in the communication and emotional regulatory processes between IPV perpetrators and nonperpetrators (49), and even between types of perpetrators (50), but no work exists examining those developing processes in children that may lead to IPV perpetration.

Finally, preventive interventions for youth violence (and other risk behaviors that emerge during adolescence) have begun to focus on the promotion of positive, prosocial behaviors and skills that have broad applicability during adolescence and adulthood for avoiding a variety of negative outcomes (28). This focus grew out of a recognition that many problem behaviors (e.g., aggression, delinquency, early sexual risk behavior, substance use, school failure) tended to co-occur and tended to have similar environmental risk and protective factors (44,51,52). Programs that address the core cognitive, emotional, and behavioral skills necessary to avoid problem behaviors, as well as perform positive behaviors have grown in popularity. Many of these programs tend to operate in multiple domains (e.g., schools and community, community and families) to promote generalization of skills and to address the key environments that may influence adolescents (28). For example, the Seattle Social Development Project included interventions for teachers, parents, and first-grade children and focused on altering children's context and enhancing their basic cognitive and social skills. Long-term follow-up of the children exposed to the intervention has found that it affected school performance, violent crime, sexual behavior, and heavy drinking (53). For IPV prevention, it is possible, and even likely, that such programs may also impact adolescent teen dating violence, given the connection between violence perpetrated toward peers and toward partners.

ISSUES IN A DEVELOPMENTAL, SOCIAL-ECOLOGICAL MODEL OF INTIMATE PARTNER VIOLENCE PREVENTION

Understanding Early Risk Factors

As already noted, most current primary prevention efforts for IPV (or dating violence) have targeted middle or high school students. Targeting middle school students makes sense from the perspective that the middle school years (12–14) are when romantic attachments begin to form. However, interventions that target adolescents for behaviors that begin during adolescence miss opportunities for prevention by failing to consider important influences that occur prior to that point. Although children do not have intimate partners prior to adolescence, there may be behaviors that serve as markers to indicate who is likely to develop into a perpetrator of IPV, and there may be environmental risk factors that reliably predict the later onset of IPV.

Until very recently, most predictive work on dating violence was cross-sectional, but a recent series of longitudinal analyses have begun to examine early predictors of IPV perpetration. There is some convergence of findings from these studies. For instance, five prospective studies have shown that early behavioral problems (including antisocial behavior problems and conduct disorder) predict later IPV perpetration (54–58). Additionally, many studies have found that a variety of family variables predict later perpetration, including harsh discipline or physical abuse (54,56,57,59,60), poor supervision (59,61), negative family communication patterns (54,55,60,62), and exposure to marital violence or conflict (54,56,57,59,60,63). Other prospective studies have found that peer variables (e.g., approval of violence) longitudinally predict dating violence perpetration (64,65). Finally, some prospective studies have shown that relationship or dyadic variables are predictive of the later onset of IPV (although many of these studies are with adults). These include variables such as premarital cohabitation (55), assortative partnering or the tendency of individuals who are likely to engage in violence to partner together (58), conflict resolution styles (66), and use of psychological aggression (67).

These longitudinal studies should lay a foundation on which to base new intervention efforts. They strongly suggest that preventing conduct disorders or more generally, behavior problems could be a fruitful early strategy for preventing the onset of IPV. This is encouraging, as effective strategies for preventing conduct problems exist through working with parents (e.g., 68) and schools (69). These studies also place a clear focus on family variables, as many family variables including discipline, monitoring, and communication show relationships to later IPV perpetration. Many pieces are still missing however. For example, although the studies just cited show prospective relationships between variables studied and later IPV perpetration, still too few studies examine different trajectories of IPV perpetration, types of IPV perpetration (physical versus sexual; more versus less severe), and which variables are important during specific developmental time periods.

Becoming More Social Ecological—With Data

As already noted, many of the major theories of IPV are social-ecological in nature, but remarkably little data exist on many of those levels, and even fewer data speak to how IPV develops (critical information for primary prevention of IPV). Of the prospective research available, most focuses on individual and family-level variables. More work is clearly needed on dyadic factors, peer groups, and broader community-level variables. Perhaps the biggest gap between theory and data is for the influence of community- or societal-level variables. For instance, although many accept that societal norms regarding patriarchy are a root cause of IPV against women (e.g., 22,70), relatively few rigorous empirical studies confirm this notion. And the studies that do exist have mixed findings regarding the role of inequality at the societal level. For instance, Yodanis (71) used cross-national data from 27 countries and found that social levels of inequity were related to men's sexual violence against women, but not their physical violence. Yllo and Straus (72) found a curvilinear relationship between women's social status and violence toward women within the 50 states; states in which women's relative status was the lowest and the highest had the highest rates of violence. Yllo and Straus also found a linear relationship between patriarchal family norms and violence against wives. Another study found that gender role stress was significantly related to a male's use of violence against a female partner, especially when these males held values associated with a traditional masculine ideology (73). Whaley and Messner (74) found that gender equality was related to lesser male-to-female homicide in some areas of the country, but greater male-to-female homicide in others, and suggested there may be a backlash effect as societies become more equitable. If patriarchy and societal norms about gender roles are contributing factors toward IPV perpetration, the questions still remain as to how to intervene upon those variables in a developmentally appropriate way (i.e., at what time and through what sphere of influence).

Other community- and societal-level factors that have been studied include poverty (75), community response to IPV, and use of violence to resolve conflicts. It is not clear whether poverty in and of itself increases risk, or if there are conditions associated with poverty that increase risk, such as crowding or males' sense of frustration at being unable to fulfill a provider role (76). One cross-national study found lower rates of male-to-female physical IPV in countries with legal and/or community sanctions against partner violence and in places where women could find support, such as in shelters or with family (77). Higher rates of IPV have been found in communities where adults regularly use violence to resolve conflicts (78). Further research is needed to understand how to create change at this level of the social ecology to prevent IPV.

Other ecological factors deserving further attention and study are peer variables and dyadic variables. The impact of negative peer groups on teens has been demonstrated for a number of risk behaviors including delinquency and violence (79,80), sexual risk behavior (81), and substance use (82). Lipsey and Derzon (45) identified social ties and involvement with antisocial peers as the strongest predictors of later youth violence among 12–14-year-olds. The influence of peer groups on IPV is less well studied. As noted, a few prospective studies have found that peer norms or beliefs about what peers think relate to IPV perpetration (64, 65). Capaldi and Clark (59) suggest that individuals who are likely to perpetrate IPV form peer groups with others who are also likely to perpetrate IPV (i.e., assortative partnering). Capaldi and Crosby (58) found that antisocial boys are more likely to have antisocial romantic partners, and that both partners tend to be psychologically and physically aggressive.

Non-intimate peers may also provide normative support for IPV. That is, they may either explicitly or implicitly endorse (or sanction) the use of aggression in relationships. Studies have linked perceived peer group norms and behavior for a variety of adolescent risk behaviors such as alcohol use (83) and sexual risk behavior (84). Thus, another intervention point may be to alter group norms that exist among peer groups in which IPV is present. This use of popular group leaders has been successful in some fields such as HIV prevention (85), but not others, such as youth violence prevention. Thus, its utility with the prevention of IPV remains to be seen.

With regard to dyadic factors, there is considerably more literature supporting the association of dyadic factors to IPV. Dyadic approaches to prevention may be most relevant for primary prevention before violence has occurred; in cases where severe, controlling IPV is ongoing, dyadic approaches are not recommended. A dyadic perspective suggests that the behavior of both partners in a relationship is important to the occurrence of IPV, that is, the context of the relationship must be considered in examining IPV. In addition to assortative partnering, as discussed earlier, considerable evidence suggests that other dyadic factors may be important in producing IPV. Relationship variables such as relationship discord (3,86), conflict (87,88), communication patterns (49,89,90), and power differences (91,92) have been shown to relate to IPV. Well-developed interventions, such as the PREP program (93), are available for changing relationship behaviors, and these have been shown to be effective at improving communication and conflict, and in at least one case, reducing violence (94). Protocols for changing relationship behaviors almost always involve both partners (with the appropriate precautions and plans for safety); however, this may be difficult with adolescents who have sporadic partnerships that may be short in duration. What may be more appropriate for primary prevention and for teens is to identify how key relationship skills develop, and work to improve those skills prior to youth engagement in relationships. Wolfe and Feiring (95) argue that processes around power, reciprocity, and intimacy are developmentally important for adolescents and should be focal points for understanding the formation of intimate relationships and violence within those relationships. But little is known about the processes and skills involved in the development of normal, healthy adolescent relationships (96,97).

We have touched on several domains of influence and some of the potentially important variables that might reside within those domains. Many other spheres of influences can be better understood in a developmental context, and many other important variables we have not discussed. For instance, there is much talk about media messages negatively affecting children and teens, particularly with regard to gender roles and violence. Yet, almost no empirical research examines how media leads to IPV or influences the variables that lead to IPV (98). Our goal was to illustrate the kinds of variables that can be viewed in a developmental context, rather than to provide an exhaustive literature review of influences of IPV.

Understanding the Development and Etiology of Types of Intimate Partner Violence—Not One Process?

To this point, we have discussed IPV as a single phenomenon. But several types of behaviors are included in the definition of IPV (psychological aggression, physical aggression, sexual aggression, and even stalking), and it is quite possible that there are different developmental precursors to the perpetration of these different behaviors. Much of the literature has focused on physical IPV, and a strong relationship has been demonstrated between psychological aggression and physical aggression in longitudinal studies, with the former predicting the latter (99). Much less is known about the development of sexual aggression in intimate relationships. Sexual IPV usually occurs with physical aggression (100), but most relationships with physical IPV do not contain sexual IPV (100,101). Thus, unique processes may be involved in the development of sexual IPV that must be understood in order to prevent that form of IPV from developing.

Many authors have also discussed typologies of IPV based on the severity of IPV (102), motivational context (103,104), and the traits and generality of the violence (105). For example, Johnson's typology (103,106) hypothesizes at least two forms of violence, *situational violence* and *intimate terrorism*. Situational violence is characterized by low-level physical IPV perpetrated by both members of a couple, and arises from conflicts and disagreements. In contrast, intimate terrorism is hypothesized to be motivated by control motives, and is characterized by repeated severe physical IPV perpetration with a great deal of psychological

abuse and control. Another well-known typology is Holtzworth-Munroe's typology of male perpetrators, who are referred to in the typology as batterers (105,107,108). In this typology, male batterers are differentiated by their psychological characteristics and the generality of their violence. The typology includes antisocial batterers, who tend to perpetrate severe physical violence against both intimate and nonintimate victims; borderline-dysphoric perpetrators, whose violence is moderate in severity and limited to intimate partners; and family-only perpetrators, who perpetrate low-level physical IPV that is limited to intimate partners. Although typologies such as these have great intuitive appeal, data supporting them are fairly limited, and some inconsistencies have been found in published studies. For example, in a longitudinal study, Holtzworth-Munroe colleagues (108) found that many abusers tended to change "types" over time; that is, the nature of their violence changes. In Johnson's model, intimate terrorism is hypothesized to be largely a one-way phenomenon, with men perpetrating intimate terrorism toward their female partners. However, a large Canadian study (109) found both men and women experience intimate terrorism from their spouses (although women more frequently than men, 60% to 40%), and Ehrensaft and colleagues (54) have shown that even among the most severe cases of IPV, physical aggression is usually perpetrated by both members of the relationship, although not necessarily during the same incidents.

Much more data are needed on the types of IPV and types of perpetrators—most of these typologies have been developed and applied to adult IPV and not teen dating violence (110). However, it is useful to consider them when thinking about primary prevention of IPV as it helps clarify that there are likely multiple processes involved in the development of IPV. As we better understand the development of IPV, it is necessary to ask *what kind* of IPV is developing.

The Sex/Gender Issue

One of the most controversial topics in the study of IPV is the role of sex and gender in IPV perpetration. Anderson (111) advocates for a more sophisticated approach to the study of IPV by recognizing that biological sex is very different from the social construct of gender. Sex refers to the biological and physiological aspects of being male or female, while gender refers to culturally and socially determined aspects (112). Thinking about gender as a phenomenon that is socially constructed and that "exists" outside individuals (e.g., gender places expectations on the ways that individuals do and do not behave, think, and interact often despite what individuals want) allows us to explain why men's and women's use of physical violence is often viewed differently. There are many findings in the literature on sex differences in IPV use (i.e., differences between men's and women's use of IPV) but fewer on role of gender and IPV, and even less on how sex and gender may interact. Disentangling these constructs may allow for a more sophisticated dialog, and may help advance prevention approaches.

Regarding sex differences, some findings seem reasonably clear: (a) among community samples of teens and young adults, males and females perpetrate acts of physical aggression toward intimate partners at about the same rate (113); (b) women experience greater harm from physical IPV than men (113); and (c) findings of equal victimization rates (or "sex-symmetry") have not been widely shown for forms of IPV such as sexual violence and stalking. Many other issues regarding sex and IPV perpetration are unclear, however. Do the precipitants, motives, and context for IPV perpetration differ by sex and gender? Does fear induction differ by sex and gender? Do the consequences of IPV differ by sex and gender? Do acts of IPV have different meanings according to the sex and gender of the perpetrators and victims? How do other forms of IPV (i.e., sexual and psychological) differ by sex and gender? Many have raised these questions (114), and a discussion of these issues is beyond the scope of this chapter; however, we believe it is critical that they be included in the study of IPV development. Many authors focus on one sex or the other (typically female victims and males perpetrators), but it is only by studying *both* sexes and gender-related constructs that we will understand whether different or similar processes are involved by sex and gender. Additionally, those taking a dyadic approach (115) argue that without studying the dyad, we will not fully understand the development and course of IPV. Intimate partner violence occurs within a context, and only by studying the context will we understand the development and course of IPV. By studying relational context, we can learn what relationship factors protect against IPV, which will be crucial in informing primary prevention efforts.

HOW VARIOUS SECTORS CAN WORK TOWARD PRIMARY PREVENTION OF INTIMATE PARTNER VIOLENCE

Although we have raised many questions that need answers to inform the primary prevention of IPV, current programmatic efforts to conduct primary prevention must continue. Knowledge will never be complete, and prevention activities must proceed on the current state of the science, whatever that state may be. In this section, we highlight some of the ways various "sectors" can work toward primary prevention of IPV based on a developmental ecological model.

Families

The study and prevention of any behavior that begins in childhood or adolescence must include the role of the family. Parents or other primary caregivers are the primary influences on the basic social, emotional, and behavioral competencies children develop. This can occur either by directly interacting and influencing children, or by modeling behavior with other adults, including romantic partners. Although the literature on the development of IPV is relatively small, it has strong implications for family-based prevention efforts. As reviewed earlier, a host of family variables have been implicated in longitudinal studies predicting dating violence. Family processes including communication, punishment, conflict, and monitoring have been found to be predictive of later dating violence perpetration. Perhaps more importantly, as already noted, conduct disorder has been shown to be predictive of later onset of dating violence. Family-based interventions to prevent conduct disorder are well-established; a number of evidence-based parenting programs have been shown to reduce problem behaviors in children including The Incredible Years (116), Triple P (68,117), Parent-Child Interaction Therapy (118), and others. To date, the idea of preventing IPV by intervening as early as preschool with evidence-based parenting programs has not been widely considered. The difficulties with such an approach in a research setting are many, including the very long follow-up time required to observe the onset of dating violence. Still, the data suggest that family-based interventions that prevent conduct disorder could be a very effective way to prevent later dating violence.

Schools

The role of school-based curricula in the primary prevention of IPV is probably the most well-defined of the various sectors described here. The importance of the successes of school-based programs such as Safe Dates cannot be understated, and it is critical that schools continue to conduct dating violence prevention activities for middle and high school students. However, in line with a developmental and social-ecological perspective, schools (like families) may influence dating violence behavior long before children reach the age of dating, by influencing factors that may not obviously be related to dating violence. As with families, school-based interventions targeting very young children are effective at preventing conduct problems that can lead to later violence, including dating violence. Two recent meta-analyses of school-based interventions (69,119) find they are effective at addressing behavior problems in schools. Again, the link between early behavior problems and later onset of dating violence has only recently received attention, and thus the notion of using early prevention of behavior problems to address dating violence has not been adequately explored in the scientific literature. But it is certainly possible that early school-based interventions targeting problem behaviors may also serve as effective intervention for the onset of later dating violence. School-based interventions may affect the intermediate processes that allow children to develop healthy, nonviolent relationships (although little research suggests what those processes may be). Here again, it would be very difficult to show this from a research perspective as a very long follow-up would be needed.

Interventions that seek to change the school environment itself, so that the school culture is less tolerant of fighting and aggression could similarly have an impact on later dating aggression, if those programs reduce the mediators of dating aggression (e.g., conduct problems). The Olweus bullying program is one such example that seeks to change the school environment, and it has been shown to reduce episodes of bullying/peer violence among school-aged children (120). Again, to our knowledge, no studies have examined whether such programs also lead to reduced dating aggression as children mature into teenagers.

Medicine and Health

One healthcare-based approach to addressing IPV recommended by many professional medical associations, including the American Medical Association, is universal screening of patients for IPV; that is, assessing all patients for IPV experiences regardless of their presenting symptoms. Studies show that universal IPV screening is acceptable and feasible (121,122), but it is not clear whether universal screening prevents violence or improves health outcomes and thus it has not been recommended by the U.S. Task Force for Preventive Medicine at this time (123). It is certainly important for physicians, nurses, and other health professionals to be aware of the range of symptoms, injuries, and health effects that can result from IPV, and to assess for IPV experiences during diagnostic questions regarding the etiology of a condition. However, both universal screening and assessment for diagnostic purposes fall outside the realm of primary prevention of IPV.

The developmental, ecological perspective that we have described would shift the focus of attention from adults to children and adolescents. Medical and healthcare organizations and providers that deal with children and families prior to the onset of dating can become aware of the risk factors associated with dating violence and be proactive in addressing those families. Some organizations do this. For example, the American Academy of Pediatrics (AAP) has a series of brochures designed to help parents talk with their children about potential risk factors for violence, such as anger management. The Society for Adolescent Medicine (SAM), in their position paper on bullying and peer violence (124), advocates for policies and practices to reduce bullying and peer violence by making physicians familiar with the signs of bullying. The SAM also recommends preventive services for adolescents, including counseling focused on health risk behaviors and health lifestyles (125). The World Medical Association adopted a statement on violence and health that includes training, prevention, research, and policy recommendations for national medical associations (http://www.wma.net/e/policy/v1.htm). Other medical and health organizations can form similar policy statements on violence generally and dating violence in particular, and those statements should be based on the latest knowledge of the developmental and ecological predictors of dating violence.

Professionals in the health arena are also members of the larger community and, as respected sources of health information, have the opportunity to engage in primary prevention efforts within their communities. Examples of these efforts include giving community talks on IPV, its health impacts, and available intervention and prevention resources at local hospitals, as well as teaching about IPV and health impacts when supervising and training students. Finally, health professionals can work within their professional organizations to assist with position statements and other efforts to ensure accuracy in media portrayals of violence. A recent similar example is the AAP statement asking a television network not to televise a show that suggested that vaccines cause autism. The mass media is a powerful source of information, and helping to ensure the accuracy of what is portrayed is an important social service that health professionals can provide.

Communities

Communities can do much to prevent IPV, from raising awareness to establishing prevention programs, to implementing policy changes that make IPV less likely. In fact, community responses to IPV have been extremely important in developing the IPV prevention movement. Historically, those efforts have focused mostly on secondary and tertiary prevention efforts, and thus include policy changes such as mandatory arrest laws and increased funding for violence against women to support community-based services such as shelters, hotlines, and rape crisis centers. These are absolutely essential services and appropriate secondary and tertiary prevention goals, and they need continued support and strengthening. At the same time, a concerted effort is needed that prevents violence from occurring in the first place. Community efforts to prevent IPV can take many forms, and can and should be coordinated with other sectors of influence (families, schools, medicine). This coordination will likely increase effectiveness, as well as make better use of resources.

One way in which communities can address primary prevention of IPV is by instituting policy changes to assist the groups considered at risk for IPV. One example of this is a recent state-wide initiative in Rhode Island to mandate dating violence prevention programs in middle school. Still, much more

can be done at the community level. As noted earlier, children who experience maltreatment, who live in poverty, and who experience poor family environments are at increased risk for later IPV involvement. Community-based efforts to promote services for at-risk populations are important. From a developmental perspective, it is critical that these services address populations at-risk for IPV *early*, before they become engaged in IPV.

CONCLUSION

The primary prevention of IPV is a critical issue for protecting the health and well-being of the population. Some interventions have shown promise, but a broad expansion of theory and practice regarding IPV prevention is needed, one that takes into account developmental considerations and a wider range of ecological influences. Such an expansion will create new opportunities for preventing IPV and will allow for targeting interventions to those most appropriate to receive them. Intimate partner violence is everyone's problem, and it will take a combined and coordinated effort from individuals, families, schools, communities, and other sectors such as medicine, business, and policy to affect real change.

IMPLICATIONS FOR POLICY, PRACTICE, AND RESEARCH

Policy

- Intimate partner violence should be considered a problem that develops over time, and thus preventive solutions to that problem must be developmentally rooted.
- Policies that influence broad risk and protective factors (e.g., poverty, social norms) may influence IPV.

Practice

- School-based primary prevention efforts for teen dating violence should continue and should be modeled after empirically supported data.
- Efforts to prevent IPV can begin in early childhood by focusing on family processes and reducing children's conduct problems.

Research

- Much more work is needed to understand the development of IPV. Specifically, information on the behavioral precursors of later IPV, how different forms of IPV develop, and how boys' and girls' behaviors regarding IPV develop differently (or similarly).
- More data are needed on social-ecological risk and protective factors for IPV, especially risk and protective factors at the outer rings of a social-ecological model (e.g., broad social influences).

References

1. U.S. Preventative Services Task Force. *Guide to clinical preventative services*, 2nd ed. Baltimore, MD: Williams & Wilkins, 1996.
2. Saltzman LE, Fanslow JL, McMahon PM, Shelley G. *Intimate partner violence surveillance: Uniform definitions and recommended data elements*. Atlanta, GA: Centers for Disease Control and Prevention, 1999.
3. O'Leary KD, Barling J, Arias I, et al. Prevalence and stability of physical aggression between spouses: A longitudinal analysis. *J Consult Clin Psychol.* 1989;57(2):263–268.
4. Whitaker DJ, Le B, Niolon PH. Persistence and desistance of perpetration of physical partner violence across relationships: Results from a national study. Under review.
5. Capaldi DM, Shortt JW, Crosby L. Physical and psychological aggression in at-risk young couples: Stability and change in young adulthood. *Merrill-Palmer Quarterly.* 2003;49(1):1–27.
6. Wekerle C, Wolfe DA. The role of child maltreatment and attachment style in adolescent relationship violence. *Developm Psychopathol.* 1998;10(3): 571–586.
7. Catalano S. *Intimate partner violence in the United States*. Washington DC: Bureau of Justice Statistics, U.S. Department of Justice, 2007.
8. Avery-Leaf S, Cascardi M. Dating violence education: Prevention and early intervention strategies. In: Schewe P, ed. *Preventing violence in relationships: Interventions across the life span*. Washington, DC: American Psychological Association; 2002:79–105.
9. Hickman LJ, Jaycox LH, Aronoff J. Dating violence among adolescents: Prevalence, gender distribution, and prevention program effectiveness. *Trauma Violence Abuse.* 2004;5(2):123–142.
10. Whitaker DJ, Morrison S, Lindquist C, et al. A critical review of interventions for the primary prevention of perpetration of partner violence. *Aggression Violent Behav.* 2006;11(2):151–166.

11. Wolfe DA, Wekerle C, Scott K, et al. Dating violence prevention with at-risk youth: A controlled outcome evaluation. *J Consult Clin Psychol.* 2003;71(2): 279–291.
12. Foshee VA, Bauman KE, Ennett ST, et al. Assessing the effects of the dating violence prevention program "Safe Dates" using random coefficient regression modeling. *Prevent Sci.* 2005;6(3):245–258.
13. Foshee VA, Bauman KE, Ennett ST, et al. Assessing the long-term effects of the Safe Dates program and a booster in preventing and reducing adolescent dating violence victimization and perpetration. *Am J Pub Health.* 2004; 94(4):619–624.
14. Jaycox LH, McCaffrey D, Eiseman B, et al. Impact of a school-based dating violence prevention program among Latino teens: Randomized controlled effectiveness trial. *J Adolesc Health.* 2006;39(5): 694–704.
15. ICF International. Final report: Experimental evaluation of gender/violence harrassment prevention programs in middle schools. Washington DC: National Institute of Justice, 2008.
16. Wakefield M, Flay B, Nichter M, Giovino G. Effects of anti-smoking advertising on youth smoking: A review. *J Health Commun.* 2003;8(3):229–247.
17. Bronfenbrenner U. *The ecology of human development: Experiments by nature and design*. Cambridge, MA: Harvard University Press, 1979.
18. Jessor R, Jessor SL. *Problem behavior and psychosocial development: A longitudinal study of youth*. New York: Academic Press, 1977.
19. Dutton DG. An ecologically nested theory of male violence toward intimates. *Int J Women's Studies.* 1985;8(4):404–413.
20. Crowell NA, Burgess AW. *Understanding violence against women*. Washington DC: National Academy Press, 1996.
21. Riggs DS, O'Leary KD. A theoretical model of courtship aggression. In: Pirog-Good MA, Stets JA, eds. *Violence in dating relationships: Emerging social issues*. New York: Praeger Publishers; 1989:53–71.
22. Heise LL. Violence against women: An integrated, ecological framework. *Violence Against Women.* 1998;4(3):262.
23. Tolan PH, Guerra N. *What works in reducing adolescent violence*. Boulder, CO: The Center for the Study and Prevention of Violence, 1994.
24. Henggeler SW. Multisystemic therapy: An overview of clinical procedures, outcomes, and policy implications. *Child Psychol Psychiatry Rev.* 1999;4(01):2–10.
25. Nation M, Crusto C, Wandersman A, et al. What works in prevention: Principles of effective prevention programs. *Am Psychologist.* 2003;58(6/7): 449–456.
26. Horne AM. The multisite violence prevention project: Background and overview. *Am J Prevent Med.* 2004;26:3–11.

27. Bierman KL. Implementing a comprehensive program for the prevention of conduct problems in rural communities: The Fast Track experience. *Am J Comm Psychol.* 1997;25(4):493–514.

28. Catalano RF, Berglund JA, Ryan HS, et al. Positive youth development in the United States: Research findings on evaluations of positive youth development programs. *Prevent Treat.* 2002;5:ArtID15.

29. Wilkinson RG, Kawachi I, Kennedy BP. Mortality, the social environment, crime and violence. *Sociol Health Illness.* 1998;20(5):578–597.

30. Messner SF. Research on cultural and socioeconomic factors in criminal violence. *Psychiat Clin N Am.* 1988;11(4):511–525.

31. Paik H, Comstock G. The effects of television violence on antisocial behavior: A meta-analysis. *Commun Res.* 1994;21(4):516.

32. Wood W, Wong FY, Chachere JG. Effects of media violence on viewers' aggression in unconstrained social interaction *Psychol Bull.* 1991;109(3): 371–383.

33. Ludwig J, Duncan GJ, Hirschfield P. Urban poverty and juvenile crime: Evidence from a randomized housing-mobility experiment. *Q J Econ.* 2001;116(2):655–679.

34. Moffitt TF. Life-course-persistent and adolescence-limited antisocial behavior: A 10-year research review and a research agenda. In: Lahey BB, Moffitt TE, Caspi A, eds. *Causes of conduct disorder and juvenile delinquency.* New York: Guilford; 2003:49–75.

35. Loeber R, Farrington DP. *Child delinquents: Development, intervention, and service needs.* Thousand Oaks, CA: Sage Publications, 2001.

36. Dahlberg LL, Simon TR. Predicting and preventing youth violence: Developmental pathways and risk. In: Lutzker JR, ed. *Preventing violence: Research and evidence-based intervention strategies.* Washington, DC: American Psychological Association, 2005: 97–124.

37. Côté S, Vaillancourt T, LeBlanc JC, et al. The development of physical aggression from toddlerhood to pre-adolescence: A nation wide longitudinal study of Canadian children. *J Abnorm Child Psychol.* 2006;34(1):68–82.

38. Tolan PH, Gorman-Smith D. Development of serious and violent offending careers. In: Loeber R, Farrington DP, eds. *Serious and violent juvenile offenders: Risk factors and successful interventions.* Thousand Oaks, CA: Sage; 1998:68–85.

39. U. S. Department of Health and Human Services. *Youth violence: A report of the Surgeon General.* Rockville, MD: U.S. Government Printing Office, 2001.

40. Farrington DP. Key Results from the first forty years of the Cambridge study in delinquent development. In: Thornberry TP, Krohn MD, eds. *Taking stock of delinquency: An overview of findings from contemporary longitudinal studies.* New York: Kluwer Academic/Plenum Publishers, 2003.

41. Loeber R, Farrington DP, Waschbusch DA. Serious and violent juvenile offenders. In: Loeber R, Farrington DP, eds. *Serious and violent juvenile offenders: Risk factors and successful interventions.* Thousand Oaks, CA: Sage 1998:13–29.

42. Farrington DP. Early developmental prevention of juvenile delinquency. *Crim Behav Mental Health.* 1994;4(3):209–227.

43. Karoly LA, Greenwood PW, Everingham SS, et al. *Investing in our children: What we know and don't know about the costs and benefits of early childhood interventions.* Santa Monica, CA: Rand, 1998.

44. Mrazek PB, Haggerty RJ. *Reducing risks for mental disorders: Frontiers for preventive intervention research.* Washington DC: National Academy Press, 1994.

45. Lipsey MW, Derzon JH. Predictors of violent and serious delinquency in adolescence and early adulthood: A synthesis of longitudinal research. In: Loeber R, Farrington DP, eds. *Serious and violent juvenile offenders: Risk factors and successful interventions.* Thousand Oaks, CA: Sage;1998: 86–105.

46. Patterson GR. *Coercive family processes.* Eugene, OR: Castilia Press, 1982.

47. Patterson GR. The early development of coercive family processes. In: Reid JB, Patterson GR, eds. *Antisocial behavior in children and adolescents: A developmental analysis and model for intervention.* Washington, DC: American Psychological Association; 2002:25–44.

48. Reid JB, Patterson GR, Snyder JJ. *Antisocial behavior in children and adolescents: A developmental analysis and model for intervention.* Washington DC: American Psychological Association, 2002.

49. Margolin G. Affective responses to conflictual discussions in violent and nonviolent couples. *J Consult Clin Psychol.* 1988;56(1):24–33.

50. Gottman JM, Jacobson NS, Rushe RH, et al. The relationship between heart rate reactivity, emotionally aggressive behavior, and general violence in batterers. Comments. Reply. *J Fam Psychol.* 1995;9(3):227–279.

51. Dryfoos JG. *Adolescents at risk: Prevalence and prevention.* New York: Oxford University Press, 1990.

52. Durlak JA. Common risk and protective factors in successful prevention programs: Prevention science research with children, adolescents and families: Introduction. *Am J Orthopsychiatry.* 1998;68(4): 512–520.

53. Hawkins JD, Catalano RF, Kosterman R, et al. Preventing adolescent health-risk behaviors by strengthening protection during childhood. *Arch Pediat Adolesc Med.* 1999;153(3):226–234.

54. Ehrensaft MK, Moffitt TE, Caspi A. Clinically abusive relationships in an unselected birth cohort: Men's and women's participation and developmental antecedents. *J Abnorm Psychol.* 2004;113(2): 258–271.

55. Magdol L, Moffitt TE, Caspi A, Silva PA. Developmental antecedents of partner abuse: A prospective-longitudinal study. *J Abnorm Psychol.* 1998;107(3):375–389.

56. Lavoie F, Hebert M, Tremblay R, et al. History of family dysfunction and perpetration of dating violence by adolescent boys: A longitudinal study. *J Adolesc Health.* 2002;30(5):375–383.

57. Ehrensaft MK, Cohen P, Brown J, et al. Intergenerational transmission of partner violence: A 20-year prospective study. *J Consult Clin Psychol.* 2003;71(4):741–753.

58. Capaldi DM, Crosby L. Observed and reported psychological and physical aggression in young, at-risk couples. *Soc Developm.* 1997;6(2):184–206.

59. Capaldi DM, Clark S. Prospective family predictors of aggression toward female partners for at-risk young men. *Developm Psychol.* 1998;34(6):1175–1188.

60. Linder JR, Collins WA. Parent and peer predictors of physical aggression and conflict management in romantic relationships in early adulthood. *J Fam Psychol.* 2005;19(2):252–262.

61. Brendgen M, Vitaro F, Tremblay RE, Lavoie F. Reactive and proactive aggression: Predictions to physical violence in different contexts and moderating effects of parental monitoring and caregiving behavior. *J Abnorm Child Psychol.* 2001;29(4):293–304.

62. Andrews JA, Foster SL, Capaldi D, Hops H. Adolescent and family predictors of physical aggression, communication, and satisfaction in young adult couples: A prospective analysis. *J Consult Clin Psychol.* 2000;68(2):195–208.

63. Lichter EL, McCloskey LA. The effects of childhood exposure to marital violence on adolescent gender-role beliefs and dating violence. *Psychol Women Q.* 2004;28(4):344–357.

64. Arriaga XB, Foshee VA. Adolescent dating violence: Do adolescents follow in their friends,' or their parents,' footsteps? *J Interpers Violence* 2004;19(2):162–184.

65. Foshee VA, Linder F, MacDougall JE, Bangdiwala S. Gender differences in the longitudinal predictors of adolescent dating violence. *Prevent Med* 2001;32(2):128–141.

66. Leonard KE, Senchak M. Prospective prediction of husband marital aggression within newlywed couples. *J Abnorm Psychol.* 1996;105(3):369–380.

67. O'Leary K, Malone J, Tyree A. Physical aggression in early marriage: Prerelationship and relationship effects. *J Consult Clin Psychol.* 1994;62(3):594–602.

68. Sanders MR. Triple P-Positive Parenting Program: Towards an empirically validated multilevel parenting and family support strategy for the prevention of behavior and emotional problems in children. *Clin Child Family Psychol Rev.* 1999;2(2):71–90.

69. Wilson SJ, Lipsey MW. School-based interventions for aggressive and disruptive behavior update of a meta-analysis. *Am J Prevent Med.* 2007;33(2S):130–143.

70. Dobash RE, Dobash RP. *Violence against wives.* New York: Free Press, 1979.

71. Yodanis CL. Gender inequality, violence against women, and fear: A cross-national test of the feminist theory of violence against women. *J Interpers Violence.* 2004;19(6):655.

72. Yllo, K. A., & Straus, M. A. (1990). Patriarchy and violence against wives: The impact of structural and normative factors. In M. Straus & R. J. Gelles (Eds.), *Physical violence in American families: Risk factors and adaptations to violence in 8,145 Families* (pp. 383-399). New Brunswick, NJ: Transaction Publishers.

73. Jakupcak M, Lisak D, Roemer L. The role of masculine ideology and masculine gender role stress in men's perpetration of aggression and violence in relationships. *J Men Masculinity.* 2002:3(2)97–106.

74. Whaley RB, Messner SF. Gender equality and gendered homicides. *Homicide Studies.* 2002;6(3):188.

75. Byrne CA, Resnick HS, Kilpatrick DG, et al. The socioeconomic impact of interpersonal violence on women. *J Consult Clin Psychol.* 1999;67(3):362–366.

76. Heise L, Garcia-Moreno C. *Violence by intimate partners.* World report on violence and health. Geneva: World Health Organization;2002:89–121.

77. Counts DA, Brown JK, Campbell JC. *Sanctions and sanctuary: Cultural perspectives on the beating of wives.* Westview Press, 1992.

78. Levinson D. *Violence in cross-cultural perspective.* Thousand Oaks, CA: Sage, 1989.

79. Dodge KA, Lansford JE, Burks VS, et al. Peer rejection and social information-processing factors in the development of aggressive behavior problems in children. *Child Developm.* 2003;74(2):374–393.

80. Thornberry TP, Huizinga D, Loeber R. The prevention of serious delinquency and violence: Implications from the program of research on the causes and correlates of delinquency. In: Howell JC, Krisberg B, Hawkins JD, Wilson JJ, eds. *Sourcebook on serious, violent, and chronic juvenile offenders.* Thousand Oaks, CA: Sage;1995:213–237.

81. Diclemente RJ. Predictors of HIV-preventive sexual behavior in a high-risk adolescent population: The influence of perceived peer norms and sexual communication on incarcerated adolescents' consistent use of condoms. *J Adolesc Health.* 1991;12(5):385–390.

82. O'Donnell J, Hawkins JD, Abbott RD. Predicting serious delinquency and substance use among aggressive boys: Prediction and prevention of child and adolescent antisocial behavior. *J Consult Clin Psychol.* 1995;63(4):529–537.

83. Simons JS. Differential prediction of alcohol use and problems: The role of biopsychological and social-environmental variables. *Am J Drug Alcohol Abuse.* 2003;29(4):861–880.

84. Santelli JS, Kaiser J, Hirsch L, et al. Initiation of sexual intercourse among middle school adolescents: The influence of psychosocial factors. *J Adolesc Health.* 2004;34(3):200–208.

85. Kelly JA, St. Lawrence JS, Stevenson LY, et al. Community AIDS/HIV risk reduction: The effects of endorsements by popular people in three cities. *Am J Pub Health.* 1992;82(11):1483–1489.

86. Pan HS, Neidig PH, O'Leary K. Predicting mild and severe husband-to-wife physical aggression. *J Consult Clin Psychol.*1994;62(5):975–981.

87. Sagrestano LM, Heavey CL, Christensen A. Perceived power and physical violence in marital conflict. *J Soc Issues.* 1999;55(1):65–79.

88. Cascardi M, Vivian D. *Context for specific episodes of marital violence: Gender and severity of violence differences.* Vol. 10. New York: Springer; 1995: 265–293.

89. Babcock JC. Power and violence: The relation between communication patterns, power discrepancies, and domestic violence. *J Consult Clin Psychol.* 1993;61(1):40–50.

90. Cordova JV, Jacobson NS, Gottman JM, et al. Negative reciprocity and communication in couples with a violent husband. *J Abnorm Psychol.* 1993;102(4):559–564.

91. Coleman DH, Straus MA. Marital power, conflict, and violence in a nationally representative sample of American couples. *Violence Vict.* 1986;1(2): 141–157.

92. Babcock JC, Waltz J, Jacobson NS, Gottman JM. Power and violence: The relation between communication patterns, power discrepancies, and domestic violence. *J Consult Clin Psychol.* 1993;61(1):40–50.

93. Stanley SM, Blumberg SL, Markman HJ. Helping couples fight for their marriages: The PREP approach. *Preventive approaches in couples therapy.* 1999:279–303.

94. Markman HJ, Renick MJ, Floyd FJ, et al. Preventing marital distress through communication and conflict management training: A 4-and 5-year follow-up. *J Consult Clin Psychol.* 1993;61(1):70–77.

95. Wolfe DA, Feiring C. Dating violence through the lens of adolescent romantic relationships. *Child Maltreatment.* 2000;5(4):360–363.

96. Furman W, Brown BB, Feiring C. *The development of romantic relationships in adolescence.* New York: Cambridge University Press, 1999.

97. Brown BB, Feiring C, Furman W. Missing the Love Boat: Why researchers have shied away from adolescent romance. In: Furman W, Brown BB, eds. *The development of romantic relationships in adolescence.* New York: Cambridge University Press;1999:1–16.

98. Manganello JA. Teens, dating violence, and media use: A review of the literature and conceptual model for future research. *Trauma Violence Abuse.* 2008;9(1):3.

99. Murphy CM, O'Leary K. Psychological aggression predicts physical aggression in early marriage. *J Consult Clin Psychol.* 1989;57(5):579–582.

100. Tjaden P, Thoennes N. *Extent, nature, and consequences of intimate partner violence: Findings from the National Violence Against Women Survey.* Washington DC: US Department of Justice, 1998.

101. Coker AL, Smith PH, McKeown RE, King MJ. Frequency and correlates of intimate partner violence by type: Physical, sexual, and psychological battering. *Am J Pub Health.* 2000;90(4):553–559.

102. O'Leary KD. Through a psychological lens personality traits, personality disorders, and levels of violence. In: Gelles RJ, Loseke DR, eds. *Current controversies on family violence.* Newbury Park, CA: Sage;1993:7–30.

103. Johnson MP. Patriarchal terrorism and common couple violence: Two forms of violence against women. *J Marriage Family.* 1995;57(2):283–294.

104. Tweed RG, Dutton DG. A comparison of impulsive and instrumental subgroups of batterers. *Violence Vict.* 1998;13(3):217–230.

105. Holtzworth-Munroe A, Stuart GL. Typologies of male batterers: Three subtypes and the differences among them. *Psychol Bull.* 1994; 116(3):476–497.

106. Johnson MP, Leone JM. The differential effects of intimate terrorism and situational couple violence: Findings from the National Violence Against Women Survey. *J Fam Issues.* 2005;26(3):322–349.

107. Holtzworth-Munroe A, Meehan JC, Herron K, et al. Testing the Holtzworth-Munroe and Stuart (1994) batterer typology. *J Consult Clin Psychol.* 2000;68(6):1000–1019.

108. Holtzworth-Munroe A, Meehan JC, Herron K, et al. Do subtypes of maritally violent men continue to differ over time? *J Consult Clin Psychol.* 2003;71(4):728–740.

109. Laroche D. *Aspects of the context and consequences of domestic violence–Situational couple violence and intimate.* Quebec: Institut de la statistique du Quebec, 2005.

110. Foshee VA, Bauman KE, Linder F, et al. Typologies of adolescent dating violence: Identifying typologies of adolescent dating violence perpetration. *J Interpers Violence.* 2007;22(5):498–519.

111. Anderson KL. Theorizing gender in intimate partner violence research. *Sex Roles.* 2005;52(11): 853–865.

112. Unger RK. Toward a redefinition of sex and gender. *Am Psychol.* 1979;34(11):1085–1094.

113. Archer J. Sex differences in aggression between heterosexual partners: A meta-analytic review. *Psychol Bull.* 2000;126(5):651–680.

114. Hamberger LK. Men's and women's use of intimate partner violence in clinical samples: Toward a gender-sensitive analysis. *Violence Vict.* 2005;20(2):131–151.

115. Capaldi DM, Kim HK. Typological approaches to violence in couples: A critique and alternative

conceptual approach. *Clin Psychol Rev.* 2007; 27(3):253–265.

116. Reid MJ, Webster-Stratton C, Hammond M. Follow-up of children who received the incredible years intervention for oppositional-defiant disorder: Maintenance and prediction of 2-year outcome. *Behav Ther.* 2003;34(4):471–491.

117. Sanders MR, Markie-Dadds C, Turner KMT. *Theoretical, scientific and clinical foundations of the Triple P-Positive Parenting Program: A population approach to the promotion of parenting competence.* Brisbane: The Parenting and Family Support Centre, 2003.

118. Eyberg SM, Funderburk BW, Hembree-Kigin TL, et al. Parent-child interaction therapy with behavior problem children: One and two year maintenance of treatment effects in the family. *Child Fam Behav Ther.* 2001;23(4):1–20.

119. Hahn R, Fuqua-Whitley D, Wethington H, et al. Effectiveness of universal school-based programs to prevent violent and aggressive behavior: A systematic review. *Am J Prevent Med.* 2007;33(2S): 114–129.

120. Limber SP. The Olweus Bullying Prevention Program: An overview of its implementation and research basis. In: Jimerson SR, Furlong MJ, eds. *The handbook of school violence and school safety: From research to practice.* New York: Routledge; 2006:293–307.

121. Coker AL, Flerx VC, Smith PH, et al. Partner violence screening in rural health care clinics. *Am J Pub Health.* 2007;97(7):1319–1325.

122. Black MC, Kresnow MJ, Simon TR, et al. Telephone survey respondents' reactions to questions regarding interpersonal violence. *Violence Vict.* 2006;21(4):445–459.

123. Nelson HD, Nygren P, McInerney Y, Klein J. Screening women and elderly adults for family and intimate partner violence: A review of the evidence for the US Preventive Services Task Force. *Ann Intern Med.* 2004;140(5):387.

124. Eisenberg ME, Aalsma MC. Bullying and peer victimization: Position paper of the Society for Adolescent Medicine. *J Adolesc Health.* 2005; 36(1):88–91.

125. Rosen DS, Elster A, Hedberg V, Paperny D. Clinical preventive services for adolescents: position paper of the Society for Adolescent Medicine. *J Adolesc Health.* 1997;21(3):203–214.

Chapter 22

Acute Intervention for Intimate Partner Violence in the Medical Setting

Gregory Luke Larkin and Jennifer Parks

KEY CONCEPTS

- Acute care creates opportunities for intervention that can reduce both immediate and downstream harms to patients exposed to intimate partner violence (IPV).
- The Harm Reduction Framework may be applied to IPV as a means to construct multivalent strategies that reduce harms to victims at a variety of levels, even when threats of violence cannot be completely eliminated.
- The initial medical assessment must include a thorough review of systems, relationship and social history, and a detailed obstetric and gynecologic evaluation.
- Proper injury and trauma care must include a detailed evaluation of neurologic status, cervical spine and neck trauma, and a high index of suspicion for traumatic brain injury (TBI).
- Psychological symptoms must be aggressively managed to enhance the victim's level of function.

- The risk of occult or overt suicidality should be routinely determined in all patients.
- The appropriate intervention is greatly informed by the lethality assessment or the dangerousness of a given situation, including attempted strangulation, firearm access, escalation of violence, relationship termination, threats to pets and/or children, and threats of homicide/suicide.
- Referrals and interventions that are stage-based, customized, and responsive to the victim's individual readiness for change are more likely to be successful.

Intimate partner violence (IPV) may take the form of physical, psychological, and/or sexual abuse, but most of the time, IPV constitutes a pattern of behavior used to establish power and control over another person through fear and intimidation, often including the threat or use of violence (1). Although IPV may include emotional abuse, economic abuse, using children, verbal threats, using male privilege, intimidation, isolation, and a variety of other behaviors used to maintain fear, intimidation, and power (2), our focus in this chapter is on medical interventions for victims of physical abuse. Intimate partner violence is extremely common in the both the clinical and general population (3,4), with approximately one-third of American women (31%) reporting physical or sexual abuse by a husband or boyfriend at some point in their lives. Although low-income women are at somewhat higher risk, IPV is a problem cutting across all socioeconomic, racial, and ethnic strata (3).

The medical encounter has the potential to play a significant role in violence prevention. According to the U.S. Department of Justice, approximately four in 10 female victims of IPV seek professional medical treatment (4). A study by Frank and Rodowski conservatively estimates that one in six women seeking emergency care for any reason describe abuse by someone they know within the past year (5). Furthermore, it has been shown that nearly one-half of all women who were victims of an IPV-related homicide had been in the emergency department within 2 years prior to their death (6). It is estimated that 5%–25% of women seen in a primary care setting are battered (7). Approximately 28% of women injured during their most recent physical assault by an intimate partner receive some type of medical care (8).

We cannot afford to ignore IPV in the clinical setting. A study by Wisner and colleagues found that health plans spent $1,775 (92%) more in healthcare costs for victims of IPV compared to general female enrollees. Victims of IPV are significantly younger (by 3 years) and had more hospitalizations, general clinic use, and out-of-plan referrals than a random sample of general female health plan enrollees (9). Furthermore, the study concluded that mental healthcare costs for victims of IPV were 800% higher than in their nonvictimized counterparts. In 1993, Koss and colleagues compared severely victimized women with nonvictims and found that victimized women made physician visits twice as frequently and generated outpatient costs that were 2.5 times greater (10).

Although such findings have resulted in many studies recommending the use of routine screening for abuse in all women presenting to hospitals and other medical care providers, a comparable number of studies detailing the actual implementation and outcomes of such programs are lacking. Most of the research and published literature pertaining to IPV to date has focused on epidemiology, barriers to identification, and the use of training programs to eliminate barriers to routine screening. Few studies have addressed or tested acute treatment interventions for victims in a randomized or rigorous fashion. Given this dearth of evidence, this chapter seeks to answer the question, "I've identified a patient with IPV exposure . . . so now what?" Healthcare workers across the nation may now find themselves in the position of trying to recognize the signs and symptoms of IPV and offer services to those victims, without adequate resources or even an understanding of what treatment and resources to offer.

Optimal intervention strategies for addressing family violence, battering, IPV, and/or relationship violence depend greatly on the immediate needs of a particular patient and the corresponding expertise, resources, and systems of care available in the emergency or acute care setting. In this chapter, our discussion of interventions will presume that both providers and processes for routine inquiry, identification, referral, and treatment are already somewhat in place. Indeed, setting up and maintaining such systems through ongoing education and enrollment of relevant administrators, providers, and stakeholders at all levels is a central challenge, vital to the acute care intervention enterprise; however important, due to space considerations, such macro-level process issues and the vertical and horizontal integration of care will not be the focus here but are addressed elsewhere in this text.

Instead, we will concentrate on the manifold micro-level acute care issues that are very much dependent on the nature of the threats and injuries to a given patient being evaluated. We will consider a novel application of the harm reduction (HR) framework that will allow expansion of addressable component harms to both direct and indirect victims, as well as the medical and nonmedical treatment needs of exposed patients more generally.

HARM REDUCTION FRAMEWORK

Although originally developed for use in smoking cessation programming, the HR model acknowledges that reducing or lowering collective harm is a worthy goal and valuable outcome, even when it may not be possible to simply eliminate harm altogether. For example, one may not be able to instantly quit smoking, but the HR model still legitimizes

Total Harm =	Prevalence ×	Frequency ×	Intensity
Harms/population/year	Victims/population/year	# Acts/victim	Mean harm/act

Figure 22.1 Calculating total harm.

interventions that lead to reduced smoking as also being useful. With some minor adaptation and nuanced extrapolation, this same harm reduction versus harm elimination approach may be applied to IPV as well. It is well established that victims cannot always "just leave" or abstain from the abuser altogether; there are often serious resource and dependency issues, and dramatic moves, such as leaving a relationship, may be fraught with considerable danger for the victim, being a time of high lethality.

The perspective from which we divine our calculus of harms that we seek to reduce is societal, not merely individual, recognizing that individual harms have "splash effects" that affect children, families, police, healthcare workers, and other members of society. We can sum up the total harm over a period of time as a product of prevalence, frequency, and intensity (Figure 22.1). Hence, a reduction in any one of the three components on the right-hand side of the equation leads to a net reduction in overall or total harm.

Prevention strategies are well known to be the most efficient way to achieve harm reduction, with primary, secondary, and tertiary prevention efforts impacting prevalence, frequency, and intensity, respectively. Intervention strategies, our emphasis here, are a well-suited means to practice tertiary prevention and exert their impact through a reduction in recidivism (frequency) and/or a reduction in the accumulated damage or intensity of each harm to victims already exposed to injury. When we operationalize harms and victims more broadly, we find we are then in a position to include multiple stakeholders, children, families, and communities, so that any intervention then reduces net harms to the greater whole and can be construed as worthwhile.

INITIAL ASSESSMENT IN THE ACUTE SETTING

Cases of confirmed or suspected IPV require a thorough assessment of the nature and severity of the abuse, in order to customize an optimal intervention strategy for a given patient. The initial evaluation should include immediate stabilization, addressing the need for resuscitation in the case of major trauma. After assuring the absence of any immediate life- or limb-threatening emergencies and assuring stable vital signs, the provider should proceed to a complete history and physical examination. It is essential that such interviews be conducted in a safe, private setting, without partners or the threat of unwanted visitors. If the use of an interpreter is required to obtain the history, it is preferable to use a trained interpreter or professional interpreting services rather than family members or friends, as the victim may be embarrassed to disclose abuse in their presence. Providers should sit down, provide non-glaring eye contact, maintain an open posture, and keep an appropriate distance. Touch should only be considered on the hand or the upper limbs, but should be used cautiously and sparingly, if at all, to reassure the patients. Although the gender of the assessor need not matter, our work has shown that female patients are more likely to disclose to another woman (11). The demeanor of the assessor is important, and questions should be asked in a professional, matter-of-fact, nonjudgmental manner. Empathic listening is useful and interruptions should be kept to a minimum in order to build rapport with traumatized patients.

Past medical and surgical histories should be elicited, with special emphasis on prior trauma, as well as reproductive and psychological histories. Social histories should include family histories of abuse and neglect as well as a review of intimate relationships, both current and past, including those that pose potential threats currently. Social risks and potential resources should be documented, including the use of tobacco, drugs, and alcohol. Employment status and family resources can suggest the presence of key support systems and opportunities for assistance and informal protection.

Most IPV cases are identified when the patient is not acutely injured. Regardless of whether the patient is injured or not, a thorough review of systems is required, recognizing that many IPV victims frequently are unable to access routine care and have long-term sequelae from previous trauma and abuse. For female patients, the dates and locations of their last PAP smear and breast exams, for example, would be appropriate to document access to care and possible neglect. A history of recurrent illnesses may also signal a pattern of abuse, as our work with IPV victims demonstrates a relative immunodeficiency; beyond the nearly universal risk of HIV, recurrent infections are common.

OBSTETRIC AND GYNECOLOGIC ASSESSMENT

All cases of IPV in women mandate a thorough menstrual history and assessment for pregnancy, given the fact that IPV may escalate in pregnancy, putting both fetus and mother at risk. The outcomes of previous pregnancies should also be documented, as should the status of any children. Cases of IPV that may also involve children directly or even indirectly may necessitate a referral to child protective services if either the well-being or safety of any children is in question.

Pregnant women should be assessed for abdominal/pelvic trauma and should be considered for fetal heart monitoring in the third trimester, particularly in the case of blunt abdominal trauma or falls. Fetal heart tones must be documented. The risk of abruption and any other source of vaginal bleeding must be thoroughly evaluated with a pelvic exam and ultrasonography when appropriate. Routine serum testing with the Kleihauer-Betke test for the presence of fetal blood cells in the maternal circulation is not recommended due to its poor sensitivity and specificity. However, Rh testing in pregnancy-related IPV trauma is important. Likewise, screening for sexually transmitted diseases, especially in cases of sexual IPV, should be strongly considered.

For cases of intimate partner rape, testing for HIV, hepatitis, and syphilis should be considered, and prophylactic treatment for *Gonorrhea*, *Chlamydia*, and *Trichomonas* should be offered as well. After sexual assault, women who are not known to be pregnant should have pregnancy tests performed, and oral contraceptive prophylaxis should be offered to those women who are confirmed to be nonpregnant. Forensic specimen collection in cases of intimate partner

rape should be preceded with a thorough explanation of what will happen, to minimize arousal and reactivation or re-experiencing of the trauma. Evidence collection should follow standardized protocols.

Many human rights organizations consider various forms of female circumcisions to be another form of sexual abuse against women. Healthcare providers (HCPs) may encounter physical signs of prior genital trauma in patients from certain parts of the Middle East and Africa. The World Health Organization estimates the total number of females who have undergone female genital mutilation (FGM) at 100 million to 140 million (12). Societies perform FGM for cultural, religious, and other reasons, and the practice is often perpetrated by family members, as they believe that the operation ensures that their daughters will have ready suitors and a satisfactory bride price. The immediate and long-term effects of the procedure on the women's physical health can be severe and include bleeding, infection, postoperative shock, dysmenorrhoea, scar tissue, and childbirth obstruction. Psychological effects include severe depression, anxiety, and sexual dysfunction. Such cases should be referred to specialists in gynecology, plastic surgery, and psychiatry, as needed.

INJURY CARE

The treatment of fractures, lacerations, dental injuries, and other wounds from IPV should follow routine standards of care. However, a few types of injuries require particularly close attention. Human bites, for example, are at high risk for infection and, unless superficial, will routinely require oral broad-spectrum antimicrobial therapy. Attempted strangulation is another example of a high-risk injury that can cause damage to the larynx and other vital structures in the neck, as well as hypoxic brain damage; strangulation mandates a careful workup to rule out vascular, airway, cervical spine injuries, and brain damage. Motor vehicle crashes in the wake of an argument or fight may involve intoxication, overdose, pregnancy, attempted escape, and may have been precipitated by IPV-related impulsiveness or suicidality.

Before any treatment, repair, or minor surgery, care must be taken to document the injury in sufficient detail, using body maps, drawings, and photographs when possible. Such forensic information is crucial to the documentation and ultimately the prosecution of IPV injury cases. In all cases of suspected IPV, complete clothing removal is vital, in order to facilitate the examination of the entire skin, including the external genitalia, and the identification of all injuries. If clothes have been soiled in the course of the physical assault, law enforcement may request they be collected in a paper bag as physical evidence.

HEAD INJURY

Mild traumatic brain injury (TBI) is recognized as a serious public health problem. The national burden of mild TBI is significant, and the incidence is higher than that previously reported at 503.1 per 100,000 (95% confidence interval [CI] 445.4–560.7). Annual incidence of emergency department visits for mild TBI due to assault is 62.6 per 100,000 (95% CI 47.3–78.0) (13). Repetitive head injury can have lasting neurologic and cognitive effects. Cells of the hippocampus may be susceptible to cumulative damage following repeated mild traumatic insults. Both glial cells and neurons appear to exhibit increased signs of damage after repetitive injury (14). Memory and learning deficits may result. Victims of IPV often incur head injury through direct or indirect trauma. Loss of consciousness may not be disclosed due to loss of awareness or subsequent posttraumatic amnesia. Head trauma can also lead to impaired judgment, and these patients should be considered for neuroimaging and possible admission if the threat of IPV cannot be ruled out and safety assured. Traumatic brain injury in IPV is discussed in more detail elsewhere in this text.

INTIMATE PARTNER VIOLENCE-RELATED MENTAL ILLNESS

Suicidal Behaviors

Although cutting, piercing, jumping, and attempted suffocation and hanging are not uncommon, the most typical suicidal gesture among women is that of attempted self-poisoning (15). Depending on the timing of an overdose, gastric decontamination with lavage and/or activated charcoal may or may not be indicated. Although activated charcoal has few downsides, it is ineffective in cases (such as lithium) that

do not bind well to the charcoal, and whole bowel irrigation is more useful in these cases. In the case of a rare, life-threatening overdose presenting within 1 hour of ingestion, gastric emptying with lavage may still be appropriate. In the case of unknown agents, screening for acetaminophen, salicylates, and substances of abuse are all reasonable, although many agents will not be detected on routine toxicological screens. Instances of intentional poisoning by a partner, although rare, constitute another form of IPV; when the partner is acting overly attentive and controlling, the patient, if awake, must be interviewed alone; herein, the role of heavy metals and a broader differential must be considered. Many overdoses are cries for help and constitute an important opportunity to get a patient into psychiatric treatment for IPV-related depression or anxiety.

Often, IPV is associated with suicidal thoughts, but both the IPV and the suicide can be occult (16). Hence, all cases of suspected IPV must include screening for suicidality. Simple and direct questioning is important. The practitioner should never worry that asking about suicide will suddenly trigger self-harm behavior in a patient. In the context of IPV, cases of suicidal ideation in either the victim or the partner should routinely be admitted, regardless of the presence or absence of a specific plan. The lethality of IPV-related suicidality, explicit or occult, is impossible to manage on an outpatient basis. However, psychosocial interventions for discharged nonsuicidal patients may be useful, including friendly letters or postcards. This is an important area for future study.

Managing Psychological Symptoms

Patients with preexisting mental illness are at higher risk of being abused, and the abuse itself may lead to mental illness. Beyond the considerable risks for overdose and suicide, IPV victims are a risk for depression, posttraumatic stress disorder (PTSD), substance abuse, and other mental illnesses. Screening victims for depression, substance misuse, and suicidal thoughts is an important part of the overall assessment. All patients with mental health symptoms should be referred to psychiatric services for further evaluation and treatment.

Specific agents have been approved in the treatment of both PTSD and depression (e.g., Sertraline) and may have a role to play in select patients. Those who use drugs and/or alcohol should also be evaluated for dangerous drinking behaviors and offered brief intervention and referral when appropriate (17). A brief intervention is a motivational interview, sometimes called a brief negotiated interview (BNI), which seeks to instill willingness for change in the participant.

There is currently much interest in developing interventions that will target traumatic memory and help reduce the development of posttraumatic illness and PTSD, but these therapies are purely experimental at this point. The role of psychotherapy, both cognitive behavioral and other forms, has yet to be fully determined in this high-risk group of patients. Doing therapy with patients in the throes of crisis has many attendant risks, and may cause hyperarousal and instigate decompensation from which the patient should ideally be protected. Debriefing and other forms of acute therapy are potentially too harmful for widespread recommendation at this time, and such treatment should be relegated to experts in psychiatry.

Mental health interventions are discussed in more detail elsewhere in this text.

MEDICAL/SURGICAL REFERRALS AND FOLLOW-UP

When patients are referred to other health professionals, care must be taken to explain privacy concerns and safety considerations, given the fact that few consultants will have the same IPV training as those in acute care settings. It is important to explain when making the referral the possible mechanism of injury and the need for the consultant to err on the conservative side of admission, when feasible, to assure an optimal medical outcome.

In addition, wound care is an opportune way to insist that the patient return to the emergency department or office where the initial care was rendered in order to assure both good wound healing and to assure the patient is safe in other ways. The medical need for follow-up will also give the HCPs license to call the patient at home to check on her status.

LETHALITY ASSESSMENT

One of the first answers to the question, "OK, I discovered intimate partner violence, now what?" is simply this: Keep the patient safe. To keep the patient safe,

one has to know exactly how much and what type of danger she is in. So, one could also answer the query of "What to do?" with the imperative, "Assess lethality!" Indeed, the recognition of IPV alone is never adequate. Once an HCP has identified a victim, the level of danger existing in the abusive relationship must also be assessed before an appropriate intervention can be realized. Perpetrator's threats of homicide, suicide, strangulation, access to firearms, escalation in the frequency and intensity of physical violence, and threats to pets and children are all signals of lethality, mandating a different level of response. The Danger Assessment tool, developed by Campbell, incorporates these factors and provides one way to systematically assess lethality in the medical setting. The tool has good psychometric properties, is available in Spanish and English, uses both dichotomous "yes/no" items, and includes a recall calendar to help overcome denial; however, it is not brief, taking about 20 minutes to complete. The research and application of this tool is discussed in detail elsewhere in this text.

A study of IPV-related femicide characterized several significant lethality risk factors, including the victim having left for another partner, having a child living in the home who was not the abusive partner's biological child, unemployment of the perpetrator, the perpetrator's threatened use of a gun, stalking, forced sex, and abuse during pregnancy (18). Based on these findings, the revised Danger Assessment tool has a weighted scoring system, with ranges of scores indicating greater or lesser acute danger for the victim. This same study also revealed that never living together and prior IPV-related arrests were both independently associated with lowered risk for lethality in this cohort.

Victims of attempted or completed femicide are more likely to be seen in the healthcare system rather than by the community of IPV advocates (19). It has been estimated that 41% of femicide victims killed by intimate partners sought medical treatment during the year prior to their death (20). Healthcare providers can thus play an important role in the prevention of femicide. In instances in which those factors placing women at increased risk are present, the intervention must include a discussion with the patient emphasizing the presence of increased danger, as well as a more aggressive attempt at persuading the victim to accept shelter placement.

Whenever possible, patients in high lethality circumstances should be admitted to the hospital for safety reasons alone. Intimate partner violence patients should be admitted under an alias when their safety is a concern. In rare cases, victims may admit to planning the retaliatory murder against their aggressor; this too must be taken seriously. Under the precedent of Tarasoff, named, identifiable, potential homicide victims must be warned; would-be perpetrators must be reported and restrained, where necessary (21). Coexisting risks for suicide and homicide must also be managed aggressively through the use of isolation and, where necessary, physical restraint and mandated treatment.

VICTIM ADVOCACY PROGRAMS

Approximately half of all battered women report negative experiences in the acute care setting of the emergency department, such as feeling humiliated and ashamed, not being given sufficient referrals to social service organizations, having abuse minimized, and not being identified as battered (22). Hospital-based intervention programs have the potential to be very beneficial for victims of IPV. Deleterious effects may also be related to these programs, such as giving false hope, inducing re-experiencing of the violence, and suffering retributive violence if the intervention is not conducted discretely. However, as with many IPV interventions, the pros and cons of these programs have not been adequately evaluated. There is a need to look at the efficacy of victim advocacy programs in order to optimize an evidenced-based approach to be taken by HCPs in treating victims of IPV. Our work in Pennsylvania shows that the impact of fully funded advocacy programs is difficult to measure; the only randomized controlled trial to date (11) revealed no advantage of advocacy over standard social service interventions.

One nonrandomized quasi-experimental study in urban Kansas City, Missouri, examined the impact of advocacy referrals from emergency departments on community resource utilization (23). Researchers hypothesized that if an IPV victim advocate met with identified victims in the emergency department, the victim would be more likely to use social service resources available in the community. The "Bridge" program provided an advocate to the emergency department 24 hours a day to conduct safety assessments, patient education, and act as a link between the hospital and community IPV service agencies.

An analysis of the data comparing the control and postintervention groups at 1 year revealed the following (23):

- No difference in the numbers of police calls at the time of the index visit, in the number of women obtaining protective orders, or in the number of women returning to the emergency department for any injury after the index visit
- A statistically significant increase in the number of women in the postintervention group who called police after the initial index visit (18% versus 39%, 95% CI on the difference: 1%–40%)
- A statistically significant increase in the number of women in the postintervention group who sought shelter (11% versus 28%, 95% CI on the difference: 6%–27%)
- A statistically significant increase in the number of women in the postintervention group who sought counseling (1% versus 15%, 95% CI on the difference: 7%–21%)

The study concluded that women going to the emergency department as a result of domestic abuse rarely make use of the community resources available to them. It is suggestive that further steps must to be taken beyond the training of healthcare workers to improve outcomes of IPV victims. Further work in the area of on-site advocacy and follow-up are needed for IPV intervention programs to reach their full potential.

A comprehensive review of IPV programs was undertaken by researchers in Canada (24). The study examined 22 published reports and included studies that attempted interventions to which a primary care clinician could refer a patient. Researchers rated the articles using the Canadian Task Force on Preventive Health Care Levels of Evidence and Quality Ratings of Individual Studies, assigning both a research design rating and a quality rating. Studies were grouped into those that compared treatment intervention with non-treatment controls and those that included treatment interventions involving batterers. They found that there were no IPV intervention programs to which a primary care physician could refer a patient that had been adequately evaluated and found to be effective in decreasing the violence.

These reviewers were unable to find strong evidence for or against routine "screening" for IPV leading to improved health outcomes for the victim, due to the dearth of well-designed outcome-based studies. Although studies demonstrate the need for ongoing training and supportive environments to sustain what has shown to be a consistent initial improvement in the rates of identification and referral, the ultimate outcome of such referrals remains an area for further research. Settings that provide on-site, 24-hour advocacy, media outreach campaigns, community collaboration building, adoption of protocols for routine inquiry, and ongoing multidisciplinary training indicate an initial and continuing elevation in rates of routine inquiry, case finding, referrals, provider self-efficacy, and patient satisfaction (23,25–29). A long-term commitment to addressing IPV must be sustained in the development and implementation of interventions if success is to be achieved (30–32).

REFERRALS TO CRIMINAL JUSTICE AND SHELTER SERVICES

Although only a minority of states in the United States have statutory IPV reporting requirements to law enforcement by health practitioners, most clinicians prefer a policy that is based primarily on the patient's autonomous desire to involve law enforcement except when weapons or child exposure to violence is involved. In addition, there is very little evidence for or against reporting mandates as a strategy to achieve greater health and safety for IPV patients. Even where reporting is discretionary, thorough documentation should be made and maintained, presuming that many victims may change their minds at a later date or records may become germane in a criminal or civil proceeding.

Overall, the data on the impact of police referrals are mixed. Nonrandomized data from Kentucky suggest that restraining orders, for example, were useful in helping victims feel safe, and increased satisfaction and feelings of security. Restraining orders in a Manhattan-based study of African Americans, however, resulted in increased fears of retaliation and had the opposite effect (33). Hence, the role of criminal justice referrals and interventions is still unclear. Many victims distrust the police, and protection orders are easily violated and poorly enforced in many communities. On the other hand, it is only through criminal prosecution that the perpetrator can be brought to justice and, in some cases, rehabilitated. Healthcare workers should understand, however, that they

may play a pivotal role in overcoming the inertia of fear and ambivalence clouding a victim's thinking, and they may contact law enforcement themselves in order to initiate the process of obtaining an emergency protective order.

Similarly, referrals to family violence shelters are also an unproven but frequently endorsed strategy. Shelters may provide a safe haven for victims, but referrals from the acute healthcare system are seldom the primary way patients get into shelter. Shelters come in all shapes and sizes, and some are better equipped than others. Many patients feel stigmatized in a shelter and are either unwilling or unready to live there. Future studies need to include evidence-based research regarding the long-term impact that such well-intended but routinely untested referrals and interventions have on the incidence of and outcomes from IPV.

STAGES OF CHANGE

One possible reason that most suggested interventions to date have been unable to show significant impact is that a one-size-fits-all approach is frequently employed. Instead, a more tailored approach to intervention and treatment may be warranted. More recent research by Hyman and Larkin (34) suggests that victim interventions and referrals should be tailored to the particular stage that a given victim is in at the time of acute care evaluation. Similar to Prochaska and DiClemente's Transtheoretical Model of Behavior Change (35), Jody Brown has explored a stage-based approach to victims, which was further refined by Hyman and Larkin. Similar to the stages of readiness for smoking cessation, there appears to be at least three stages that victims occupy with respect to their willingness to change their relationship: precontemplation, ambivalence, and readiness for action. In the first stage, patients are often in denial and are not ready to confront the problem directly. Intimate partner violence patients in the second stage are in the process of weighing the pros and cons (36) and are unsure of their next move; in many cases, they report emotional numbing. Victims in the later stages of willingness to change are in the action mode, willing to affirmatively do things to better their circumstances. Only those in this last group are going to be interested in referrals to shelter, police, or other outside resources. Referring someone to shelter, for example, who is still in denial, is a meaningless gesture. Better to give precontemplators messages of empathic listening and education that affirm who they are and that help them appreciate the potential danger of the situation; that is, get them thinking. Moving them from precontemplation to ambivalence would be considered a successful intervention. As has been tested in patients with high-risk drinking (37,38), it is possible to use BNIs to effect stage movement. A motivational interview may help victims be willing to move from early stages to later stages, but in all cases, they must be allowed to move at their own pace. Forcing victims into treatment is fraught with problems and will likely do more to harm than to help their trust in the medical enterprise.

SAFETY PLANNING

Vital information must to be conveyed to victims of IPV prior to their discharge. Merely giving victims the choice of shelter placement or police involvement is not enough. These options are infrequently selected, as leaving and making a police report often go hand in hand. Safety planning with victims who decline shelter placement and police involvement is a pragmatic form of harm reduction. In safety planning, the future harm posed by the abuser is addressed through a discussion of strategies individualized for each victim. These strategies offer practical safety tips and also often provide victims with increased feelings of control and connectedness to resources, despite their decision not to utilize shelters or police.

Safety planning involves tips for safety in the home, what to do when tension is building, steps to take when leaving, items to take along, and safety after leaving. Such tips include developing a plan with neighbors; teaching them to recognize signs of distress (lights on/off); training the children to call 911; and packing a flight bag that contains birth certificates, driver's license, social security card, insurance documents, money, car registration, medical and school records, medications, clothing, extra keys to vehicles and home, address book, calling cards, and IPV resource hotline numbers. Information on how to obtain a protective order should also be provided to the victims prior to discharge.

Safety planning should leave the victims feeling empowered with strategies and connected to community resources. It is a lengthy process that is best conducted by trained family violence advocates.

CONCLUSION

Other issues in acute care are not addressed in this chapter, but may be found elsewhere in this text. For example, the forensic needs of patients and the provider's parallel duty to properly document those signs and symptoms is critical to the successful prosecution of perpetrators in areas that have passed laws allowing charges to be filed without the cooperation of the abuse victims. There has been much discussion about the healthcare profession's responsibility in inquiring about perpetration as well as victimization and what its expanded role is beyond treating immediate physical injuries. Constitutive of the physician and provider role, in all circumstances, is ensuring the immediate safety and security of the patient. This, above all else, is paramount. Acute treatment and referral is an area of intense investigation, and more evidence-based approaches to acute crisis intervention are forthcoming. Tailoring interventions to patients' specific needs will be the state of the art in IPV intervention for the foreseeable future.

IMPLICATIONS FOR POLICY, PRACTICE, AND RESEARCH

Policy

- Underresourced and underappreciated, acute interventions in the medical setting have a significant but largely unrealized potential to impact the lives of IPV victims.
- However well intended, routine reporting, police referral, or protection-from-abuse orders have the potential to backfire, and reflect the more general concern that one-size-fits-all approaches are fraught with potential dangers. These policies should be reassessed in light of little to no data substantiating an improved outcome for IPV victims who have been reported.
- To be maximally responsive to the needs of victims, policies should be somewhat flexible to allow for provider and patient discretion, and to balance privacy with patient safety.
- These cases can be complex and occupy considerable time by practitioners. A diagnosis of IPV (or adult maltreatment as defined in the International Classification of Diseases) should be appropriately valued and procedural codes appropriately defined for IPV intervention.

Practice

- Tailored approaches offer the most promise, and examining a victim's stage or readiness for change may be a useful way to determine how best to intervene.
- Standard social service interventions by licensed social workers may be more cost effective than special victim or women's advocacy services.
- Have some sort of victim consultation services available 24/7 to address the immediate health threats of the patient, develop safety plans, and ensure adequate follow-up.

Research

- Medical and psychosocial interventions for IPV victims are only now being considered in earnest, and properly designed, sufficiently powered, randomized trials may yield new options for treatment in the near term.
- Further research is needed to address the concerns of the U.S. Preventative Health Task Force regarding the role of screening and routine assessments for IPV in the general patient population.
- Biomarkers and other assessments may help predict who is most resilient and who is most at risk for developing posttraumatic stress, depression, suicide, or other IPV-related sequelae.

References

1. Centers for Disease Control and Prevention. *Costs of intimate partner violence against women in the United States.* Atlanta: Author, 2003.
2. Warshaw C, Ganley A. *Improving the health care response to domestic violence: A resource manual for health care providers.* San Francisco: Family Violence Prevention Fund, 1998.
3. Collins K. *Health concerns across a woman's lifespan: The Commonwealth Fund 1998 survey of women's health.* New York: Commonwealth Fund Press, 1999.
4. U.S. Department of Justice, Office of Justice Programs. *Bureau of Justice Statistics special report: Intimate partner violence.* Washington DC: U.S. Government Printing Office, 2000.
5. Frank JB, Rodowski MF. Review of psychological issues in victims of domestic violence seen in emergency settings. *Emerg Med Clin North Am.* 1999;17(3):657–677, vii.
6. Wadman MC, Muelleman RL. Domestic violence homicides: ED use before victimization. *Am J Emerg Med.* 1999;17(7):689–691.
7. Valente SM. Evaluating and managing intimate partner violence. *Nurse Pract.* 2000;25(5):18–19, 23–16, 29–30 passim; quiz 34–15.
8. U.S. Department of Justice, Office of Justice Programs, National Institute of Justice. *Extent, nature, and consequences of intimate partner violence.* Washington DC: U.S. Government Printing Office, 2000.
9. Wisner CL, Gilmer TP, Saltzman LE, Zink TM. Intimate partner violence against women: Do victims cost health plans more? *J Fam Pract.* 1999;48(6): 439–443.
10. Koss M. The impact of crime victimization on women's medical use. *J Women's Health.* 1993;2:67.
11. Larkin GL, Hyman KB, Mathias SR, et al. Universal screening for intimate partner violence in the emergency department: Importance of patient and provider factors. *Ann Emerg Med.* 1999;33(6): 669–675.
12. World Health Organization study group on female genital mutilation and obstetric outcome. *Lancet.* 2006;367:1835–1841.
13. Bazarian J, McClung J, Shah MN, et al. Mild traumatic brain injury in the United States 1998–2000. *Brain Injury.* 2005;19(2):85–91.
14. Slemmer JE, Matser EJ, DeZeeuw CI, Weber JT. Repeated mild injury causes cumulative damage to hippocampal cells. *Brain.* 2002;125: 2699–2709.
15. Institute of Medicine. *Reducing suicide.* Washington DC: The National Academies Press, 2002.
16. Claassen CA, Larkin GL. Occult suicidality in an emergency department population. *Br J Psychiatry.* 2005;186:352–353.
17. D'Onofrio G, Berstein E, Woolard R, et al. Patients with alcohol problems in the emergency department, part 2: Intervention and referral. *Acad Emerg Med.* 1998;5:1210–1217.
18. Campbell J, Webster D, Koziol-McLain J, et al. Risk factors for femicide in abusive relationships: Results from a multistate case control study. *Am J Pub Health.* 2003;93:1089–1097.
19. Campbell JC. Helping women understand their risk in situations of intimate partner violence. *J Interpers Violence.* 2004;19(12):1464–1477.
20. Sharps PW, Koziol-McLain J, Campbell J, et al. Health care providers' missed opportunities for preventing femicide. *Prev Med.* 2001;33(5): 373–380.
21. *Tarasoff v. Regents of University of California.* Vol. 131: California Reporter; 1976:551.
22. Campbell JC, Pliska MJ, Taylor W, Sheridan D. Battered women's experiences in the emergency department. *J Emerg Nurs.* 1994;20(4):280–288.
23. Muelleman RL, Feighny KM. Effects of an emergency department-based advocacy program

for battered women on community resource utilization. *Ann Emerg Med.* 1999;33(1):62–66.

24. Wathen N, MacMillan H. Interventions for violence against women: Scientific review. *JAMA.* 2003;289:589–600.

25. Short LM, Hadley SM, Bates B. Assessing the success of the WomanKind program: An integrated model of 24-hour health care response to domestic violence. *Womens Health.* 2002;35(2–3):101–119.

26. Fanslow JL, Norton RN, Robinson EM. One-year follow-up of an emergency department protocol for abused women. *Aust N Z J Public Health.* 1999;23(4):418–420.

27. McCaw B, Berman WH, Syme SL, Hunkeler EF. Beyond screening for domestic violence: A systems model approach in a managed care setting. *Am J Prev Med.* 2001;21(3):170–176.

28. Thompson RS, Rivara FP, Thompson DC, et al. Identification and management of domestic violence: A randomized trial. *Am J Prev Med.* 2000; 19(4):253–263.

29. Campbell JC, Coben JH, McLoughlin E, et al. An evaluation of a system-change training model to improve emergency department response to battered women. *Acad Emerg Med.* 2001;8(2): 131–138.

30. Feighny KM, Muelleman RL. The effect of a community-based intimate-partner violence advocacy program in the emergency department on identification rate of intimate-partner violence. *Mo Med.* 1999;96(7):242–244.

31. Furbee PM, Sikora R, Williams JM, Derk SJ. Comparison of domestic violence screening methods: A pilot study. *Ann Emerg Med.* 1998; 31(4):495–501.

32. Waller AE, Hohenhaus SM, Shah PJ, Stern EA. Development and validation of an emergency department screening and referral protocol for victims of domestic violence. *Ann Emerg Med.* 1996; 27(6):754–760.

33. Logan T, Shannon L, Walker R, Faragher T. Protective orders: Questions and conundrums. *Trauma, Violence Abuse.* 2006;7:175–205.

34. Burkitt, K.H., Larkin, G.L. The transtheoretical model in intimate partner violence victimization: Stage changes over time. *Violence Vict* 2008;23(4):411–431.

35. Prochaska JO, DiClemente CC. Stages of changes in the modification of problem behaviors. *Prog Behav Modif.* 1992;28:183–218.

36. Brown J. Working toward freedom from violence. The process of change in battered women. *Violence Against Women.* 1997;3(1):5–26.

37. D'Onofrio G. The prevention of alcohol use by rural youth. *NIDA Res Monogr.* 1997;168: 250–363.

38. D'Onofrio G, Nadel ES, Degutis LC, et al. Improving emergency medicine residents' approach to patients with alcohol problems: A controlled educational trial. *Ann Emerg Med.* 2002;40(1): 50–62.

Chapter 23

Safety Planning, Danger, and Lethality Assessment

Jacquelyn Campbell and Nancy Glass

KEY CONCEPTS

- Homicide is a leading cause of premature death for all women in the United States, especially African-American and Native-American women.
- The majority of women killed in the United States and around the world are killed by intimate partners, husbands, boyfriends, or ex-partners.
- The leading risk factor for intimate partner homicide (IPH) of both female and male partners is prior intimate partner violence (IPV) against the female partner.

- Other important risk factors include guns in the home, estrangement, stepchildren (woman's biological child, not male partner's child) in home, male partner unemployment, threats to kill, and threats with a weapon, forced sex, and abuse during pregnancy.
- Needed areas of research related to IPH include interventions to decrease IPH, causes of ethnic disparities in IPH, IPH as a leading cause of maternal mortality, IPH among same-sex partners, and children affected by IPH.
- The Danger Assessment (DA) is a validated lethality risk assessment instrument that can be used in healthcare systems and other victim services as the basis for safety planning with abused women.

Note: Funding from National Institutes of Health (NIH: NIDA, NIMH, NIA)/Centers for Disease Control and Prevention (CDC)/National Institute of Justice (NIJ) (R01 DA/AA11156, J. Campbell, PI); *Risk Factors for Homicide in Violent Intimate Relationships* and NIJ (2000WTVX0011, J. Campbell, PI); *Evaluation of Domestic Violence Risk Assessment Instruments*).

Even though the rates of intimate partner homicide (IPH) have decreased substantively in the United States over the past 20 years (1), each homicide is unnecessary, and each haunts and harms the families left behind. Intimate partner homicide is defined as a homicide perpetrated against a current or former spouse, cohabitant, or romantic partner by his or her intimate partner. We have well established that the leading risk factor for IPH is prior intimate partner violence (IPV) perpetrated against the female partner, no matter if it is a male or female who is killed (2–4). In our recent national femicide study, we found that approximately 80% of the women had been the victim of physical and/or sexual IPV or stalking prior to their murder, and close to half (42%) of the women were seen in the healthcare system during the year before they were killed (5). If we, as healthcare professionals, first assessed for IPV routinely among women, and then had a valid and practical means of identifying those women who were most at risk to be killed, we might have saved some of those lives. This chapter synthesizes the latest research on IPH and attempted homicide, and describes the development, validity assessment, and suggestions for use of the Danger Assessment (DA) as part of a process of safety planning that can be used in the healthcare system (Figure 23.1).

Although abused women are often good predictors of their own risk of reassault in abusive relationships (6–8), they tend to underestimate their risk (9). In fact, in the national femicide study, only about 47% of the women killed accurately perceived how dangerous their perpetrator was (5). Thus, it is clear that women need help in realistically assessing their danger.

One of the most widely recommended interventions for abused women in the healthcare system or elsewhere is safety planning. Although the elements in recommended safety planning procedures vary, and no clinical trial has yet tested the efficacy of safety planning, this process is widely accepted among advocates and practitioners as helping to keep abused women safe. The one form of safety planning that has been tested, in a quasi-experimental design, is the McFarlane and Parker "brochure-driven" safety planning process (10,11). This safety planning process starts with a lethality assessment, taken from the DA (12,13), which gives women a more realistic sense of the risk factors for homicide that are present in their situations. Since the brochure intervention was developed, the DA has been revised with a weighted scoring developed based on the national femicide study and further tested in subsequent research. The DA is one strategy available to healthcare professionals as a way of working with abused women so that safety planning is based on a realistic appraisal of degree of danger and thereby helping to prevent IPH and near homicide.

INTIMATE PARTNER HOMICIDE: INCIDENCE AND PATTERNS

Approximately 1,200 women have been killed by their current or former intimate partner in the United States during each year of the 21st century, and approximately 300 males were killed by their intimate partners during those same years (1,14). The United States continues to lead the industrialized world in homicide overall and IPH specifically (15). These numbers are down, from close to 1,600 of both male and female intimate partners in 1976. Somewhat ironically for those of us in the IPV field, the trajectory of decline has been much steeper for male than for female victims, from a close to 1:1 ratio in 1976 to a 4:1 ratio of females killed by intimate partners for every male.

These figures are based on the Supplemental Homicide Reports (SHR) and the analysis conducted by the Bureau of Justice Statistics (of the U.S. Department of Justice) on that data (1,14) which reports homicide between spouses, ex-spouses, and girlfriend-boyfriends. There is no category for ex-girlfriend/boyfriend. In the data from the national intimate partner femicide study, 19.3% of the victims, identified by a hand search of homicide records, were ex-girlfriends of the perpetrator (16). Therefore, the yearly total for the past 5 years is likely closer to 1,400 women and 400 male intimates killed.

This underreporting is important to keep in mind when examining the proportion of homicides that are officially placed in the intimate partner category. American women are most often killed by a husband or lover, or ex-husband or ex-lover (17–19). Thus, IPH is the largest category of murders of women, or femicide, accounting for approximately 30%–40% of murders of women according to the National Institute of Justice (20). The SHR misclassifies as many as 13% of IPHs of women in addition to the uncounted ex-boyfriends/girlfriends (21). A recent analysis of state data on homicides of women in 2001 found that husbands and intimates perpetrated in 51% of cases (22), a proportion supported by the addition of the ex-boyfriend perpetrator category found in the intimate partner femicide study. In contrast to homicides of women, homicides by intimate partners account for a relatively

Several risk factors have been associated with increased risk of homicides (murders) of women and men in violent relationships. We cannot predict what will happen in your case, but we would like you to be aware of the danger of homicide in situations of abuse and for you to see how many of the risk factors apply to your situation.

Using the calendar, please mark the approximate dates during the past year when you were abused by your partner or ex-partner. Write on that date how bad the incident was according to the following scale:

1. Slapping, pushing; no injuries and/or lasting pain
2. Punching, kicking; bruises, cuts, and/or continuing pain
3. "Beating up"; severe contusions, burns, broken bones, miscarriage
4. Threat to use weapon; head injury, internal injury, permanent injury, miscarriage
5. Use of weapon; wounds from weapon
   (If any of the descriptions for the higher number apply, use the higher number.)

Mark Yes or No for each of the following:
("He" refers to your husband, partner, ex-husband, ex-partner, or whoever is currently physically hurting you.)

Yes	No		
		1.	Has the physical violence increased in severity or frequency over the past year?
		2.	Does he own a gun?
		3.	Have you left him after living together during the past year?
			3a. (If have never lived with him, check here _____)
		4.	Is he unemployed?
		5.	Has he ever used a weapon against you or threatened you with a lethal weapon?
			5a. (If yes, was the weapon a gun? _____)
		6.	Does he threaten to kill you?
		7.	Has he avoided being arrested for domestic violence?
		8.	Do you have a child that is not his?
		9.	Has he ever forced you to have sex when you did not wish to do so?
		10.	Does he ever try to choke you?
		11.	Does he use illegal drugs? By drugs, I mean "uppers" or amphetamines, "meth," speed, angel dust, cocaine, "crack," street drugs or mixtures.
		12.	Is he an alcoholic or problem drinker?
		13.	Does he control most or all of your daily activities? (For instance: does he tell you who you can be friends with, when you can see your family, how much money you can use, or when you can take the car?
			(If he tries, but you do not let him, check here: _____)
		14.	Is he violently and constantly jealous of you? (For instance, does he say "If I can't have you, no one can.")
		15.	Have you ever been beaten by him while you were pregnant? (If you have never been pregnant by him, check here: _____)
		16.	Has he ever threatened or tried to commit suicide?
		17.	Does he threaten to harm your children?
		18.	Do you believe he is capable of killing you?
		19.	Does he follow or spy on you, leave threatening notes or messages on answering machine, destroy your property, or call you when you don't want him to?
		20.	Have you ever threatened or tried to commit suicide?

	Total "Yes" Answers
Thank you. Please talk to your nurse, advocate, or counselor about what the Danger Assessment means in terms of your situation.	

Figure 23.1 Danger assessment.
Source: Johns Hopkins University, School of Nursing, 2004 (www.dangerassessment.com).

small proportion of murders of men in the United States, approximately 5%–8% in 2000 (20,23).

As noted, the U.S. IPH rates overall have declined (24,25). One possible explanation for this trend is that the concurrent lower marriage rates in recent decades have decreased women's exposure to legally sanctioned spouses. However, although there has been a decrease in murders of married women by their husbands, there has been an increase in murders of nonmarried women by their boyfriends (25). Another reason for the decline appears to be lowered handgun availability, at least in some cities (20,26). A third possibility is that whatever is precipitating the risk of homicide overall to decrease is affecting the IPH rate in the same way. However, for female victims, the decrease in nonintimate partner victims has been far steeper than that for intimate partners.

As previously described, the largest decreases in IPH have been for male victims. Consequently, the *proportion* of male homicides by female intimate partners has decreased and the proportion of femicides by male intimate partners has increased. From 1976 to 1996, the percentage of IPHs with female victims increased from 54% to 70% (20,27). The decrease in the number of men killed by female partners coincided with the development of services for battered women and the enhancement of the criminal justice response, and it is in states where legal and advocacy resources are the strongest that the rates of male victims being killed have decreased the most (4). Since the vast majority (approximately 75%) of women who kill their abuser have been beaten by the victim before he was killed, we can deduce that these IPV resources and laws are facilitating women to take other alternatives to address the violence rather than feeling like "the only way out" is to kill. The contextual analysis by Rosenfeld (25) and his colleagues (24) has supported these connections on a local level, as well as indicating that divorce availability and female economic resources also have contributed to the decline in IPH for both men and women.

AREAS OF NEGLECT IN KNOWLEDGE RELATED TO INTIMATE PARTNER HOMICIDE

Despite a fairly robust analysis of IPH in general, several areas of inquiry have been neglected. Clear racial/ethnic disparities exist in rates of IPH, with Native-American and African-American women at increased risk (17,28). Although a significant proportion of this variation can be explained by increased rates of unemployment among African-American men (16), few investigations have tried to delineate what accounts for these discrepancies. In our intimate partner femicide study, although the majority of risk factors were similar for the African-American, White, Hispanic, and mixed race couples, we found different strengths of risk factors in certain groups and some risk factors not applying for some groups (29). For instance, prior arrest was found to be strongly protective against intimate partner femicide for White and mixed race couples but not protective at all for African-American and Hispanic couples. When looking at the data more closely, this was related to the fact that minority ethnic group males who killed their partners were more frequently arrested than the White male killers, and those ethnicity minority men were equally often arrested among both the lethal and abusive control groups.

Another understudied group is same-sex intimate partners. Nine cases (five actual, four attempted) of same-sex IPH were examined using a case series analysis (30) from the national intimate partner femicide study. The same-sex femicides represented approximately 2% of the overall cases of femicide and attempted femicide. In all but one of the cases, prior IPV against the victim of a lethal or potentially lethal act was revealed, and in that case, the victim was reported as having been violent toward her partner before she was killed. Three of the other female victims had also used violence in the relationships, both in self-defense and as primary aggressor. The risk factors for homicide identified in the larger study were common in this sample, with extreme control and jealousy on the part of the perpetrator nearly universal. However, this is the only published study of IPH among same-sex couples and this is of female same-sex couples only. The prevalence of IPV among male same-sex couples is apparently higher (up to 12 times the rate) than among females (6.2% of IPH are male couples versus 5% for female) (1).

A third area of neglect in terms of research is intimate partner femicide as a major cause of maternal mortality, or death during pregnancy, childbirth, or in the first year after delivery. As other medical causes of maternal mortality have decreased, the proportion of deaths caused by homicide has increased. In several U.S. cities and the entire state of Maryland, homicide is the leading cause of maternal mortality, causing as many as 20% of maternal deaths (31,32). In a national analysis, homicide was the second leading cause of maternal mortality (1.7 per 100,000 deaths) after automobile accidents (33). The lack of linkages between criminal justice and medical examiner records on maternal deaths has resulted in undercounts of maternal mortality due to homicide in any national database and limited the study of the association between maternal mortality and IPV, with the nature of the perpetrator–victim relationship unknown. Population-based studies have also not investigated the association between maternal mortality and abuse during pregnancy, although the 12-city femicide study demonstrated that abuse during pregnancy was a risk factor for IPH of women (34). In that investigation, 25.8% of 494 women killed or almost killed by their husband, boyfriend, or ex-partner had been abused during pregnancy (versus 8.4% of abused controls; AOR = 3.8) and 13 women (4.2%) were killed while they were pregnant. Eleven of those 13 women had been physically or sexually abused by their partners before those men killed or attempted to kill the women.

RISK FACTORS FOR INTIMATE PARTNER HOMICIDE

The dynamics of IPH are so distinct from general homicide that almost all experts agree that the risk factors need to be considered separately (17). Several studies over the last three decades have identified risk factors for IPH, especially for intimate partner femicide. Risk factors for IPH of male partners have been less well studied. The next section summarizes research on the most important and well-substantiated risk factors.

Battering

As previously described, prior IPV is most often a precursor of IPHs, whether the victim is the male or female partner. The majority (67%–75%) of IPHs involve battering of the female by the male intimate, no matter which partner is killed (2,3,16–18,35–37). Two early American studies in different jurisdictions demonstrated that two-thirds of the intimate partner femicide cases had a documented history of battering of the female partner (2,3). The recent 12-city femicide study found that 72% of the femicide cases were preceded by physical violence by the male partner

before he killed the woman (16). Battering characterized by increasing severity and threats with a weapon are hallmarks of increased risk.

Intimate partner homicides of men by women are also characterized by a history of battering of the female homicide perpetrator by the male partner in as many as 75% of the cases (2,38). It has long been noted that female-perpetrated IPHs are often characterized by self-defense, when the male partner is the first to show a weapon or strike a blow and is subsequently killed by his victim (2,4,39–43).

Stalking

Stalking may be an even more common precursor of IPH than abuse. McFarlane, Campbell, and Watson (44) reported that stalking and harassment occurred in 70%–90% of 200 actual and attempted femicides in the 12 U.S. cities. The strongest association with stalking was the combination of estrangement and prior abuse. Yet stalking also occurred in the majority of femicides in intact marriages and relationships in which there was no history of violence, and it also occurred frequently among the women in the same cities who were abused but not killed. Therefore, although stalking scores were significantly higher among women who were killed than abused women in the bivariate analysis, they were not significant in the multivariate analysis when other risk factors were entered into the equation (16).

Estrangement

An association has also been found between IPH involving husbands and wives and a history of estrangement (37,45–47). The estrangement may take the form of physical leaving or starting legal separation procedures. In an analysis of spousal homicide data from Canada, Chicago, and the United Kingdom, Wilson and Daly (46) found that the combination of physical and legal separation posed the most risk. From these studies and clinical experience with battered women, it has been theorized that male partners are threatened by loss of control over the relationship when women announce their decision to separate, and some men will stop at nothing to regain control, including femicide. Although it is clear that the period after separation is a time of increased risk, this danger has not been compared with the risk of staying in an abusive relationship. It has also been difficult to calculate whether separation increases risk in unmarried couples, since the proportion of separated to intact couples is not known. In studies in North Carolina and Ontario, two to three times as many couples (married and not) were intact as were estranged when the woman was killed (39,47). Close to the same proportion (70% intact, 30% estranged) was found in the data analysis of the femicides from the U.S. 12-city study. However, in 20% of the "intact" couples, the woman had left and returned at least once in the prior year (44). If one considers separation at least once during the prior year as a more precise measure of estrangement, then 55% of the intimate partner femicide victims in the final study were estranged from their partners when killed (16). In the final model, estrangement increased the risk of femicide (in comparison to abused women) by an adjusted odds ratio (OR) of 3.64. When the perpetrator was highly controlling *and* there was separation, the OR increased to 5.52.

Demographic Characteristics Associated with Intimate Partner Homicides

Like perpetrators of other homicides, male perpetrators of IPHs in the United States are mostly poor, young, a member of an ethnic minority group, have a history of other violence, and have a history of substance abuse (48). Resource theory of domestic abuse from sociology may offer a partial explanation. This theory suggests that when a man's personal resources, such as education, income, job prestige, and community standing, are lower than his spouse's, he may use violence to decrease the perceived status difference (49–51). Often young ethnic minority males are poorly educated, unemployed, or underemployed in comparison with their female partners (20,52,53). As a result, a small percentage may resort to violence and eventually murder as a means of exerting power and control to elevate or equalize their status in their intimate relationships. In the 12-city intimate partner femicide study, unemployment was the only demographic characteristic that was significant in the final model, increasing the risk of intimate partner femicide by an OR of 4.42.

Guns

Retrospective and case control studies have associated the use of guns and substance abuse (both drugs and alcohol) with IPH (4,54). Access to and availability of firearms in the United States greatly increases the risk of homicide in general, as well as the risk of IPH (55). Bailey and associates (18) reanalyzed the results of two population-based case-control studies and found that prior IPV and gun ownership were strongly associated with femicide in the home. In a study of 134 homicides of Native American, Hispanic, and non-Hispanic White women in New Mexico, researchers also found that firearms were nearly two times more likely to be used in "domestic" (intimate partner) femicides than other femicides (56). In most cities, handguns are the weapon of choice for IPHs (26) although in Chicago (43) knives (37%) were the most commonly used weapon from 1993 to 1996, with firearms a close second (37%). Male perpetrators were more likely than female perpetrators to beat an intimate partner to death and slightly more likely to use a handgun. In the 12-city femicide study (16), perpetrator access to a gun increased the risk of femicide by an OR of 5.38, and the use of a gun drastically increased the risk of the worst incident of abuse being fatal (incident level risk factor, OR = 41.38).

Alcohol and Drug Use

It is generally difficult to identify substance abuse in homicide perpetrators with certainty unless they have committed suicide and blood alcohol levels are thus available. There may also be differential risk depending on the substance used (drugs versus alcohol), general substance abuse versus intoxication at the time of the homicide, whether the victim or perpetrator or both were substance abusers, and sex of the victim and perpetrator. Males are more likely to be alcohol abusers as victims of IPH than as perpetrators, but male victims and perpetrators are more likely to abuse alcohol than are females in either category (2,39,57). Furthermore, alcohol use is not uniquely associated with IPH for women. Both Wilt (26) and Moracco (3) found alcohol use in as many women killed by intimate partners as killed by others. Persuasive evidence about drug abuse was found in two large data sets (Chicago and North Carolina) where significantly *less* drug abuse was found in cases of IPH than other homicides (3,58). Although both were significant at the bivariate level, neither perpetrator problem drinking nor perpetrator illicit drug use were significant predictors of femicide in the final models of the 12-city femicide study (16). Illicit drug use was a stronger predictor than problem drinking and remained a significant predictor until perpetrator aggressive behavior toward the partner was added into the model. Although subsumed by more powerful predictors, a remarkable 70% of the male perpetrators were using drugs or alcohol at the time of the homicidal incident (59). Neither victim drug nor alcohol use before or during the femicide were significant predictors after controlling for demographics (60).

Mental Illness

Zawitz (27) reported that 13% of perpetrators (12% of males, 15% of females) in 540 IPHs in the United States had a history of mental illness, compared to 3% (not reported by gender) of nonfamily murderers. In other data, approximately one-third of the 200 perpetrators in the 12-city study of attempted and actual femicides were described as being in poor (versus fair, good, or excellent) mental health (5). Forty-six percent of the male perpetrators had had at least one contact with a mental health professional, as compared to 29% of the victims; 33% had had some contact with an alcohol or drug treatment program, as compared to 25% of victims. In the comparative analysis, perpetrator mental health was a significant predictor on the bivariate level but not in multivariate analysis. It was, however, significant for the 29% of the cases of femicide that were followed by suicide by the male perpetrator (61). Few other studies have found mental illness to be a significant risk factor for IPHs, but few have been able to use adequate operationalization.

Differential Risk by Gender: Homicide–Suicide, Overkill, Forced Sex, and Abuse During Pregnancy

Homicide–suicides represent a significant proportion (27%–32%) of intimate partner femicides. This pattern is almost never seen when women kill a male intimate. Only 0.1% of such cases occurred in the North Carolina and Chicago studies (3,58). Intimate partner homicide–suicides follow different patterns than other intimate partner femicides. In this type of femicide, Whites are disproportionately represented (37,62,63).

Buteau and associates (63) in Canada as well as U.S. researchers (28,62) have divided homicide–suicides into "mercy killings" or "suicide pacts" that involve older couples afflicted by physical illness or other serious problems, and the more common case of IPH that is involuntary on the part of the victim,

followed by suicide of the perpetrator. In the much larger category of involuntary homicides involving younger perpetrators and victims (accounting for 90% of such cases in North Carolina), risk factors for perpetrators included being male, jealousy, current or past depression, a longstanding relationship with the victim, a history of physical abuse or separation/reunion episodes, personality disorder, and alcohol abuse (28,63). Separation was a factor in 45% of the North Carolina homicide–suicides (28). A significant proportion of the male perpetrators (15% in NC; 21% in Quebec) in the two major studies of the phenomenon had consulted mental health services in the year prior to the event (28,63). Depression was reported in 46% and substance abuse in 23% of perpetrators in Quebec. In North Carolina, 38% of the homicide–suicide perpetrators had ingested alcohol before death, but this was a slightly lower percentage than for partner femicides without suicide (3,28). In the analysis of the 29% of femicides that were homicide–suicides in the 12-city femicide study, perpetrator threats of suicide and perpetrator history of poor mental health were unique predictors of this form of femicide (61).

Overkill is another characteristic of intimate partner femicide that is not usually present when a female kills a male partner (2,4). Overkill was first described by Wolfgang in 1958 (42) as two or more acts of shooting or stabbing or beating the victim to death. Several North American studies have found that the majority (46%–90%) of women in IPHs are the victims of overkill, compared to 12% or less of males (4).

Data from the 12-city controlled-analysis study, as well as earlier descriptive studies, show associations of forced sex and abuse during pregnancy with intimate partner femicide (12,16,64–66). Forced sex was a significant risk factor in the final model of the 12-city femicide study (OR = 1.9), but abuse during pregnancy was significant on a bivariate level only. Particularly violent and dangerous men may be those who also force their partners into sex and beat them during pregnancy. In addition, jealous and controlling men may suspect or have evidence that the unborn child is not their biological progeny and therefore may kill their partners out of male sexual competitiveness (67). This theoretical approach was supported by evidence linking heightened risk of intimate partner femicide (uxoricide) and the presence of stepchildren in Canadian data as well as data from Chicago (67). The importance of this risk factor was also found in the 12-city intimate partner femicide study, with an increased risk of OR of 2.4 (16). However, the findings can also be explained through a power and control framework. Regardless, this finding, along with the abuse during pregnancy and forced sex findings, all have important implications for health providers. It is particularly important to asses for IPV among women who are being seen for gynecological problems and/ or prenatal care, since these women, if abused, are at particular risk. The same is true of mothers whose intimate partners are not the biological father of one or more of their children.

ATTEMPTED HOMICIDE

The other area of need for further research is attempted homicides. It is extremely difficult to determine just how common this phenomenon is since there is no separate database to access, but from our estimates in the national intimate partner femicide study and from gun injury data, it appears that there are approximately nine near-lethal (gunshot or stab wound to head, neck, or torso; strangulation or immersion in water to the point of unconsciousness; severe head injuries with a blunt object weapon) incidents for every IPH. Intimate partner violence is the most common cause of nonfatal injuries to young women in the United States (68,69). Intimate or ex-intimate partners use a variety of weapons, including guns, knifes, and their own hands to inflict severe injury (69,70). We do know that of the estimated 4.9 million intimate partner sexual and physical assaults perpetrated against women annually, approximately 2 million (41.5%) of the assaults will result in an injury to the woman, and 28% of the injured women will seek care in a healthcare setting (71). In the Tjaden and Thoennes (71) population-based survey, 16.7% of the women who sought care in the healthcare system were injured severely enough to be hospitalized at least overnight, and 17% said they had a head or spinal cord injury or a knife wound. An analysis of National Victim Survey data from 1992 to 1996 shows that 51% of abused women report that they have been injured from an IPV incident, with 7% treated in the emergency department, 3% treated in an outpatient setting, and fewer than 1% hospitalized (72). Of those treated in the emergency department, 21% were injured by a weapon, and 25% were diagnosed with a head injury, stab wound, or internal injury. Without intervention, these cases are most likely to continue to escalate, with potentially

fatal outcomes (70). Therefore, opportunities exist in healthcare settings to identify and intervene with women who are at risk for lethal and near-lethal assaults by intimates. In our study of attempted femicide, we found that very few (<10%) of the victims had been referred to IPV services even though they spent considerable time in emergency department and hospital settings, including trauma and rehabilitation centers.

Although we found the risk factors for intimate partner attempted femicide substantially the same as for actual femicide (including approximately 75% prior DV), we also found some interesting differences (16). In the multivariate analysis, perpetrator race (minority ethnicity: African American and Hispanic) was significant, rather than unemployment, and college education was protective in terms of demographics. Prior "choking" (attempted strangulation), forced sex, and threats to harm the children were stronger risk factors (OR = 2.9, 3.4, and 10.5, respectively). The major limitation of the attempted femicide analysis was that the population was difficult to identify and locate and therefore the sample was less representative. It was skewed toward poor and minority ethnicity victims, since those were the victims who had not been able to change locales after the attempted murder, as those who had resources tended to do. However, the advantage of this sample was that it avoided relying on police reports and/or proxies for information, and therefore there was less missing data and fewer concerns about validity. Our study of attempted IPHs is the only systematic controlled study of this phenomenon. More research clearly is needed in this area, and in terms of practice, more IPV services offered to the victims while they are recovering in the healthcare system.

Attempted Strangulation

The finding of attempted strangulations as a significant risk factor for attempted femicide also has extremely important implications for healthcare providers. There is a growing body of knowledge about attempted strangulation as a common abusive tactic by batterers and a potentially lethal act (73–75). The signs of strangulation can be detected by skilled medical or forensic nursing exam but are usually missed by non–healthcare professional providers (76–78). It is therefore important that these women are seen in the healthcare system, and the signs carefully documented both for potential future criminal justice proceedings but also because serious health consequences can result.

CHILDREN INVOLVED IN INTIMATE PARTNER HOMICIDE

Intimate partner homicide is at least occasionally accompanied by homicide of one or more of the couple's children, and rarely, children are killed in an IPV incident in which the mother is not killed. These events involving children being killed are far more common for intimate partner femicides than IPH of male partners, although there is only one systematic study of these incidents, a statewide study in Florida, that we could locate (37). In that study, 17% of the IPH cases in Florida also involved a child being killed and, in 49% of the cases, prior child abuse had occurred. This is another area of needed research, especially in terms of risk factors specific to children being killed.

In the 12-city intimate partner femicide study, we collected and analyzed data related to children who were in the homes of these cases of homicide and attempted homicide (79). Children younger than 18 years old were present in more than half (59%) of the femicide cases and 74% of the attempted cases. Of those cases with children, among the actual and attempted femicide cases, 32% and 58% of the cases respectively, a child witnessed the femicide, and in an additional 43% and 37% of the cases respectively, a child was the first to find the body. These are severely traumatized children, with 75% having witnessed IPV before the lethal or near-lethal event and 8% being the victims of reported child abuse. Even so, the majority of these children either never received any counseling or mental health services or only saw a professional once related to this trauma. Even though the majority of femicide cases ended with the mother's kin having custody of the children, many custody battles occurred and some children (26%) ended up in foster homes or with the perpetrator's kin. Clearly, all pediatric practices should inquire as to what was the precipitating event if a family member and not the biological parent is raising a child, with appropriate referrals in mind for children traumatized by direct child abuse, parental substance abuse, or homicide of a parent, the most common reasons for such living arrangements—and all traumatic for children. In the cases of attempted femicide, careful attention needs to be paid to appropriate referrals to child psychological

services and/or programs for children. These are also clearly areas for additional research.

LETHALITY ASSESSMENT

Recent studies of reassault suggest that battered women are the best predictors of their own risk of reassault (7,8), or at least in conjunction with a risk assessment instrument (6). Yet, existing research such as the 12-city femicide study (16) and other studies of IPH suggest that the risk factors for femicide and IPV reassault, although overlapping, are not exactly the same. It may be that women are better predictors of risk of reassault than of lethality; in fact, the recently completed National Institute of Justic (NIJ)-funded Risk Assessment Validation (RAVE) study, involving 1,307 battered women in New York City and Los Angeles, found some support for this, with abused women slightly better predictors of any reassault (0.572 accuracy with ROC analysis) than severe reassault (0.551) (80). The women also tended to underestimate rather than overestimate their risk. Thus, there is support for the contention that abused women who perceive their partner to be extremely dangerous are indeed correct about that perception, but that at least some and perhaps as many as half of those who do not perceive him to be extremely dangerous are underestimating their risk. The finding from the intimate partner femicide study that 54% of the actual femicides and 47% of the attempted victims did not accurately assess him (or her) as capable of killing continues to be persuasive in demonstrating the need for other means of helping battered women more accurately perceive their risk.

Several validated risk assessment instruments are primarily designed to be used in the criminal justice system to address risk of reassault (9,81–83). Continued research is needed to conduct wider and independent validation studies of these instruments.

THE DANGER ASSESSMENT

In contrast to the instruments designed to address risk of reassault, the DA is a clinical and research instrument designed to assist battered women in assessing their danger of being murdered by their intimate partner. The DA was originally developed with consultation and content validity support from battered women, shelter workers, law enforcement officials, and other clinical experts on battering (12). The initial items on the DA instrument were developed from retrospective research studies of IPH or serious injury (84–87). It was designed to assess risk of lethality for women killing male intimate partners as well as women being killed.

The first portion of the measure assesses severity and frequency of battering by presenting the woman with a calendar of the past year. The woman is asked to mark the approximate days when physically abusive incidents occurred, and to rank the severity of the incident on a 1 to 5 (1 = slap, pushing, no injuries and/or lasting pain through 5 = use of weapon, wounds from weapon) scale. The calendar portion was conceptualized as a way to raise the consciousness of the woman and reduce the normal minimization of IPV, especially since using a calendar increases accurate recall in other situations (100). In the original scale development, 38% of women who initially reported no increase in severity and frequency changed their response to "yes" after filling out the calendar (12).

The second part of the original DA was a 15-item yes/no dichotomous response format of risk factors associated with IPH, which has been expanded to 20 items based on the 12-city femicide study (88). Both portions of the instrument take a total of approximately 20 minutes to complete. The woman can complete the instrument by herself, with professionals from the healthcare, criminal justice, or victim advocate systems assisting in the interpretation of the instrument within the context of her situation. The DA can be scored by counting the "yes" responses with no classification or cutoff score, with a higher number indicating that more of the risk factors for femicide are present in the relationship. The original DA has published data on construct validity (54), but all studies thus far except for the original homicide study (2,84) address issues of risk with women as victims and men as perpetrators.

The initial studies using the DA instrument are described in detail elsewhere (12,100). In the 10 research studies (12,89–91,100) in which the DA was used, internal consistency reliability ranged from 0.60 to 0.86) without significant differences in different ethnic groups. In two studies in which test-retest reliability was assessed, it ranged from 0.89 to 0.94 (92,100). All samples include a substantial portion of minority women (primarily African American) and women from a variety of settings (100). Construct validity was supported by significant differences in mean scores among contrasting groups of women. The lowest mean score was found in the nonabused sample, with the highest score among the sample of women in the emergency department (54).

Convergent construct validity has been supported in the majority of the studies, with moderate to strong correlations with instruments measuring severity and frequency of IPV, including the Index of Spouse Abuse, the Conflict Tactics Scale, and injury from abuse (54). Since the last overall description, at least five additional independent studies have been conducted with additional reliability support (internal consistency of .69–.78). In further support of construct validity, the DA had significant correlations (.56–.62) as expected with instruments measuring symptoms of posttraumatic stress disorder (PTSD) (.93) and severity and frequency of IPV (.75) (66). In addition, in both of these studies, the DA successfully discriminated between groups of abused and nonabused women.

The DA instrument has been utilized in a variety of settings including battered woman's shelters and healthcare settings. The criminal justice system also is using the DA as a means of increasing victim safety, deterring perpetrators, and using limited resources effectively. In several jurisdictions, the DA has become a requirement for presentencing investigations, to develop appropriate sentences and probation conditions for IPV offenders in at least one jurisdiction (82). The Delaware State Police also use a revised version of the DA to evaluate perpetrator dangerousness.

The original DA measured the total number of "yes" responses by the battered woman on the 15 risk factors associated with IPH and is scored by counting the "yes" responses; a higher number indicates that more of the risk factors for homicide are present in the relationship. There is substantial concurrent construct validity support for the original DA, and now two independent predictive validity studies at least partially support the instrument's ability to predict reassault (6,7). The 12-city study also provided support for the risk factors on the DA being important risk factors for intimate partner femicide (94). The multivariate analysis of the risk factors for femicide from the 12-city study was used to revise the DA (four items added, one "double-barreled" item divided into two for a total of 20) and the weights used to develop a scoring algorithm with levels of risk (9). These levels of risk were then tested with the attempted femicide sample, producing a final outcome of .90 of the cases included in the ROC curve.

In more recent assessment of the DA in terms of reassault, the DA was found to be more predictive than three other systems of risk assessment—the DVSI, a 12-item assessment of risk of recidivism for use in offender-related decisions such as supervision and probation/parole; the K-SID, a 10-item risk assessment for recidivism used for offender charges and supervision decisions; and the DV-MOSAIC, a computer-assisted 46-item assessment of short- and long-term risk of severe and lethal violence in abusive relationships—primarily used to assist the victim in safety planning, as well as in determining women's perception of risk in a multiethnic, multisite study of relatively severely abused women seeking help for IPV or reported to the criminal justice system (9). In that analysis, the predictive accuracy of the revised DA was .687 (ROC curve analysis) for severe reassault, taking into account women's protective actions, compared to .647 for the DV-MOSAIC (95,96), .622 for the K-SID (97,98), .619 for the victim's perception, and .616 for the DVSI (99). Using the Wald statistic, which models the strength of the association of the method with the outcomes of severe reassault, again taking victim protective actions into account, the DA was again the most predictive. The comparative Wald statistics were 27.64 for the DA, 20.01 for victim perception, 8.61 for the DVSI, 4.80 for the DV-MOSAIC, and .34 (nonsignificant) for the K-SID. The DV-MOSAIC threat assessment system performed better than any of the other systems for prediction of stalking (Wald statistic 16.27 versus 15.14 for the DA, 13.38 for the DVSI, and 7.91 for victim perception, all significant at $p < .001$; K-SID nonsignificant). The DA attained the only significant Wald statistic (9.58) for mild to moderate reassault.

In summary, the DA is meant to be a collaborative exercise between an IPV advocate, healthcare professional, and/or criminal justice practitioner and the abused woman herself. It is meant to give both the woman and the practitioner information that may be useful for the criminal justice, advocacy, social welfare, substance abuse, batterer intervention, and/or healthcare systems as the woman navigates those systems. It is also meant to give a voice to abused women and to give their perceptions of risk credence, as it includes an item asking for the woman's perception of risk (6–8). Finally, the DA is designed to be used in conjunction with and to improve upon practitioner wisdom (100).

USE OF LETHALITY ASSESSMENT AS BASIS OF SAFETY PLANNING

Safety planning is the cornerstone of advocacy interventions for abused women, yet safety planning needs to be individualized according to the degree of violence and what the abused woman is planning. Women who are planning to leave or have already left the relationship need very different strategies for safety than do women who are planning to stay. We must also recognize that these choices may change over time, and that women may go back and forth among their choices, as well as back and forth in their relationship, and this is a normal part of the process of dealing with IPV and trying different strategies to make the violence end. The majority of abused women eventually do leave the violent relationship or manage to make it end (101), but this is a process that takes time. Our challenge is to help them stay safe during that time.

Safety planning also needs to be based on the degree of danger the perpetrator presents to the woman. Conducting the DA with her helps her come to a more realistic appraisal of the lethality risk and makes her much more engaged in safety planning. Another approach is to appeal to her mothering concerns. The majority of abused women have children, and the majority of abused women are indeed good mothers (102). Saying something like, "Let's talk about ways to keep you and the children safe" is an excellent entry into safety planning.

One safety planning strategy has been validated as increasing safety behaviors and decreasing postpartum violence using a quasi-experimental design in an ethnically diverse (African American, Anglo, and Hispanic) prenatal clinic sample (35,10). Often called "the brochure-driven intervention," the complete protocol can be obtained from the March of Dimes (11). It uses a brochure that can be made community-specific, individualized to the particular abused woman. It is meant to be a guide for the healthcare professional. It starts with an abbreviated version of the DA and then proceeds through safety planning strategies based on the woman's "choices" of whether she is planning to leave or stay, wants to use the criminal justice system or shelter services (residential and/or in the community), or other resources, as well as basic safety strategies for all women and space for the woman and healthcare provider to mutually generate additional strategies. The brochure may be kept in the woman's chart as a record of the safety planning process and to return to at the next visit for continuity. Rather than take an abuse-specific brochure or other IPV literature home, where it may be found by the abusive partner and create more danger, we recommend creating a community-specific list of "Women's Resources" that includes many (20–30) referral phone numbers for nonabuse-related services (e.g., WIC, the community mental health center, poison control, other women's health clinics, etc.) as well as, buried in the middle somewhere, the local DV hotline and the National DV Hotline (1–800–799-SAFE). This can be taken home without fear of reprisal.

The purpose of safety planning in the healthcare system is to use the process to determine a lethality assessment and bridge the woman to specialized IPV services if at all possible. Domestic violence (DV) program advocates in shelters, court programs, community-based programs, or other settings are well versed in comprehensive safety planning strategies. For those in healthcare settings, getting abused women in personal contact with DV advocates is one of the most effective means of making sure they have appropriate plans for keeping themselves and their children safe. Just giving a woman a referral number is not enough to get her there; we must take more proactive actions. A frequent method of control over abused women is for her abuser to provide her with only a cell phone; in this way, he can monitor the phone bills and see all outgoing and incoming phone numbers. Therefore, giving a woman access to a phone and privacy may allow her to reach out to advocates while she is in the healthcare setting. Making that phone call with her is often even more effective. Actually reaching out for assistance is a huge step; it feels stigmatizing, frightening, and a leap into the unknown. All the assistance and facilitation we can give her to make that first contact can be crucial in making sure she is in touch with IPV specialists.

The brochure-driven safety planning intervention can be used in the emergency department, primary or prenatal care settings, home visitation programs, pediatric clinics, or anywhere in the healthcare system where women are seen. It can take as little as 10 minutes to complete, depending on the complexity of the situation and the degree of risk. If the brief DA that is part of this intervention indicates more than half of the items present, a full DA is definitely warranted, with the calendar assessment and the weighted scoring determining levels of risk. Certification for using the weighted scoring of the DA and advice to give women

depending on the level of risk can be obtained at the DA website (www.dangerassessment.com).

CONCLUSION

Intimate partner homicide and attempted homicide continue to be a major threat to women's safety and health. Abuse against women is the major risk factor for IPH. The other most important risk factors that significantly elevate danger over prior abuse are estrangement, perpetrator gun ownership, perpetrator unemployment, a highly controlling abuser, threats to kill, threats with a weapon or use of a weapon, forced sex, a stepchild in the home (her biological child, not his), and the perpetrator avoiding arrest for DV. The woman having a separate domicile ("a place of her own") is protective against intimate partner femicide. Attempted intimate partner femicide is also an important issue, particularly for healthcare professionals, as these severely injured women are usually treated in the healthcare system and need intensive safety planning. The DA can be used as the basis for safety planning, so that women have a realistic appraisal of their level of risk.

IMPLICATIONS FOR POLICY, PRACTICE, AND RESEARCH

Policy

- Develop stricter policies for gun removal in homes where there is IPV and prior convictions for IPV assault or active protective orders under which gun ownership is prohibited.
- Promote systematic identification of children affected by IPH in every community, with proactive case management and mental health service and safety planning.

Practice

- Incorporate assessment of lethality risk for IPV victims in the healthcare system, with safety planning based on this danger assessment.
- Assess for IPV in victims of attempted homicide in the healthcare system, and require through practice guidelines and monitor through quality improvement measures to provide appropriate intensive safety planning with these victims.

- In homes where there is IPV and children, provide gun-safe storage materials and teaching.

Research

- A neglected area of research related to IPH includes determining risk factors for IPH when a male partner is killed, same-sex IPH, risk factors for attempted homicide, and maternal mortality and IPH.
- Also needed is clinical trial testing of safety planning interventions for abused victims in the healthcare system, to determine the value of lethality assessment as part of the safety planning process, and the development and validity testing of a brief version of the DA.

References

1. Fox GL, Jawitz MW. *Homicide trends in the United States.* Washington, DC: US Department of Justice: Bureau of Justice Statistics, 2004.
2. Campbell JC. "If I can't have you, no one can": Power and control in homicide of female partners. In: Russell JR, ed. *Femicide: The politics of woman killing.* New York: Twayne; 1992:99–113.
3. Moracco KE, Runyan CW, Butts J. Femicide in North Carolina. *Homicide Studies.* 1998;2:422–446.
4. Browne A, Williams KR, Dutton DG. Homicide between intimate partners: A 20-year review. In Smith, Dwayne M, Zahn MA, eds. (1999). *Homicide: A sourcebook of social research*; 1998.
5. Sharps PW, Koziol-McLain J, Campbell J, et al. Health care providers' missed opportunities for preventing femicide. *Prev Med.* 2001;33(5):373–380.
6. Heckert DA, Gondolf EW. Battered women's perceptions of risk versus risk factors and instruments in predicting repeat reassault. *J Interpersonal Violence.* 2002;19:778–800.
7. Goodman LA, Dutton MA, Bennett L. Predicting repeat abuse among arrested batterers: Use of the Danger Assessment Scale in the criminal justice system *J Interpersonal Violence.* 2000;15:63–74.
8. Weisz A, Tolman R, Saunders DG. Assessing the risk of severe DV: The importance of survivors' predictions. *J Interpersonal Violence.* 2000;15: 75–90.
9. Campbell JC, O'Sullivan C, Roehl J, Webster DW. *Intimate partner violence risk assessment validation study: The RAVE study. Final report to the National Institute of Justice.* (NCJ 209731–209732). Washington, DC: US Department of Justice, Office of Justice Programs, Bureau of Justice Statistics, 2005.
10. Parker B, McFarlane J, Soeken K, et al. Testing an intervention to prevent further abuse to pregnant women. *Res Nurs Health.* 1999;22(1):59–66.

11. McFarlane J, Parker B, Moran B. *Abuse during pregnancy: A protocol for prevention and intervention,* 3rd edition. White Plains, NY: March of Dimes, 2006.
12. Campbell JC. Nursing assessment for risk of homicide with battered women. *ANS Adv Nurs Sci.* 1986;8(4):36–51.
13. Campbell JC. Assessing dangerousness. 1995.
14. Durose MR, Harlow CW, Langan PA, et al. *Family violence statistics: Including statistics on strangers and acquaintances.* (No. NCJ 207846). Washington, DC: US Department of Justice, Office of Justice Programs, Bureau of Justice Statistics, 2005.
15. Krug EG, Dahlberg LL, Mercy JA, et al, eds. *World report on violence and health.* Geneva: World Health Organization, 2002.
16. Campbell JC, Webster D, Koziol-McLain J, et al. Risk factors for femicide in abusive relationships: Results from a multisite case control study. *Am J Public Health.* 2003;93(7):1089–1097.
17. Mercy JA, Saltzman LE. Fatal violence among spouses in the United States, 1976–85. *Am J Public Health.* 1989;79(5):595–599.
18. Bailey JE, Kellermann AL, Somes GW, et al. Risk factors for violent death of women in the home. *Arch Intern Med.* 1997;157(7):777–782.
19. Bachman R, Saltzman LE. *Violence against women: Estimates from the redesigned survey.* Washington, DC: US Department of Justice, 1995.
20. National Institute of Justice. *A study of homicide in eight US cities: An NIJ intramural research project (Research in Brief).* Washington, DC: US Department of Justice, 1997.
21. Langford L, Isaac NE, Kabat S. Homicides related to intimate partner violence in Massachusetts. *Homicide Studies.* 1998;2(4):353–377.
22. Brock K, Stenzel A. *When men murder women: An analysis of 1997 homicide data. Females murdered by males in single victim/single offender incidents.* Washington, D.C.: Violence Policy Center, 1999.
23. Lattimore PK, Linster RL, MacDonald JM. Risk of death among serious young offenders. *J Res Crime Delinquency.* 1997;34(2):187–209.
24. Dugan L, Nagin D, Rosenfeld R. Do domestic violence services save lives? *Natl Instit Justice J* 2003;250:20–25.
25. Rosenfeld R. Changing relationships between men and women. A note on the decline of IPH. *Homicide Studies.* 1997;1(1):72–83.
26. Wilt SA, Illman SM, Brodyfield M. *Female homicide victims in New York City.* New York: New York City Department of Health, 1995.
27. Zawitz MW. *Violence between intimates.* Washington, DC: Bureau of Justice Statistics, 1994.
28. Morton E, Runyan CW, Moracco KE, Butts J. Partner homicide victims: a population based study in North Carolina, 1988–1992. *Violence & Victims.* 1998;13(2):91–106.
29. Walton-Moss B, Campbell JC, Sharps PW. Ethnic group specific risk factors for intimate partner femicide. *Homicide Studies.* In press.

30. Glass N, Koziol-McLain J, Campbell J, Block CR. Female-perpetrated femicide and attempted femicide. *Violence Against Women.* 2004;10(6):606–625.

31. Krulewitch CJ, Pierre-Louis ML, de Leon-Gomez R, et al. Hidden from view: Violent deaths among pregnant women in the District of Columbia, 1988–1996. *J Midwifery Womens Health.* 2001;46(1):4–10.

32. Horon IL, Cheng D. Enhanced surveillance for pregnancy-associated mortality—Maryland, 1993–1998. *JAMA.* 2001;285(11):1455–1459.

33. Chang J, Berg CJ, Saltzman LE, Herndon J. Homicide: A leading cause of injury deaths for pregnant and postpartum women in the US, 1991–1999. *Am J Public Health.* 2005;95:1–7.

34. McFarlane J, Campbell JC, Sharps P, Watson K. Abuse during pregnancy and femicide: Urgent implications for women's health. *Obstet Gynecol.* 2002;100(1):27–36.

35. McFarlane J, Parker B, Soeken K, et al. Severity of abuse before and during pregnancy for African American, Hispanic, and Anglo women. *J Nurse Midwifery.* 1999;44(2):139–144.

36. Pataki G. *Intimate partner homicides in New York State.* Albany: State of New York, 1998.

37. Websdale N. *Understanding domestic homicide.* Boston: Northeastern University Press, 1999.

38. Hall-Smith P, Moracco KE, Butts J. Partner homicide in context. *Homicide Studies.* 1998;2(4):400–421.

39. Smith PH, Moracco KE, Butts J. Partner homicide in context: A population based perspective. *Homicide Studies.* 1998;2:400–421.

40. Crawford M, Gartner R. *Woman killing: Intimate femicide in Ontario: 1974–1990.* Ontario, Canada: Women We Honor Action Committee, 1992.

41. Jurik NC, Winn R. Gender and homicide: A comparison of men and women who kill. *Violence & Victims.* 1990;5:227–242.

42. Wolfgang ME. *Patterns in criminal homicide.* Philadelphia: University of Pennsylvania Press; 1958.

43. Block CR, Ovcharchyn Devitt C, Fugate M, et al. *The Chicago Women's Health Risk Study (Final Report).* Washington, DC: United States Department of Justice, National Institute of Justice, 2000.

44. McFarlane J, Campbell JC, Watson K. Intimate partner stalking and femicide: urgent implications for women's safety. *Behav Sci Law.* 2002;20 (1–2):51–68.

45. Wilson M, Daly M. Spousal homicide risk and estrangement. *Violence & Victims.* 1993;8(1):3–15.

46. Wilson M, Johnson H, Daly M. Lethal and nonlethal violence against wives. *Can J Criminol.* 1995;37:331–362.

47. Dawson R, Gartner R. Differences in the characteristics of intimate femicides: The role of relationship state and relationship status. *Homicide Studies.* 1998;2:378–399.

48. Weiner NA, Zahn MA, Sagi RJ, Merton RK. *Violence: Patterns, causes, public policy.* San Diego: Harcourt, Brace, Jovanovich, 1990.

49. Walker LE. *The battered woman syndrome.* New York: Springer, 1984.

50. Howard M. Husband-wife homicide: An essay from a family law perspective. *Law Contemp Probl.* 1986;49(1):63–88.

51. Jaynes GD, Williams RM. *A common destiny: Blacks and American society.* Washington, DC: National Academy Press, 1989.

52. Smith MN, Brewer VE. Female status and the "Gender Gap" in US homicide victimization. *Violence Against Women.* 1990;1(4):339–350.

53. Bowman PJ. The impact of economic marginality among African American husbands and fathers. In: McAdoo HP, ed. *Family ethnicity: Strength in diversity.* Thousand Oaks, CA: Sage; 1993: 120–140.

54. Campbell JC. Prediction of homicide of and by battered women. In: Campbell JC, Milner J, eds. *Assessing dangerousness: Potential for further violence of sexual offenders, batterers, and child abusers.* Newbury Park, CA: Sage; 1995:95–113.

55. Kellerman AL, Rivara FP, Rushforth NB. Gun ownership as a risk factor for homicide in the home. *N Engl J Med.* 1993;329:1084–1091.

56. Arbuckle J, Olson L, Howard M, et al. Safe at home? Domestic violence and other homicides among women in New Mexico. *Ann Emerg Med.* 1996;27(2):210–215.

57. Block CR, Block RL, Illinois Criminal Justice Information Authority. Homicides in Chicago, 1965–1995 [computer file], 4th ICPSR version. Chicago, IL: Illinois Criminal Justice Information Authority and Inter-university Consortium for Political and Social Research, 1998.

58. Block CR, Christakos A. Intimate partner homicide in Chicago over 29 years. *Crime & Delinquency.* 1995;41(4):406–526.

59. Sharps PW, Campbell JC, Campbell DW, et al. Risky mix: Drinking, drug use, and homicide. *NIJJ.* 2003;250:8–13.

60. Sharps PW, Campbell JC, Campbell DW, et al. The role of alcohol use in intimate partner femicide. *Am J Addictions.* 2001;10:122–135.

61. Koziol-McLain J, Webster D, McFarlane J, et al. Risk factors for femicide-suicide in abusive relationships: Results from a multi-site case control study. *Violence & Victims.* In press.

62. Stack S. Homicide followed by suicide: An analysis of Chicago data. *Criminology.* 1997;35(3): 435–453.

63. Buteau J, Lesage AD, Kiely MC. Homicide followed by suicide: A Quebec case series, 1988–1990. *Can J Psychiatry.* 1993;38(8):552–556.

64. Campbell JC, Soeken K, McFarlane J, Parker B. Risk factors for femicide among pregnant and nonpregnant battered women. In: Campbell JC, ed. *Empowering survivors of abuse: Health care for battered women and their children.* Thousand Oaks, CA: Sage; 1998:90–97.

65. Campbell JC, Soeken K. Forced sex and intimate partner violence: Effects on women's health. *Violence Against Women.* 1999;5(9):1017–1035.

66. McFarlane J, Soeken K, Campbell JC, et al. Severity of abuse to pregnant women and associated gun access of the perpetrator. *Public Health Nurs.* 1998;15(3):201–205.

67. Daly M, Wiseman KA, Wilson M. Women with children sired by previous partners incur excess risk of uxoricide. *Homicide Studies.* 1997 1(1):61–71.

68. Grisso JA, Wishner AR, Schwarz DF, et al. A population-based study of injuries in inner-city women. *Am J Epidemiol.* 1991;134(1):59–68.

69. Kyriacou DN, Anglin D, Taliaferro E, et al. Risk factors for injury to women from domestic violence. *N Engl J Med.* 1999;341(25):1892–1898.

70. Crowell NA, Burgess AW. *Understanding violence against women.* Washington, DC: National Research Council, 1996.

71. Tjaden T. *Extent, nature, and consequences of physical violence: Findings from the National Violence Against Women Survey.* Washington, D.C.: National Institute of Justice and Centers for Disease Control and Prevention, 2000.

72. Greenfeld LA, Rand MR, Craven PA, et al. *Violence by intimates: Analysis of data on crimes by current of former spouses, boyfriends and girlfriends* (Bureau of Justice Statistics Factbook, NCJ 167237). Washington, DC: Department of Justice, Bureau of Justice Statistics, 1998.

73. Strack GB, McClane GE, Hawley D. A review of 300 attempted strangulation cases Part I: Criminal legal issues. *J Emerg Med.* 2001;21:303–309.

74. Wilbur L, Higley M, Hatfield J, et al. Survey results of women who have been strangled while in an abusive relationship. *J Emerg Med.* 2001;21:297–302.

75. Glass NE, Laughon K, Campbell JC, et al. Strangulation as a risk factor for attempted and completed intimate partner femicide. *J Emerg Med.* In press.

76. Sheridan DJ. Treating survivors of intimate partner abuse: Forensic identification and documentation. In: Olshaker JS, Jackson MC, Smock WS, eds. *Forensic emergency medicine.* Philadelphia: Lippincott Williams, & Wilkins; 2001:203–228.

77. Sheridan DJ. Forensic nursing of family violence. In: Humphreys JC, Campbell JC, eds. *Family violence in nursing practice.* Philadelphia: Lippincott, Williams, & Wilkins; 2004.

78. Smith DJ, Mills T, Taliaferro E. Violence: Recognition, management, and prevention-Frequency and relationship of reported symptomology in victims of intimate partner violence: the effect of multiple strangulation attacks. *J Emerg Med.* 2001;21: 323–329.

79. Lewandowski LA, McFarlane J, Campbell JC, et al. He killed my mommy: Children of murdered mothers. *J Family Violence.* 2004;19(4):211–221.

80. Roehl J, O'Sullivan C, Webster D, Campbell JC. *Intimate partner violence risk assessment validation study (The RAVE Study): Practitioner summary and recommendations.* Report to the National Institute of Justice. At http://www.ncjrs.org/pdffiles1/nij/grants/209732.pdf 2005. Accessed 11/1/2008.

81. Dutton DG, Kropp PR. A review of DV risk instruments. *Trauma Violence & Abuse.* 2000;1: 171–181.

82. Roehl J, Guertin K. *Current use of dangerousness assessments in sentencing domestic violence offenders.* Pacific Grove, CA: State Justice Institute; 1998.

83. Roehl J, Guertin K. Intimate partner violence: The current use of risk assessments in sentencing offenders. *Justice Syst J.* 2000;21(2):171–198.

84. Campbell JC. Misogyny and homicide of women. *Adv Nurs Sci.* 1981;3:67–85.

85. Browne A. When battered women kill. In: Bergen RL, Edleson JL, Renzetti CL, eds. *Violence against women: Classic papers (2005).* Boston: Allyn & Bacon; 1987:xiv, 400.

86. Berk RA, Berk SF, Loseke DR, Rauma D. Mutual combat and other family violence myths. In: Gelles RJ, Hotaling G, Straus MA, Finkelhor D, eds. *The dark side of families.* Beverly Hills, CA: Sage Publishing; 1983.

87. Fagan J, Stewart DE, Hansen K. Violent men or violent husbands? Background factors and situational correlates. In: Gelles RJ, Hotaling G, Straus MA, Finkelhor D, eds. *The dark side of families.* Beverly Hills, CA: Sage Publications; 1983:49–68.

88. Campbell JC, Webster D, Koziol-McLain J, et al. Assessing risk factors for IPH. *Natl Instit Justice J.* 2003;250:14–19.

89. McFarlane J, Parker B, Soeken K, Bullock L. Assessing for abuse during pregnancy. Severity and frequency of injuries and associated entry into prenatal care. *JAMA.* 1992;267(23):3176–3178.

90. McFarlane J, Parker B, Soeken K. Abuse during pregnancy: Associations with maternal health and infant birth weight. *Nurs Res.* 1996;45(1):37–42.

91. McFarlane J, Gondolf E. Preventing abuse during pregnancy: A clinical protocol. *MCN Am J Matern Child Nurs.* 1998;23(1):22–26; quiz 27.

92. Stuart EP, Campbell JC. Assessment of patterns of dangerousness with battered women. *Issues Ment Health Nurs.* 1989;10(3–4):245–260.

93. Silva C, McFarlane J, Soeken K, Parker B, Reel S. Symptoms of post-traumatic stress disorder in abused women in a primary care setting. *J Womens Health.* 1997;6(5):543–552.

94. Campbell JC, Koziol-McLain J, Glass NE, et al. Risk factors for attempted femicide: Results from a cross national case control study. (Paper presented at Annual Meeting of the Homicide Research Work Group). 2003.

95. De Becker G. *The gift of fear.* Boston: Little, Brown, & Co., 1997.

96. De Becker GA. Domestic Violence Method (DV MOSAIC). At http://www.mosaicsystem.com/dv.htm; 2000. Accessed 11/1/2008.

97. Gelles R. Lethality and risk assessment for family violence cases. Paper presented at the 4th International Conference on Children Exposed to Family Violence. San Diego, CA, October 1998.

98. Lyon E. *The Revised K-SID: Analysis of reliability and relationships to new arrests after one year (An interim report).* The Office of Policy and Management, State of Connecticut; May 1998.

99. Williams KR, Houghton AB. Assessing the risk of DV re-offending: A validation study. *Law Hum Behav.* 2004;28(4):437–455.

100. Campbell JC, Sharps P, Glass NE. Risk Assessment for IPH. In: Pinard GF, Pagani L, eds. *Clinical assessment of dangerousness: Empirical contributions.* London: Cambridge University Press, 2001.

101. Campbell JC, Rose L, Kub J, Nedd D. Voices of strength and resistances: A contextual and longitudinal analysis of women's responses to battering. *J Interpersonal Violence.* 1998;13(6): 743–762.

102. Sullivan CM, Nguyen H, Allen NE, et al. Beyond searching for deficits: Evidence that physically and emotionally abused women are nurturing parents. *J Emotional Abuse* 2000;2(1):51–70.

Chapter 24

Mental Health Treatment for Survivors of Intimate Partner Violence

Carole Warshaw and Phyllis Brashler

KEY CONCEPTS

- Physical and emotional safety are primary concerns for survivors of intimate partner violence (IPV).
- Becoming knowledgeable about the dynamics of IPV and the strategies batterers use to control their partners is essential for working with survivors of IPV.
- Survivors face many obstacles in trying to leave an abusive relationship and/or to maintain their safety, credibility, and connections with others in the face of ongoing abuse.
- A combined IPV–trauma framework is potentially most helpful for understanding mental health symptoms in the context of ongoing trauma, entrapment, and danger.
- Respecting survivor self-determination and choice are key elements of both DV advocacy and trauma-informed treatment.

- Issues of culture, context, community, and spirituality play important roles in survivors' lives and need to be taken into account. Services should be culturally sensitive and relevant, as well as fully accessible.
- Maintaining confidentiality within the confines of the law and attending to DV-appropriate documentation are critical to survivors' safety.
- Intimate partner violence is not a psychiatric condition. No single treatment modality will meet the needs of all survivors.
- Limited research exists on mental health treatment in the context of ongoing IPV. Current best practice approaches involve combining core principles of IPV advocacy work with evidence-informed (and in some cases, evidence-based) trauma treatment. Research is needed to assess the types of interventions and treatment modalities that will be most helpful to survivors of IPV.

> • Recognizing the need to play an advocacy as well as a clinical role may be a new concept for clinicians, but supporting individual survivors and influencing policy and practice is integral to improving mental health care and preventing future violence.

Because intimate partner violence (IPV) victimization is not, itself, a psychiatric condition, mental health treatment for survivors of IPV involves a combination of IPV-specific interventions related to safety, confidentiality, and access to resources, as well as treatment for the range of symptoms that can arise in the context of ongoing abuse. Although important strides have been made in addressing the general healthcare response to IPV, little research has specifically addressed treatment outcomes for the mental health sequelae of IPV. Over the past 30 years, recommendations for responding to IPV have evolved into consensus models of care that can be integrated into appropriate evidence-based and/or emerging multidimensional treatment approaches. This chapter reviews currently available intervention and treatment research, discusses the strengths and limitations of existing evidence-based models for addressing the range of issues faced by IPV survivors, and describes current consensus recommendations for IPV-specific interventions and trauma treatment.

This is review has several limitations. First, no evidence-based treatments exist for addressing mental health issues in the context of ongoing IPV, although a small number of intervention studies targeting safety and/or providing post-shelter advocacy have demonstrated efficacy in reducing mental health symptoms (1–3). Second, only two studies exist on posttraumatic stress disorder (PTSD) treatment for survivors of IPV — one pilot study of women in shelters and one randomized controlled trial of cognitive behavioral therapy (CBT) for women who were no longer in an abusive relationship (4,5). Third, few controlled studies exist of complex trauma treatment in general, and none specifically designed for survivors of IPV, although a number of trauma treatment trials have included women who had experienced physical abuse as adults in addition to other lifetime trauma (6–10). Given that IPV survivors have a wide variety of life experiences with a range of mental health effects, no single treatment model will fit the needs of all survivors.

PREPARING TO ADDRESS INTIMATE PARTNER VIOLENCE: ISSUES TO CONSIDER

Although evidence-based interventions for IPV are still needed, "best practice" models have emerged to address the particular concerns of individuals dealing with ongoing violence and abuse (11–13). Key elements include integrating questions about IPV and other lifetime trauma into mental health assessments, discussing the impact of the abuse along with survivors' strengths and goals, addressing immediate and long-term safety needs, providing information about trauma and IPV, and discussing options, priorities, and choices. Documenting in ways that do not place survivors in further jeopardy, incorporating IPV- and trauma-specific issues into clinical treatment, and helping link survivors to community resources are also important components of a IPV-specific response.

A number of issues must be kept in mind when working with a person who is being abused by her (or his) partner; these that have been identified through the collective experience of survivors, clinicians, and advocates over the past 30 years. They can be attended to in conjunction with a range of treatment modalities to provide a consensus-based framework for addressing the potential, but avoidable, dangers that IPV survivors may face in seeking mental health care (13–18).

Attending to Physical and Emotional Safety

Recommendations for creating safe and welcoming practice environments reflect the convergence of experience from a number of different fields, including IPV literature, with its emphasis on physical safety and confidentiality (19); trauma literature, with its attention to emotional safety and the creation of trauma-informed services (16); cultural competency literature that focuses on creating culturally welcoming environments and culturally relevant services (20); disability literature that stresses the importance of universal accessibility and inclusive design (21); and the mental health peer support recovery movement that highlights self-determination, noncoercive practices, and choice (22).

Specific elements of welcoming practice environments include displaying visual materials that reflect the range of cultures and communities being served, providing written information about trauma and IPV in multiple languages as well as large print and

Braille, hiring multilingual and multicultural staff and American Sign Language (ASL) interpreters, employing assistive technology, and working in collaboration with community-based groups to ensure that services reflect the needs of their communities. Establishing practice environments and policies that support clinicians' efforts to address complex issues, provide adequate supervision and peer support, and that reimburse more time-intensive treatment modalities, advocacy, and collaboration are also key to institutionalizing culturally effective responses to trauma and IPV (23).

For all survivors of abuse, the issue of safety is paramount. This means considering a survivor's physical and emotional safety while in the clinical setting, as well as helping to assess options for safety when leaving. Although the traditional focus of mental health interventions has been on safety from self-harm, ongoing danger from a current or former partner and prevention of revictimization are also critical safety issues. Abusers are typically skilled at manipulating both their partners and the systems to which their partners turn for help, so all possible interventions should be considered through the lens of safety, looking for practices that can potentially put survivors at risk.

Women consistently report that the quality of the clinical interaction is an important factor in their response to questions about abuse (24,25). For a person living with ongoing threats and intimidation, the experience of being treated with respect and feeling free to make choices without fear of judgment or retaliation can be therapeutic in itself and is often central to the healing process (26,27). Clinical interactions can provide an opportunity for survivors to experience other people as trustworthy and safe, to counter abuse-related dynamics they may have internalized, and to regain a sense of connection to themselves and others. For some survivors of IPV, any manifestation of themselves as an autonomous human being is met with further abuse and retaliation, forcing them to psychologically disappear from view. Creating an atmosphere of acceptance and validation can help to counter the batterer's ability to control and undermine a woman's perceptions of herself and can provide a safe place for her to reemerge. It can diminish shame and reduce the likelihood of retraumatization in the therapeutic encounter and provides a vehicle through which survivors can access information, resources, and support, and then build on existing strengths and develop new skills. For some survivors, particularly those whose trust has continually been betrayed, reestablishing trust may be part of a much longer therapeutic process.

The power imbalances inherent to clinical interactions also require conscious attention. Survivors of abuse are particularly vulnerable to reinjury and often are very attuned to relational dynamics. This is of particular concern for clinicians who have been trained in more directive treatment modalities or work in settings that require adherence to a specific treatment plan. Being able to tolerate feelings of fear and uncertainty that may arise when a person is in danger and chooses not to leave an abusive relationship can be particularly challenging. It is incumbent on clinicians to be aware of their own responses and manage them in ways that are not distancing or judgmental to the person seeking care.

Numerous studies have demonstrated that the manner in which clinicians ask about abuse and the nature of their responses to a disclosure impact women's level of comfort in discussing these issues (28–31). In addition, the clinical and research literature on trauma-informed services corroborates the importance of creating emotionally safe practice environments, particularly for survivors of abuse (9,10,16,32–34). Clinicians can facilitate this process by attending to the environment itself for potential ways a survivor could be retraumatized. For example, it is critical to establish privacy before inquiring about current IPV and to assure patients that what they say will remain confidential within the limits of the law. However, for a person who has experienced abuse, particularly if they were abused by someone in a caregiving role, being alone in a room with another person behind a closed door may evoke earlier experiences that were unsafe. Telling a patient "what goes on between us will not leave the room," may be frightening, rather than reassuring to someone who was sexually abused as a child (16). For others, routine history taking may feel too much like interrogation. Discussing these issues at the outset can help to mitigate some of these concerns.

Another set of issues germane to emotional safety is communicating in ways that help to destigmatize mental health symptoms, normalize responses to abuse, and offer information, choices, and hope. Survivors frequently report that one of the things they find most helpful in talking with advocates is learning that they aren't "crazy." There are a number of ways one can communicate respect and understanding, by how questions are asked and framed and by conveying the following information:

- Abuse experiences are common.
- You are willing to listen.
- You believe her and are concerned.
- The abuse is not his fault; no one deserves to be treated that way.
- Resources are available to help them if they are currently in danger.
- They will not be judged or stigmatized as a result of what they have said to you.
- All information will be confidential within the confines of subpoenas and mandatory reporting laws (inform patients about the limitations of confidentiality in your state) (11,35).

Understanding the Dynamics of Abuse and Perpetrator Accountability

Understanding the dynamics of IPV and recognizing that abusive behavior is the responsibility of the perpetrator, not the victim, is another area in which mental health treatment models have had to be reexamined, particularly psychodynamic and family systems approaches. Actively counter the notion that the abuse is or was the fault of the person being victimized and make clear that, regardless of any seeming provocation, the perpetrator is ultimately responsible for his (or her) abusive behavior and also responsible for stopping it (15). Until the 1980s, the psychiatric literature generally viewed domestic violence (DV) as resulting, at least in part, from women's pathology (e.g., masochism), or from problematic dynamics within the relationship (36,37). This is no longer considered a legitimate understanding.

Although experiencing or witnessing abuse in childhood may place women at greater risk for being abused as adults, the major risk factor for partner abuse is living in a society that tolerates gender-based violence. Growing up in a situation in which protecting oneself was not an option or never having learned that a woman has rights in a relationship does not make a person responsible for another's criminal behavior. The use of abuse and violence is a choice of the perpetrator to maintain coercive control over an intimate partner. Although taking responsibility for *one's own behavior* is one of the hallmarks of a mental health recovery, if a woman is continually being told that she is responsible for *her partner's behavior*, hearing this in

treatment is not only confusing but can be undermining and dangerous as well (e.g., helping survivors to understand why they unconsciously "chose" an abusive partner or labeling survivors as "codependent" or "enabling"). Working with a survivor to understand the psychological roots of her current feelings, symptoms, and situations, or working with patients on changing cognitions and behaviors that they feel are getting in their way, can be helpful in the right context. In the context of ongoing IPV, this is often problematic, particularly when a survivor's options for changing her situation are limited or the risks she faces are too great. The influence of earlier abusive relationships on survivors' ability to find safe, mutually respectful relationships as adults is best addressed in later phases of treatment when survivors are no longer worried about their immediate safety, being bullied by a partner, negotiating the legal system, or blaming themselves for experiences that were beyond their control.

Freeing oneself from the tyranny of the past *is* empowering. Timing and sensitivity are critical. That is why certified batterer intervention programs, accompanied by criminal sanctions rather than individual or couples therapy, are the preferred mode of intervention for abusers, where the need for ongoing accountability and attention to victim safety are always in the forefront (38).

Utilizing an Intimate Partner Violence-informed Trauma Framework

There is a growing consensus that mental health treatment is best delivered within a framework that incorporates an understanding of the pervasive experience of trauma among people seeking mental health services. This includes the ways in which a history of trauma can affect survivors' symptoms and presentations, their experience of clinical relationships, and their responses to treatment (16,39). Trauma theory offers a perspective that acknowledges strengths, views individuals as survivors rather than victims, and recognizes symptoms as adaptive responses to intolerable experiences when real protection is unavailable and coping mechanisms are overwhelmed or never had a chance to develop (27,40). Although efforts to infuse a trauma perspective into mental health services have mainly focused on the long-term effects of childhood abuse, a trauma framework is also useful for understanding the mental health effects of IPV. The recognition that external events can have a psycho-physiological impact has helped alleviate survivor concerns about a diagnostic system that did not take into account the context in which symptoms developed. When viewed through a trauma lens, symptoms are understood, at least in part, as responses to repetitive trauma that affects a person's expectations about human relationships and causes both physical and psychological harm.

Ongoing abuse and violence can also induce feelings of shock, disbelief, confusion, terror, isolation, and despair, and can undermine a person's sense of self. This, in turn, can manifest as psychiatric symptoms and disorders. For those who have also experienced abuse in childhood, the ability to manage painful internal states (affect regulation) may be disrupted, leaving survivors with coping mechanisms (e.g., self-cutting, suicide attempts, risky behavior, substance use) that incur further harm. Trusting others, particularly those in caretaking roles, may be especially difficult.

However, for a person who is still at risk, symptoms may also reflect a realistic response to ongoing danger and entrapment. For example, from a trauma perspective, an "overreaction" to minor stimuli is seen as symptomatic of a trauma-related psychiatric disorder (e.g., PTSD) rather than an appropriate response to ongoing threats, danger, and terrorization. What may be interpreted as "triggering" through a trauma lens, might, from an advocacy perspective, reflect a response to ongoing victimization. When dealing with ongoing abuse, operating from a framework that addresses both internal and external threats is essential. Although wariness, lack of trust, or seemingly paranoid reactions may be a manifestation of previous abuse and/or a response to the trauma of current victimization, heightened sensitivity may also be a necessity for survival.

Other, seemingly passive behaviors may represent survival strategies as well. For example, over the course of an abusive relationship, survivors often exhibit considerable strength and ingenuity, attempting to remedy their situations through talking, seeking help, fighting back, and trying to change the conditions that they either perceive or are told cause the abuse. When those attempts fail, however, they may retreat into a mode that appears more passive and "compliant" but which actually reflects strategies designed to reduce their immediate danger by meeting the coercive demands of an abusive partner (41). A primary example of this is the decision to stay in an abusive relationship: although some mental health models conceptualized this as passive dependent behavior, leaving an abusive partner can involve great risk to the victim. In fact, the majority of IPV homicides occur after the victim has left the relationship (42). Choosing to remain in an abusive relationship is often based on a strategic analysis of safety and risk.

Responses such as dissociation, avoidance, and/or use of drugs or alcohol may protect against feelings that have become unbearable, particularly if survivors' options are limited. Although these responses may make it possible to survive intolerable conditions, they can also restrict a person's capacity to reach out for help. Societal constraints, such as the ongoing trauma of social discrimination, lack of basic resources, and revictimizing experiences within the systems a survivor turns to and/or the legacies of historical or cultural trauma, are other factors that affect a survivor's ability to heal from the abuse and mobilize the resources necessary to create safety and stability in her life. Utilizing a IPV-informed trauma framework to address coping strategies such as substance abuse or seeming passivity in the face of ongoing threats not only provides perspective for survivors on behaviors they may experience as shameful, but also reduces the likelihood of responding in ways that are unintentionally judgmental or pathologizing.

In addition, trauma theory affords a more balanced approach to treatment—one that focuses on resiliency and strengths as well as psychological harm. Trauma-focused interventions help survivors to recognize their own abilities, develop new skills, and enhance their capacities to manage previously overwhelming feelings. A trauma framework regards collaborative therapeutic relationships as central to the process of healing, requiring that providers be attuned to the impact of their own responses on the person seeking help. Utilizing a trauma framework enhances the prospect for therapeutic success by fostering an awareness of the impact of this work on providers. Self-awareness, consultation, and peer support are hallmarks of this approach.

Attending to Issues of Culture, Community, and Spirituality

Intimate partner violence affects people across cultures, communities, races, sexual orientations, gender identities, religions, spiritual and political beliefs, ages, abilities, socioeconomic status, educational backgrounds, and occupations (43). There is general consensus among the mental health, trauma, and IPV fields that to be effective, interventions need to be sensitive to the range of experiences and values survivors bring to treatment (39,44). Clearly, many factors affect personal choices and realistic options, including how individuals view mental health and mental illness, the types of stressors they encounter, the decisions they make in seeking help, the symptoms and concerns presented to clinicians, and their coping styles and sources of social support (45). Recognizing these concerns and addressing them directly can help reduce some of the barriers survivors face in obtaining help. There may also be specific sources of support survivors can access through their membership in particular communities. Understanding how particular cultures and communities uniquely affect each survivor entails talking with them about how their experience of culture, as they define it, affects their perceptions of abuse, access to services, response to interventions, perspective on staying with an abusive partner, and the constraints they may face in leaving. For male victims, these issues may be more complicated.

Attending to Privacy and Confidentiality

Although assessment is often looked upon as the first phase of treatment, it is also an ongoing component of the treatment process. Even when IPV is present, survivors may have compelling reasons for not disclosing the abuse. A woman could lose custody of her children if she is identified as having mental health problems—or if it is discovered that she lives in a violent household. Her partner may have threatened to kill her or her children if she reports the abuse or tries to leave. A woman may also experience intense guilt and shame, particularly about sexual assault and abuse. This can make it difficult for her to raise or discuss these issues until she feels safe in a therapeutic relationship or more secure in her own life. Thus, it is important that providers continue to be mindful of IPV as a possibility and inquire about it periodically even when abuse is not initially reported.

Because disclosure of abuse carries the risk of retaliatory violence, asking about IPV requires that every measure be taken to maintain privacy and confidentiality. Consensus guidelines are clear with regard to not asking about abuse in the presence of a possible perpetrator, or in the presence of another person whom

a patient has not privately identified as someone she or he can trust, with that information, including an untrained translator, a personal assistant, guardian, a friend, or a child. In addition, these questions should not be asked during a couple's therapy session, or in the presence of a person who is providing collateral information—even if a patient is unable to respond herself at the time. It is common practice when a person is being evaluated for a psychiatric emergency to try to obtain additional information from the accompanying party or a family member, who may, turn out to be abusing them. It is better to ask patients whom they would prefer information be obtained from and whom they trust the clinician to talk with about their situation. Questions about abuse also should not be included in forms that are sent to a patient's home. Online questions about abuse are also potentially unsafe, as abusers can track their partners Internet activity. Patients should be told that the information they give is confidential and, within the confines of the law, will not be revealed to their partner or anyone else without their permission. For those clinicians who practice in states with mandatory reporting laws for DV, it is essential to inform clients of this requirement in the beginning of the evaluation, preferably before they have discussed the abuse, so that they can determine whether it will be safe to disclose. It is also important to discuss reporting obligations before inquiring about child abuse (46).

In addition, because batterers are often resistant to being separated from their partners, strategies for safely separating clients from abusers should be developed in advance, so that inquiry can take place. If there does appear to be an immediate threat from a client's abusive partner, clinicians should be prepared to notify the police or security, outlining any potential risk. If a patient calls on the phone, it is prudent to establish whether or not it is safe for them to discuss these issues before inquiring about abuse. Once initial safety is established, however, a patient's wish to have another person present should be respected.

Incorporating an Advocacy Approach and Emphasizing Survivors' Goals and Concerns

Incorporating an advocacy stance adds an important dimension to traditional clinical interactions—one that is consistent with recovery approaches (47). For example, advocacy involves facilitating rather than directing change by actively helping survivors to become aware of their options, gain access to community resources, make their own choices about how to best reduce their exposure to ongoing violence, and mitigate the impact of abuse on their lives. Awareness of both the internal and external barriers survivors face in ending abuse and recovering from its traumatic effects is necessary to advocate with other systems. Clinicians can also play a critical role in preventing future violence by participating in professional, community, and public policy activities that address these issues.

To clarify priorities, plan treatment, and determine advocacy needs, it is also important to understand survivors' immediate concerns and long-term goals, how they envision achieving those goals, and the assistance and resources they feel would be helpful. Some authors have found it useful to apply the transtheoretical "stages of change" model (e.g., precontemplation, contemplation, preparation, action, maintenance), developed by Prochaska and DiClimente for treating addictions, to the process of leaving an abusive relationship (48–50). The original model was based on the assumption that changing—that is, stopping—the harmful behavior is the desired goal and that the barriers to doing so reside within the patient. In situations of ongoing IPV, this is often not the case (e.g., a survivor may not want to leave or options for doing so may be limited or possible only at great cost).

A number of concepts derived from this model can be useful to consider in this context (e.g., decisional balance, process of change). The goal of the transtheoretical model was to examine how change takes place and what helps patients in that process. The danger of applying this model directly to work with IPV survivors is that they do not control the dangerous behavior, nor is it their responsibility to change it. The recognition that relapse is often an integral part of the process of change is also both useful and problematic. Domestic violence survivors frequently leave abusive relationship multiple times before gathering the internal and external resources to support a permanent separation. Understanding this process helps reduce frustration and blame. However, framing these decisions as "relapses" implies that the problem is located in the woman's ability to change, rather than in circumstances that may in fact be out of her control. More recent adaptations of this concept, however, have been used to foster recognition that deciding to leave can be a longer process, that

"precontemplation" may actually be a survival mechanism, and that moving from "contemplation" to "action" involves many factors that are not always under a survivor's control (51).

For a person faced with multiple, complex survival issues, the abuse they are currently experiencing may not be their most immediate concern. Being able to understand how a woman feels about her relationship and to discuss this openly and nonjudgmentally will ideally make it safer for her to reassess her situation over the course of treatment. Although the choice of whether or not to leave an abusive partner may seem like a clear-cut decision, it is often a lengthy process filled with enormous barriers—one that involves continually weighing a complex set of risks and concerns that a survivor may have little ability to change. Thus, decision-making is not just a question of whether she wants to stay in the relationship, but a complex process of careful risk assessment. Issues such as negotiating safety and retaining custody of children are constantly in the balance. Davies, Lyon, and Monti-Catania developed a conceptual framework for addressing these issues that allows practitioners to help a survivor sort through the complex and potentially competing demands she faces (19).

ROUTINE INQUIRY AND ASSESSMENT

Because presentations of IPV vary widely, inquiring only when abuse is suspected will miss significant numbers of individuals who are at risk. Although some controversy persists over routine screening for IPV in healthcare settings, consensus documents in the United States continue to recommend routine inquiry of all women patients and, although less studied, men who may be at risk—men with disabilities, older men, and men in gay relationships (11,14,18,52–56). It is important to note that many survivors are still in danger at the time they seek help, and if they decide to leave, the danger may increase significantly. Some are at increased risk because they have left or their partner is aware of their intention to leave. Assessing ongoing safety and risk for harm is an essential component of working with IPV survivors and should be incorporated into both the initial and ongoing assessment process. An in-depth review of research on danger assessment is addressed elsewhere in this text, and can also be found in the well-regarded volume on safety planning by Davies, Lyon, and Monti-Catania (19).

Mental Health Crisis Calls or Phone Intakes

Although routine inquiry about IPV in healthcare settings is addressed elsewhere in this volume, a number of specific issues arise in mental health settings. How initial inquiry and assessment take place will vary by setting, but attention to immediate safety is always a priority. Integrating IPV inquiry into emergency mental health assessments may necessitate the revision of standard intake procedures. For example, typical mental health crisis assessment involves determining whether a patient is *a danger to* herself or others. Crisis evaluation should also assess whether or not a person is *in danger from* others. If a person does state they are in imminent danger from another person, addressing immediate safety needs take precedence. Asking questions that can be answered with a "yes" or "no" may be safer under these circumstances

Integrating Questions About Intimate Partner Violence into Mental Health Assessments

Introducing the subject of abuse may feel awkward, particularly if there are no obvious indications a patient has been victimized. There are many ways to frame abuse-related questions that let patients know that this is a common experience and that you are interested in knowing (e.g.,"I don't know if this has happened to you, but because so many women experience abuse and violence in their lives, it's something I always ask about," or "Tell me about your relationship."). It is, however, important to ask explicit questions about specific abusive experiences. Simply asking a woman "Have you ever been abused?" places her in the doubly difficult position of having to evaluate her assailant's behavior, as well as report it. For an example of an IPV assessment tool, see the *National Consensus Guidelines on Identifying and Responding to Domestic Violence Victimization in Health Care Settings* (11).

Because abusers frequently use mental health issues to control and undermine their partners, these issues need to be addressed specifically. Clients who are currently experiencing IPV should be asked the following:

- Has your partner ever used mental health issues against you? Does your partner try to control your medication or your treatment? Does he blame you for his abusive behavior by telling you you're "crazy"? Does he tell you that no one will believe you? That you'll lose your children if you try to leave? Has he used your mental health condition as a way to undermine you with other people? Does he tell people that your claims of abuse are delusional, or that you aren't to be trusted? Has he ever forced you to take an overdose or kept you from routines that are healthy for you (eating, sleeping, resting, seeing other people, exercising)? Has he ever lied about your condition to have you involuntarily committed? Has he strangled or otherwise assaulted you and then claimed that you were out of control and needed to be restrained? Has he engaged in behaviors that were designed to play on your particular vulnerabilities or undermine your sense of reality (e.g., lies, distortion, doing and saying things and then denying them, taunting, abandoning, trying to turn the children against you, threatening to take or harm your children, or telling you that you should kill yourself)?
- Does your partner try to prevent you from stopping drinking or using drugs? Does he try to keep you from attending treatment or going to meetings?

As well as eliciting a history of physical assaults and sexual violation, obtain a more detailed history of the forms of psychological abuse and the level of control the abuser has over a survivor's life, including social isolation, stalking and harassment, economic abuse, destruction of property, use of children, and abuse of animals or pets. It is also helpful to ask survivors about the *pattern* of abuse they've been subjected to, such as when it started; its duration, frequency, severity, pace of escalation; and its relation to events such as pregnancy, separations, unemployment, or substance abuse. Working collaboratively to identify patterns related to the use of and degree of control, isolation, and fear, as well as identifiable signs of impending violence and other criminal behaviors, can be particularly useful. Discussing these patterns can help to clarify the ongoing nature of the abuse both for the clinician and survivor, and reduce some of the denial, avoidance, or dissociation a woman may have needed to survive.

Keep in mind that women seeking help who are currently being abused by an intimate partner may have already been asked to provide detailed accounts of their experience to emergency room personnel and to the police. It is important to assess the nature of the trauma that may have precipitated treatment; however, acquiring more detailed information should be paced to the survivor's needs. Asking about a patient's experience of IPV can serve a number of important functions beyond informing treatment. It allows clinicians to document critical information for women seeking legal protection, redress, or custody and provides a safe opportunity to examine the ongoing nature of the abuse and its impact. In addition, asking a woman what she has done to try to remedy her situation and how others have responded to her efforts creates a chance to explore new options and to acknowledge the resourcefulness she has exhibited in coping with her situation.

The same caveats apply to asking about previous trauma. Traumatic childhood experiences may also play a significant role in patients' current mental health symptoms, increasing their risk for revictimization and affecting how they experience current abuse. Over time, understanding and demystifying the long-term effects of prior abuse can be both freeing and empowering. In general, inquiry about childhood abuse and other lifetime trauma should be part of a comprehensive mental health assessment, preferably in the context of an ongoing clinical relationship in which trust has been established. During the initial assessment process, asking a general question about the relationship of previous trauma to current symptomatology can be helpful. For example, "Are there other painful or frightening experiences you've had recently or in the past that you think may be related to what you are feeling now?"

Previous Trauma History

The timing of questions about abuse experiences should be geared toward an individual's ability to respond without being flooded or overwhelmed, particularly if currently experiencing a crisis. Although the symptoms or issues that emerge during an assessment may seem to point to a history of trauma, an individual survivor may not see it that way. Although some women may seek treatment for symptoms or issues explicitly related to a particular traumatic experience, not everyone will link their current distress to such events. Many will not recall earlier traumas until later in the course of treatment, and survivors may avoid thinking and talking about trauma-related topics because the feelings associated with the trauma can be overwhelming (57).

General consensus from the trauma field suggests that it is incumbent upon clinicians to keep an open mind about the potential presence of trauma in a patient's history, to attend to abuse-related information as it arises, and to validate those perceptions without "digging" for memories or assuming that because a woman has a particular constellation of symptoms she has been sexually abused as a child. Similar to inquiry about current IPV, questions about previous trauma should be designed not to uncover, but to let patients know that these experiences are common, and that they can discuss them, if and when they feel comfortable doing so. Inquiry should take place at a time when there is room for patients to talk about how they were affected by those experiences, whether or not they are experiencing symptoms currently, and what would be most helpful to them now.

Because conducting a trauma history can in itself be traumatizing, informing patients of what will be asked and why, checking to see if they are comfortable with proceeding, attending to signs (such as increased anxiety or dissociation) that prior traumatic experiences are being triggered, and ensuring that they have someone to talk with should the need arise after they leave, are critical (58,59). A number of tools are available for obtaining a trauma history that have primarily been used for research purposes (60–64). In clinical practice, this type of information is often better elicited by asking more general questions accompanied by gentle probing when indicated. Questions embedded in self-administered general health questionnaires have also been found acceptable (65). Often this information emerges gradually during the narrative retelling of an individual's life history. The aim is to let patients know that many people have experienced trauma in their lives, that these experiences may have some bearing on their health and well-being, and that the clinician is interested in knowing about the things in their life that have affected them (Table 24.1).

ASSESSING SAFETY

Immediate Safety and Risk of Future Harm

For any patient who is at risk, safety issues should be addressed during the initial interview, and access to a

Table 24.1 Previous Trauma History: Questions to Consider

- Has this person experienced abuse prior to her/his current relationship?
- Was she/he physically, sexually, or emotionally abused, bullied, or neglected as a child? Was she ever removed from her home?
- Was she/he sexually assaulted or harassed as an adult?
  - Have you had other experiences that left you feeling frightened and alone? For example, have you ever been physically or sexually assaulted by someone other than your partner? With who? When? What happened?
  - How did that affect you, and how are you now?
  - Have you ever been pressured to engage in sexual activities that made you uncomfortable or been forced to have sex against your will, such as unwanted kissing, hugging, touching, nudity, exposure, attempted intercourse, trading sex for drugs?)
- Has she/he experienced other types of trauma in the past?
  - Have you had other painful or frightening experiences, such as:
  - Living through a disaster?
  - Being the victim of a crime?
  - Having someone close to you die or seeing someone being abused, injured, or killed?
  - Having had a family member who used drugs or alcohol, who committed or attempted suicide, or who was incarcerated?
  - Having been homeless, incarcerated, or institutionalized?
  - Having had your children taken from you?
  - Been harassed or discriminated against in any way? Been a combat veteran, lived through war as a civilian, or experienced acts of political torture, terrorism, or other violations of your human rights?
  - Experienced discrimination or harassment? Experienced seclusion and/or physical or chemical restraint in a hospital, institution, or other setting?
- If a person is here as an immigrant or refugee, has she/he has ever experienced torture, terrorism, or other violations of her human rights either at home or in the process of coming to this country?
  - Did you ever live in a refugee camp?
  - Were you ever separated from your family, clan, or other close social network?
- How does she/he feel these experiences have affected her/him? At the time? Now?

DV hotline should be ensured before they leave the clinical setting. Patients who are in imminent danger are likely to require assistance in finding a safe place to go, either by the mental health provider or through referral to a DV program or hotline. At the same time, many women do leave abusive relationships, although this may be a long and complicated process. For women who choose to stay, interventions can help to increase their safety. Domestic violence advocates can be a critical resource in helping survivors to conduct a risk analysis. (Again, see the book by Davies and colleagues [19] for more information on safety planning and risk assessment, as well as other chapters in this volume.)

Suicide Risk

Another critical safety issue is the relationship between IPV and suicidality. Being battered by an intimate partner places women at increased risk for attempted and completed suicide (66–69). For example, 13% of women who committed suicide in the state of Washington in 2003 had a court-documented history of experiencing domestic abuse. Other states are reporting similar findings from their DV fatality reviews (70). Some women do not feel they have any other options for ending the abuse and pain they are experiencing. They may have made multiple attempts to protect themselves, to stop the abuse, or to leave, without success. For other women, the risk of suicide may increase after they have left the relationship, before they have had a chance to recover their sense of self-worth and ability to function on their own. Whether the separation is by choice or because the batterer has left them for another partner, the experience of abandonment and loss may become too painful to tolerate (14). Women with early trauma histories, particularly those who meet criteria for complex PTSD/disorders of extreme stress not otherwise specified (DESNOS) may have particular difficulty with threats of abandonment, even in the face of ongoing abuse. For survivors who are also dealing with a mental illness that carries increased risks for suicide, being abused by a partner (and/or experiencing abuse in childhood) adds to these risks. Although some suicide attempts may reflect a considered response to untenable circumstances, others may reflect a more spur-of-the- moment attempt by a survivor to alter her immediate situation and/or state of mind.

For some survivors, a suicide attempt may lead to the help they need (i.e., recognition of what they are experiencing, access to support, safety, resources, and treatment). For others, feelings of depression, hopelessness, and despair may take longer to resolve. When hospitalization is indicated, care should be taken to not involve the abuser in treatment unless a survivor specifically requests otherwise. Domestic violence advocacy and safety planning should be provided prior to discharge, whether by someone on staff who is trained to do so or in collaboration with a local DV program.

For perpetrators, suicidality is strongly associated with IPV homicide and risk factors for murder–suicide include depression, pathological jealousy, and facing abandonment or separation (71–73). The presence of any one risk factor should prompt a full assessment.

Homicidality

Homicidal ideation also warrants emergency psychiatric evaluation. Actual homicide attempts by survivors against an abusive partner, are however, very rare. In the majority of cases, women who kill their partners have been severely abused for long periods of time, feel that they are in imminent danger, and see no other way out. They believe they have no other choice but to kill their partner to prevent the murder or serious injury of themselves or their children. Experienced clinicians have found that it is very rare for battered women to premeditate the murder of an abusive partner. Rather, they develop self-defense strategies (e.g., carrying a weapon) that have potentially lethal outcomes both for themselves and their partners (14). Assessing a woman's level of danger and discussing the risk of lethality, the likelihood of incarceration, and the range of other alternatives can help diffuse the immediate danger if she raises these issues.

Discussing the possibility of safety measures such as being transported to out-of-state shelters, relocation, witness protection plans, and temporary hospitalization can provide alternatives to homicide when she is in danger. In fact, as alternatives for women have become more prevalent (i.e., shelter, police/court services, etc.), homicides of male batterers have decreased significantly (74).

Try to determine if such circumstances reflect a woman's current situation. Ask her to describe how she perceives her options for safety. If homicide is a possible scenario, ask her directly if she has plans to kill or harm her partner. If she says "yes," she should be asked specifically if she has a weapon or plan for how to carry out that action. If she does have a plan, "duty to warn" considerations come into play. A clinician's duty to warn is based on state statute and case law. The Tarasoff decision (*Tarasoff vs. Regents of the University of California*, 1976) requires clinicians to take reasonable steps to protect a third party from harm, including victims of IPV and their abusers. When the patient is being abused by a current or former partner, and the intent to harm is perceived as a desperate means of self-defense, clinicians must intervene to protect *the patient* as well as their intended victim (i.e., their abusive partner). That might include hospitalization or sheltering of a victim who sees homicide as the only way to be safe. As with a suicide assessment, the clinician should assess whether the survivor has a plan and access to the means to carry out that plan. When IPV victims perceive homicide as their only option for safety, discussing other options available to them may minimize the homicide threat. Patients must be told of your intention and offered protective services. Alternate safety strategies should be discussed. Voluntary or involuntary psychiatric hospitalization may obviate the duty to warn the third party as long as they are not in danger from the patient.

In cases in which the patient is known to be a perpetrator of IPV, voluntary or involuntary commitment to a psychiatric facility is one way to achieve temporary safety until other measures can be put in place. A patient who is openly discussing his intent may be more open to intervention, but this is not necessarily the case. Temporary psychiatric hospitalization or assessment, particularly for a determined abuser, may not prevent homicidal action. Treating acute psychiatric conditions (e.g., depression, suicidality, paranoia) is an important part of intervention. However, consultation with experts in abuser treatment should be sought and legal interventions put in place as well. In addition to warning an intended victim of an abusive partner's intent to harm them, it is also critical to discuss safety planning and provide access to community resources such as DV programs, hotlines, and shelters.

ISSUES THAT AFFECT OPTIONS AND CHOICES

Although women often share similar experiences, individual responses to abuse will also differ based on a range of personal, cultural, and societal factors. For example, a woman may be reluctant to discuss abuse if she perceives this as betraying her community or likely to invoke discriminatory criminal justice responses toward the perpetrator. Cultural or religious constraints and experiences of racism may make it difficult for a woman to discuss the abuse with someone outside her community. Alternatively, women may be afraid to discuss these issues with someone from the same cultural background. Issues of privacy, shame, safety, and confidentiality can all influence a woman's decision to reveal that she is being abused. Mental health treatment may be stigmatized, thus making it more difficult for women to seek help for trauma-related symptoms. Women may face social isolation and ostracism if they attempt to leave an abusive spouse, which makes it harder for them to consider this as a possibility. The idea of breaking marriage vows may create spiritual conflicts for some women as well.

Women who are immigrants also face obstacles to treatment. Those who are undocumented may find it even more difficult to reveal a history of partner abuse, in part because they are afraid of bringing attention to their situation, and in part because batterers threaten to have them deported if they tell or threaten to leave them without resources or support. Some batterers control their wives by deliberately failing to file their petitions for permanent residency. State Domestic Violence Coalitions are usually aware of services that specifically address these issues. Women who enter the United States as refugees have often experienced "triple trauma"—the trauma and loss in their home countries that caused them to flee, trauma that occurred during their transit, and the trauma of displacement and loss of familiarity and home (75). Yet, for many survivors, talking to a stranger about personal experiences is not something they find acceptable, and talking to someone in a position of authority is not perceived as safe.

Discussing partner abuse may also be difficult for women in lesbian relationships who have experienced homophobic responses outside the gay and lesbian community and denial about IPV within. It may be more difficult for lesbians to find confidential sources of help, particularly when their abusive partner is involved in organizations that provide services to battered women. Gay and lesbian batterers may attempt to control their partners by threatening to "out" them if they reveal the abuse or try to leave, or by defining their partners' efforts to defend themselves as "mutual combat," thus undermining their efforts to get help (76–78). Internalized responses to homophobia and violence in a woman's family of origin may contribute both to perpetration and to an increased vulnerability to victimization once it occurs. Although there are couples in which the abuse or violence is mutual, or in which one partner initiates and the other fights back, for many women, the pattern of one partner systematically controlling the other is no different from that in abusive heterosexual relationships, although positions may change in a subsequent relationship (79). It is important to ask for explicit examples of what actually happens in the relationship when these questions arise. Abusers typically use tactics of denial and distortion, and do not take responsibility for their behaviors. Any therapist working with gay or lesbian couples must interview each partner separately to ask about abuse.

Clinicians should also be aware that lesbian, gay, and transgender survivors of childhood sexual abuse may have some unique concerns about the therapeutic relationship. They may be grappling, for example, with their sense of psychological safety as a lesbian or gay man within the therapy. This may manifest as a need to know about a therapist's view of homosexuality or familiarity and comfort in working with lesbian, gay, bisexual, transgender, queer, and questioning (LGBTQ) individuals. A client's sense of safety may be undermined by a therapist's refusal to disclose her own views and experiences, by a therapist's interpretation of lesbianism as a response to the incest, or by a therapist's inability to identify the homophobia faced by the client as a potential cause of trauma-related disorders (80).

As noted previously, women already diagnosed with mental health or substance abuse disorders contend with an additional set of concerns. They may fear not being taken seriously because of previous experiences with helping professionals or because abusers have convinced them this is so. These issues may affect a woman's ability to process information and sort out her options, and may limit her access to shelter.

In addition, women with physical disabilities or disabling medical conditions, some of which have been caused by the abuse, may find it even more difficult to leave a partner or family member she depends on for access to services and basic care. People who have a disability are even more likely to feel trapped in abusive relationships, particularly when jobs and transportation are limited or when their only alternative is to live in an institution or return to an abusive family. Personal assistants may also turn out to be abusers, further decreasing women's options for living independently. People with disabilities may face unique forms of abuse, such as neglect, refusal to provide essential care, manipulation of medications, withholding or destroying equipment, or preventing access to mobility or communication. In addition, women with disabilities are often perceived as asexual and de-gendered, reducing the likelihood that partner abuse will be recognized. Those relationships may also be harder to give up (81). Men with disabilities may also be at greater risk for abuse. Therapists can learn more about the specific needs of people with nonpsychiatric disabilities and find ways to make their own practice settings more accessible by contacting a disability rights advocacy group such as the Americans with Disabilities Act Technical Assistance Program, or the OVW Accessing Safety Initiative (http://www.verainstitute.org). Applying concepts of universal access/inclusive design and making sure agencies and practice settings have the appropriate assistive technology can help mitigate the barriers survivors face in accessing necessary resources.

Summary

To summarize, research and experience in the field indicate that during a routine inquiry or assessment, any mental health symptoms should be considered in relation to current or past abuse and other traumatic experiences. Developmental and biological issues should be examined from a trauma perspective as well. If a patient does disclose a history of current or past victimization, a more in-depth assessment of her situation is indicated. Additional information is also needed about the nature of a woman's traumatic experience(s) and the scope of their impact on her life; her current safety status; how the abuse has affected her and her children and how she protects her children and herself (documenting this information can be particularly helpful when custody is an issue); the presence of medical illnesses and psychiatric symptoms, particularly conditions known to be related to trauma as well as coexisting health or mental health problems; and the coping strategies she uses and how they affect her daily life (currently and at the time of the trauma).

Abuse that is targeted toward patient's mental health condition should be asked about specifically (i.e., withholding medication, coerced overdose, telling her no one will believe her because she's mentally ill), as well as the relationship of abuse to symptom exacerbation (e.g., recurrence of panic attacks, worsening depression or acute psychotic episode in the face of escalating threats or recent assault). In addition, presenting symptoms should be considered in light of any social discrimination a patient has experienced, as well as any cultural differences and language barriers that may be present. Although in some settings it may be necessary to gather large amounts of information in a relatively short period of time, clinicians can help to destigmatize the process by explaining what they are thinking and why they are asking particular questions. Engaging survivors as partners in the assessment process is generally experienced as more respectful and empowering (16,29).

ASSESSING THE MENTAL HEALTH IMPACT OF INTIMATE PARTNER VIOLENCE AND OTHER LIFETIME TRAUMA

Conceptual Issues

Although in the course of obtaining a mental health history, particular attention to trauma-related symptoms and disorders is warranted, emerging neuroscience research on the effects of trauma across the lifespan indicates that responses to trauma are best viewed along a multi-axial continuum rather than as discrete diagnoses. Briere and Spinazzola, in a 2005 review on complex trauma assessment, underscore that given the many types of trauma, the number of domains that can be affected, and the array of potential intervening factors, assessment may better achieved by looking at the range of possible posttraumatic responses in conjunction with a survivor's particular experiences and risks (e.g., impact of adult single-event trauma versus chronic severe abuse and neglect in early childhood; secure attachment and supportive caregivers versus disorganized attachment and abusive, nonattuned caregivers; no genetic vulnerabilities versus significant genetic vulnerabilities; presence or absence of resilience/mitigating factors; positive versus adverse subsequent experiences/life trajectory) (82). A survivor of IPV might fall anywhere on this continuum.

Harris and Fallot distinguish between a *PTSD/ diagnostic model* that views trauma as a discrete event (sexual assault, disaster) and responses to trauma as a discrete set of symptoms, and a *complex trauma model* that views trauma as a core set of developmental experiences around which individuals organize their identity, sense of self, and beliefs about the world, and which affects people in multiple and sometimes seemingly unrelated ways (16). Neuroscience research is beginning to corroborate these clinically based understandings by examining the effects of trauma on key brain regions, circuits, and neurotransmitters (83–89). Research also supports the long-held clinical recognition that a person's developmental trajectory is shaped by a combination of genetic endowment and life experiences (e.g., nurturing and attachment, early trauma or stress, resilience-promoting qualities of individuals and their environments, etc.). Having a developmental perspective is useful for understanding the long-term effects of childhood trauma, as well as positive adaptations to traumatic experiences (i.e., developing capacities one might not otherwise have developed) and posttraumatic growth (i.e., positive change as result of crisis such as personal strength, greater appreciation of life, renewed sense of spirituality, etc.) (90).

However, a number of issues must be considered in regard to how the relationship between previous trauma and IPV is conceptualized. Because IPV is primarily an adult (or adolescent)-onset phenomenon, survivors have raised concerns that linking IPV to earlier childhood experiences can be construed as victim blaming (something inherent to the victim that caused the abuse) or as a way to not hold batterers accountable (attributing abusive behavior to childhood trauma and its effects on the brain, conflating childhood etiology with adult responsibility). As noted earlier, research on the mental health sequelae of IPV has not applied a complex trauma lens. Whether this model will mainly prove helpful to survivors who have experienced significant childhood abuse or if its dimensional approach to a range of potential effects make it useful for assessing and responding to the consequences of adult as well as childhood trauma, remains to be determined.

Disorders of extreme stress not otherwise specified criteria formed the initial construct for current thinking on complex PTSD (also referred to as *complex developmental trauma disorder*) and complex posttraumatic self-dysregulation (58,91,92). Hallmarks of complex trauma or DESNOS include alterations in emotional (and impulse) regulation (e.g., suicide attempts, high-risk behavior, self-cutting); states of consciousness (dissociation) and self-perception (self-hatred and shame); alterations in perceptions of the perpetrator (idealizing, preoccupation with); alterations in relations with others (fear, rage, abandonment); and alterations in system of meanings (no one can be trusted). When DESNOS was initially conceptualized, it was meant to describe the changes that can take place when a person is entrapped in a longstanding abusive relationship, whether in childhood or as an adult (91). However, most subsequent research has focused on the developmental effects of trauma that begins in childhood. In some senses, DESNOS was a critical reframing of the diagnosis of borderline personality disorder—as the developmental sequelae of chronic abuse in childhood and adaptive attempts to manage intolerable feelings without optimal internal resources or psychological survival strategies that emerge when entrusted early caretakers are the ones causing the distress. Researchers have developed a number of different constructs in an attempt to organize these wide-ranging effects. For example, functional magnetic resonance imaging (fMRI) research has begun to examine the different kinds of responses survivors may have to chronic interpersonal trauma (e.g., distinguishing between responses that primarily involve fear and hyperarousal versus those that involve numbing and dissociation) (84,86).

Assessment Tools

A number of validated trauma assessment tools are available, such as the Trauma Symptom Inventory (93,94), the Clinician Administered PTSD Scale (CAPS) (95), the Interview for Disorders of Extreme Stress (SIDES) (96), Trauma and Attachment Belief Scale (TABS) (97), and Dissociative Experiences Scale (DES) (98), to name a few. They can usually be obtained by contacting the authors (99–102). Tools such as the Posttraumatic Stress Scale for Family Violence (103) provide questions that specifically link PTSD symptoms to ongoing abuse. The Posttraumatic Growth Inventory (104) offers a way to assess more positive aspects of survivors' experiences. For a review of additional screening tools associated with PTSD, see Brewin (105) or complex trauma, see Briere (82); for a review of trauma screening tools for children and adolescents, see Strand, Sarmiento, and Pasquale (82,105,106). Assessment for other commonly occurring trauma-related symptoms and conditions should be included as well (depression, other anxiety disorders, substance abuse, etc.). For clinical purposes, questions can be adapted from existing instruments and integrated into mental health assessments tailored to individual survivor responses and needs. When used for research or diagnostic purposes, however, handpicking individual questions will clearly affect the statistical reliability of these measures.

One tool for assessing the impact of more severe early trauma (The Trauma Recovery Empowerment Profile, or TREP) emerged from the work of Harris, Fallot, Beyer, and Berley as part of the Substance Abuse and Mental Health Services Administration (SAMHSA) Violence Against Women with Co-Occurring Disorders study (107). They identified 11 core skill dimensions that women in their program with histories of childhood trauma, substance abuse, and psychiatric disabilities often found themselves struggling with. These domains included basic self- and relational-capacities (self-awareness, self-protection, self-soothing, emotional modulation, relational mutuality, accurate labeling of self and others), as well as higher-order functions (such as a sense of agency and initiative taking, consistent problem solving, reliable parenting, possessing a sense of purpose and meaning, decision making and judgment). They also developed specific skill-building exercises that women could use to develop their capacities in arenas that had been affected. For some women, a lifetime of abuse and neglect had disrupted the development of fundamental aspects of themselves, what Saakvitne and her colleagues refer to as *self-capacities* or *feeling skills* (feeling internally connected over time to caring others; experiencing oneself as deserving and worthwhile); and affect regulation (recognizing, tolerating, modulating, and integrating feelings) (27). *Affect regulation* refers to being able to experience feelings without becoming overwhelmed or having to manage them in ways that are potentially harmful or restricting, that become walled off and then evoked unexpectedly, or that leave survivors without access to important parts of themselves and their experience (108). This type of information can be used to tailor both assessments

and treatment to more accurately match the arenas in which a particular survivor may have been affected and the skills that will be most helpful to her in accessing safety, recovering from trauma and/or mental illness, and rebuilding her life (14).

Another tool that has been used to assess the nature of early caregiver experiences to help explain current responses is the Trauma Antecedents questionnaire (108). In addition to identifying types of traumatic experiences, it assesses areas of competence as well as feelings of safety with potentially protective people at different stages of development as a way of determining what experiences and capacities a survivor already has and what needs to be worked on through a variety of treatment modalities. Other researchers emphasize the importance of balancing trauma assessments with assessments of resilience. The concept of resilience refers to the capacity for successful adaptation despite challenging or threatening circumstances (109).

In practice, teasing out these connections means assessing the relationship of current or past abuse to new symptoms and/or to the exacerbation of a co-existing psychiatric condition and exploring how current or past abuse has affected survivors in other relevant ways, such as how they feel about themselves, their ability to trust themselves or other people, their perceptions of others, their capacity to manage feelings, their ability to take in and process information, and the beliefs they hold about the future. In addition to the domains just mentioned, trauma can affect beliefs, spirituality, systems of meaning, and states of consciousness, as well as the ways in which individuals solve problems and protect themselves from harm. It can be helpful to both normalize and inquire about the specific kinds of feelings that may have resulted from ongoing or past abuse such as anger, fear, confusion, guilt, or despair. Discussing coping mechanisms that may be harmful (such as posttraumatic avoidance, numbing or dissociation, self-injury, and substance use) and reframing them as survival strategies rather than pathology can help reduce shame and increase openness to exploring other ways of coping. It also helps survivors to build on their own resources and strengths.

ADDITIONAL ASSESSMENT CONSIDERATIONS

The following section provides a brief overview of additional issues that would be included in a comprehensive mental health assessment for survivors of IPV, but which are discussed in greater depth elsewhere in this volume.

Substance Use Assessment in Context

Alcohol and other drugs are often used as form of self-medication to numb the pain of current or past abuse. In addition, some survivors grow up in families in which substance abuse is a problem or in communities where drug use is common, thus putting them at greater risk for early use of drugs themselves, and for exposure to violent relationships. Some abusers coerce their partners into illegal drug activity and may then exert further control by withholding or threatening to withhold the drug(s) she has become dependent on. This common scenario creates an additional layer of entrapment for the woman; by calling the police to avert a violent assault by her partner, she risks her own arrest for drug possession and/or usage. Attempts to stop using may be met with increasing threats and violence. Understanding the role of substance abuse in a particular survivor's life and its relationship to current or past abuse is essential for developing an integrated treatment approach. Standard substance abuse screening questions can also be adapted to a survivor's experience of IPV (for an example, see Figure 24–1).

A more in-depth discussion of this issue is found elsewhere in this text.

Health Impact of Intimate Partner Violence and Other Trauma

A mental health history should also include questions about the impact of IPV and previous trauma on patients' physical health. In addition to addressing the abuse-related injuries, medical problems (including chronic pain, autoimmune or cardiovascular disorders, exacerbations of previous medical conditions, symptoms associated with stress, anxiety disorders, and depression), complications of pregnancy or unprotected sex, or hospitalizations secondary to the abuse or medical conditions that might place a person at greater risk (i.e., dependency on an abuser for transportation, mobility or care) must be assessed. In assessing the health impact of abuse, careful attention should be paid to the sequelae of head and strangulation injuries, such as loss of consciousness, postconcussive syndromes, and cognitive impairment, as well as conditions that might impact the choice of psychotropic medication, as indicated (110). Not only is this information important to document for a patient's legal case, but it is also important to factor into mental health treatment—how a survivor's life has been

---

Standard substance abuse screening questions (e.g., the CAGE questionnaire) can be adapted to a survivor's experience of IPV, CAGE: "Have your ever tried to cut down on your drinking?" "Have you ever been annoyed by someone criticizing your drinking?" "Have you ever felt guilty about your drinking?" and "Have you ever had an eye-opener in the morning?" For example:

1. "Has your partner ever tried to stop you from cutting down on your drinking?"

2. "Have you ever been made to feel afraid by someone's criticizing your drinking? Has your partner used your drinking as a way to threaten you?"

3. "Have you ever felt coerced into drinking (or using drugs) or engaging in illegal activities or other behaviors you weren't okay with or that compromised your integrity, and then felt guilty about it?"

   a. "Have you ever used drugs or alcohol to manage painful feelings and/or numb yourself from pain, and then felt guilty about doing that?"

   b. "Have you ever had to trade sex for drugs, and then felt bad about that?"

   c. "Were drugs or alcohol ever involved in the abuse you experienced as an adult? As a child?"

4. "Have you ever had a drink in the morning, because things felt so hopeless or because that felt like the only way you could survive or get through the day?"

Figure 24.1 Adaptation of the CAGE questionnaire for intimate partner violence questioning.

altered by these sequelae, the extent to which they continue to serve as traumatic reminders, the effects of capacity-limiting conditions on a batterer's ability to exert control, the role of stress/depression in the development (and maintenance) of physical symptoms, and the like. A more in-depth discussion of the health impact of IPV is found elsewhere in this text.

Impact on Children

Asking a survivor about what the children have been exposed to and how they have been affected raises a number of potentially challenging issues, particularly if custody is a concern. Taking an informed-consent approach to asking about IPV and other abuse means letting women know upfront about mandatory reporting requirements. At the same time, children often play a primary role in women's decision-making, and creating a safe place for women to talk about their concerns is critical (111,112). Questions about whether she has noticed changes in her children or in her relationship with them and what fears she may have about her children's safety, behavior, or emotional states can be asked in a way that invites collaboration. Inquiring about and documenting what a woman does to protect the children's safety and attend to their needs can be particularly helpful in building her custody case, as well as supporting her as a parent (113). Ultimately, being able to support the parenting capacity of and attachment to the nonabusive parent is most helpful to children's development (114,115). Other questions include whether the children have developed any medical or behavior problems or psychiatric symptoms that might be related to the abuse or if young children have regressed from a previous level of development. A more in-depth discussion of the impact of IPV on children is found elsewhere in this text.

Coping Mechanisms and Survival Strategies

A key component of empowerment-based interventions involves discussing a survivor's sources of strength and support, as well as the additional skills and resources a survivor may need. One way to do this is to help survivors identify the strengths they rely on to survive and resist the abuse, access the capacities that have been buried or undermined by their abusive partner (and possibly others), and reframe perceived weaknesses as abuse-related coping strategies or sequelae and/or actual survival strategies. A strengths-based assessment provides a fuller picture of the individual and of her potential. It also provides an opportunity to discuss and acknowledge patients' spiritual beliefs and practices, their hopes for creating a better life, and their persistence and determination in the face of uncertainty and fear. A detailed review of the literature on coping styles and IPV is beyond the scope of this chapter.

Considerations for Survivors Who Are Living with a Chronic Mental Illness

The stigma of mental illness is often used by the abuser and internalized by the person being victimized, particularly if her sense of self has been organized around experiences of abuse and mental illness (e.g., she is the problem, she is being paranoid, no one will believe her, she deserves it, she does not have any rights). In addition to safety, treatment should be designed to address stigma as well as abuse-related issues. As discussed by Harris and her colleagues, when a survivor's very sense of self has been undermined by a combination of stigmatized conditions and circumstances, these issues need to be attended to gradually but directly (16). Treatment in this context attends to aspects of the self that have been undermined and capacities that a survivor may not yet have had the opportunity to develop.

For women who are living with a mental illness, abuse may come at the hands of people in their social networks, not necessarily a partner (e.g., someone in their residential setting, a family member, a "friend"). Women who are homeless are at even greater risk for abuse by both strangers and acquaintances. Intimate relationships may be transient and may involve high-risk activities such as trading sex for drugs, cigarettes, food, or housing. Working with survivors to recognize and name the abuse and to develop alternate social networks can be a critical part of the work (16).

Psychotic episodes may reflect a crisis in a woman's network, such as abuse or abandonment. If these are recognized and addressed proactively, it may prevent crises from occurring (16). With the exception of a few model programs across the country, virtually no trauma- and IPV-sensitive crisis or transitional housing is available for women with a serious mental illness (116). The Americans with Disabilities Act and Fair Housing laws require DV shelters to serve women who have psychiatric disabilities and who do not present a danger to themselves or other people. Most shelters will take in women with psychiatric histories providing they are relatively stable and ongoing psychiatric support is available. Alternatively, with sufficient staff training, local respite or crisis beds could become safe havens for women who are currently in danger and experiencing psychiatric or abuse-related mental health crises.

Women who have a mental illness often face significant custody hurdles that are exacerbated by the abuse and manipulated by abusers. Women with mental illness can be capable parents, particularly if they have adequate supports. Yet, stigma associated with mental illness makes this more difficult to achieve and increases the ability of an abuser to control his partner through custody-related threats. Parenting support is a critical component of mental health interventions.

Psychiatric hospitalization can be made more empowering by providing an opportunity for women to refuse calls or visits from an abusive partner and by providing advocacy interventions and safety planning onsite. Encouraging women to maintain phone contact with children, when possible, helps demonstrate their commitment and capacity to parent. Having women notify employers of their absence increases the likelihood of retaining their jobs post hospitalization (117). All patients should be asked about abuse and safety issues on admission and at discharge from psychiatric hospitalizations. Abusers should not be given information as to their partner's whereabouts or involved in treatment unless the patient indicates this is what she wants.

Issues of Documentation

Any information that becomes available to the batterer can increase a woman's danger and can be used to control her or be used against her in court around custody issues, thus making sensitivity to the nuances of documentation essential. It is important to document women's descriptions of abusive experiences in their own words, particularly when the potential for legal action exists. Guidelines have been developed by a number of responsible professional and advocacy organizations to help clinicians negotiate this complex terrain (Family Violence Prevention Fund; American Psychiatric Association; American Psychological Association; International Society for Traumatic Stress Studies; AMA Guidelines on Mental Health Consequences of Family Violence) (11,13,113,118).

Documenting symptoms that result from or are aggravated by abuse, and the potential for them to subside once a woman is safe, can be particularly helpful to survivors in custody battles, with attention to how information about diagnoses and medications might be used. For example, one might consider using "acute stress disorder" or "adjustment disorder NOS" rather than "PTSD" if a woman is still being abused and is dealing with custody issues. On the other hand, careful documentation, regardless of diagnosis, can be helpful to a survivor in court, depending on her legal representation. Discussion should be framed around the relationship of symptoms to the abuse and should describe a woman's strengths, her coping strategies, her ability to care for her children, and the efforts she has made to protect them. Indications of her parenting ability and the children's attachment to their mother (e.g., observations of interactions with her children, discussions that demonstrate her attunement and concern) should also be clearly documented.

For clinicians involved in custody evaluations, it is important to recognize the appropriateness of a woman's anger toward the abuser and her reluctance to expose her children to a violent, abusive parent. Women are often penalized in these situations for being the less cooperative parent. Clinicians must also take care not to be fooled by the seeming health of an abuser, whose partner may look more symptomatic than the person who has been abusing them for years (119). Abusers frequently use custody battles and visitation as ways to control a partner who is attempting to leave. Prolonged custody battles are particularly devastating to survivors and their children. Abusers often continue to drag their partners to court, depleting their legal funds and threatening the safety and well-being of their children.

APPROACHES FOR WORKING WITH INTIMATE PARTNER VIOLENCE SURVIVORS

This section provides an overview of current approaches for working with survivors of IPV and lifetime trauma. Included in this overview are IPV-specific interventions, trauma treatment interventions (both therapeutic and pharmacological), substance abuse treatment in the context of IPV, potentially harmful interventions, and legal issues that need to be considered by clinicians and other service providers when working with survivors.

INTIMATE PARTNER
VIOLENCE-SPECIFIC INTERVENTIONS

Providing Information

Many battered women are either numb or in a state of terror and confusion at the time they seek help, and have not had room to do more than survive. Providing information about the dynamics of abuse; about typical battering tactics; about common sequelae; about the pattern of abuse and likelihood that it will continue; about the impact of abuse on children; about risk, danger, and safety planning; and about available options and resources, is also a powerful intervention tool. It helps decrease isolation and shame, helps women gain perspective, aids in decreasing psychological entrapment, and offers a sense of hope and connection.

If a woman is seeking help for her abusive partner, discuss what is known about perpetrators, about the limits of treatment programs, the possibility of his continued controlling behavior even if he stops his violence, and his need for long-term commitment to counseling and change. The importance of a genuine commitment to change cannot be overestimated. When a women's abusive partner is in counseling, she may stay with him longer in the hope that he will stop the abuse. Many batterers enter counseling solely to keep their partners from leaving. It may be necessary to revisit these issues during the course of therapy ensure her safety.

In addition, by explaining the common traumatic sequelae of abuse, clinicians can mitigate the effect of abusers' undermining behaviors and impart relief to survivors who truly fear they are going crazy. Information about trauma and its impact also helps survivors gain perspective on their own responses, anticipate potential difficulties, and develop tools to manage feelings, behaviors, and states of consciousness that may interfere with their ability to achieve desired goals.

Women often want their children to grow up in intact homes, but are deeply concerned about their children's safety. They may wish to remain in the relationship with the abuser if the children are not at risk for physical harm and if they believe that their partner is essentially a good father. Discussing the long-term traumatic effects of witnessing one parent perpetrate violence against the other (e.g., developmental regression, behavior problems, poor school performance, social withdrawal, psychiatricsymptomatology, increased risk of becoming a victim or perpetrator) can help a survivor weigh her options about whether to stay or leave. If the children are in need of treatment, plan the treatment in partnership with her, rather than just making a referral. Try to ensure access to a child therapist who understands the issues faced by both children and their mother, and who works in ways that support her capacities as a parent (120).

Discuss what written material will be safe for a woman to take home. Many batterers check the odometers on their partners' cars and go through their partners' purses, briefcases, pockets, and drawers. Insurance information sent to the home may also put her in danger. It is also important to ask if precautions need to be taken to avoid having written information about the abuse on materials he may see. She may need to write important phone numbers on scraps of paper or memorize them, or she may be able to leave the information at work or with a friend.

Safety Planning: Building Collaboration
to Enhance Safety

Safety planning strategies are based on the consensus experiences of survivors and advocates over the past 30-plus years. Research on this issue is limited, but some randomized controlled trials have indicated positive effects (121). This issue is discussed in greater depth elsewhere in this text. Some dimensions of safety are best addressed by advocates, others by mental health providers, and some clearly by both. Most clinicians are already familiar with helping patients develop strategies for keeping themselves safe at times when mental health symptoms place them in jeopardy (i.e., when they are feeling suicidal, experience triggers that are likely to evoke overwhelming feelings, are starting to feel destabilized, etc.). A person who is being victimized by an intimate partner can also benefit from having someone to work with in analyzing her situation, identifying risks and thinking through specific strategies to increase her and her children's safety.

Advocates who work for a local DV program can be particularly helpful in this area. For example, advocates are best able to provide linkages to immediate shelter and discuss a range of safety options, including legal protections, alternatives to shelter, options for LGBTQ and immigrant survivors, and ways to be safer if the survivor remains at home. They actively participate in the process of negotiating with bureaucratic sysems, including child protective services,the welfare system, and the courts. In addition toconsiderable experience assisting women to increase safety through shelter, relocation, and legal interventions, DV programs are also knowledgeable about other safety issues, such as the responses of law enforcement and judges in a community.

Clinicians, however, should be skilled at helping patients assess their danger, discuss their options, and access advocacy resources, particularly when advocates are not immediately available. For example, if a patient is in immediate danger, DV hotlines are accessible 24 hours a day and can assist with safety planning. If state or local hotlines are not readily available, the National Domestic Violence Hotline can always be accessed [1–800–799-SAFE (7233), 1–800–787–3224 (TTY)].

Patients currently in danger should be encouraged to develop safety and escape plans if they are staying with an abusive partner or he has access to them, and to consider options for safety if leaving. It is helpful for survivors to rehearse their plans, so that they will be in place when needed. Survivors can do a number of things in addition to calling the police or a crisis line or getting a protective order from the courts. They can review previous episodes for information that identifies predictable patterns and locations that may be dangerous, think about how to anticipate and reduce danger if possible, make provisions for their children (rehearse escape strategies, places to stay, numbers to call); locate (in advance) a safe place to go in an emergency; and make provisions for leaving quickly and have necessary items and papers packed, accessible, and if at all possible, hidden from the abuser. Police can escort a woman back to her home if she needs to gather belongings but if an abuser suspects his partner is leaving, he may destroy valuable items and papers. A woman can also develop and rehearse an escape plan, and develop a plan for getting help when she cannot escape (signal to neighbors, teach the children to dial 911).

It is important that safety planning be seen as a process that a survivor adjusts in response to changing circumstances, rather than as an actual document or work product. In addition, creating a written safety plan that is incorporated into formal treatment planning and placed in the clinical record can be used against a woman in custody cases or other situations if she has not followed the steps outlined in her safety plan. Therefore, while having a written plan may be useful for a given survivor to make for herself, at her discretion, documentation in the mental health record should be more circumspect (e.g., "Strategies for increasing safety were discussed, they included . . . Janna will continue to weigh the risks and benefits over time").

For survivors who are living with a psychiatric disability, there are a number of additional dimensions to consider. For example, safety planning should address safety from ongoing abuse by members of their social network (i.e., friends, roommates, family members, staff, or others in residential settings) as well as by a partner. In addition to addressing physical, emotional, and sexual safety, it should attend to mental health–specific forms of abuse, such as withholding medication, sleep deprivation, coerced treatment, custody threats, threats of commitment, control of finances, guardianship, and advance directives. Plans should be adapted to a survivor's cognitive abilities and her ability to process information during a crisis (i.e., account for symptoms of dissociation, anxiety, depression, psychosis, mania, developmental disabilities, traumatic brain injury, etc.). Examples of this include using simpler, more concrete language; adjusting the pace of talking; checking in to make sure information is understood; asking a patient if she can let you know what she heard, so that you can make sure you are conveying information in a way that is most effective for her; helping a survivor recognize when she is with you and when she has dissociated, and identifying strategies she can use to bring herself back (i.e., grounding techniques); or helping the person develop ways to calm herself if anxiety is making it difficult to concentrate—in other words, helping survivors stay connected to themselves and to the clinician while engaging in a way that is optimally paced for them. Safety issues need to be addressed before an IPV survivor is discharged from an inpatient unit or leaves a community mental health setting.

Intimate partner violence safety planning can also be incorporated into existing mental health recovery, self-help/peer support tools that survivors may be using. One example is the Wellness Recovery Action Plan ™ (WRAP; Mary Ellen Copeland, PhD), which was "developed by and for people with mental health difficulties to take charge of their own recovery and well-being." It is designed to "decrease and prevent intrusive or troubling feelings and behaviors, increase personal empowerment, improve quality of life, and assist people in achieving their own life goals and dreams" through a structured system of "planned responses that includes responses from others when individuals need help to make a decision, take care of themselves, or keep themselves safe" (122). Although the focus of WRAP™ is on achieving and maintaining wellness from mental health symptoms, much like IPV safety plans, it is structured to enable people to notice, anticipate, and plan for potential threats to their well-being, and to create and modify as needed an action plan for themselves and for the people they can safely rely on for support. It is currently undergoing a randomized control trial as a peer support tool. An IPV safety planning version is also being developed (123). Individual safety plans should also include survivors' preferred methods of calming themselves during a crisis to reduce the likelihood that an abuser will be able to exert control in those situations and to reduce the use of coercive interventions by mental health personnel.

Psychiatric advance directives offer another tool that can be utilized in conjunction with IPV safety planning to make provisions for who survivors do or do not want informed about and/or involved in their treatment, and who they want named as the attorney-in-fact to make decisions on their behalf at a time when they are unable to do so. Psychiatric advance directives also delineate treatment modalities that are or are not acceptable to them (i.e., medications, hospitals, electroshock therapy, etc.) if they are ever in a position in which they are not able to make competent decisions for themselves. As part of safety planning, it is important to find out if a survivor does have an existing psychiatric advance directive and, if so, who is the designated attorney-in-fact and what their relationship is to the abusive party. If a survivor does not have a psychiatric advance directive, it might be worth considering one as a way to ensure that the abuser is not involved in treatment or decision-making or is not informed about her location if she is hospitalized and she wishes her whereabouts to remain unknown.

Working with Local Domestic Violence Programs

Local DV programs, as well as online DV resources can also play an important role in a survivor's overall strategy for accessing safety and support, which in turn has salutary effects on mental health. The majority of research on nonclinical interventions for survivors (as opposed to perpetrators) of DV has focused on shelter and/or post-shelter services. Several studies, including one randomized controlled trial, have found that DV advocacy

counseling reduced violence, increased quality of life, enhanced safety and well-being, and helped women expand their networks of support (124). Other studies have found significant reductions in depression among women who were able to end the violence and some reductions even among women who were still exposed (125–129).

In one longitudinal randomized control study, Sullivan and colleagues found women who received free services from trained college student-advocates for 10 weeks post-shelter experienced less physical violence over time and reported increased quality of life, greater social support, less emotional attachment to the abuser, fewer depressive symptoms, less fear and anxiety, and increased effectiveness in obtaining resources, although differences in anxiety and depression were not sustained over time (3,130). Social support, however, has been associated with better self-perceived mental health status, lower psychological distress, and lower rates of psychiatric disorders among survivors of IPV, including anxiety, depression, PTSD, and suicide attempts (131,132). One additional series of studies found brief nursing interventions delivered during prenatal visits to be effective in increasing safety behaviors for IPV survivors (133). Methodological designs limit generalizing to some extent but do provide preliminary evidence that both hospital- and shelter-based interventions can be effective for some women (124). Overall, studies have begun to demonstrate that flexible, survivor-centered interventions providing advocacy and social support may be more effective strategies for improving quality of life and helping women to be safe (134,135).

Domestic violence advocacy programs and shelters provide a variety of services for battered women and their children, as well as public education and training for service providers. They are the major source of support for many survivors. Others may feel most safe when connected to a mental health provider, with advocacy playing an important but adjunctive role, and still others, in peer support groups. The majority of DV survivors do not stay in shelters, either because of insufficient resources or because they have other options, but they do utilize a wide range of services available through DV programs.

Typical offerings include a 24-hour hotline and crisis intervention counseling; assistance in evaluating options, resources, safety planning, and referrals; information about legal remedies and legal and court advocacy (such as assistance with protective orders, etc.); emergency shelter, hotel vouchers, safe homes; counseling, support groups, and referrals for therapy; immigrant rights information advocacy with child protective services; literacy programs, job training, and transitional housing; and referrals for perpetrators/abusers. It is important to note that some of theses services may not be available in the woman's community. Culturally specific DV services and services designed for lesbian, gay, bisexual, and transgender survivors exist across the country but are much fewer in number. Developing a working relationship with community DV programs can offer support to clinicians as well, and can increase the likelihood that women will receive the range of services they need. For example, not all DV programs have the resources to shelter women with more acute mental health symptoms. However, working closely with a mental health provider who can provide consultation, access to referrals, backup support for shelter staff, and/or access to medication and mobile crisis services can make a difference in the extent to which shelters are able to serve women who are also dealing with a mental illness or more severe trauma related symptoms.

EXISTING TRAUMA TREATMENT APPROACHES

Recognition of the impact of abuse and violence against women has led to the emergence of a number of approaches to trauma treatment, only a handful of which are specific to IPV. And, although some PTSD treatment studies have included survivors of IPV, trauma models generally target symptoms associated with abuse that occurred in the past. Complex trauma treatment models address many, but not all, of the dimensions of trauma just discussed. This section will focus on the trauma treatment/recovery component of these approaches by reviewing existing research, controversies, and consensus on treatment for PTSD and complex trauma (DESNOS/complex traumatic stress) and discussing their applicability for survivors of IPV. Women experiencing ongoing IPV are generally excluded from clinical trials due to safety and accessibility concerns and because these treatment modalities may be less appropriate when a person is still under siege. The richest literature on the intersection of trauma and IPV, although not yet evidence-based, derives from the combined experience of advocates and clinicians working with survivors over time and

from survivors themselves (14,17). These approaches interweave the IPV-specific interventions discussed earlier with elements of empowerment-based trauma recovery models described next.

The trauma treatment literature is essentially divided into two categories (although a number of models are starting to bridge this gap): evidence-based treatment for PTSD, and a combination of controlled, promising, and consensus-based treatments for complex trauma.

Evidence-based treatments for PTSD was originally developed for survivors of single-event trauma (e.g., sexual assault) and have since proven effective in treating PTSD among survivors of IPV who are no longer in an abusive relationship, for female combat veterans, and for some survivors of childhood abuse. Evidence-based treatment includes medication and protocol based CBT. Forms of CBT with the strongest evidence are prolonged exposure (PE), cognitive processing therapy (CPT), eye movement desensitization reprocessing (EMDR), and cognitive trauma therapy for battered women (CTT-BW), all of which involve working through memories of the traumatic event. More recently, several hybrid models have emerged that combine affect regulation and interpersonal skills training with attenuated exposure interventions for adult or adolescent survivors of childhood abuse (6,136,137). These models evolved to address concerns that exposure techniques may further disrupt pathways that have been chronically dysregulated by early trauma (138).

Current consensus approaches to treating complex trauma or DESNOS incorporate evidence-based techniques into a variety of multidimensional phased treatment models that attend to the domains affected by chronic, interpersonal trauma, particularly the developmental effects of childhood neglect and abuse. Research has not yet begun to explore the differential impact of trauma, such as IPV, that is experienced primarily as an adult or adolescent versus abuse that occurs during critical developmental periods in childhood. Therefore, these models may be most applicable for the subset of IPV survivors who are also experiencing the long-term effects of childhood trauma. However, since complex trauma models offer a more comprehensive framework for understanding and responding to the various effects of chronic abuse as well as a more flexible multimodal treatment approach, they may ultimately prove to be more useful to IPV survivors as well, particularly those whose experiences of abuse were more prolonged and severe.

In other words, complex trauma models attend to many of the domains that can be affected by interpersonal trauma that are not addressed by the PTSD diagnosis or PTSD treatment, although they do not address IPV-specific concerns.

COGNITIVE BEHAVIORAL THERAPIES FOR POSTTRAUMATIC STRESS DISORDER IN GENERAL

Until relatively recently, published PTSD treatment studies mainly focused on cognitive behavioral interventions following single-event sexual assaults (139,140). These modalities have demonstrated considerable success in preventing or reducing the severity of PTSD and, to some extent, associated depression and anxiety. Focal short-term psychodynamic therapies have also demonstrated some efficacy in treating PTSD (141). Research looking specifically at whether and under what circumstances these models are helpful to IPV survivors is still needed; the current research literature includes one randomized controlled trial of CBT for survivors of IPV and a handful of quasi-experimental studies.

Cognitive Processing Therapy

Cognitive processing therapy provides survivors with controlled exposure to traumatic memories and trains them to recognize and modify "maladaptive" cognitions (meanings and "lessons" one has taken from the traumatic experience such as "walking outside is dangerous") that cause unnecessary pain and constrict women's lives. Participants are encouraged to write about the traumatic event and are taught how to reconfigure their thinking about the trauma in ways that modify its impact on daily functioning. This technique has been effective in reducing PTSD and depression (8,140,142–145). It was designed to address inaccessible cognitive beliefs generated by the trauma as well as rape-related fears. Compared to controls, women who received this intervention had a significantly greater reduction in symptoms 3 months following the training.

Prolonged Exposure Therapy

Prolonged exposure (PE) therapy is based on Foa and Kozak's emotional processing theory, in which memories of a traumatic event are encoded in pathological fear structures that, once formed, generalize to other situations (146). Physiologic arousal and avoidant responses are then evoked by harmless stimuli which, in turn, interfere with the ability to place the experience in perspective and recover from its traumatic effects. Prolonged exposure therapy involves education about PTSD, breath retraining, imaginal exposure (detailed recounting of the rape and its aftermath plus discussion of responses with opportunities to correct fear-related cognitions within a highly structured intensive treatment program), and in vivo exposure to safe but feared (and avoided) stimuli (repetitive descriptions of the traumatic event) (147). Its effectiveness has been examined in several studies applying PE to victims of rape who were suffering from PTSD immediately after an assault (63,139,148,149). Foa and colleagues compared the effectiveness of stress inoculation training (SIT) to the use of PE techniques and supportive counseling (150). They found that all three led to posttreatment improvement. Stress inoculation training was most effective in reducing fear, anxiety, and depression, but exposure was most effective for reducing PTSD at 3 months. In another 1999 study, Foa and colleagues compared PE, SIT, and combined PE/SIT. In this study, PE alone demonstrated superior results (139). Any contact with a therapist was found to reduce many forms of rape-induced distress, but active treatment seems to be necessary to prevent PTSD (119).

Eye Movement Desensitization Reprocessing

Eye movement desensitization reprocessing involves the deconditioning of anxiety through reactivation and reexposure to traumatic memories and the transformation of pervasive abuse-related beliefs about one's self and one's world into more adaptive cognitions (151). In EMDR treatment, exposure is under the control of the patient. This is designed to engender a sense of mastery in the face of the traumatic experience. Some studies have suggested unusually rapid therapeutic responses using three to four sessions of therapy to treat isolated trauma. Although a growing body of research supports the efficacy of EMDR (152–156), others have questioned these findings, citing studies that suggest that the eye movements do not contribute to the therapeutic effects (157,158). More recently, Rothbaum, Astin, and Marsteller compared

PE treatment to EMDR for sexual assault survivors with PTSD. Both treatments led to clinically and statistically significant improvements immediately following treatment; 95% of PE participants and 75% of EMDR participants no longer met the criteria for PTSD at the conclusion of treatment (138). The difference between the two treatment groups was not statistically significant. These gains were maintained at a 6-month follow-up, although PE participants reported better end-state functioning than EMDR participants. The authors of the study suggest that EMDR and PE are both exposure techniques that simply diverge in administration and instructions for work between sessions.

COGNITIVE BEHAVIORAL THERAPY SPECIFIC TO SURVIVORS OF INTIMATE PARTNER VIOLENCE

Only two studies have examined the efficacy of PTSD treatment for battered women. Johnson and Zlotnick conducted a small pilot study of CBT for women living in DV shelters (4). Although they did not have a control group for comparison, they found that the women who participated in treatment experienced significant decreases in PTSD and depression symptoms, as well as significant increases in the level of social functioning and effective use of resources. The most significant improvement occurred between women's stay at the shelter and 1 week after their departure, but gains were maintained up to 6 months later. Because of the small sample size and the lack of a control group, however, it is unclear whether these gains are due specifically to their participation in treatment or to advocacy services utilized during their shelter stay. Some gains could represent participants' successful use of shelter resources or reflect a natural course of PTSD for battered women.

Kubany and co-workers, in the only rigorously controlled treatment study specifically focused on survivors of IPV, also tested the efficacy of cognitive trauma therapy for PTSD (CTT-BW) (5). Their model, along with more standard modalities such as psychoeducation about PTSD, stress management, and exposure (talking about the trauma, homework), includedcomponents to address four unique areas of concern they had identified as salient to battered women. These included (a) trauma-related guilt that many survivors reported (guilt about failed marriage, effects on children, decisions to stay or leave); (b) histories of other traumatic experiences; (c) likelihood of ongoing stressful contact with the abuser in relation to parenting; and (d) the risk for subsequent revictimization. Modules were designed to address these concerns (assessing and reframing negative beliefs about the self and inaccurate cognitions that help to maintain trauma symptoms; assertiveness and self-advocacy skills training; and strategies for managing contact with former partners, particularly around custody and visitation, and strategies for identifying and avoiding potential perpetrators in the future).

Women were assigned to either immediate or delayed treatment groups. The researchers found that 87% of women who completed immediate treatment no longer met diagnostic criteria for PTSD at the final assessment at the conclusion of treatment, whereas PTSD and depression among women in the delayed treatment group did not diminish during the 6-week period prior to the start of their treatment. These improvements were maintained at 3- and 6-month follow-up assessments. Sixty-nine percent of participants no longer met the criteria for both PTSD and depression, which is comparable to the findings of Resick and colleagues (140). Of particular note, 85% of women who completed treatment no longer met the Diagnostic and Statistical Manual of Mental Health Disorders (*DSM-IV*) PTSD criterion for numbing/avoidance. This is significant because PTSD treatments have generally been less successful in eliminating this symptom constellation. The authors also reported that the treatment was effective in an ethnically and educationally diverse group of women, and worked equally well when delivered by clinically and non–clinically trained therapists.

To participate in the study, however, women had to have been out of an abusive relationship for at least 30 days, with no intention of reconciling, and to have not experienced physical or sexual abuse or stalking during that time. The mean time since last physical abuse among women in this study was 5 years. The authors note that this limited the study's generalizability to women who are still being abused by a partner, for whom interventions may need to focus more on increasing safety and accessing resources. They also note that for women who develop chronic PTSD, the symptoms, if untreated can persist for many years, even after they are safe.

In addition, several small studies have examined innovative strategies to reduce mental health symptoms and improve well-being among survivors of IPV. Koopman and colleagues conducted a small randomized controlled study assessing the impact of expressive writing (writing about traumatic experiences) compared to writing about a neutral topic on depression, pain, and PTSD (159). They found a reduction in symptoms of depression, although overall effects were not significant. In another study with a quasi-experimental design, music therapy plus progressive relaxation reduced anxiety and improved self-reported sleep quality (160).

In sum, only a handful of PTSD treatment studies are specific to survivors of IPV. The only randomized controlled trial was designed for women who were no longer in an abusive relationship. Cognitive trauma therapy for battered women however, was effective in treating IPV-related PTSD, reducing IPV-associated feelings of guilt, and addressing several key post-abuse issues. In addition, this model was developed and delivered in conjunction with advocates and survivors and did not require previous clinical training to administer. It demonstrates the potential for developing replicable treatment models that combine evidence-based techniques with interventions designed to address specific concerns of IPV survivors. Determining which, if any, elements of this approach would be helpful to survivors still involved with an abusive partner and/or survivors who have experienced abuse in childhood as well, would be useful next step.

EFFICACY OF CBT FOR SURVIVORS OF CHRONIC INTERPERSONAL TRAUMA: ISSUES AND CONTROVERSIES

Although CBT models appear to be effective in treating PTSD among selected survivors of adult-onset trauma, the use of prolonged exposure techniques has raised a number of concerns that are potentially relevant to survivors of IPV, including reports of negative effects (161,162) and lack of tolerability (163,164) among a subset of survivors, particularly those who have experienced childhood abuse. In addition, studies indicate that exposure therapy appears to be more appropriate for women who are physically safe, who do not have dissociative symptoms, and who are not primarily depressed (161,165). In one study,

participants exhibited a poorer response if they felt defeated during a traumatic experience, alienated following the event, and had developed a sense that their lives would never be the same (166). For survivors of chronic childhood abuse who have not developed the internal capacity to modulate affect and arousal, symptoms may be exacerbated by exposure. The distress associated with confronting traumatic memories may make these modalities unacceptable to many survivors, particularly if they are still living in fear or, as Levitt and Cloitre note, if they have difficulty managing feelings of anger or anxiety or establishing a therapeutic relationship (166). In addition, research indicates that people with childhood exposure to interpersonal violence who experience symptoms of PTSD plus other conditions (such as bipolar disorder, suicidality, substance abuse, dissociation, or depression) often do not respond to conventional treatment for these conditions but are generally screened out of trials for PTSD treatment (162). As mentioned previously, randomized controlled studies assessing treatment for women who have been abused by an intimate partner, experienced the lasting effects of childhood abuse, and/or who have comorbid conditions, are still limited (58,82,92).

These issues have generated considerable controversy within the trauma field (164). In response to these concerns, Foa and colleagues investigated the impact of exposure on survivors with chronic PTSD (167). In this study, imaginal exposure did not exacerbate symptoms in the majority of participants and did not lead to treatment dropout. In addition, the minority whose symptoms were exacerbated by exposure still benefited from treatment. However, only 10% of the sample had histories of abuse in childhood, and women experiencing substance abuse, bipolar disorder or schizophrenia, or exposure to ongoing IPV were excluded. Assessment for complex trauma/ DESNOS was not reported.

Another study that compared cognitive processing therapy (CPT) and PE therapies for victims of sexual assault did note that within the sample of rape survivors, 85% had experienced at least one other major crime victimization (140). Forty-eight percent had also experienced sexual abuse as a child. In this study, both CPT and PE were found to be successful in treating PTSD, but the authors report a slight advantage in effect sizes and functioning for CPT. Cognitive processing therapy was also better at addressing issues of guilt. In addition, CPT incorporated cognitive processing designed to modify trauma-related beliefs and employed a less intensive version of trauma recall. The large majority of participants in the two treatment groups were no longer diagnosed with PTSD at the end of treatment, and their improvement was maintained at a 9-month follow-up. Although CPT had been generally conducted in the context of group therapy, this study demonstrated its efficacy in the context of individual therapy, as well.

Russell and Davis, after reviewing over 40 studies of PTSD treatment for rape survivors, claim that none of the criticisms of PE are supported by research data (145). These studies, however, still leave questions about which therapies are most effective for and amenable to survivors of other types of trauma. For example, the persistent danger and coercive control associated with current IPV also makes it difficult to engage in this type of treatment for obvious reasons: the inability to participate safely and consistently, the lack of emotional safety to access feelings while still under siege, and the challenges of treating PTSD via exposure modalities when the trauma is ongoing. Cognitive behavioral therapy appears to be effective in treating PTSD in survivors of various types of abuse, but is not applicable to all survivors, particularly those experiencing greater affect dysregulation or significant comorbidity, or who are still in danger.

Modifications to CBT to Address Controversies: Affect Dysregulation and Complex Trauma

Several researchers have attempted to address these concerns by modifying their treatment approach to include affect regulation and interpersonal skills training prior to introducing exposure techniques. Cloitre and colleagues investigated the efficacy of a modified CBT for PTSD related to child abuse (physical or sexual) (6). Their model, Skills Training in Affect and Interpersonal Regulation with Modified Prolonged Exposure (STAIR-MPE) consists of two eight-session phases: the first involves teaching skills to improve regulation of mood and emotions and the ability to tolerate distress; the second involves the attenuated exposure regimen. Participants showed significant improvement in three specifically targeted domains, including affect regulation, interpersonal skills, and PTSD symptoms. Gains were maintained, and some were enhanced, at the 3- and 9-month follow-up.

The authors found that the development of a positive therapeutic alliance and the improvement in negative mood regulation were significant predictors of PTSD reduction.

In another study, McDonagh-Coyle and co-workers adapted an exposure-oriented CBT model originally developed for rape survivors to survivors of child sexual abuse (136). The treatment was more effective than the control condition and present-centered therapy in improving PTSD symptoms and self-dysregulation; gains were maintained at 6- and 12-month follow-ups. However, many participants dropped out of treatment (43%), and treatment outcomes for these participants were not assessed. In sum, these adaptations generally involve strategies that enhance a survivor's capacity to manage the level of arousal induced by imaginal exposure (i.e., cognitive information about trauma and PTSD, cognitive reframing of trauma-related beliefs, and interpersonal and affect regulation skills) followed by less intensive exposure. Both of these models were framed by the authors as treating chronic PTSD among survivors of interpersonal abuse (and in some instances, substance abuse, as well), rather than as treating complex trauma, per se.

In a review of treatment for complex trauma (complex posttraumatic dysregulation), Ford and associates view the hybrid models just described as part of a broader category of interpersonal self-regulation and affect regulation therapy models (IAT) (58). They suggest that, unlike CBT, these models teach specific skills for social problem-solving and affect regulation; may use current stressor experiences and more recent memories as vehicles for examining and dealing with interpersonal difficulties and problematic emotions; and emphasize therapeutic attachment as a vehicle for enhancing survivors' capacities for self-regulation.

As Ford and associates describe, many of protocol-based treatments for PTSD plus chronic affect dysregulation utilize a partial phase-oriented approach—one that focuses on skill development and the establishment of a positive therapeutic relationship as precursor to traumatic memory work, although they point out that little empirical guidance exists on how to determine when a survivor has developed sufficient self-regulatory capacity to move safely from phase I to II. They note that with careful preparation, these modalities can be both effective and safe for some survivors and provide empirical support for the consensus-based phase-oriented approach described next. They also note that some evidence indicates that trauma recovery work may not be necessary to this process (168,169). Rather, these particular models focus more on helping survivors to understand the relationship between current distress and adaptations needed to survive previous trauma, develop new skills and capacities, and achieve a new sense of purpose and meaning.

Although research has not specifically addressed the efficacy of these approaches for survivors of IPV who have experienced other lifetime abuse, a number of studies have demonstrated promising results for a range of violence survivors experiencing complex trauma. Although some survivors respond to short-term interventions to reduce or eliminate symptoms, for others it may take a number of years and a variety of resources to recover from the traumatic effects of longstanding abuse. From an IAT perspective, safety includes stabilizing suicidality, impulsive, risky behavior, affect lability, dissociation, substance use, and dangerous relationships. It is unclear whether dangerous relationships are viewed as a symptom to be addressed rather than a situation over which a survivor may have little control. However, incorporating an understanding of the dynamics of IPV and attention to IPV safety concerns could extend the usefulness of these modalities for survivors of IPV.

OVERVIEW OF COMPLEX TRAUMA TREATMENT

As clinicians, researchers, and survivors came to recognize the distinct and often pervasive developmental impact of chronic abuse, more complex treatment models evolved. Although it appears that the majority of people who develop complex traumatic stress experienced chronic abuse or neglect in childhood, it is not clear what percentage of people who have experienced childhood abuse go on to develop its more serious sequelae (e.g., DESNOS/complex posttraumatic self-dysregulation/DID). Exposure to abuse in childhood does not necessarily lead to the development of complex trauma disorders. However, a complex trauma framework may be more useful in addressing the multiple domains affected by current and past abuse of various sorts.

These approaches combine emerging data on the neurobiology of trauma with developmental relational perspectives, CBT for managing overwhelming affect states, skill-building strategies to address

developmental disruptions, and in some cases, a feminist emphasis on empowerment and social context. Some incorporate non–cognitively based modalities (e.g., meditation, dance, music, or body-centered therapies), as well. Some involve traumatic memory recovery work after preparation; others do not. All address safety as a priority, recognize that symptoms may be coping strategies, and stress the importance of the survivor–therapist relationship to the process of healing, particularly its role supporting personal and relational experiences that facilitate the reinstatement of disrupted developmental processes, including trust (27,170).

A key difference in approaches to complex trauma versus PTSD treatment is the emphasis on rebuilding, reinstating, and repairing aspects of development that were disrupted by early trauma and subsequent life trajectories, coming to terms with the impact of those experiences, and creating new meaning and purpose as one moves forward in life. Complex trauma models incorporate symptom-focused PTSD treatment as part of a larger array of interventions that help restore a survivor's sense of self, connections to others, and feelings about the world. They tend to view symptom management as a necessary precursor to deeper intra- and interpersonal work. Although designed specifically for survivors of childhood abuse and neglect, many of these domains can also be affected by severe chronic traumatization as an adult, such as torture and IPV (84).

Complex Trauma: Phase-Based Treatment Approach

The primary consensus-based approach to complex trauma treatment incorporates many of the aspects described above into a flexible three-phased model (safety and stability, trauma processing and recovery, reintegration and rebuilding) (26,58,171,172). This model again draws from a combination of evidence-based treatments targeted toward PTSD symptoms, attention to issues of ongoing safety, skill-building training to address capacities that have been derailed by early trauma, and emotional and cognitive reprocessing of feelings and thoughts associated with or stemming from traumatic experiences. This reprocessing includes nonverbal techniques to access experiences that were not verbally stored, all of which are embedded within a relational framework designed to heal the interpersonal bonds disrupted by abuse and betrayal by a trusted caregiver (and/or person or system that should have been trustworthy). Part of the healing process involves fostering survivors' sense of mastery and control through the development of skills to regulate affect and manage symptoms. And, like the hybrid IAT models, the emphasis is on establishing safety and stability, building a collaborative therapeutic relationship and other supports, and developing a sense of self-efficacy before proceeding (in some versions) to trauma-focused work.

In more developed complex trauma models, however, building a working alliance when trustworthy relationships were never part of a survivor's experience may be critical focus of the initial work, and stabilization may be a longer process. Phase II work involves developing a more integrated and "emotionally modulated" autobiographical narrative and gradual reorientation to the present and future that is no longer dominated by the past (173). Phase III, not addressed in the IAT models, involves integrating new skills, capacities, and traumatic memories (being able to separate past from present) and rebuilding a meaningful, engaging life (no longer defined by trauma and its effects). Other shared components include psychoeducation to help survivors accurately label the abuse and reduce self-blame (i.e., to counter abusers' distortions about blame and responsibility) and destigmatize responses to trauma by recognizing symptoms as adaptations to psychically overwhelming situations.

These models are strength-based, viewing individuals as survivors rather than as victims and promote empowerment, therapeutic collaboration, and choice. They are also attentive to survivors' cultural and spiritual values. They are designed to support survivors' ability to function (i.e., do not promote regression) and to master rather than avoid the effects and/or actual memories of previous trauma (58). Final stages of treatment involve the integration of memories into a coherent narrative, the development of new capacities, reconnecting to others, developing a new sense of meaning and purpose, and rebuilding (14,174). This process is not linear but rather one in which work proceeds and is then revisited from more recent vantage points.

In sum, trauma is complex, individual responses are unique and social context makes a difference. Therefore, treatment needs to be flexible, multimodal, and individually tailored, as well as evidence-informed and, where possible, evidence-based.

Complex Trauma: Research-Based Treatment Models and Approaches

Given these caveats, the limited number of randomized controlled trials on treatment for complex trauma is not surprising. Establishing an evidence base for addressing trauma in the context of ongoing IPV raises a number of additional challenges. For example, a tension exists between the on-the-ground need for flexible, multidimensional survivor-driven models in addition to the fixed, manualized treatments that are easier to evaluate in randomized controlled trials. And, because the harm of interpersonal trauma occurs in the context of relationships, healing often takes place in the context of relationships, as well, which again is more difficult to quantify (e.g., restoring trust in oneself and others through the experience of a nonjudgmental, accepting therapeutic relationship or peer support). In addition, treatment in the context of IPV needs to address realities that often are not under survivor's control. Finally, addressing parenting and attachment issues adds further layers of complexity to incorporate into research designs. Thus, while numerous evidence-based "techniques" are available for treating PTSD, they are generally geared toward addressing specific sets of symptoms, rather than healing from the interpersonal and developmental effects of abuse and violence—a process that, as noted earlier, may require the safety, consistency, caring, and respect of ongoing healing relationships; the development of internal capacities and external supports, including restoring a sense of community; and, in the context of ongoing IPV, access to safety and resources (26,58). The models discussed next, however, are beginning to demonstrate efficacy in combining these core elements in a variety of different configurations.

For example, given the efficacy of evidence-based treatments for acute and chronic PTSD, clinicians have begun to combine pertinent elements into more individually tailored treatment regimes. Many of the techniques utilized in treatment for PTSD have also been incorporated into multidimensional treatment programs designed specifically for women with severe trauma histories and complex PTSD, serious mental illness, and/or substance abuse (8–10,85,169,170,175–181). Several also involve a deeper level work in integrating trauma memories, grieving losses, and establishing a new sense of self and/or meaning (26,27,182). Some are now evidence-based, some have proven efficacy in open trials, and others are more general approaches to this work.

Several of these models, when combined with IPV-specific interventions, may be particularly applicable to survivors of IPV who have experienced multiple forms of trauma beginning in childhood. For example, the trauma recovery empowerment model (TREM) is a 33-week psycho-educational outpatient group intervention designed to assist women in recovering from long-term effects of childhood abuse. It addresses many of the domains that can be affected by early trauma, including intrapersonal skills (e.g., self-knowledge, self-soothing, self-esteem, self-trust) and interpersonal skills (e.g., self-expression, social perception and accurate labeling, self-protection, self-assertion, relational mutuality), as well as more global skills (e.g., identity formation, initiative taking, problem solving). In addition to skill development, it also focuses on countering feelings of powerlessness and rebuilding connections to oneself and others that were lost in the face of trauma. It also helps women develop the sense of self, skills, and supports needed to prevent future victimization. The TREM was evaluated as part of the SAMHSA Women, Violence and Co-Occurring Disorders Study (quasi-experimental design), which involved integrated mental health, trauma, and substance abuse treatment within a comprehensive array of trauma-informed services (including individual therapy, case management, psychiatric care, supported housing, and peer support). It was one of several treatment modalities that demonstrated modest efficacy compared to controls. Although not specifically reported, for many of the women in this study, although not exposed at the time, IPV was one aspect of the long continuum of trauma they had experienced over the course of their lives.

Trauma recovery and skill-building interventions are also successful for women diagnosed with more severe mental illness, but require increased supports and slower pacing. Again, for a survivor of IPV who is also experiencing a psychiatric disability, these treatments could be adapted to address both safety and trauma symptoms. Mueser and Rosenberg developed a PTSD treatment model designed specifically for survivors experiencing a serious mental illness (183). Their initial model involved brief cognitive-behavioral intervention (psychoeducation followed by modified exposure) designed for people diagnosed with schizophrenia. It focused more narrowly on treating symptoms of PTSD. More recently, they report

on a 21-week mixed-group intervention model for addressing PTSD among people with severe mental illness that was piloted at a community mental health center with promising results (137). The Trauma Recovery Group is a CBT intervention comprised of breath retraining, psychoeducation about PTSD, cognitive restructuring, learning to cope with symptoms, and making a recovery plan. In their pre-/post design, participants who completed the program (59% retention rate) had significant improvement in PTSD symptoms, depression, and trauma-related cognitions compared to people who dropped out. Their rationale for using cognitive restructuring rather than PE was based, in part, on the body of positive experience using CBT to treat other symptoms among people who have mental illness, which is not the case for PE. In addition, people who have a mental illness appear to have greater sensitivity to stress, which PE treatment can increase. Again, the authors note that this type of treatment is best embedded within a more comprehensive array of treatment and supports (e.g., meds, case management, and other supports). For example, a survivor may have many other concerns and needs (comorbid symptoms, substance use, issues of managing daily living, medication-related concerns, and the need for skill development in a variety of domains). For survivors of IPV, safety concerns and abusers' use of mental health issues as tactics of control also become priorities. What this and other research point to is the need to recognize both the strengths of evidence-based PTSD treatment models, particularly symptom reduction and prevention of PTSD, as well as their limitations, for someone experiencing affect dysregulation and/or other disruptive mental health symptoms.

Other complex trauma treatment models and approaches that could be adapted for working with survivors of IPV include Trauma Adaptive Recovery Group Education and Therapy (TARGET), the Sanctuary model, and risking connection, among others (27,176,182). TARGET is also designed to address complex trauma among people with serious mental illness; it is a strengths-based model, teaching a set of practical skills to enable participants to gain control of PTSD symptoms. The Sanctuary model, a residential trauma treatment model for creating healing environments, is designed to address the long-term sequelae of chronic abuse (182). It was initially developed for use on inpatient psychiatric units but has been applied in DV shelters and residential treatment programs for children and adolescents. It is a four-stage model (SAGE) addressing Safety, developing Affect regulation skills, processing Grief, and supporting Emancipation (freedom from the effects of trauma, developing new capacities and meaningful connections, and reinvesting in life). The Risking Connection curriculum is an individual complex trauma treatment approach developed for use in the public mental health systems in Maine and New York; it addresses both provider and survivor issues, particularly transference, countertransference, and vicarious trauma. It too emphasizes the importance of a collaborative therapeutic relationship that provides information; fosters respect, connection, and hope; and supports the development of new self-capacities. Several of these models have been tested through the SAMHSA Women, Violence and Co-Occurring Disorders Study (TREM, Seeking Safety) and have demonstrated efficacy as part of a broader array of trauma-informed mental health and substance abuse services (10,34,184,185). None of these models specifically address IPV. More research is needed to determine if and how they can best be used in conjunction with IPV-specific interventions when safety and coercion are still a concern.

There are several additional studies of promising and/or evidence-based group treatment modalities for survivors of childhood abuse (91,186–190), as well as evidence-based interventions designed specifically for managing the symptoms and self-harming behavior of women with complex trauma who have been diagnosed with borderline personality disorder, a high percentage of whom have experienced abuse in childhood (7,191). Although many initial reports were descriptive in nature, featured nonstandardized approaches to care, and/or demonstrated relatively modest positive results, recent studies (e.g., trauma-focused group therapy) have been more rigorously designed but need to be specifically evaluated to assess their applicability for survivors of IPV who have also experienced childhood abuse (188,192).

Complex Trauma Treatment in the Context of Intimate Partner Violence

Thus, despite the emergence of the models for treating complex traumatic stress, little research has addressed complex trauma in the context of ongoing IPV, where legal, safety, and custody issues abound. And, although each of these models has moved forward our understanding of what is and is not helpful in healing the long-term effects of childhood trauma, none attend to the social context in which IPV takes place, nor do they address the social conditions in which violence and inequality are condoned and supported (18,193). They do, however, provide a treatment framework that could be adapted for survivors of ongoing IPV. And, because complex trauma treatment models stem from work with survivors of gender-based violence (childhood sexual abuse, sexual assault, IPV), they can be offered in ways that incorporate feminist and advocacy perspectives. For example, feminist approaches explicitly address the role of power dynamics, both within a woman's life and within therapeutic encounters, that has been a concern of advocates and survivors. Mental health peer support recovery models promote collaboration and power sharing between consumers and providers, as well (22). In addition, DV advocacy models attend to the social reality of ongoing danger and entrapment and the impact of social institutions, culture, and communities on a survivor's ability to change her or his life. Again, although flexible survivor-centered treatment approaches are more difficult to study than shorter-term protocol-based models, they nonetheless reflect current consensus in this area.

Although the issues that are unique to IPV were described earlier, many survivors have experienced multiple forms of abuse and are dealing with both past and current trauma—trauma that may affect their ability to deal with the ongoing abuse in their lives. In addition, many of the aspects of interpersonal trauma that survivors of IPV report are better addressed by complex trauma models (e.g., betrayal of trust; feelings about oneself, other people, and the world; feelings of shame, guilt, grief, loss, fear, hurt, anger, sadness, emptiness, despair, confusion, etc.).

Regardless of type of trauma, the first priority of treatment is establishing safety, no matter where the threat originates. In the context of ongoing IPV, this means attending to safety from an abusive partner. If a survivor is also experiencing trauma- or mental health-related symptoms, those also need to be addressed, both in terms of how they affect a survivor's ability to be safe from an abusive partner and how they affect a survivor's ability to be safe from potentially dangerous coping strategies and/or symptoms.

Treatment also involves establishing a collaborative working alliance. If a woman is a survivor of childhood abuse and has had no safe, nurturing attachment relationships in her life, then establishing trust can be much more challenging for her and becomes a central aspect of early work. This phase of treatment may also focus on supporting a survivor in dealing with the many practical issues that arise in establishing safety and economic stability and parenting children who have also been affected by IPV, legal, and custody issues, as well as the myriad of other concerns she is facing, including immigration and potential loss of her community. It also involves providing information and access to resources, creating a safe place for survivors to think clearly and evaluate their situations and options.

At the same time, therapy may include working to decrease fear and isolation, assisting with symptom management and skill acquisition, helping survivors to assess and reformulate any abuse-related perceptions of themselves while making and trusting their own decisions, identifying and building on strengths, establishing networks of support, and working in collaboration with community DV programs. Later phases may involve the processing of traumatic memories and abuse-related feelings and integrating them into the next stage of a survivor's life. Expert clinicians note a number of issues that may emerge during this time, including feelings of anger, fear, betrayal, sadness, and loss, as well as concerns about safety, intimacy, and trust (14,17). Although phase-based models for complex trauma view trauma memory processing as part of phase II with reintegration and rebuilding as the third phase, for survivors of IPV, establishing a safe, secure life may need to occur before it is possible to process the full impact and meaning of their experiences. For others, some of this work may be an important precursor to other steps they will take to create lives that are both safe from abuse and no longer haunted previous trauma.

In summary, the mental health effects of IPV vary widely. Some resolve with safety and support; others require longer-term treatment. A range of modalities may be applicable to victims of IPV. Evidence-based PTSD treatment for single-event trauma includes CBT and medication. Hybrid treatments for chronic PTSD and/or adult survivors of child abuse incorporate affect and interpersonal skill-building techniques prior to trauma memory processing. Complex trauma treatments are comprehensive and phase-based models that incorporate evidence-based affect regulation, skill-building techniques, and traumatic memory work into individualized treatment approaches. Treatment for survivors of IPV includes IPV-specific care, care of acute symptoms, and longer-term trauma recovery.

Treatment must also attend to a range of psychological sequelae related to IPV, as well as to ongoing stressors due to stalking, harassment, or prolonged legal battles. Working with community DV advocacy programs to provide concrete and emotional support is vital. From a phase-based perspective, clinical work with survivors who remain in danger should focus on issues of safety, stability, and support, saving trauma recovery work for when it is safe to do so. Research is needed to determine which modalities are most appropriate to individual survivors and which are most helpful to survivors who are experiencing ongoing abuse and violence.

PHARMACOLOGICAL TREATMENT

In their initial work on the healthcare system response to IPV, Stark, Flitcraft, and Frazier found that battered women were more likely to be prescribed psychotropic medication than nonbattered women, even when the abuse went unrecognized (194). Intimate partner violence survivors have also voiced concerns about medications not being paired with attention to abuse-specific issues, including the emotional effects of abuse, abusers' use of medication to undermine and control their partners, safety concerns, and access to resources (116). Although research in this area is limited, a number of issues must be considered when prescribing psychotropic medication in the context of ongoing IPV. They involve (a) the ways in which an abuser is likely to respond to the partner's use of medication, and, more specifically, the potential for an abuser to use medication to control or undermine the partner; (b) the direct effects of an abuser's behavior on the development and exacerbation of symptoms (e.g., being kept from sleeping or maintaining adequate hydration, etc.); (c) the importance of enhancing a survivor's sense of options and choice; (d) the interaction between the effects of current abuse with previous trauma and other mental health symptoms; and (e) the likelihood that a given medication will improve symptoms and enhance safety.

For example, medication should be offered in ways that enhance a survivor's sense of control over her life, ideally in the context of treatment that attends to both IPV and trauma-specific concerns. This can be done by discussing the pros, cons, and possible impact of taking medication and making certain survivors know that deciding whether or not to take psychotropic medication is a choice. It is also important to work with survivors to try to ensure that they will not be defined or controlled by their use of medication. For example, an abuser may use his partner's prescription for psychotropic medication as evidence that she is "crazy" and/or incapable of caring for their children. Discussing these issues directly can help a woman counter those perceptions and reduce an abusive partner's ability to define her reality. A batterer may also control her partner's access to medication (e.g., withholding medication), or coerce her partner to overdose or to ingest food or medication that is contraindicated. These issues should be addressed as part of safety planning and also factored into medication choice as it pertains to potential toxicity.

In addition, care should be taken so that medication does not lower the vigilance that may be important to a survivor's safety. Sedation, cognitive impairment, and reduced alertness can all impinge on previously honed mechanisms a survivor has used to keep herself safe in the past. Again, these issues need to be taken into account when making medication decisions, in conjunction with considerations about drug interactions and side effects. If a survivor is not able to make decisions for herself at a given point in time, then having discussed these issues in advance (whether or not there is a formal advance directive or other type of plan in place) will help inform clinical decisions and increase the likelihood that they will be consistent with her wishes and not controlled by her partner. At the same time, reducing symptoms while minimizing risks can clearly be of help to a survivor in his efforts to access safety and regain control over his life.

Although initial research on the mental health effects of IPV focused on depression and anxiety, more recent studies have focused on PTSD and/ or commonly accompanying comorbidities, most notably depression and anxiety disorders and, to a lesser extent, suicidality and substance abuse. Survivors of IPV may experience a range of mental health symptoms consequent to the abuse. In addition to the issues noted earlier, attention to trauma-related symptoms and concerns may provide the most useful overall approach to psychopharmacologic treatment in the context of IPV. Since virtually no research specifically addresses the use of psychotropic medication in the context of ongoing IPV or for treating complex trauma, this section will draw from research on pharmacotherapy for PTSD and for depression plus PTSD and/or childhood abuse.

Pharmacological Treatment for Posttraumatic Stress Disorder: Conceptual Issues

A number of studies have found significant comorbidity between depression and PTSD, in general and among survivors of IPV (195,196). Trauma exposure appears to be a risk factor for major depression as well as for PTSD (197,198). Each may constitute a risk for the other or, alternatively, may reflect a shared vulnerability (195,199). More significantly, several studies have found differential responses to treatment for depression among women experiencing comorbid PTSD (195) and/or childhood abuse (85,88), causing researchers to speculate that early life stress (childhood trauma) may set processes in motion (e.g., alterations in the hypothalamic-pituitary-adrenal [HPA] axis) that lead to a neurobiologically different subtype of depression—one for which psychotherapy may be more effective than medication (88).

In contrast, the study by Green and colleagues found that women with depression plus comorbid PTSD are more likely to have experienced assaults in childhood and/or as adults (including IPV), and to be more symptomatic at the outset and end of treatment than women without PTSD. Both groups, however, had a significantly better response to treatment (medication [paroxetine] or CBT) than did controls (195). These findings, albeit in different ways, are consistent with research supporting the construct of complex trauma/DESNOS as a "better fit" diagnosis than the notion of PTSD plus comorbidities. Green and colleagues hypothesized that the comparable response to CBT among women with depression plus PTSD was due, in part, to the fact that their depression-focused CBT had an additional trauma component. In other words the "comorbidities" that develop in the context of interpersonal trauma appear to be part of a larger constellation of trauma symptoms that may be neurobiologically distinct from their nontrauma-associated counterparts. They also appear to respond differently to treatment (i.e., are more challenging to treat and do not respond as well when trauma is not specifically addressed). Although work in this area is still preliminary, it does begin to provide both a theoretical and research basis for examining how trauma affects the development and treatment of a range of psychiatric conditions.

Research has yet to tease out the respective impact of early life stress versus chronic interpersonal trauma that occurs later in life on neural circuitry and subsequent mood and anxiety disorders, nor has it delineated what the implications might be for pharmacological (or other) treatment. Developing an evidence-base in this area has been challenging because people experiencing ongoing trauma (such as IPV), as well as individuals with comorbid conditions, are often excluded from clinical trials (92,162,172). And, trauma is not often factored into treatment studies for other co-occurring conditions. This raises questions about the efficacy of pharmacological (and other) treatment for people experiencing complex trauma. Spinnazola suggests the need for broadening inclusion criteria to ensure representation of people experiencing diverse types of trauma and multiple comorbidities, as well as providing detailed reporting on exclusion criteria, study declension, and attrition. Studies on treatment efficacy for individuals who are still in danger from an abusive partner, although critical, will be more difficult to devise and will have to factor in (i.e., assess for and report) abuser-related factors noted earlier, as well.

Although no psychopharmacology is specific to survivors of abuse, medication targeted toward symptoms of PTSD has demonstrated some efficacy in the reduction of core PTSD symptoms of intrusiveness, avoidance, psychic numbing, and hyperarousal; reduction of associated disability and vulnerability to stress; treatment of comorbid symptoms (e.g., depression, anxiety, panic, etc.); reduction of psychotic or dissociative symptoms; improved impulse control; and reduction of self-harming behaviors (200). The treatment recommendations that follow, however, are based on a limited number of randomized clinical trials for PTSD conducted with combat veterans and/or a variety of civilian samples, as well as promising open-label trials for drugs that have not yet moved to the randomized clinical trial stage. Medication studies for the most part have not specifically targeted complex trauma/DESNOS, and only one (pharmaceutical industry-sponsored study) has focused explicitly on survivors of IPV (201). Despite the dearth of controlled trial research, clinicians have been able to draw on the treatment literature for associated disorders (depression, anxiety, panic, bipolar disorder, psychotic disorders) and the ongoing treatment experience of national trauma centers. Few studies have examined response differences for victims of single versus multiple traumas, acute versus chronic PTSD (202), or childhood versus adult-onset trauma, and

few specifically examine gender differences in treatment response (203).

Current options for treatment include antidepressants, mood stabilizers, atypical antipsychotics, α-adrenergic inhibitors and, to a lesser extent, anxiolytics. Early PTSD studies mainly focused on the use of tricyclic antidepressants (TCAs) and monoamine oxidase inhibitors (MAOIs) (204,205). Data emerging from double-blind, placebo-controlled clinical trials, however, support the use of selective serotonin reuptake inhibitor (SSRI) antidepressants (paroxetine, sertraline, fluoxetine) as first-line treatment for PTSD. In many, but not all studies, SSRIs have demonstrated greater efficacy for women exposed to civilian trauma than for predominantly male combat veterans (206,207). In some studies, both TCAs and SSRIs were found to be useful for patients with depression plus PTSD, but SSRIs were associated with better outcomes than agents primarily affecting norepinephrine reuptake (208). However, some TCAs (imipramine, amitriptyline), MAOIs (phenelzine, moclobemide), and novel agents (mirtazapine) have demonstrated efficacy in reducing PTSD symptoms (209).

In a meta-analytic review of randomized controlled medication trials for PTSD, antipsychotic medications (olanzapine, risperidone), the anticonvulsant lamotrigine, and the MAOI brofamine did not show demonstrable treatment efficacy, nor did alprazolam, inositol, desipramine, and phenelzine, although they did in open label studies. These results may be due to small sample sizes and short durations of treatment, or, in the case of desipramine, noradrenergic stimulation (210). Although heightened anxiety is characteristic of PTSD, benzodiazepines have not proven useful in controlled trials, and may be associated with rebound anxiety when discontinued. Use of benzodiazepines in the immediate aftermath of trauma is still controversial. In one small placebo-controlled study, subjects given a benzodiazepine (clonazepam or alprazolam) 1 week post-trauma were more likely to develop PTSD than those who had received placebo (211). However, they have received cautious recommendation in some consensus reviews (150,210,212).

In addition, several recent studies have examined the hypothesis that β-blockers and corticosteroids may be useful in preventing the consolidation of traumatic memories if administered shortly after the trauma occurs (PTSD prophylaxis) (213–215), although these findings have not been consistently replicated (210). Despite advances over the past 10 years, less than 60%

of people with chronic PTSD respond to medications, although women who have experienced interpersonal trauma appear to be more medication-responsive than male combat veterans. This points to the need for combining pharmacotherapy with psychotherapy, as well as the need for longitudinal, larger scale, and more nuanced research. The next section describes the more robust research in this area.

Antidepressants: A Focus on Selective Serotonin Reuptake Inhibitors

Antidepressants have been the most well-studied medications for PTSD and have the greatest empirical support, with SSRIs making up the majority of large randomized clinical trials. They have demonstrated efficacy in reducing all three PTSD symptom clusters and increasing the number of treatment responders, based on cut-off scores on the Clinician Administered PTSD Scale (CAPS). They are also effective in treating comorbid depression and improving quality of life, as well as treating other commonly co-occurring conditions (e.g., anxiety disorders). Although other antidepressants, such as TCAs, MAOIs, and novel agents like mirtazapine have also showed some efficacy, those findings appear to be less robust, and TCAs have been mainly studied among veterans with chronic, severe PTSD, whereas SSRI trials have included civilians as well (210,216,217).

Posttraumatic stress disorder affects a number of neuroendocrine and neurotransmitter systems, including serotonin pathways, which appear to have a modulating effect on the processing of external stimuli and on noradrenergic activity through their connections to the locus ceruleus (216,218). The SSRIs have been effective in reducing PTSD symptoms in open-label and double-blind randomized controlled trials (219–224). Many of these studies have included women with longstanding PTSD secondary to childhood abuse, rape, or physical assault (225). One randomized double-blind, placebo-controlled study comparing fluoxetine, EMDR, and placebo found EMDR to be superior to fluoxetine in reducing symptoms of PTSD and depression at 6 months, but more so for people who had experienced trauma as adults (75% remission) versus as children (33% remission). Overall, neither treatment led to complete symptom remission for survivors of childhood trauma (226).

Sertraline and paroxetine have shown efficacy in both open and randomized controlled trials, as well

(219,220,223,224,227). In one small ($n = 5$), open, 12-week clinical trial, Rothbaum and co-workers found that sertraline significantly reduced PTSD among women who had been raped (228). Two randomized placebo-controlled trials have confirmed these results (219,220). In both studies, over 70% of the participants were women, medication was well-tolerated, and treatment response was significantly better for the sertraline group than for controls. In the first study, sertraline was more effective at reducing symptoms of increased arousal and avoidance/numbing than intrusive reexperiencing. A reanalysis of data from these two studies found sertraline to be more effective than placebo for people who had experienced child abuse or interpersonal (versus non-interpersonal) trauma (207). Effect sizes, although significant, were also modest (216). One randomized controlled double-blinded study of a predominantly male population with combat-related PTSD conducted at an outpatient VA clinic did not find sertraline to be more effective than placebo in treating PTSD (229). Two randomized controlled trials of paroxetine (12-week, fixed-dose studies with predominantly female participants) also found significant reductions in all three symptom clusters for those taking the drug versus placebo (223,227). In these studies, results did not differ by gender (230).

In the Stein and colleagues' meta-analytic review, 12 SSRI randomized clinical trials demonstrated significant reductions in symptom severity on all three subscales of the CAPS for both paroxetine and (to a slightly lesser extent), sertraline (210). The authors postulated that the lack of demonstrable treatment effects for venlafaxine, fluoxetine, and citalopram was due to small sample size and insufficient power in their analysis. In their numbers needed to treat (NNT) analysis, compared to placebo, the likelihood of becoming a treatment responder was 23%, 22%, and 16.5%, respectively, for paroxetine, sertraline, and fluoxetine. A randomized controlled study of extended-release venlafaxine found it superior to placebo in reducing reexperiencing and avoidance/numbing, but not hyperarousal cluster scores on the CAPS (231). It was also superior to placebo on measures of depression, quality of life, functioning, and global illness severity.

The SSRIs, unlike other drugs that have been studied for this disorder, seem to address both the psychic numbing associated with PTSD and comorbid depression (232,233). They may also provide additional efficacy for reducing alcohol consumption, as well as a range of possible serotonergically mediated symptoms associated with PTSD such as rage, impulsivity, suicidal intent, depression, panic, and obsessional thinking (232,234). On the other hand, SSRIs have been less effective than MAOIs and TCAs in treating comorbid anxiety (210).

Longer-term Selective Serotonin Reuptake Inhibitor Treatment Studies

Although initial randomized controlled trials were designed to assess short-term treatment responses (12 weeks), several additional studies have examined longer-term treatment effects examining two primary questions: (a) Do response rates improve with longer-term treatment, and (b) does longer term treatment prevent relapse? Two open-label 24-week extensions to 12-week randomized clinical studies found continued improvement in CAPS scores for paroxetine and sertraline, as well as ongoing improvement in depression and quality of life for sertraline during the extension phase (220,235,236). In addition, two double-blind placebo-controlled extension studies found increased relapse rates for subjects who were switched to placebo from fluoxetine and sertraline (220,237). The majority of subjects in the sertraline study were women who had experienced physical or sexual assault. Subjects in the paroxetine study (urban adults, the majority of whom were Latinas who had experienced a range of interpersonal trauma) also had significant reductions in dissociative symptoms and self-reported interpersonal problems. In another 9-month open-label paroxetine study, in which the predominant type of trauma was childhood sexual abuse (9 men and 14 women), in addition to improvement in CAPS scores, subjects also demonstrated improvement in verbal declarative memory and increases in hippocampal volume, although these findings did not correlate with PTSD symptomatology or with each other. They do lend support to the hypothesis that SSRIs may increase neurogenesis in the hippocampus (238).

These findings highlight several important points. First, many survivors, particularly those with more severe symptoms, may take longer to respond than the time allotted for standard short-term (12 weeks) treatment trials or the 3–4 weeks generally thought of as the time needed for SSRIs to work. Second, in these studies, the majority of participants who did not respond during the acute treatment phase did become treatment responders during the 24-week extension,

and approximately a third of the treatment response occurred during this period. It was not entirely clear what portion of this response was due to natural course or other benefits that accrue from participation in a clinical trial. In addition, one study reported drop-out rates of close to 40% (239). The role of IPV (i.e., abuser control) in study declension or attrition, to our knowledge, has not been specifically addressed. Nonetheless, these findings highlight the importance of a therapeutic relationship in helping to sustain treatment when responses are delayed and is consistent with research demonstrating superior results with nonpharmacological and/or combined pharmacological and nonpharmacological treatment modalities. Because none of these studies specifically addressed issues of ongoing violence, there is no way to know what role an abuser's behavior and or safety interventions may have played in a survivor's response to treatment.

Other Psychopharmacological Treatments for Posttraumatic Stress Disorder: A Theory-Driven Approach

A number of theory-driven approaches to psychopharmacological treatment of PTSD have yet to demonstrate efficacy in randomized controlled trials (e.g., anticonvulsants, adrenergic-inhibiting agents benzodiazepines, antipsychotics, and cortisol). However, a brief discussion of current thinking in this area may be helpful in guiding treatment choices when initial modalities are not successful, as well as illuminating future research.

Kindling and Anticonvulsants

Kindling (lowering of the excitability threshold after repeated electrical stimulation, leading to oversensitization of the limbic system, manifesting in physiologic hyperarousal) has been posited as one theoretical model for the development of PTSD. Kindling and sensitization have also been viewed as a possible mechanism for the repeated activation of fear memories leading to flashbacks and intrusive reexperiencing and therefore may be useful in preventing the development of sensitization of these pathways in the aftermath of trauma (216). This has led to several trials of anticonvulsants, which have demonstrated some beneficial effects in people with chronic PTSD, although their efficacy is yet to be fully demonstrated in randomized controlled trials (240,241).

Dysregulation and Adrenergic Inhibition

Dysregulation of adrenergic and noradrenergic systems and their mediating effects on cortisol production is thought to be a core component of PTSD and has been implicated in the over-consolidation of traumatic memories, and subsequent intrusive reexperiencing and hyperarousal. Theoretically, α_2-blockade of presynaptic norepinephrine release or β-blockade of postsynaptic norepinephrine receptors would reduce cortisol-enhanced memory consolidation and fear conditioning and could potentially prevent or reduce these effects, although results from clinical trials have been mixed (242).

γ-Aminobutyric Acid/Glutamine Dysregulation and Benzodiazepines

Because benzodiazepines potentiate the inhibitory effects of γ-aminobutyric acid (GABA) receptors that are found throughout the brain and appear to counter excitatory glutaminergic transmission and modulate the increased arousal associated with PTSD, theoretically they should be useful treatment modalities for PTSD. However, recommendations for the use of benzodiazepines for acute and chronic PTSD remain unclear, and studies have yielded mixed results, as well. Benzodiazepines appear to reduce anxiety, arousal, irritability, and insomnia in people with PTSD and in a small number of those with dissociative identity disorder. They have not been found to be effective for intrusive symptoms or for avoidance and numbing.

Endogenous Opioid Dysregulation and Narcotic Antagonists

The use of narcotic antagonists, studied because they should theoretically reduce endogenous opioid-induced numbing, has also met with mixed results, showing improvement in some studies and worsening in others (243).

Dopaminergic, Serotonergic and α-Adrenergic Pathways, and Antipsychotics

The rationale for using antipsychotic medication was the similarity between flashbacks and the visual and auditory hallucinations seen in schizophrenia, as well as their potential action on dopaminergic,

serotonergic, and α-adrenergic pathways (239,244). Current thinking is that these agents may be of benefit for people who have chronic PTSD that is more treatment-resistant and/or for treating concomitant psychotic symptoms, but larger randomized clinical trial research is needed to determine their efficacy (216,245,246). The potential for developing metabolic syndrome also makes these medications a less desirable option unless psychotic symptoms are part of the clinical picture.

Hypothalamic-Pituitary-Adrenal Axis and Cortisol

Several preliminary studies report theory-driven efforts to prevent the development of PTSD through medications that might prevent the consolidation of fear-based memories and chronic hyperarousal. One set of studies is based on the role of cortisol in the retrieval and consolidation of traumatic memories (elevated cortisol inhibits memory retrieval in animals and healthy humans). These were conducted with small samples of patients who had chronic PTSD, were experiencing septic shock, and/or were undergoing cardiac surgery (213,215,245,247–249). Results in the prevention of the consolidation of traumatic memories were mixed. Although these preliminary findings are of interest, more research is needed before this strategy can be recommended.

Pharmacological Management of Posttraumatic Stress Disorder with Comorbid Conditions

Although a complex trauma framework may be more useful for understanding the psychological effects of chronic interpersonal trauma, medication trials generally focus on single disorders and few have specifically addressed comorbidity in the context of PTSD treatment. Given the high rates of comorbidity associated with PTSD (most notably affective disorders, anxiety disorders, and substance abuse), as well as treatment for PTSD in the context of other psychiatric conditions (e.g., bipolar disorder, schizophrenia), choice of medication needs to be tailored to address co-occurring conditions as well. For example, SSRIs can be used to effectively treat both PTSD and major depression, although responses appear to be less robust when they co-occur (216,223). Sertraline and paroxetine have also demonstrated effectiveness, compared to placebo, in comorbid anxiety and sleep disturbances (250,251). Associated insomnia can also be treated with low-dose trazodone at bedtime or prazosin for nightmares, and acute or persistent agitation with clonidine or small regular doses of a benzodiazepine such as clonazepam. Mood stabilizers can also be used to treat agitation or co-occurring bipolar disorder, as can atypical antipsychotics, which can also be used to treat psychotic symptoms or disorders. For acute trauma, reduction of autonomic arousal with propranolol or corticosteroids might theoretically prevent the development of chronic PTSD, although replication studies have not yet borne this out. Schoenfeld and colleagues present a useful set of recommendations for pharmacological treatment of comorbid conditions in the presence of PTSD (216). However, expert consensus guidelines recommend a combination of psychotherapy and pharmacotherapy under these circumstances (150).

Gender Differences in Treatment Response

Seedat and colleagues provide a summary of research on gender differences in treatment response to for depression and PTSD (225). Several studies have found SSRIs, MAOIs, and to a lesser extent selective norepinephrine reuptake inhibitors (SNRIs) to be more effective for women than men, while finding the opposite true for TCAs (252–255). Other studies of SSRIs, TCAs, and MAOIs failed to demonstrate any gender effects (256–258). Hamilton and Jensvold were among the first to point out that fluctuations in hormone levels can alter antidepressant pharmacokinetics and pharmacodynamics, potentially necessitating dosage alterations (259). Estrogen may also influence responses of the key neurotransmitter systems involved in PTSD, including serotonin receptors (260). Seedat and colleagues also point out that other gender-related metabolic factors may affect SSRI metabolism through the cytochrome P450 system (256). Although the research is not sufficiently developed to provide clear guidelines in this area, it is important to keep in mind in tailoring medication for individual women. Again, most important for women experiencing ongoing IPV, is to be sure that medication does not undermine the need to remain vigilant when safety is at stake. Even medications that are not overtly sedating (e.g., paroxetine, sertraline, venlafaxine) can cause people to feel like they've "lost their edge." Sometimes this is desirable. Other times it is not.

Summary of Pharmacologic Therapy for Posttraumatic Stress Disorder

In summary, SSRIs appear to be the most effective medications for post-assault or abuse-related PTSD among civilian trauma survivors and have the most favorable side-effect profile. Sertraline and paroxetine are the only two medications approved by the U.S. Food and Drug Administration (FDA) for treatment of PTSD, although fluoxetine has shown some efficacy as well. The SNRIs also show promise in this area but have not been well-studied. Full treatment response may take up to 9 months or longer, and longer-term treatment appears to prevent relapse. Additional medications should be targeted toward specific unresponsive symptom constellations or comorbidities. Potential gender-related drug level alterations need to be taken into account. However, there is a limited evidence-base in this area and further study is needed. Differences in response to medication by type and duration of trauma, gender, race, culture, ethnicity, and age, as well as specific abuser behaviors also need to be taken into account. Attending to safety issues is a critical factor in recommending a course of medication and evaluating drug response.

SUBSTANCE ABUSE AND TRAUMA TREATMENT IN THE CONTEXT OF INTIMATE PARTNER VIOLENCE

Achieving sobriety may be difficult if underlying issues of abuse are not addressed, whether they are related to ongoing coercion and danger, in which a survivor's use of drugs or alcohol and her efforts to stop, may be controlled by an abusive partner, or to feelings associated with current or previous trauma. Understanding the role of trauma and abuse in initiating and sustaining a woman's use of substances, as well as the role substance use plays in a survivor's life, are important to developing a treatment plan that is tailored to her needs. In addition, not all substance abuse is associated with experiences of abuse or other trauma. Initial use may relate more to the availability and social acceptance of drugs or alcohol in one's family, neighborhood, or peer group. Using, however, places women at increased risk for being abused. Many authors view these as two separate but frequently interconnected phenomena that require individualized treatment to address the particular constellation of issues a survivor is facing (261). While describing how to conduct substance abuse treatment in the context of IPV is beyond the scope of this chapter, a number of models are available for treating substance abuse in the context of previous trauma, some of which have been adapted to work with survivors experiencing ongoing IPV. Evidence that integrated models may be more effective is beginning to emerge. For example, treatment models that address trauma (PTSD) and substance abuse together appear to be more effective for women experiencing both conditions (169,175,181). Trauma-enhanced residential substance abuse programs have higher retention rates for women trauma survivors who experiencing co-occurring disorders (184). The SAMHSA's treatment intervention protocol (TIP) on substance abuse and IPV offers guidance for substance abuse providers working with both victims and perpetrators of IPV (262). Combining IPV advocacy services and substance abuse treatment appears to be effective in improving self-efficacy and reducing use of drugs and alcohol, but may lead to more painful awareness of the effects of abuse (IPV) (261). Research from the SAMHSA-funded Violence Against Women and Co-Occurring Disorders Study, also indicates that an integrated approach (i.e., one that incorporates attention to both trauma and substance use—as well as ongoing safety and other mental health concerns) is likely to be more helpful than any single approach (9,10,34,168,263). Substance abuse recovery among women who have experienced multiple forms of trauma can be challenging and may require a combination of supports and skill development strategies (174).

Integrated treatment plans should address issues of safety, sobriety, and trauma recovery. Models for which there is some evidence base include Trauma Recovery Empowerment Model (TREM) a 33-week psychoeducational group intervention that addresses basic life skills as well as trauma and substance use issues (170); Seeking Safety, a 25-topic cognitive behavioral group intervention that addresses both PTSD and substance abuse (initially designed for women in groups, although it has since been adapted for men and for individual treatment formats as well, and includes 80 coping skills) (179); and the Addiction, Trauma, Recovery Integration Model (264). Two additional models, Helping Women Recover: A Program for Treating Addiction and Beyond Trauma: A Healing Journey for Women, which integrate trauma recovery and substance abuse treatment, again through a combination of empowerment and support, psycho-education, identification of relapse triggers, and the fostering of new coping skills development, are still being evaluated (265,266). For a more detailed description of these treatment models see the survey by Finkelstein and colleagues (267).

Again, when a woman is contending with ongoing IPV, safety issues need to be attended to along with other IPV-specific concerns. These include issues such as the abuser's role in undermining a survivor's efforts to achieve sobriety; isolating her from sources of support and using her dependence as a way to control her; threats that undermine custody or credibility, or that implicate a survivor in illegal activities that limit her ability to access law enforcement; realistic options for creating a different life, including economic support, and job and financial skills; stigma; and social support, as well as trauma related-feelings that are likely to emerge.

POTENTIALLY HARMFUL INTERVENTIONS FOR INTIMATE PARTNER VIOLENCE SURVIVORS

Because of the ongoing dangers battered women face, it is important to be aware of interventions that can potentially increase their risk of harm, such as confronting a batterer with the intention of getting him to change. In some cases, a batterer's violence may escalate while he (or she) is in treatment or participating in a batterer intervention program. Therefore, it is generally not recommended that programs for batterers without supports for battered women begin until women have access to adequate shelter and advocacy (38). In addition, many agencies offer anger control groups that fail to confront underlying issues of power and control. A batterer may then feel entitled to "lose control" to reprimand or punish his partner. Anger management alone is a potentially problematic intervention unless it also challenges a batterer's need to control his partner and his right to use violence against her (268). Anger management is not considered an appropriate intervention for a variety of reasons. First, it assumes that the individual cannot control his anger, when in fact abusers control their anger very well—their violence is targeted to a very specific victim (their partner). Second, anger management courses ask participants to identify things that "trigger" their anger. In doing so, these programs blame the victim for the violence perpetrated against her, and suggest that the violence is something the batterer cannot control. Although some controversy exists about these issues, both experienced advocates and batterer intervention practitioners concur that IPV is always a choice—the batterer's choice to use violence and abuse to exert power and control over his partner. Finally, survivors report that having a partner in treatment creates the illusion of safety, which may not turn out to be realistic.

Referral to couples' counseling in situations of ongoing violence, threats, or intimidation is another potentially harmful intervention. Any disclosure of abuse during a counseling session is highly unsafe for the victim and can precipitate violent retaliation. Couples therapy also assumes equal power in the relationship and equal contribution to the couple's problems, and thus can reinforce the victim-blaming that occurs. Again, in considering couples therapy, it is important to remember that IPV, by definition, is about a systematic abuse of power by one partner over another. Partners in these situations do not have equal power, and victims are not responsible for the violence that is committed against them. Because of these concerns, victim advocates have felt strongly for some time that clinicians should never recommend couples therapy when there is ongoing IPV. Assessing for these dynamics is critical before proceeding with any couples work.

Some survivors may request a referral for couples therapy because they feel this is the only way to get help for their partner. At a minimum, couple's counseling is indicated only when violence and coercive tactics have ceased for longer than the longest period the batterer has stopped before, when both parties request this form of treatment, and after the perpetrator has successfully completed a batterer intervention treatment program, the abusive pattern has been successfully altered, and the couple is committed to repairing the damage. Conjoint therapy should not occur when there is ongoing violence, threats and intimidation, stalking, fear expressed by the victim, continued use of alcohol or drugs, or a high level of danger.

To engage in couples counseling, the survivor needs to feel that the therapist is on her side and the perpetrator must be ready to take full responsibility for his actions; refrain from further violence, harassment, and stalking; and understand that maintenance of safety takes priority over the resolution of relationship issues (269). This requires a careful assessment of many factors, including the woman's safety, her

understanding of the risks involved, what she wants, what she thinks will happen, when her partner was last violent to her or someone else, threats the abuser has made, and whether she has procured a protective order and whether or not the abuser has violated it. For example, couples counseling would be contraindicated if there has been a recent assault or if the woman has a protection order from a court. Whether or not she has been coerced into seeking couples therapy is also important to assess. Additional requirements for the perpetrator include having stopped all obsessive thoughts about the survivor, having learned skills to manage his need for control, having learned to manage anger and conflict in nonabusive ways, having addressed key family-of-origin issues, having learned new sex-role socialization patterns and, as noted a moment ago, having been violence-free for longer than the time between two past incidents. Stopping the abuser's violence and controlling behavior should not be the focus of couples therapy (14,268). Working to rebuild the relationship and repair the damage will only be helpful if that dynamic has truly changed. Because of the many significant factors that must be in place before engaging in conjoint therapy, it will not often be an optimal choice. In essence, couples work should not be attempted, even when these conditions appear to have been met, without having had very specific training and supervision on these issues. These considerations apply to work with gay and lesbian couples also.

Court mediation is also problematic in cases of DV. It is based on the assumption of equal parties who can negotiate in good faith and solve problems together. Abusers, by definition, manipulate, intimidate, and bully their partners and do not negotiate responsibly. Given this scenario, battered women should be encouraged to seek legal assistance from an attorney who is knowledgeable about DV before discussing divorce, child custody, visitation, and other issues with their partners (268).

LEGAL ISSUES PERTINENT TO MENTAL HEALTH INTERVENTION

Information to Present to Patients about Legal Rights and Remedies

A range of legal issues, both criminal and civil, may emerge in working with patients who are being abused by a current or former partner. Particular concerns include custody decisions, divorce settlements, immigration issues, enforcement of protection orders, testifying against the abuser, and other ramifications of DV. These issues are very complex, vary by jurisdiction, are continually in flux, and are best addressed by DV programs and/or lawyers knowledgeable about DV. The best way to support patients who are dealing with complicated legal situations is through relationships with local DV programs. Patients involved in DV-related cases can refer their attorneys to national DV organizations for assistance (e.g., National Council on Juvenile and Family Court Judges, Battered Women's Justice Project, National Center on Domestic Violence, Trauma & Mental Health, Legal Momentum).

Although survivors of abuse face a multitude of legal situations, the issues tend to fall into two categories: (a) understanding the laws, the options for utilizing the criminal and civil system to enhance safety, and a victim's rights under such laws; and (b) advocating within the legal system to have the laws enforced, survivors' rights upheld, and their safety needs considered. The latter category represents the unique challenges faced by victims of DV and illustrates the necessity of clinicians to link effectively with advocacy organizations. Knowing the law, calling the police, filing for divorce—such remedies that one might traditionally think of are not necessarily simple solutions. Inconsistent enforcement of laws and the biases of court systems can have devastating effects on the safety and well-being of DV victims and their children. It will often be necessary to consult with DV programs and DV legal specialists to obtain accurate information when these complex issues arise. Information is also available from the National Resource Center on Domestic Violence (1–800–537–2238), State Domestic Violence Coalitions, and websites such as the National Coalition Against Domestic Violence (http://www.ncadv.org), the National Network to End Domestic Violence (http://www. nnedv.org), and the American Bar Association Commission on Domestic Violence (http://www.abanet.org/domviol/).

Supporting Patients Facing Retraumatizing Experiences in the Judicial Process

In addition, going through prolonged legal battles with an abusive partner can be traumatic in itself. The court may minimize the abuse a woman has experienced, and the abuser may not receive appropriate consequences for the abuse, be it jail time or restricted visitation rights. A survivor may be pressured to testify against the abuser, which can put her at increased risk for retaliatory abuse. Batterers are known to use the system to control their partners, often through prolonged court battles. The stress for a woman trying to navigate the legal system to protect herself and her children from further abuse cannot be overestimated. Furthermore, having to repeatedly tell the story of the abuse to strangers and often with the abuser present can be particularly difficult and retraumatizing. It can be an eye-opening experience for mental health providers to learn about the court process in criminal and civil DV cases. For those without prior experience with DV court proceedings, it might be shocking to learn about some of the policies and practices in handling such cases (of course, court systems vary widely in this regard). Societal biases and stereotypes still have a strong influence on the legal process, and victims often find that the court did not effectively mete out justice or offer adequate protection to them and their children. Again, referring a patient to a DV advocacy program may be the most helpful way for her to obtain the resources and expert advice that will be most beneficial. At the same time, working with a survivor to manage these additional stressors can be an important aspect of treatment.

Mandated Reporting: Adult Victims

Because healthcare providers in some states are required by law to report injuries they suspect resulted from a battering incident, it is important to become familiar with state reporting laws. Although these requirements generally refer to patients seen after an acute injury, statutory reporting mandates vary greatly from state to state regarding who is required to report, what kind of injuries need to be reported, penalties for failure to report, and/or immunity from liability.

Liability can also attach to providers who fail to respond appropriately to the DV experiences and injuries of their patients. Clinicians can be held liable for subsequent injuries sustained by a patient who returns to an abusive situation if no inquiries about abuse were made when they were initially seen or treated. Documenting discussions of DV in a patient's record, including any referrals to other services is critical. Remembering that records may be discoverable in a legal proceeding, it is also important not to include unnecessary information such as the patient's denial of need for services or attributions of self-blame. On the other hand, documenting the specific ways a survivor is taking care of herself and her children can be quite helpful.

Mandated Reporting: Child Victims

State laws require mental health professionals to report known or suspected child abuse to their local child protective services authority, a mandate that is generally quite familiar to clinicians. Although some states classify the witnessing of DV as a form of child *abuse or neglect*, in other states definitions of exposure and risk are less clear, allowing clinicians greater discretion over reporting. The most helpful interventions are those that support the nonabusive parent to keep her and her children safe.

Many child trauma experts question the effectiveness of addressing children's exposure to DV as a form of child abuse (270). Given the wide range of experiences, varying levels of protective factors, and diversity of effects among children who witness DV, standardization of criteria for defining and reporting child witnessing of DV becomes an unwieldy task. Reporting to child protective services under these circumstance can, and often does, have devastating consequences for both the children and the abused parent because it risks the possibility that an abused woman will be viewed as "failing to protect" her children. This may lead to removal of the children from the home, rather than efforts to work with the mother to create a safer environment or steps to ensure the perpetrator is held accountable. Because the nonoffending parent is sometimes the only legal parent, she also becomes an easier target for public sector interventions.

Reporting children as being directly physically abused or at serious risk of harm presents difficult tasks for the clinician as well. Providers must inform the abused parent about the potential consequences of involving child protective services, such as investigation, retaliation by the abuser, losing children to protective custody, and advocating for their needs and safety with the system, while also discussing the hazards of children continuing to live in a home where they are being abused. It is a complicated and often painful challenge to uphold one's legal and ethical obligations and to maintain a working alliance with the nonabusive parent. If an abused woman is also abusing her children, efforts to support the woman and protect the children must be made, difficult as that can be. Working with battered women to understand ways in which their own experiences of current or past abuse have affected their ability to parent and helping them to develop new skills and capacities to address these issues, appears to be helpful to some women.

Whenever the clinician involves the child protection system, the safety of the woman and her children again becomes a critical factor. If a woman feels that reporting will put her in danger from her partner, discuss and help arrange a safe place for her and her children to go. Children's protective services should also be warned of the risk of danger posed by the abuser. Particularly if the children are being abused by someone other than the patient, it may be preferable for her to make the report to children's services herself. It can help her retain a sense of control over the situation and can become a collaborative endeavor between clinician and patient. Making the report herself can also demonstrate to the child protective system that she is taking steps to protect the children and herself from abuse, potentially shielding her from "failure to protect" charges. However, this may not be the best practice for every survivor, or in every community. Mental health providers should consult with local DV experts about the most effective procedures for reporting child abuse/neglect when there is concurrent DV, in order to elicit the most helpful, and least punitive, response from the local children's protective services agency.

Subpoena of Records and Testimony

Mental health records may be subpoenaed by the patient's lawyer, the abuser. or by the court. Without a subpoena, however, records do not have to be released, even if the patient has signed a release. In general, patients do not know what is in their records and the potential ways they could be harmful in court. Providers should discuss with the patient the possible ramifications, and benefits, of releasing records, so that the person is able to make informed decisions. Careful documentation may preclude some of the dangers but, as noted earlier, private information can be always be used by an abuser to further control his partner. The laws of many states protect clients from unnecessary release of mental health records through a formal court process. Receiving a subpoena is the first step of this process, and records should never be released at this stage. Mental health providers should consult an attorney familiar with the rules of civil procedure before releasing any information. Consulting with DV programs or lawyers who specialize in DV is advisable in these situations (17).

Good documentation of IPV and its mental health consequences can be of help to clients if a client's mental health becomes an issue in a legal case, particularly in custody battles, divorce settlements, civil damages, or immigration. Clinicians can offer general clinical information to the attorney (e.g., educating about PTSD) that could be very helpful to the case. Clinicians may be asked to testify as to their opinions about their client's mental health, the relationship of symptoms to abuse, and/or their ability to be a good parent. The testimony of a professional can do a great deal to enhance the credibility of a woman who is being battered, and this testimony is viewed by the judge as valuable evidence on relevant issues. Thorough discussion with the client about the proposed testimony is a necessity. When it is determined that the clinician will provide evidence in court, the lawyer should prepare the clinician to testify. If the patient's legal counsel does not provide adequate pretrial coaching, consultation with a lawyer experienced in these issues is advisable.

Custody disputes are common in cases involving DV. Very often, the court orders an evaluation to determine where the child's best interests lie, and the evaluator seeks the release of the battered woman's treatment records for use in the evaluation. Again, good documentation in the treatment file can play a crucial role in a successful litigation outcome for the client, playing much the same role for the evaluator as for the judge. The clinician should confer with the patient, and perhaps the lawyer, to determine if the information contained in the file would be helpful, as well as the possible negative ramifications of the file's release. The clinician can assist the patient in making informed decisions on these issues.

Protecting the patient–therapist relationship will be of concern to the clinician under these circumstances. Keeping the client informed about the clinician's interactions with the evaluator or the lawyer, ensuring the client is involved and giving consent to any communications, and explaining the ramifications of these activities are key. Clear parameters must be drawn between the role of the treating therapist who must maintain his alliance with his client and a nontreating expert witness who interviews the client for the sole purpose of evaluating the issue in question. The clinician must also be careful to maintain clear boundaries with the patient's lawyer, while also collaborating and advising whenever necessary. The therapist's involvement in the court case poses risks to his relationship to the client, particularly if the case does not turn out as hoped. Clinicians must be prepared to discuss these issues with the client in advance of any court proceedings, as well as processing their feelings afterwards.

CONCLUSION

Working collaboratively with other systems to create the kind of society that will stop violence against women and prevent its traumatic sequelae is of vital importance for all clinicians. important. Mental health providers have a significant role to play in voicing concerns about the impact of abuse and violence on the lives of individuals they work with clinically. Working with people who have survived unthinkable trauma teaches us about the complexity and unpredictability of human life; the intersections among individual biology, human development, social and cultural contexts, and larger societal norms; and the importance of caring, respectful human interactions. In working toward social justice, it is also necessary to incorporate an understanding of how the traumatic effects of social *injustice* can play out in both individual and social/institutional/political forms. When we do not address the denial of intolerable feelings at a personal level, we are in danger of recreating them not only in individual relationships, but also on social and political levels as well, and when we do not acknowledge the impact of social forms of abuse of power, they are often internalized and reproduced through individual interactions. Mental health providers can play a critical role in preventing IPV in addition to treating its consequences by beginning to address the social as well as psychological conditions that create and support this kind of violence in the first place.

Offering mental health treatment in the context of IPV also raises a number of practice and policy concerns. First is the need to ensure that any mental health treatment incorporates an understanding of the dynamics of IPV and the range of issues survivors face related to safety, confidentiality, coercive control, parenting, custody, legal issues, immigration, social support, economic independence, and more, all of which influence how a survivor is affected and what her or his options are. Second is the need to change the way that symptoms and disorders are currently viewed, documented, and reimbursed, and to incorporate recognition of the direct impact of abuser behaviors, as well as the traumatic effects of abuse. Although trauma models focus on the impact of abuse and healing from its traumatic effects, advocacy approaches focus on social context and on changing the conditions that place survivors in jeopardy. Responding to a person who is experiencing the mental health effects of IPV and other trauma clearly requires attention to both of these domains. This, in turn, will necessitate changes in practice, research, and policy.

IMPLICATIONS FOR POLICY, PRACTICE, AND RESEARCH

Policy

- Support cross-sector collaboration among mental health and substance abuse providers, mental health peer support services, DV advocacy and legal organizations, and other community groups to ensure a wider range of options for survivors. This could take a number of different forms, such as: (a) establishing individual relationships with local DV resources for consultation and referral; (b) brokering existing resources through the development community task forces to examine existing services, needs, resources, gaps, barriers, and potential strategies; (c) establishing mechanisms for interagency cross-training, cross-consultation and referral, and providing mental health backup to DV shelters; or (d) creating pro bono or sliding scale mental health services for survivors without adequate insurance coverage.
- An obvious need exists for additional funding to support research, training, and services. Funding cuts to DV services are dire and reflect the loss of a critical element of support for both survivors and practitioners. Advocacy programs work not only to provide safety, justice, and redress for individual survivors but also to eliminate key sources of ongoing trauma, stress, and despair, including unresponsive court systems, retraumatizing custody practices, punitive immigration laws, lack of economic opportunities or social safety nets, and ultimately to develop strategies to reduce IPV. Having a broader base from which to mobilize may also help in the process of garnering the necessary funding to improve existing clinical services, develop new institutional capacities (education, training, supervision, and consultation) and create new resources for survivors (new onsite services, linkages with other health and mental health agencies.)
- Facilitate the development and dissemination of resolutions and practice recommendations from mental health professional associations related to IPV that reflect the perspectives of advocates and survivors, as well as cutting-edge research and practice
- Support efforts to reduce stigma associated with mental illness, promote recovery-oriented practices, and establish mental health parity.
- There is sufficient consensus to warrant integration of training on core principles of working with survivors of IPV and other lifetime trauma into clinical and advocacy training. Integrated training materials need to be created and strategies for incorporation into graduate and postgraduate health and mental health training to be developed.
- In addition, concepts of vicarious trauma, elements of transference and countertransference, and the likelihood of one's own experiences of trauma being evoked, also need to be carefully attended to, and opportunities for support and processing are essential.

Practice

- Ensure that mental health treatment incorporates an understanding of the dynamics of IPV and the range of issues survivors face.
- Influence the ways psychiatric symptoms and disorders are currently viewed, documented, and reimbursed to incorporate recognition of the direct impact of abuser behaviors, as well as the traumatic effects of abuse.
- Ensure attention to the ways mental health information can be misused by abusers and other systems by developing policies for documentation, confidentiality, and information sharing, and new levels of protection for electronic health information technology systems.

- Support the creation of institutional and practice environments that are IPV, trauma-, and culture-informed. Elements of creating safe, welcoming services for IPV survivors were discussed earlier. Creating trauma-informed practice environments also requires institutional or agency commitment to equalizing power imbalances, ensuring provider trustworthiness, maximizing survivor control and choice, and establishing the necessary hiring practices, training, supervision, policies, and administrative support to change agency culture in this regard. Funding streams are also needed to support this type of agency and institutional work.
- Another important element for integrating complex IPV–trauma treatment into practice is the need for ongoing mentoring, supervision, and peer support. It is notoriously difficult to translate research into practice when practitioners often work under severe time constraints and patients have messy, complicated lives not necessarily under their own control. Institutional or agency commitment to provide regular consultation and/or supervision is also key. This can also be accomplished through distance expert consultation accompanied by local peer support.

Research

- One of the overarching gaps in existing research on mental health, trauma, and IPV is the need to develop a better understanding of the range of ways survivors of IPV are affected, given the vastly different circumstances of their lives and, consequently, what types of treatment modalities and community interventions are likely to be most effective and for whom.
- Research is needed to determine the extent to which a complex trauma framework is useful for understanding the traumatic effects of IPV or only so for some survivors: For example, survivors of childhood abuse; survivors of multiple types of trauma; survivors whose experience of IPV is prolonged, severe, and more akin to torture; survivors who are dealing with a mental illness as well as IPV where stigma, abuser manipulation, and institutionalization bring additional layers of trauma; or survivors who are trapped in prolonged custody battles and visitation experiences who live in constant fear for their children.

- Studies could be designed to inquire about unmet mental health needs; what has and has not been helpful, and what might have been helpful at the time; sources of healing and support; and what survivors would find both compelling and safe—not only after being out of an abusive relationship, but also while they are still under siege.
- Additional steps might include developing comprehensive intervention and treatment models along with strategies to evaluate specific core elements, as well as the flexible delivery of an individually tailored menu of services and treatment modalities with or without an additional set of community-based resources and supports—guided by survivors' experience, goals, and priorities.
- Research is also needed to examine inclusion criteria for study participation (who is excluded and why, what treatment works best for survivors who are excluded) and to assess study attrition (who leaves, why, to what extent does this relate to safety, tolerability, or efficacy). There is also a need for longitudinal studies that can assess changes over time, studies that examine the interactions among a wider range of factors that influence women's experiences and responses, and studies that look at the variations in responses to trauma and to treatment interventions
- Research is needed to examine the applicability of a complex trauma framework for understanding the traumatic effects of IPV.
- It is essential to evaluate combined IPV-, culture-, and trauma-informed treatment and intervention models that can be individually tailored and flexibly applied in a range of practice and community settings.

References

1. McFarlane A, Schrader G, Bookless C, Browne D. Prevalence of victimization, posttraumatic stress disorder and violent behaviour in the seriously mentally ill. *Aust N Z J Psychiatry.* 2006;40(11–12):1010–1015.
2. McFarlane J, Malecha A, Gist J, et al. An intervention to increase safety behaviors of abused women: Results of a randomized clinical trial. *Nurs Res.* 2002;51(6):347–354.
3. Sullivan CM, Bybee DI. Reducing violence using community-based advocacy for women with abusive partners. *J Consult Clin Psychol.* 1999;67(1):43–53.

4. Johnson DM, Zlotnick C. A cognitive-behavioral treatment for battered women with PTSD in shelters: Findings from a pilot study. *J Trauma Stress.* 2006;19(4):559–564.

5. Kubany ES, Hill EE, Owens JA, et al. Cognitive trauma therapy for battered women with PTSD (CTT-BW). *J Consult Clin Psychol.* 2004; 72(1):3–18.

6. Cloitre M, Koenen KC, Cohen LR, Han H. Skills training in affective and interpersonal regulation followed by exposure: A phase-based treatment for PTSD related to childhood abuse. *J Consult Clin Psychol.* 2002;70(5):1067–1074.

7. Linehan MM, Tutek DA, Heard HL, Armstrong HE. Interpersonal outcome of cognitive behavioral treatment for chronically suicidal borderline patients. *Am J Psychiatry.* 1994;151(12):1771–1776.

8. Resick PA, Nishith P, Griffin MG. How well does cognitive-behavioral therapy treat symptoms of complex PTSD? An examination of child sexual abuse survivors within a clinical trial. *CNS Spectr.* 2003;8(5):340–355.

9. Morrissey JP, Ellis AR, Gatz M, et al. Outcomes for women with co-occurring disorders and trauma: Program and person-level effects. *J Subst Abuse Treat.* 2005;28(2):121–133.

10. Morrissey JP, Jackson EW, Ellis AR, et al. Twelve-month outcomes of trauma-informed interventions for women with co-occurring disorders. *Psychiatr Serv.* 2005;56(10):1213–1222.

11. *National consensus guidelines on identifying and responding to DV victimization in health care settings.* San Francisco, CA: Family Violence Prevention Fund, 2004.

12. *Comprehensive accreditation manual for behavioral health care.* Oakbrook Terrace, IL: Joint Commission on the Accreditation of Health Care Organizations, 2005.

13. Goldman LS, Horan D, Warshaw C, et al. Diagnostic and treatment guidelines on mental health effects of family violence. At http://www.ama-assn.org/ama1/pub/upload/mm/386/mentaleffects.pdf. Accessed 11/04/2008.

14. Dutton MA. *Empowering and healing the battered woman: A model for assessment and intervention.* New York: Springer, 1992.

15. Ganley AL. Understanding DV. In: Warshaw C, Ganley AL, Salber PR, eds. *Improving the health care response to DV: A resource manual for health care providers.* San Francisco: Family Violence Prevention Fund and the Pennsylvania Coalition Against Domestic Violence, 1995.

16. Harris M, Fallot RD, eds. *Using trauma theory to design service systems.* San Francisco: Jossey-Bass, 2001.

17. Walker L. *Abused women and survivor therapy: A practical guide for the psychotherapist.* Washington, DC: American Psychological Association, 1994.

18. Warshaw C. Women and violence. In: Stotland NL, Stewart DE, eds. *Psychological aspects of women's health care: The interface between psychiatry and obstetrics and gynecology,* 2nd ed. Washington, DC: American Psychiatric Press;2001:477–548.

19. Davies J, Lyon E, Monti-Catania D. *Safety planning with battered women: Complex lives/difficult choices.* Thousand Oaks, CA: Sage, 1998.

20. Lu FG, Lim RF, Mezzich JE. Issues in the assessment and diagnosis of culturally diverse individuals. *Am Psychiatric Press Rev Psychiatry.* 1995;14: 477–510.

21. Garcia-Moreno C. *WHO Multi-country study on women's health and DV against women: Initial results on prevalence, health outcomes, and women's responses.* Geneva: World Health Organization, 2005.

22. Mead S, MacNeil C. Peer support: A unique approach. 2003. At http://www.mentalhealthpeers.com. Accessed 11/04/2008.

23. Masaki B, Kim M, Chung L. *The multilingual access model: A model for outreach and services in non-English speaking communities.* Philadelphia, PA: National Resource Center on Domestic Violence, 1999.

24. Coker AL, Flerx VC, Smith PH, et al. Partner violence screening in rural health care clinics. *Am J Public Health.* 2007;97(7):1319–1325.

25. Thackeray J, Stelzner S, Downs SM, Miller C. Screening for intimate partner violence: The impact of screener and screening environment on victim comfort. *J Interpers Violence.* 2007;22(6):659–670.

26. Pearlman LA, Courtois CA. Clinical applications of the attachment framework: Relational treatment of complex trauma. *J Trauma Stress.* 2005;18(5): 449–459.

27. Saakvitne KW, Gamble SG, Pearlman LA, Lev BT. *Risking connection: A training curriculum for working with survivors of childhood abuse.* Lutherville, MD: Sidran Foundation and Press, 2000.

28. Chang JC, Cluss PA, Ranieri L, et al. Health care interventions for intimate partner violence: What women want. *Womens Health Issues.* 2005;15(1):21–30.

29. Feder GS, Hutson M, Ramsay J, Taket AR. Women exposed to intimate partner violence: Expectations and experiences when they encounter health care professionals: A meta-analysis of qualitative studies. *Arch Intern Med.* 2006;166(1):22–37.

30. Rhodes KV, Frankel RM, Levinthal N, et al. "You're not a victim of DV, are you?" Provider patient communication about domestic violence. *Ann Intern Med.* 2007;147(9):620–627.

31. Warshaw C. Domestic violence: Changing theory, changing practice. *J Am Med Womens Assoc.* 1996;51(3):87–92.

32. Clark C, Young MS, Jackson E, et al. Consumer perceptions of integrated trauma-informed services among women with co-occurring disorders. *J Behav Health Serv Res.* 2008;35(1):71–90.

33. Markoff LS, Finkelstein N, Kammerer N, et al. Relational systems change: Implementing a model of change in integrating services for women with

substance abuse and mental health disorders and histories of trauma. *J Behav Health Serv Res.* 2005;32(2):227–240.

34. Markoff LS, Reed BG, Fallot RD, et al. Implementing trauma-informed alcohol and other drug and mental health services for women: Lessons learned in a multisite demonstration project. *Am J Orthopsychiatry.* 2005;75(4):525–539.

35. *Firearms and mental illness: State and territorial code provisions.* Chicago: National Center on Domestic Violence, Trauma Mental Health, 2008.

36. Bograd M. Family systems approaches to wife battering: A feminist critique. *Am J Orthopsychiatry.* 1984;54(4):558–568.

37. Shainess N. Vulnerability to violence: Masochism as process. *Am J Psychother.* 1979;33(2):174–189.

38. Gondolf EW. *Batterer intervention systems: Issues, outcomes and recommendations.* Thousand Oaks, CA: Sage, 2001.

39. *NASMHPD position statement on services and supports to trauma survivors.* Washington, DC: National Association of State Mental Health Program Directors, 2005.

40. McCann IL, Pearlman LA. Constructivist self development theory: A theoretical model of psychological adaptation to severe trauma. In: Sakheim DK, Devine SE, eds. *Out of darkness: Exploring satanism and ritual abuse.* New York: Lexington Books;1992:185–206.

41. Grigsby N, Hartman B. The barriers model: An integrated strategy for intervention with battered women. *Psychotherapy.* 1997;34(4):485–497.

42. Campbell JC, Glass N, Sharps PW, et al. Intimate partner homicide: Review and implications of research and policy. *Trauma Violence Abuse.* 2007; 8(3):246–269.

43. Tjaden P, Thoennes N. Prevalence and consequences of male-to-female and female-to-male intimate partner violence as measured by the National Violence Against Women Survey. *Violence Against Women.* 2000;6(2):142–161.

44. *Mental health: A report of the Surgeon General.* Rockville, MD: US Department of Health and Human Services, National Institutes of Health, 1999.

45. *Mental health: Culture, race, and ethnicity: A supplement to Mental Health: A report of the Surgeon General.* Rockville, MD: Center for Mental Health Services, Substance Abuse and Mental Health Services Administration, 2001.

46. Warshaw C, Ganley AL. *Improving the health care response to DV: A resource manual for health care providers.* San Francisco: Family Violence Prevention Fund and the Pennsylvania Coalition Against Domestic Violence, 1995.

47. *Achieving the promise: Transforming mental health care in America.* Rockville, MD: New Freedom Commission, US Department of Health and Human Services, 2003.

48. Brown J. Working toward freedom from violence. The process of change in battered women. *Violence Against Women.* 1997;3(1):5–26.

49. Edwards TA, Houry D, Kemball RS, et al. Stages of change as a correlate of mental health symptoms in abused, low-income African American women. *J Clin Psychol.* 2006;62(12):1531–1543.

50. Prochaska JO, DiClemente CC. Transtheoretical therapy: Toward a more integrative model of change. *Psychotherapy Theory Res Pract.* 1982;19:276–288.

51. Cluss PA, Chang JC, Hawker L, et al. The process of change for victims of intimate partner violence: Support for a Psychosocial Readiness Model. *Womens Health Issues.* 2006;16(5):262–274.

52. Flitcraft AH. Violence, values, and gender. *JAMA.* 1992;267(23):3194–3195.

53. Hamberger LK, Phelan MB. *Domestic violence screening and intervention in medical and mental healthcare settings.* New York: Springer, 2004.

54. McCloskey LA, Lichter E, Ganz ML, et al. Intimate partner violence and patient screening across medical specialties. *Acad Emerg Med.* 2005;12(8):712–722.

55. Samuelson SL, Campbell CD. Screening for DV: Recommendations based on a practice survey. *Prof Psychol Res Pr.* 2005;36(3):276–282.

56. Sohal H, Eldridge S, Feder G. The sensitivity and specificity of four questions (HARK) to identify intimate partner violence: A diagnostic accuracy study in general practice. *BMC Fam Pract.* 2007;8:49.

57. Briere J. *Child abuse trauma: Theory and treatment of the lasting effects.* Newbury Park: Sage, 1992.

58. Ford JD, Courtois CA, Steele K, et al. Treatment of complex posttraumatic self-dysregulation. *J Trauma Stress.* 2005;18(5):437–447.

59. Jennings A. Policy regarding the prevention of seclusion and/or restraint informed by the client's possible history of trauma in facilities operated by BDS. In: Services MDoBaD, ed. Maine Department of Behavioral and Developmental Services, 2002.

60. Briere J, Johnson K, Bissada A, et al. The Trauma Symptom Checklist for Young Children (TSCYC): Reliability and association with abuse exposure in a multi-site study. *Child Abuse Negl.* 2001;25(8):1001–1014.

61. Elliott DM, Briere J. Sexual abuse trauma among professional women: Validating the Trauma Symptom Checklist-40 (TSC-40). *Child Abuse Negl.* 1992;16(3):391–398.

62. Falsetti SA, Resnick H, Kilpatrick DG, Freedy JR. A review of the Potential Stressful Events Interview: A comprehensive assessment instrument of high and low magnitude stressors. *Behavior Therapist.* 1994;17:66–67.

63. Foa EB, Hearst-Ikeda D, Perry KJ. Evaluation of a brief cognitive-behavioral program for the prevention of chronic PTSD in recent assault victims. *J Consult Clin Psychol.* 1995;63(6):948–955.

64. Goodman LA, Corcoran C, Turner K, et al. Assessing traumatic event exposure: General issues and

preliminary findings for the Stressful Life Events Screening Questionnaire. *J Trauma Stress.* 1998; 11(3):521–542.

65. Felitti VJ, Anda RF, Nordenberg D, et al. Relationship of childhood abuse and household dysfunction to many of the leading causes of death in adults. The Adverse Childhood Experiences (ACE) Study. *Am J Prev Med.* 1998;14(4):245–258.

66. Golding JM. Chicago: Domestic Violence and Mental Health Policy Initiative, 2000.

67. Kaslow NJ, Price AW, Wyckoff S, et al. Person factors associated with suicidal behavior among African American women and men. *Cultur Divers Ethnic Minor Psychol.* 2004;10(1):5–22.

68. Kaslow NJ, Sherry A, Bethea K, et al. Social risk and protective factors for suicide attempts in low income African American men and women. *Suicide Life Threat Behav.* 2005;35(4):400–412.

69. Stark E, Flitcraft A. Killing the beast within: Woman battering and female suicidality. *Int J Health Serv.* 1995;25(1):43–64.

70. Mitchell C. Personal communication, 2007.

71. *If I had one more day: Findings and recommendations from the Washington State DV fatality review.* Seattle: Washington State Coalition Against Domestic Violence, 2006.

72. Koziol-McLain J, Webster D, McFarlane J, et al. Risk factors for femicide-suicide in abusive relationships: Results from a multisite case control study. *Violence Vict.* 2006;21(1):3–21.

73. Morton E, Runyan CW, Moracco KE, Butts J. Partner homicide-suicide involving female homicide victims: A population-based study in North Carolina, 1988–1992. *Violence Vict.* 1998;13(2):91–106.

74. Browne A, Williams K. Gender, intimacy, and lethal violence: Trends from 1976 through 1987. *Gend Soc.* 1993;7(1):78–98.

75. Fabri M. Personal communication, 2008.

76. Hart B. Lesbian battering: An examination. In: Lobel K, ed. *Naming the violence* Seattle: Seal Press;1986:173–189.

77. Renzetti CM. Violence in lesbian and gay relationships. In: O'Toole LL, Schiffman JR, eds. *Gender violence: Interdisciplinary perspectives.* New York: New York University Press;1997:285–293.

78. West CM. Leaving a second closet: Outing partner violence in same-sex couples. In: Jasinski JL, Williams LM, eds. *Partner violence: A comprehensive review of 20 years of research.* Thousand Oaks, CA: Sage;1998:163–183.

79. Marrujo B, Kreger M. Definition of roles in abusive lesbian relationships. In: Renzetti C, Miley CH, eds. *Violence in gay and lesbian domestic partnerships.* New York: Haworth, 1996.

80. Pintzuk T. Personal communication, 1998.

81. Gill CJ, Kirschner KL, Panko-Reis J. Health services for women with disabilities: Barriers and portals. In: Dan AJ, ed. *Reframing women's health.* Thousand Oaks, CA: Sage Publications;1994:357–366.

82. Briere J, Spinazzola J. Phenomenology and psychological assessment of complex posttraumatic states. *J Trauma Stress.* 2005;18(5):401–412.

83. Bremner JD. Traumatic stress: Effects on the brain. *Dialogues Clin Neurosci.* 2006;8(4):445–461.

84. Classen CC, Pain C, Field NP, Woods P. Posttraumatic personality disorder: A reformulation of complex posttraumatic stress disorder and borderline personality disorder. *Psychiatr Clin North Am.* 2006;29(1):87–112,viii-ix.

85. Heim C, Plotsky PM, Nemeroff CB. Importance of studying the contributions of early adverse experience to eurobiological findings in depression. *Neuropsychopharmacology.* 2004;29(4): 641–648.

86. Lanius RA, Bluhm R, Lanius U, Pain C. A review of neuroimaging studies in PTSD: Heterogeneity of response to symptom provocation. *J Psychiatr Res.* 2006;40(8):709–729.

87. Lanius RA, Frewen PA, Girotti M, et al. Neural correlates of trauma script-imagery in posttraumatic stress disorder with and without comorbid major depression: A functional MRI investigation. *Psychiatry Res.* 2007;155(1):45–56.

88. Nemeroff CB. Neurobiological consequences of childhood trauma. *J Clin Psychiatry.* 2004;65 (Suppl 1):18–28.

89. Yehuda R. Advances in understanding neuroendocrine alterations in PTSD and their therapeutic implications. *Ann N Y Acad Sci.* 2006;1071: 137–166.

90. Cobb AR, Tedeschi RG, Calhoun LG, Cann A. Correlates of posttraumatic growth in survivors of intimate partner violence. *J Trauma Stress.* 2006;19(6):895–903.

91. Herman JL. *Trauma and recovery: The aftermath of violence: Domestic abuse to political terror.* New York: Basic Books, 1992.

92. van der Kolk BA, Roth S, Pelcovitz D, et al. Disorders of extreme stress: The empirical foundation of a complex adaptation to trauma. *J Trauma Stress.* 2005;18(5):389–399.

93. Briere J. *Trauma Symptom Inventory Professional Manual.* Odessa, FL: Psychological Assessment Resources, 1995.

94. Briere J, Elliott DM, Harris K, Cottman A. Trauma Symptom Inventory: Psychometrics and association with childhood and adult trauma in clinical samples. *J Interpers Violence.* 1995; 10:387–401.

95. Blake DD, Weathers FW, Nagy LM, et al. The development of a Clinician-Administered PTSD Scale. *J Trauma Stress.* 1995;8(1):75–90.

96. Pelcovitz D, van der Kolk B, Roth S, et al. Development of a criteria set and a structured interview for disorders of extreme stress (SIDES). *J Trauma Stress.* 1997;10(1):3–16.

97. Pearlman LA. *Trauma and Attachment Belief Scale.* Los Angeles: Western Psychological Services, 2003.

98. Bernstein EM, Putnam FW. Development, reliability, and validity of a dissociation scale. *J Nerv Ment Dis.* 1986;174(12):727–735.

99. Briere J, Woo R, McRae B, et al. Lifetime victimization history, demographics, and clinical status in female psychiatric emergency room patients. *J Nerv Ment Dis.* 1997;185(2):95–101.

100. Carlson EB. *Trauma assessments: A clinician's guide.* New York: Guilford Press, 1997.

101. Norris FH, Riad JK. Standardized self-report measures of civilian trauma and posttraumatic stress disorder. In: Wilson JP, Keane TM, eds. *Assessing psychological trauma and PTSD.* New York: Guilford;1997:7–42.

102. Wilson JP, Keane TM, eds. *Assessing psychological trauma and PTSD.* New York: Guilford, 1997.

103. Saunders DG. Posttraumatic stress symptom profiles of battered women: A comparison of survivors in two settings. *Violence Vict.* 1994; 9(1):31–44.

104. Tedeschi RG, Calhoun LG. The Posttraumatic Growth Inventory: Measuring the positive legacy of trauma. *J Trauma Stress.* 1996;9(3):455–471.

105. Brewin CR. Systematic review of screening instruments for adults at risk of PTSD. *J Trauma Stress.* 2005;18(1):53–62.

106. Strand VC, Sarmiento TL, Pasquale LE. Assessment and screening tools for trauma in children and adolescents: A review. *Trauma Violence Abuse.* 2005;6(1):55–78.

107. Harris M, Fallot RD, Beyer L, Berley RW. *Trauma Recovery and Empowerment Profile (TREP) and Skill Building Strategies Menu.* Washington, DC: Community Connections, 2003.

108. Van der Kolk B. The assessment and treatment of complex PTSD. In: Yehuda R, ed. *Traumatic stress.* Washington, DC: American Psychiatric Press, 2001.

109. Waller MA. Resilience in ecosystemic context: Evolution of the concept. *Am J Orthopsychiatry.* 2001;71(3):290–297.

110. Jackson H, Philp E, Nuttal RL, Diller L. Traumatic brain injury: A hidden consequence for battered women. *Professional psychology, research and practice.* 2002;33(1):39–45.

111. Zink T, Regan S, Jacobson C, Pabst S. Cohort, period, and aging effects: A qualitative study of older women's reasons for remaining in abusive relationships. *Violence Against Women.* 2003;9(12):1429–1441.

112. Zink TM, Jacobson J. Screening for intimate partner violence when children are present: The victim's perspective. *J Interpers Violence.* 2003;18(8):872–890.

113. Markham DW. Mental illness and DV: Implications for family law litigation. *J Poverty Law Policy.* 2003;May-June:23–35.

114. Lieberman AF. Traumatic stress and quality of attachment: Reality and internalization in disorders of infant mental health. *Infant Ment Health J.* 2004;25(4):336–351.

115. Van Horn P, Blumenthal S, Warshaw C. *Children exposed to DV: A curriculum for DV advocates.* Chicago: Domestic Violence Mental Health Policy Initiative, 2008.

116. Warshaw C, Moroney G. *Mental health and DV: Collaborative initiatives, service models, and curricula.* Chicago: Domestic Violence Mental Health Policy Initiative, 2002.

117. Tiberio P. Safety planning with battered women in inpatient and drug treatment programs *Family Violence Prevention Fund Health Care Conference.* Atlanta, GA, 2002.

118. Markham DW. Legal issues. In: Warshaw C, Pease T, Markham DW, et al., eds. *Access to advocacy: Serving women with psychiatric disabilities in DV settings.* Chicago: Domestic Violence Mental Health Policy Initiative, 2007.

119. Koss MP, Goodman LA, Browne L, et al., eds. *No safe haven: Male violence against women at home, at work, and in the community.* Washington, DC: American Psychological Association, 1994.

120. Lieberman AF, Van Horn P. *Don't hit my mommy: A manual for child-parent psychotherapy with young witnesses of family violence.* Washington, DC: Zero to Three, 2004.

121. McFarlane J, Malecha A, Gist J, et al. Increasing the safety-promoting behaviors of abused women. *Am J Nurs.* 2004;104(3):40–50; quiz 50–41.

122. Copeland ME. Mental Health Recovery WRAP. At http://www.mentalhealthrecovery.com/. Accessed 4/8/2008.

123. Warshaw C, Pease T, Markham DW, et al. *Access to advocacy: Serving women with psychiatric disabilities in DV settings.* Chicago: Domestic Violence Mental Health Policy Initiative, 2007.

124. Wathen CN, MacMillan HL. Interventions for violence against women: Scientific review. *JAMA.* 2003;289(5):589–600.

125. Campbell DW, Campbell J, King C, et al. The reliability and factor structure of the Index of Spouse Abuse with African-American women. *Violence Vict.* 1994;9(3):259–274.

126. Campbell JC, Kub J, Belknap RA, Templin TN. Predictors of depression in battered women. *Violence Against Women.* 1997;3(3):271–293.

127. Campbell JC, Lewandowski LA. Mental and physical health effects of intimate partner violence on women and children. *Psychiatr Clin North Am.* 1997;20(2):353–374.

128. Follingstad DR, Brennan AF, Hause ES, et al. Factors moderating physical and psychological symptoms of battered women. *J Fam Violence.* 1991;6(1):81–95.

129. Kernic MA, Holt VL, Stoner JA, et al. Resolution of depression among victims of intimate partner

violence: is cessation of violence enough? *Violence Vict.* 2003;18(2):115–129.

130. Sullivan CM, Rumptz MH. Adjustment and needs of African-American women who utilized a DV shelter. *Violence Vict.* 1994;9(3):275–286.

131. Coker AL, Davis KE, Arias I, et al. Physical and mental health effects of intimate partner violence for men and women. *Am J Prev Med.* 2002;23(4): 260–268.

132. Constantino R, Kim Y, Crane PA. Effects of a social support intervention on health outcomes in residents of a DV shelter: A pilot study. *Issues Ment Health Nurs.* 2005;26(6):575–590.

133. McFarlane J, Soeken K, Reel S, et al. Resource use by abused women following an intervention program: Associated severity of abuse and reports of abuse ending. *Public Health Nurs.* 1997;14(4): 244–250.

134. Coker AL, Watkins KW, Smith PH, Brandt HM. Social support reduces the impact of partner violence on health: Application of structural equation models. *Prev Med.* 2003;37(3):259–267.

135. Goodman L, Dutton MA, Vankos N, Weinfurt K. Women's resources and use of strategies as risk and protective factors for reabuse over time. *Violence Against Women.* 2005;11(3):311–336.

136. McDonagh A, Friedman M, McHugo G, et al. Randomized trial of cognitive-behavioral therapy for chronic posttraumatic stress disorder in adult female survivors of childhood sexual abuse. *J Consult Clin Psychol.* 2005;73(3):515–524.

137. Mueser KT, Bolton E, Carty PC, et al. The Trauma Recovery Group: A cognitive-behavioral program for post-traumatic stress disorder in persons with severe mental illness. *Community Ment Health J.* 2007;43(3):281–304.

138. Rothbaum BO, Astin MC, Marsteller F. Prolonged Exposure versus Eye Movement Desensitization and Reprocessing (EMDR) for PTSD rape victims. *J Trauma Stress.* 2005;18(6): 607–616.

139. Foa EB, Dancu CV, Hembree EA, et al. A comparison of exposure therapy, stress inoculation training, and their combination for reducing posttraumatic stress disorder in female assault victims. *J Consult Clin Psychol.* 1999;67(2):194–200.

140. Resick PA, Nishith P, Weaver TL, et al. A comparison of cognitive-processing therapy with prolonged exposure and a waiting condition for the treatment of chronic posttraumatic stress disorder in female rape victims. *J Consult Clin Psychol.* 2002;70(4):867–879.

141. Marmar CR. Brief dynamic psychotherapy of PTSD. *Psychiatr Ann.* 1991;21:405–414.

142. Bradley R, Greene J, Russ E, et al. A multidimensional meta-analysis of psychotherapy for PTSD. *Am J Psychiatry.* 2005;162(2):214–227.

143. Resick PA. The psychological impact of rape. *J Interpers Violence.* 1993;8(2):223–255.

144. Resick PA, Schnicke MK. Cognitive processing therapy for sexual assault victims. *J Consult Clin Psychol.* 1992;60(5):748–756.

145. Russell PL, Davis C. Twenty-five years of empirical research on treatment following sexual assault. *Best Pract Ment Health.* 2007;3(2):21–37.

146. Foa EB, Kozak MJ. Emotional processing of fear: Exposure to corrective information. *Psychol Bull.* 1986;99(1):20–35.

147. Foa E, Hembree E, Rothbaum B. *Prolonged exposure therapy for PTSD: Emotional processing of traumatic experiences therapist guide.* New York: Oxford University Press, 2007.

148. Foa EB, Hembree EA, Cahill SP, et al. Randomized trial of prolonged exposure for posttraumatic stress disorder with and without cognitive restructuring: Outcome at academic and community clinics. *J Consult Clin Psychol.* 2005;73(5):953–964.

149. Foa EB, Rothbaum BO, Riggs DS, Murdock TB. Treatment of posttraumatic stress disorder in rape victims: A comparison between cognitive-behavioral procedures and counseling. *J Consult Clin Psychol.* 1991;59(5):715–723.

150. Foa EB, Jaycox LH. Cognitive-behavioral theory and treatment of posttraumatic stress disorder. In: Spiegel D, ed. *Efficacy and cost-effectiveness of psychotherapy (clinical practice, 45).* Washington, DC: American Psychiatric Press;1999:23–61.

151. van der Kolk BA, McFarlane AC, van der Hart O. A general approach to treatment of posttraumatic stress disorder. In: van der Kolk BA, McFarlane AC, Weisaeth L, eds. *Traumatic stress: The effects of overwhelming experience on mind, body, and society.* New York, NY: Guilford Press;1996:417–440.

152. Boudewyns PA. Posttraumatic stress disorder: Conceptualization and treatment. *Prog Behav Modif.* 1996;30:165–189.

153. Carlson JG, Chemtob CM, Rusnak K, et al. Eye movement desensitization and reprocessing (EDMR) treatment for combat-related posttraumatic stress disorder. *J Trauma Stress.* 1998;11(1):3–24.

154. Marcus S, Marquis P, Sakai C. Eye movement desensitization and reprocessing: A clinical outcome study for post-traumatic stress disorder. Annual Meeting of the American Psychological Association. Toronto, 1996.

155. Rothbaum BO. A controlled study of eye movement desensitization and reprocessing in the treatment of posttraumatic stress disordered sexual assault victims. *Bull Menninger Clin.* 1997;61(3):317–334.

156. Scheck MM, Schaeffer JA, Gillette C. Brief psychological intervention with traumatized young women: The efficacy of eye movement desensitization and reprocessing. *J Trauma Stress.* 1998;11(1):25–44.

157. Lohr JM, Kleinknecht RA, Tolin DF, Barrett RH. The empirical status of the clinical application of eye movement desensitization and reprocessing. *J Behav Ther Exp Psychiatry.* 1995;26(4):285–302.

158. Lohr JM, Tolin DF, Lilienfeld S. Efficacy of eye movement desensitization and reprocessing: Implications for behavior therapy. *Behav Ther.* 1998;29:123–156.

159. Koopman C, Ismailji T, Holmes D, et al. The effects of expressive writing on pain, depression and posttraumatic stress disorder symptoms in survivors of intimate partner violence. *J Health Psychol.* 2005;10(2):211–221.

160. Hernandez-Ruiz E. Effect of music therapy on the anxiety levels and sleep patterns of abused women in shelters. *J Music Ther.* 2005;42(2):140–158.

161. Pitman RK, Altman B, Greenwald E, et al. Psychiatric complications during flooding therapy for posttraumatic stress disorder. *J Clin Psychiatry.* 1991;52(1):17–20.

162. Spinazzola J, Blaustein M, van der Kolk BA. Posttraumatic stress disorder treatment outcome research: The study of unrepresentative samples? *J Trauma Stress.* 2005;18(5):425–436.

163. Cloitre M, Koenen KC. The impact of borderline personality disorder on process group outcome among women with posttraumatic stress disorder related to childhood abuse. *Int J Group Psychother.* 2001;51(3):379–398.

164. Rothbaum B. Cognitive-behavioral therapy. In: Foa E, Keane TM, Friedman M, eds. *Effective treatments for PTSD: Practice guidelines from the International Society for Traumatic Stress Studies.* New York: Guilford;2000:320–325.

165. Ehlers A, Clark DM, Dunmore E, et al. Predicting response to exposure treatment in PTSD: The role of mental defeat and alienation. *J Trauma Stress.* 1998;11(3):457–471.

166. Levitt JL, Cloitre M. A clinician's guide to STAIR/MPE: Treatment for PTSD related to childhood abuse. *Cogn Behav Pract.* 2005;12:40–52.

167. Foa EB, Zoellner LA, Feeny NC, et al. Does imaginal exposure exacerbate PTSD symptoms? *J Consult Clin Psychol.* 2002;70(4):1022–1028.

168. Fallot RD, Harris M. The trauma recovery and empowerment model (TREM). *Community Ment Health J.* 2002;38:475–485.

169. Najavits LM. Clinicians' views on treating posttraumatic stress disorder and substance use disorder. *J Subst Abuse Treat.* 2002;22(2):79–85.

170. Harris M. *Trauma recovery and empowerment: A clinician's guide for working with women in groups.* New York: Free Press, 1998.

171. Courtois CA. Healing the incest wound: A treatment update with attention to recovered-memory issues. *Am J Psychother.* 1997;51(4):464–496.

172. van der Kolk BA, Courtois CA. Editorial comments: Complex developmental trauma. *J Trauma Stress.* 2005;18(5):385–388.

173. Harvey MR. An ecological view of psychological trauma and trauma recovery. *J Trauma Stress.* 1996;9(1):3–23.

174. Harris M, Fallot RD, Berley RW. Qualitative interviews on substance abuse relapse and prevention among female trauma survivors. *Psychiatr Serv.* 2005;56(10):1292–1296.

175. Brady KT, Dansky BS, Back SE, et al. Exposure therapy in the treatment of PTSD among cocaine-dependent individuals: Preliminary findings. *J Subst Abuse Treat.* 2001;21(1):47–54.

176. Ford JD, Russo E. Trauma-focused, present-centered, emotional self-regulation approach to integrated treatment for posttraumatic stress and addiction: Trauma adaptive recovery group education and therapy (TARGET). *Am J Psychother.* 2006;60(4):335–355.

177. Mueser K, Bond GR, Foster FR, Lynde D. Psychosocial and rehabilitation treatments for patients with severe mental illness. *CNS Spectr.* 2004;9(12):891.

178. Najavits LM, Gallop RJ, Weiss RD. Seeking safety therapy for adolescent girls with PTSD and substance use disorder: A randomized controlled trial. *J Behav Health Serv Res.* 2006;33(4):453–463.

179. Najavits LM, Weiss RD, Shaw SR, Muenz LR. "Seeking safety": Outcome of a new cognitive-behavioral psychotherapy for women with posttraumatic stress disorder and substance dependence. *J Trauma Stress.* 1998;11(3):437–456.

180. Toussaint D, Vandemark N, Bornemann A. Modifications to the Trauma Recovery and Empowerment Model (TREM) for substance-abusing women with histories of violence: Outcomes and lessons learned at a Colorado substance abuse treatment center. *J Community Psychol.* 2007;35(7):879–894.

181. Zlotnick C, Najavits LM, Rohsenow DJ, Johnson DM. A cognitive-behavioral treatment for incarcerated women with substance abuse disorder and posttraumatic stress disorder: findings from a pilot study. *J Subst Abuse Treat.* 2003;25(2):99–105.

182. Bloom S. *Creating sanctuary: Toward an evolution of sane societies.* New York: Routledge, 1997.

183. Mueser KT, Rosenberg SD. Treatment of PTSD in persons with severe mental illness. In: Wilson JP, Friedman MJ, Lindy JD, eds. *Treating psychological trauma and PTSD.* New York: Guilford Press;2001:354–382.

184. Amaro H, Dai J, Arevalo S, et al. Effects of integrated trauma treatment on outcomes in a racially/ethnically diverse sample of women in urban community-based substance abuse treatment. *J Urban Health.* 2007;84(4):508–522.

185. Cocozza JJ, Jackson EW, Hennigan K, et al. Outcomes for women with co-occurring disorders and trauma: Program-level effects. *J Subst Abuse Treat.* 2005;28(2):109–119.

186. Courtois CA. *Healing the incest wound: Adult survivors in therapy.* New York: Norton, 1988.

187. Lubin H, Johnson DR. Interactive psychoeducational group therapy for traumatized women. *Int J Group Psychother.* 1997;47(3):271–290.

188. Spiegel D, Classen CC, Thurston V, Butler L. Trauma-focused versus present-focused models of group therapy for women sexually abused in childhood. In: Koenig L, Doll L, O'Leary A, et al., eds.

From sexual abuse to adult sexual risk: Trauma, revictimization, and intervention. Washington, DC: American Psychological Association;2004: 251–268.

189. Talbot NL, Houghtalen RP, Cyrulik S, et al. Women's safety in recovery: Group therapy for patients with a history of childhood sexual abuse. *Psychiatr Serv.* 1998;49(2):213–217.

190. Zlotnick C, Shea TM, Rosen K, et al. An affect-management group for women with posttraumatic stress disorder and histories of childhood sexual abuse. *J Trauma Stress.* 1997;10(3):425–436.

191. Simpson EB, Pistorello J, Begin A, et al. Use of dialectical behavior therapy in a partial hospital program for women with borderline personality disorder. *Psychiatr Serv.* 1998;49(5):669–673.

192. Barnett OW, Miller-Perrin CL, Perrin RD. *Family violence across the lifespan: An introduction.* Thousand Oaks, CA: Sage, 1997.

193. Goodman L, Epstein D. *Listening to battered women: A survivor-centered approach to advocacy, mental health, and justice.* Washington, DC: American Psychological Association, 2008.

194. Stark E, Flitcraft A, Frazier W. Medicine and patriarchal violence: The social construction of a "private" event. *Int J Health Serv.* 1979;9(3): 461–493.

195. Green BL, Krupnick JL, Chung J, et al. Impact of PTSD comorbidity on one-year outcomes in a depression trial. *J Clin Psychol.* 2006;62(7): 815–835.

196. Kessler RC, Sonnega A, Bromet E, et al. Posttraumatic Stress Disorder in the National Comorbidity Survey. *Arch Gen Psychiatry.* 1995;52(12): 1048–1060.

197. Cascardi M, O'Leary KD, Schlee KA. Co-occurrence and correlates of posttraumatic stress disorder and major depression in physically abused women. *J Fam Violence.* 1999;14(3):227–249.

198. McQuaid JR, Pedrelli P, McCahill ME, Stein MB. Reported trauma, post-traumatic stress disorder and major depression among primary care patients. *Psychol Med.* 2001;31(7):1249–1257.

199. Breslau N, Lucia VC, Davis GC. Partial PTSD versus full PTSD: An empirical examination of associated impairment. *Psychol Med.* 2004;34(7): 1205–1214.

200. Davidson JR. Biological therapies for posttraumatic stress disorder: An overview. *J Clin Psychiatry.* 1997;58(Suppl 9):29–32.

201. Padala PR, Madison J, Monnahan M, et al. Risperidone monotherapy for post-traumatic stress disorder related to sexual assault and domestic abuse in women. *Int Clin Psychopharmacol.* 2006;21(5): 275–280.

202. Turkus J. Crisis intervention. In: Classen CC, Yalom I, eds. *Treating women molested in childhood.* San Francisco: Jossey-Bass;1995:35–62.

203. Seedat S, Lochner C, Vythilingum B, Stein DJ. Disability and quality of life in post-traumatic stress disorder: Impact of drug treatment. *Pharmacoeconomics.* 2006;24(10):989–998.

204. Davidson J, Kudler H, Smith R, et al. Treatment of posttraumatic stress disorder with amitriptyline and placebo. *Arch Gen Psychiatry.* 1990;47(3):259–266.

205. Frank JB, Kosten TR, Giller EL, Jr., Dan E. A randomized clinical trial of phenelzine and imipramine for posttraumatic stress disorder. *Am J Psychiatry.* 1988;145(10):1289–1291.

206. Ipser J, Seedat S, Stein DJ. Pharmacotherapy for post-traumatic stress disorder: A systematic review and meta-analysis. *S Afr Med J.* 2006;96(10): 1088–1096.

207. Stein DJ, Kaminer D, Zungu-Dirwayi N, Seedat S. Pros and cons of medicalization: The example of trauma. *World J Biol Psychiatry.* 2006;7(1):2–4.

208. Dow B, Kline N. Antidepressant treatment of post-traumatic stress disorder and major depression in veterans. *Ann Clin Psychiatry.* 1997;9(1):1–5.

209. Zhang W, Davidson JR. Post-traumatic stress disorder: An evaluation of existing pharmacotherapies and new strategies. *Expert Opin Pharmacother.* 2007;8(12):1861–1870.

210. Stein DJ, Seedat S, Iversen A, Wessely S. Post-traumatic stress disorder: Medicine and politics. *Lancet.* 2007;369(9556):139–144.

211. Gelpin E, Bonne O, Peri T, et al. Treatment of recent trauma survivors with benzodiazepines: A prospective study. *J Clin Psychiatry.* 1996;57(9): 390–394.

212. Ballenger JC, Davidson JR, Lecrubier Y, et al. Consensus statement update on posttraumatic stress disorder from the international consensus group on depression and anxiety. *J Clin Psychiatry.* 2004;65(Suppl 1):55–62.

213. de Quervain DJ. Glucocorticoid-induced inhibition of memory retrieval: Implications for posttraumatic stress disorder. *Ann N Y Acad Sci.* 2006;1071: 216–220.

214. Pitman RK, Sanders KM, Zusman RM, et al. Pilot study of secondary prevention of posttraumatic stress disorder with propranolol. *Biol Psychiatry.* 2002;51(2):189–192.

215. Schelling G, Roozendaal B, De Quervain DJ. Can posttraumatic stress disorder be prevented with glucocorticoids? *Ann N Y Acad Sci.* 2004;1032: 158–166.

216. Schoenfeld FB, Marmar CR, Neylan TC. Current concepts in pharmacotherapy for posttraumatic stress disorder. *Psychiatr Serv.* 2004;55(5):519–531.

217. Stein MB, Kerridge C, Dimsdale JE, Hoyt DB. Pharmacotherapy to prevent PTSD: Results from a randomized controlled proof-of-concept trial in physically injured patients. *J Trauma Stress.* 2007;20(6):923–932.

218. Charney DS, Deutch AY, Krystal JH, et al. Psychobiologic mechanisms of posttraumatic stress disorder. *Arch Gen Psychiatry.* 1993;50(4):295–305.

219. Brady K, Pearlstein T, Asnis GM, et al. Efficacy and safety of sertraline treatment of posttraumatic stress

disorder: A randomized controlled trial. *JAMA.* 2000;283(14):1837–1844.

220. Davidson J, Pearlstein T, Londborg P, et al. Efficacy of sertraline in preventing relapse of posttraumatic stress disorder: Results of a 28-week double-blind, placebo-controlled study. *Am J Psychiatry.* 2001;158(12):1974–1981.

221. Londborg PD, Hegel MT, Goldstein S, et al. Sertraline treatment of posttraumatic stress disorder: Results of 24 weeks of open-label continuation treatment. *J Clin Psychiatry.* 2001;62(5): 325–331.

222. Marmar CR, Schoenfeld F, Weiss DS, et al. Open trial of fluvoxamine treatment for combat-related posttraumatic stress disorder. *J Clin Psychiatry.* 1996;57(Suppl 8):66–70; discussion 71–62.

223. Marshall RD, Beebe KL, Oldham M, Zaninelli R. Efficacy and safety of paroxetine treatment for chronic PTSD: A fixed-dose, placebo-controlled study. *Am J Psychiatry.* 2001;158(12):1982–1988.

224. Zohar J, Amital D, Miodownik C, et al. Double-blind placebo-controlled pilot study of sertraline in military veterans with posttraumatic stress disorder. *J Clin Psychopharmacol.* 2002;22(2):190–195.

225. Seedat S, Stein DJ, Carey PD. Post-traumatic stress disorder in women: Epidemiological and treatment issues. *CNS Drugs.* 2005;19(5):411–427.

226. van der Kolk BA, Spinazzola J, Blaustein ME, et al. A randomized clinical trial of eye movement desensitization and reprocessing (EMDR), fluoxetine, and pill placebo in the treatment of posttraumatic stress disorder: Treatment effects and long-term maintenance. *J Clin Psychiatry.* 2007;68(1):37–46.

227. Tucker P, Zaninelli R, Yehuda R, et al. Paroxetine in the treatment of chronic posttraumatic stress disorder: Results of a placebo-controlled, flexible-dosage trial. *J Clin Psychiatry.* 2001;62(11): 860–868.

228. Rothbaum BO, Ninan PT, Thomas L. Sertraline in the treatment of rape victims with posttraumatic stress disorder. *J Trauma Stress.* 1996;9(4):865–871.

229. Friedman MJ, Marmar CR, Baker DG, et al. Randomized, double-blind comparison of sertraline and placebo for posttraumatic stress disorder in a Department of Veterans Affairs setting. *J Clin Psychiatry.* 2007;68(5):711–720.

230. Stein DJ, Davidson J, Seedat S, Beebe K. Paroxetine in the treatment of post-traumatic stress disorder: Pooled analysis of placebo-controlled studies. *Expert Opin Pharmacother.* 2003;4(10):1829–1838.

231. Davidson J, Rothbaum BO, Tucker P, et al. Venlafaxine extended release in posttraumatic stress disorder: A sertraline- and placebo-controlled study. *J Clin Psychopharmacol.* 2006;26(3):259–267.

232. Friedman MJ. Current and future drug treatment for PTSD patients *Psychiatr Ann.* 1998;28(8): 461–468.

233. van der Kolk BA, Herron N, Hostetler A. The history of trauma in psychiatry. *Psychiatr Clin North Am.* 1994;17(3):583–600.

234. Brady KT, Killeen T, Saladin ME, et al. Comorbid substance abuse and posttraumatic stress disorder: Characteristics of women in treatment. *Am J Addict.* 1994;3:160–164.

235. Marshall RD, Lewis-Fernandez R, Blanco C, et al. A controlled trial of paroxetine for chronic PTSD, dissociation, and interpersonal problems in mostly minority adults. *Depress Anxiety.* 2007;24(2):77–84.

236. Rapaport MH, Endicott J, Clary CM. Posttraumatic stress disorder and quality of life: results across 64 weeks of sertraline treatment. *J Clin Psychiatry.* 2002;63(1):59–65.

237. Martenyi F, Brown EB, Zhang H, et al. Fluoxetine versus placebo in posttraumatic stress disorder. *J Clin Psychiatry.* 2002;63(3):199–206.

238. Vermetten E, Vythilingam M, Southwick SM, et al. Long-term treatment with paroxetine increases verbal declarative memory and hippocampal volume in posttraumatic stress disorder. *Biol Psychiatry.* 2003;54(7):693–702.

239. Davis M, Barad M, Otto M, Southwick S. Combining pharmacotherapy with cognitive behavioral therapy: Traditional and new approaches. *J Trauma Stress.* 2006;19(5):571–581.

240. Lipper S, Davidson JR, Grady TA, et al. Preliminary study of carbamazepine in post-traumatic stress disorder. *Psychosomatics.* 1986;27(12):849–854.

241. Wolf ME, Alavi A, Mosnaim AD. Posttraumatic stress disorder in Vietnam veterans clinical and EEG findings: Possible therapeutic effects of carbamazepine. *Biol Psychiatry.* 1988;23(6):642–644.

242. Pitman RK, Delahanty DL. Conceptually driven pharmacologic approaches to acute trauma. *CNS Spectr.* 2005;10(2):99–106.

243. Roth AS, Ostroff RB, Hoffman RE. Naltrexone as a treatment for repetitive self-injurious behaviour: An open-label trial. *J Clin Psychiatry.* 1996;57(6): 233–237.

244. Hamner MB, Robert S, Frueh BC. Treatment-resistant posttraumatic stress disorder: strategies for intervention. *CNS Spectr.* 2004;9(10):740–752.

245. Hamner MB, Faldowski RA, Ulmer HG, et al. Adjunctive risperidone treatment in post-traumatic stress disorder: A preliminary controlled trial of effects on comorbid psychotic symptoms. *Int Clin Psychopharmacol.* 2003;18(1):1–8.

246. Saporta JAJ, Case J. The role of medication in treating adult survivors of childhood trauma. In: Paddison P, ed. *Treating adult survivors of incest.* Washington, DC: American Psychiatric Press;1991:101–134.

247. Aerni A, Traber R, Hock C, et al. Low-dose cortisol for symptoms of posttraumatic stress disorder. *Am J Psychiatry.* 2004;161(8):1488–1490.

248. Schelling G, Briegel J, Roozendaal B, et al. The effect of stress doses of hydrocortisone during septic shock on posttraumatic stress disorder in survivors. *Biol Psychiatry.* 2001;50(12):978–985.

249. Weis F, Kilger E, Roozendaal B, et al. Stress doses of hydrocortisone reduce chronic stress symptoms and

improve health-related quality of life in high-risk patients after cardiac surgery: A randomized study. *J Thorac Cardiovasc Surg.* 2006;131(2):277–282.

250. Brady KT, Clary CM. Affective and anxiety comorbidity in post-traumatic stress disorder treatment trials of sertraline. *Compr Psychiatry.* 2003;44(5): 360–369.

251. Tucker P, Beebe KL, Burgin C, et al. Paroxetine treatment of depression with posttraumatic stress disorder: Effects on autonomic reactivity and cortisol secretion. *J Clin Psychopharmacol.* 2004;24(2): 131–140.

252. Davidson LM, Baum A. Chronic stress and post-traumatic stress disorders. *J Consult Clin Psychol.* 1986;54(3):303–308.

253. Hidalgo R, Hertzberg MA, Mellman T, et al. Nefazodone in post-traumatic stress disorder: Results from six open-label trials. *Int Clin Psychopharmacol.* 1999;14(2):61–68.

254. Khan A, Brodhead AE, Schwartz KA, et al. Sex differences in antidepressant response in recent antidepressant clinical trials. *J Clin Psychopharmacol.* 2005;25(4):318–324.

255. Kornstein SG, Schatzberg AF, Thase ME, et al. Gender differences in chronic major and double depression. *J Affect Disord.* 2000;60(1):1–11.

256. Hildebrandt MG, Steyerberg EW, Stage KB, et al. Are gender differences important for the clinical effects of antidepressants? *Am J Psychiatry.* 2003;160(9):1643–1650.

257. Parker G, Parker K, Austin MP, et al. Gender differences in response to differing antidepressant drug classes: two negative studies. *Psychol Med.* 2003;33(8):1473–1477.

258. Quitkin FM, Stewart JW, McGrath PJ, et al. Are there differences between women's and men's antidepressant responses? *Am J Psychiatry.* 2002;159(11):1848–1854.

259. Jensvold MF, Hamilton JA. Sex and gender effects in psychopharmacology: Contributing factors and implications for pharmacotherapy. *Bailliere's Clin Psychiatry. Intl Pract Res.* 1996;2(4):647–665.

260. Frackiewicz EJ, Sramek JJ, Cutler NR. Gender differences in depression and antidepressant pharmacokinetics and adverse events. *Ann Pharmacother.* 2000;34(1):80–88.

261. Bennett L, O'Brien P. Effects of coordinated services for drug-abusing women who are victims of intimate partner violence. *Violence Against Women.* 2007;13(4):395–411.

262. Substance abuse treatment and DV. In: Administration SAMHS, ed. US Department of Health and Human Services, 1997.

263. Noether CD, Finkelstein N, VanDeMark NR, et al. Design strengths and issues of SAMHSA's Women, Co-occurring Disorders, and Violence Study. *Psychiatr Serv.* 2005;56(10):1233–1236.

264. Miller D, Guidry L. *Addictions and trauma recovery: Healing the body, mind, and spirit.* New York: WW Norton Company, 2001.

265. Covington S. *Helping women recover: A program for treating addiction.* Center City, MN: Hazelden, 1999.

266. Covington S. *Beyond trauma: A healing journey for women.* San Francisco: Jossey-Bass, 2003.

267. Finkelstein N, Vandemark N, Fallot RD, et al. *Enhancing substance abuse recovery through integrated trauma treatment.* Sarasota: National Trauma Consortium, 2004.

268. Schechter S. *Domestic violence guidelines for mental health practitioners in DV cases* Washington, DC: National Coalition Against Domestic Violence, 1987.

269. Harway M, Hansen M. Treatment of spouse abuse. In: Harway M, Hansen M, eds. *Spouse abuse: Assessing and treating battered women, batterers, and their children.* Sarasota, FL: Professional Resource Press;1994:57–87.

270. Edleson J. Children's witnessing of adult domestic violence. *J Interpers Violence.* 1999;14(8):839–870.

Chapter 25

Strength and Resilience in Battered Women and Their Children

Jacquelyn Campbell, Phyllis Sharps, and Kerry Parsons

KEY CONCEPTS

- A strengths or resilience framework can be helpful in explaining the responses of women and children to intimate partner violence (IPV) and designing interventions for them.
- Considerable research documents that abused women display impressive strengths, including that the majority eventually leave the abusive relationships and/or make the violence end.
- Abused women take many impressive protective actions to keep themselves and their children safe.
- Abused women are most often good and protective mothers.
- Children exposed to IPV display many detrimental effects, but many if not most of the problems are alleviated if the violence ends.
- Interventions that build upon women's strengths and children's resilience may be most effective in dealing with the consequences of abuse, but have yet to be tested.

The first decade of scholarly depictions of battered women emphasized their victim status, their needs for assistance, their injuries, and their physical and mental pathologies in order to demonstrate to a disbelieving world that intimate partner violence (IPV) was a serious problem, and that victims needed services. The psychological theory of learned helplessness [1,2] was applied to battered women with the unfortunate terminology "sticking" in the general consciousness of practitioners and researchers more so than the insights the model afforded. Some of these insights may have relevance yet today, particularly that under certain conditions, especially prior victimization and self-blame, abused women may become seriously depressed and find it difficult to see alternatives to their situation [3]. Yet, under most conditions, abused women demonstrate incredible strengths, with the majority of women experiencing IPV leaving the abusive relationship and/or managing to make the violence end [4,5]. Advocates have been emphasizing an approach of never discounting the serious dangers and effects of IPV but still appreciating and therefore facilitating the strengths of abused women. Although evidence supporting this viewpoint exists in the literature, few syntheses of this literature exist, and little attempt has been made to develop interventions and conduct research explicitly from this kind of framework.

A similar history accompanied the scholarship on the children of abused women, with an initial appropriate documentation of detrimental effects on children from exposure to parental IPV. As serious as these problems are and deserve to be taken, they were initially documented without appropriate comparison groups among children in shelters who were also affected by disruption of their regular existence and by normal anxiety about the future given their circumstances (6,7). Later studies demonstrated that, although the children of abused women did indeed show significantly more problems in a number of areas than those without such exposure to violence, such outcomes were much more serious in those who also experienced child abuse, a commonly concurrently occurring trauma (8,9). There were also indications in the few prospective studies of these children, plus studies of adults exposed to IPV during childhood, that if the violence ended, the majority of children regained normalcy in most areas (10,11). A resiliency framework helped explain these outcomes.

The purpose of this chapter is to review the existing literature specific to strength and resilience in battered women and their children and to discuss the implications of a resiliency framework for healthcare policy, practice, and research.

CONCEPTUALIZATIONS

We conceptualize resilience as a dynamic process encompassing positive adaptation within the context of significant adversity. From the work of Luthar and Chichetti (12), two conditions are implicit in this definition: (a) exposure to significant threat or severe adversity, such as IPV; and (b) the achievement of positive adaptation despite major assaults on the developmental process. These authors caution against conceptualizing resilience as a personal attribute or personality trait. They point to ego-resiliency as a construct referring to a set of traits that reflect general resourcefulness, and sturdiness and flexibility of functioning, in response to varying circumstances.

Ego-resiliency differs from resilience in that it does not presuppose adversity; resilience, on the other hand, is a process in which significant adversity is a given. Garmezy (13), Werner (14), and others (15–17) have added to our understanding of how children vary in their response to adversity and have worked to identify protective factors that distinguish adaptive or resilient from maladaptive children.

PROCESS OF DEALING WITH VIOLENCE FROM A STRENGTHS PERSPECTIVE

A resilience framework (Figure 25.1) has not yet been fully applied to adult victims of IPV. Even so, numerous studies have documented adult women's strengths in the face of the adversity of IPV, and even early nursing (18) and other research (19) labeled abused women as "survivors" rather than victims. A fairly consistent process of dealing with the violence has been described through several qualitative studies synthesized in a meta-analysis of qualitative data by Kearney (20). Various but similar "stages," "decision points," or "turnings" have been described in several different qualitative analyses of data from different ethnic groups of abused women from both shelters and the community (10,21–26). These works all emphasize the normative nature of this response rather than characterizing it as pathological. There are also similarities to a normative loss and grieving framework (3,27).

Several studies using qualitative data further explicated and primarily supported the phases of the first such process framework, Landenburger's (21) grounded theory of entrapment and recovery from an abusive relationship. The Landenburger (21,28) phase labels (binding, enduring, disengaging, and recovering) along with similar titles used by other authors will be used to describe the basic process below. Table 25.1 summarizes these findings.

Binding (Falling in Love, Commitment, Shock, and Denial)

The first phase of binding incorporates the initial development of the relationship and the beginnings of abuse within the relationship. As in any intimate relationship, the woman is trying to create a loving, long-term partnership. She has made a commitment to try to make this relationship work, and she works

Pre-event risk/protective factors	→	Responses mediated by:	Outcomes
Individual Factors • Age, socioeconomic status, ethnicity • Religious participation • Mental illness • Alcohol/drug abuse		**Resiliency Factors** • Courage and determination • Problem-solving skills • Sense of purpose, hope in the future	**Health** • Physical and mental health consequences
Relationship Factors • Marital/relationship conflict • Power and control • Divorce or separation • Economic stress, unemployment • Living/housing status	IPV Exposure	**Event-specific Factors** • Degree of personal threat/injury • Perceptions of abuse • Fighting back, self-defense • Self-blame/sense of responsibility	**Parenting** • Protecting children • Competent parenting • Mother-child relationship
Situational Factors • Exposure to other traumas • Stressful family life events • Witnessed or experienced abuse as a child		**Coping** • Effective coping skills • Social support • Help-seeking behaviors • Resourcefulness	**Relationship** • Ending abuse or leaving relationship

Figure 25.1 Conceptual model – resilience in women exposed to intimate partner violence.

very hard at that, despite warning signals that begin to develop. She concentrates on the positive aspects and chooses to interpret the controlling behavior or jealousy that is almost always present as symbols of the love, attention, and commitment she needs rather than as troublesome. When actual abuse first starts, there is often an initial period of shock and denial, similar to what follows any significant loss (3). The woman experiences a tremendous sense of loss of the idealized relationship she has dreamed about and worked to achieve. Battered woman may deny

or minimize the importance of the initial abuses in a variety of ways (5,29).

At first, the abuse is typically only a small part of the relationship (21). Other problems may seem far more important, such as unemployment, pregnancy, inadequate housing, or health problems. The woman may explain the occasional push or shove as a temporary aberration in an essentially loving relationship, or she may blame the stress that the man is currently undergoing or her own behavior. She may admit the violence, but blame it on alcohol or a temporary loss

Table 25.1 Literature Supporting and Extending Landenburger's Stages of Abuse

Binding	Enduring	Disengaging	Recovering
Falling in love, commitment, shock, and denial	Restriction, diminishing of self	Counteracting abuse, resistance, resourcefulness	Resolve, not going back
Initial period of shock and denial similar to any significant loss (3)	Putting up with behavior and trying to change it (21)	Moving from restriction to resolve; reclaiming self (29,31,32)	"Claim and maintain territory" by getting to safe place, learning to use resources, and gaining control (32)
Deny or minimize importance of initial abuse; displace blame (5,21,29)	Feeling blame and responsibility (3,21)	Resistance, resourcefulness, and active problem solving(5,33,36)	Justifying to self and others; addressing moral conflicts in decision making; negotiating with self (5,32,37)
Question what is happening as impact and meaning start to become apparent (21)	Placating and bargaining (5,19,21)	Identify and label as abuse for first time (5)	
	Loss; silencing or shrinking of self (21,37)	Actively seek help to end the abusive relationship (19,21,28,34)	Obtaining needed support and learning to survive on own (21,28,32)
	Hiding abuse not labeling as abuse (5,30)	"Releases," leaving due to safety concerns and personal growth (23)	Working through losses and searching for meaning in the experience (39)
		Anger and rage; fighting back; fantasize about killing partner (5,21)	

of control in her partner. He typically blames such factors also and minimizes his own responsibility, supporting her denial. However, once a man has used actual violence, a psychological barrier seems to have been broken, and a pattern of abuse is started.

As the violence recurs, the impact and meaning start to become apparent. She begins to question what is happening as her attempts to make things right are obviously futile (21). For the woman, this is a transitional period into the next phase. Many strong feelings may be experienced by the woman. However, the intermittent pattern of some abuser's beatings may allow the woman to return to denial during quiescent periods. The feeling that first surfaces is sometimes anger, and the woman may try to fight back, either verbally or physically. These acts of aggressiveness may be a pattern of self-defense against prior violence, even if not in an immediate sense (5). If the woman finds that fighting back only worsens the violence directed against her, she will stop her use of violence and therefore have to suppress her anger.

Enduring (Restriction, Diminishing the Self)

In Landenburger's (21) second phase, enduring, the woman sees herself as putting up with the behavior of her partner and trying to change it. Feeling responsible is an important aspect of this phase. It has been noted in much of the literature that battered women frequently blame themselves for the abuse, at least at first. Their guilt is reinforced by the psychological abuse and blame dealt out by the abusive partner. Women may not blame themselves directly for the abuse (3), although many blame themselves for other issues, such as not seeing the abuse coming. They may also feel responsible for helping their partner deal with his problems or for staying in an abusive relationship (21). Another aspect of the enduring phase Landenburger called "placating," in which the woman makes a pact, either overtly or covertly, with her husband that she will correct whatever behavior he sees as a problem in return for an absence of violence. She also bargains with him about returning to him or staying with him only if he changes his behavior or seeks treatment for the violence or substance abuse (5). Threatening to leave or actually leaving temporarily can be a very effective strategy for entering abusive men into treatment, as shown by Gondolf (19).

The feelings of helplessness, despair, and loss of control so often identified by abused women and clinically seen as depression, are a normal part of the period of enduring. It is extremely painful for the woman to struggle with her feelings of responsibility to the relationship while trying to determine why she is being abused. Women in several studies (21,23,24) have described a loss or silencing or shrinking of self as the abuse continued and escalated. The battered woman doubts her ability to cope without the man and may feel totally worthless. She usually tries to hide the abuse, and finds it difficult to disclose to anyone. This is also a normal desire to avoid the stigma associated with abuse and to protect her partner. Even to herself, she usually does not label what is happening to her as abuse or battering (5,30).

Disengaging (Counteracting Abuse, Resistance, Resourcefulness)

In Landenburger's (21) third phase, disengaging, women respond to and resist abuse using a variety of methods. Draucker (31) describe themes of first "restriction" and then "resolve." Merritt-Gray and Wuest's (29,32) theory identified reclaiming self as the central process for women leaving. Their first stage of the process, counteracting abuse, stressed women's resistance to abuse from the beginning of the violence. Similarly, Langford (33), used grounded theory to describe how battered women develop sophisticated knowledge of impending violence (such as specific changes in their partner's eyes, speech, tone of voice) and response strategies to avoid their partner's abuse, temporarily, if not permanently. In the only prospective analysis of qualitative data, Campbell and colleagues (5) identified patterns of response also demonstrating resistance and resourcefulness, with active problem solving.

Women in the disengaging phase begin to actively seek help to end the relationship (21,28). Gondolf (19) noted that women in his large sample of women in shelters more actively sought help as the abuse increased in severity and frequency. Bowker (34) also noted that women's help-seeking switched from

family and friends to more formal systems as time elapsed, and the more formal systems were found to be more helpful. In Ulrich's study, the two most frequent reasons for leaving were safety and personal growth (35). The safety category included fearing for their own, others,' or their children's physical safety, or their children's emotional safety. The personal growth category included sudden changes in awareness, having reached a personal limit, or being concerned for their own potential

During disengagement, anger often reemerges and may become rage, and the woman may fantasize about killing her partner (5,21). Her partner senses that she is close to a breaking point, and he often escalates his threats and violence to keep her in the relationship. These situations are extremely volatile, and serious injury or homicide of either partner may occur. This is the most dangerous part of the process, but also the stage at which the woman's self starts to reemerge.

An important component of research describing battered women's responses to abuse is the continued description of the women's strengths and abilities, or "creativity within severely limited options" (36). Much of the research in this trajectory is nursing research, but it has also been supported by research from other disciplines (22) and, importantly, is validated by this rich confluence of findings across studies, using a variety of methods, both retrospective and prospective. Also important is that, although several of the studies were limited by primarily White, middle-class samples (37,21,29,35), others were more ethnically diverse (5,33,38).

Recovering (Resolve, Not Going Back)

Wuest and Merritt-Gray's work (32) has been particularly important in its exploration of a phase of "not going back," when women have to "claim and maintain territory" by getting to a safe place, learning to use resources, and gaining control. They also have to go through a process of "relentless justifying" to others and, importantly, to the self, a process similar to Belknap's (37) description of addressing the moral conflicts in decision making and Campbell's (5) "negotiating with self."

Progress is seldom direct and without vacillation between stages. The recovering phase includes the initial adjustment to leaving the relationship and may encompass a temporary return to him. It takes considerable work, effort, pain, and assistance from others for a woman to survive on her own (21,28,32). Part of the recovering phase is a struggle for survival, in terms of the necessities of life, dealing with her children's losses, and justifying her leaving to her partner, children, and critical others. Idealization of the spouse may be seen during this period, which is also characteristic of grieving. This mechanism is often difficult for professionals working with the abused woman to understand, and it may lead her to return to the spouse, especially if she is having problems with survival and depression. When viewed as a normal part of a process to be worked through, it is more acceptable.

The response is also compounded by the fact that the man is not dead, even if the woman has left him, and he constantly reappears in her life when she is psychologically vulnerable. Part of this aspect of the recovery process is a search for meaning in the experience and her behavior, which includes determining why she stayed so long. Successfully working through the multiple losses and searching for meaning may well depend on the support given to the abused woman through the process (39).

During the disengaging stage, the abused woman may begin to identify with other women in similar situations through media accounts of abuse, friends or family members, or in community or shelter support groups. All are therefore important adjuncts to other kinds of intervention, and the media should be encouraged to continue informed news coverage of abuse and abuse-related entertainment programs. After seeing such media, the woman for the first time may label what is happening as abuse, and herself as an abused or battered woman. Women in Campbell's longitudinal study stated that this labeling process was accompanied by a significant change in how they thought about the relationship and what they did (5). They recounted shifts in blame from themselves to him, feeling like he was the one who had to change, not her, and deciding that the relationship would have to end.

Acceptance of the loss of their most important relationship, along with realistic plans for change, either within the relationship or outside of it, comes slowly for most women. The degree of loss, in terms of time and energy invested in the relationship, perceived ability to cope without it, and the love felt for their partner, may prolong the time needed to opt for change. Some women may never actually work through the grieving process or are so traumatized that they are immobilized.

QUANTITATIVE DATA SUPPORT FOR A STRENGTHS FRAMEWORK

Quantitative studies have also supported this strengths-based or resilience-type framework. Campbell used two separate longitudinal studies to support that the majority (67% and 56% in the two samples) of both African-American (40% and 80% sample proportions) and Anglo battered women in community volunteer samples either left the abusive relationship or managed to make the violence end (40,41). The first found no predictive factors identified for continuingrelationship violence for either the battered ($N = 51$) or nonbattered (but having serious relationship problems) comparison group ($N = 65$) in terms of the woman's demographic and personal characteristics (including childhood physical or sexual abuse, prior abusive relationship, self-care agency, self-esteem, depression, physical symptoms) or the frequency and severity of relationship violence (measured by the Conflicts Tactics Scale). The second followed 141 battered women over time and found that both physical and mental health status generally improved during the process of women becoming violence free (41), and that self-care agency (women's ability to take care of themselves) was important in protecting women from deleterious health outcomes (42). Both studies were limited by attrition (38% and 30%, respectively), lack of full ethnic diversity (other than African-American and Anglo), and the voluntary nature of the samples.

The Campbell and Soeken (42) use of self-care agency midrange theory is another strengths-based approach that can be useful in an overall resilience framework. Self-care agency was found to be protective against physical health problems and depression. The concept is similar to Lempert's concept of agency, identified in her qualitative work with abused women (22).

The recently completed Risk Assessment Validation Study (RAVE) study (43) also demonstrated that the majority (two-thirds) of abused women in a multiethnic sample of severely abused women were taking protective actions, such as getting protective orders, going to a shelter, living apart from the abuser, getting new locks, and so forth. Other research (44) has also documented the active strategic protective actions that the majority of abused women take, but often not until they have reached the disengaging stage. Although several of the studies demonstrating the strengths of abused women, both qualitative and quantitative, have been of ethnically diverse samples, few have specifically documented culturally specific contributions to women's resilience.

CULTURAL INFLUENCES ON RESILIENCE

From a cultural standpoint, it is important to take into account the cultural context, as well as individual factors that can affect resilience to IPV. In an analysis of anthropological data from primarily small-scale societies in developing countries, Counts, Brown, and Campbell (45) found that neighborhood- and/or extended family-level sanctions against severe IPV, as well as somewhere for abused women to go to escape (e.g., divorce availability or natal home access) and women having some source of power (e.g., women's work groups) in the society were all important in keeping wife beating at low levels.

In this country, African-American women have both particular challenges and particular strengths. Disproportionate rates of unemployment and incarceration in African-American men, health disparities, increased rates of prior sexual assault, and continued discrimination complicate African-American women's abilities to be resilient in the face of IPV. The historical context of the African immigrant's experiences in this country, the slavery experience and its destruction of Black families, and the oppression and discrimination that African Americans have experienced for over 200 years has led some scholars to theorize that IPV is a maladaptive behavior that evolved over time to cope with these negative experiences (46,47). These experiences may contribute to women believing that the IPV is no different than the violence they have experienced (e.g., mistrust, disrespect, rudeness, and physical threats) from helping agencies and law enforcement agents. These perceptions may contribute to African-American women being reluctant to disclose IPV. Black women may also feel as if the men in their community will be dealt with more harshly than they deserve at the hands of the criminal justice system and thus be concerned about asking for help in that arena.

Even so, African-American women display impressive strengths in the face of IPV on top of multiple discriminations. Impressive coping responses and active problem solving among African-American abused women was noted by several researchers (5,48).

Spirituality and the support of the African-American community are particularly important (49). O'Campo and colleagues (50) demonstrated that cohesive neighborhoods can be protective against abuse for urban African-American women.

Some similar observations have been made about Latina women and the importance of their community support (51,52) and those of indigenous cultures (53), but, in general, research on IPV in other ethnic communities is just beginning. There are, as yet, few studies that underscore strengths and resilience in other ethnic groups specifically.

ROLE OF SOCIAL SUPPORT

Social support has long been identified as an important "buffer" against the deleterious effects of stress in human beings. It would therefore be important in a resilience framework. Yet the research that has been conducted in the area of IPV and social support has been relatively sparse, and the few studies available suggest that the role of social support is complex in relationship to IPV for women.

For each of the "releases" from the abusive relationship in Ulrich's (35) study, a different source (friends, agencies, family) and type of social support (instrumental, emotional) was the most critical. Moss and associates (38) and Rose and associates (54) also explicated the complex role of social support for primarily African-American women's process of dealing with abuse, with their communities not always supportive of them leaving per se or naming the abuse to outsiders (e.g., the police, professionals). Even so, extended families and religious beliefs were extremely important in supporting healthy decisions. Many studies have shown that religious institutions are not always experienced as supportive to abused women. Even so, Gielen and O'Campo have found social support important as a protective factor against abuse during pregnancy for poor women (50). They also found social support important for dealing with abuse for human immunodeficiency virus (HIV)-positive women, again despite low incomes (55).

MENTAL HEALTH ISSUES

It is clear from many studies that depression is the mental health problem most likely to affect victims of

IPV (56). Other bodies of research have suggested that maternal stress and the mental health consequences associated with IPV, such as depression and anxiety, may result in deleterious mental and physical health effects and developmental outcomes for infants and children. Three longitudinal controlled studies in the United States and the United Kingdom demonstrated that mothers with higher stress and anxiety during pre- and postpartum periods are related to physiological measures of stress in infants as well as physical, mental, and behavioral problems and symptoms in children aged 2–45 months (57–59). A randomized individualized intervention designed to decrease maternal stress resulted in less maternal depression and better infant feeding in mothers of preterm infants (60). None of these studies measured IPV per se, but it is often assumed that IPV is inherent in maternal depression, resulting in difficulty parenting and leading to deleterious infant outcomes no matter what the stress and depression is in response to.

Yet, several prospective studies document that depression lifts as abuse lessens (41,61,62). Thus, the depression we see in abused women is likely to be a response to the abuse rather than a deficit among women who are victims or an inherent problem that contributes to their victimization. One of the issues with much of the cross-sectional research on women experiencing IPV is that the oft-noted correlate of depression is often described as a "risk factor" for abuse, thus leaving the impression that it precedes the violence.

Recent evidence also suggests that much if not most of the depression we have noted in abused women is actually comorbid with posttraumatic stress disorder (PTSD), that when both are measured, depression seldom exists by itself in abused women (63–65). This comorbidity has important treatment implications, as well as having the potential to change the perception of women who are abused in the eyes of the providers and the eyes of the courts. If women become depressed as a response to abuse through a traumatic response rather than a predisposition to depression, a resilience framework becomes easier to apply. Judges who are examining custody disputes are less likely to see a depressed woman (who is therefore a poor parent) and more likely to see a traumatized woman whose mental health symptoms are more likely to resolve once the violence ends. There is also evidence that PTSD mediates the relationship between IPV and other physical health problems such as chronic pain (65).

BATTERED WOMEN AS GOOD PARENTS

With evidence of an overlap of child abuse and wife abuse (both most often perpetrated by the father or father figure, but most often investigated through the mother), documentation of depression in battered women and increased prevalence of drug and alcohol abuse, evidence of deleterious effects of exposure to IPV on children, and consequent charges of "failure to protect" against abused women who stay with or are in the process of leaving their abuser, the assumption is often that abused women are poor parents. Abused mothers are very concerned with the well-being of their children, but they often report that daily survival needs are so overwhelming that the needs of their children, including emotional needs, may be overlooked or unmet (66,67).

Furthermore, when parenting is actually measured, the majority of abused mothers are shown to be nurturing parents (67). In one of the few comparison studies, Casaneuva and Martin (68) found that the abused mothers' parenting did not differ from the nonabused. Levendosky and Graham-Bermann (69) advanced a contextual model of parenting and children's adjustment that demonstrates under what conditions victimized mothers are able to parent effectively. Not surprising, it is when the mothers report less frequent and/or less severe abuse that their parenting is most effective, and when children are abused as well as exposed to IPV that their health and behavior is most severely affected (8,70). In an ethnographic analysis of data from both abused mothers and their children, Humphreys (71) showed that abused women and their children go to considerable lengths to take care of and protect each other. These behaviors make perfect sense and do not necessarily represent "enmeshment" or other pathology that had been alluded to in prior literature. Buchbinder (72) and Berman (73) also documented abused women struggling to repair their children's negative experiences. In a recent prospective study of abused women after a shelter stay, Sharps (74) demonstrated that the mothers were taking very good care of their children in terms of physical health care, school reentry and attendance, and a measure of parenting skills. The positive outcomes of these kinds of behaviors are documented by findings such as McFarlane and Soeken's (75), who found infant weight gain significantly greater in infants whose mothers had left the abusive relationship compared to mothers who stayed.

Susan Schechter's insights and tireless advocacy about ensuring the safety of abused women as the best way to keep their children safe led to important national policy change and cross-training initiatives that have fostered understanding around these issues (76). Even so, there is still a lack of appreciation of the parenting abilities and resilience of abused women and more emphasis on the problems of children exposed to IPV than on their resilience.

CHILDREN EXPOSED TO INTIMATE PARTNER VIOLENCE—DETRIMENTAL EFFECTS

There have been at least three recent reviews of research in the area of the effects of children exposed to IPV (77–79). Almost all the research reviewed has concentrated on the problems these children demonstrate, almost none have investigated resilience. The more general literature will be briefly summarized, and then the resilience conceptual framework and few studies examining resilience in these children reviewed.

About 3–10 million children witness IPV in the United States annually (80). Witnessing IPV has been associated with a wide variety of physical and mental health effects in childhood and long-term developmental sequelae (7,77). This includes negative physical (such as asthma and weight gain) and mental health effects (PTSD symptoms, IQ diminishment) for children, (7,77,81,82), as well as negative effects on adjustment in adulthood (83), adult physical health problems (9,84), and increased risk of being in an IPV relationship and abusing one's own children as adults (85). New studies on the biology of trauma and the subtle effects of trauma on the development of young children are beginning to elucidate the complex interplay of physiological and psychological influences that are seen in the behavior of young children exposed to IPV (86–88). Yet all agree that there are still significant gaps in our knowledge, especially in regards to the youngest of these children.

The degree to which children experience negative effects from witnessing IPV is influenced by contextual and individual factors. For example, families with violence may have other contextual stressors (e.g., poverty, job and family instability, residential instability, parental stress, social isolation) that affect their children's health. Multiple risk factors increase

the negative effects for children and, the longer the exposure and victimization of child abuse, the more serious the outcomes (70,89). The child's gender may also be important. Finkelhor and Wolak (90) cite several studies that found boys who have witnessed severe violence showed more aggressive behaviors, whereas girls tended to withdraw or become more introverted. However, at least three recent studies, including a meta-analysis, have found no difference in gender related to behavioral problems among these children (79,91,92).

Specific problems also may vary according to developmental stage. Infants and preschoolers have been observed to have sleep problems and separation anxiety, lower developmental scores, more physical health problems (e.g., underweight, overweight, choking, and hearing) and more behavioral problems (temper tantrums and frequent crying) by maternal report, whereas school-age children may have somatic complaints, and teenagers may become depressed or suicidal (80). Children's sensitivity to interparental anger is posed as an important link between IPV and very young children's adjustment problems (57). Other possible influences include the frequency and severity of abuse, quality of parent–child relationships, the presence of child abuse in addition to IPV, and the presence of protective factors (e.g., community supports, positive adult role models) (80). Race has not been found to be a significant factor in reviews (7,77) and in the meta-analysis (79), but in a more recent study of 167 children aged 2–17, racial background was a significant predictor of behavior problems, even controlling for income and parental education (93).

CHILDREN EXPOSED TO INTIMATE PARTNER VIOLENCE: RESILIENCE

Using Garmezy's (13) general categories of resilience, a constellation of three factors can be identified as mediating the effects of chronic stress upon children: (a) dispositional attributes in the child (temperament, personality, cognitive style); (b) family milieu (family warmth, support, organization); and (c) supportive environment (external support, sense of community identification). A study of children in domestic violence (DV) shelters found that different factors were related to resilience depending on race and ethnicity. For African-American children, better adjustment was associated with less hostility and more competent parenting on the part of their mothers, whereas for Anglo children, it was more associated with mother's mental health (94). Not being exposed to child abuse (physical and mental) was important to resilience in both groups. In that study and another by the same authors (95) with the children of battered women, approximately 30% of the children could be described as resilient. Mothers' reports of appropriate parenting in spite of the violence, and less psychological abuse of either the mother or the children, were factors associated with these children's resilience. Of note is the finding of several authors that a nurturing relationship with even one person can mitigate, although not eliminate, the effects of marital turmoil (96) and stress (97) on children. Among multiple studies using varying measurement strategies, consistent themes have recurred indicating the importance of close relations with supportive adults, effective schools, and connections with competent, prosocial adults in the wider community (12). Resilience is a function of the interaction between maturational, individual, and environmental influences and thus may be fluid over time with changing environmental or situational conditions; resilience in one area (e.g., school performance) may not be accompanied by resilience in other areas (e.g., interpersonal relations) and excellence in one area can deteriorate over time (95). A potential model of resilience in children exposed to IPV is shown in Figure 25.2.

As shown in the model, risk and protective factors are present before the IPV that can predispose or protect the children from deleterious outcomes often observed when children are exposed to parental violence. For instance, younger children in poorer homes with a history of problems and exposure to other trauma are more vulnerable to serious and persistent problems if in homes where IPV also occurs. These outcomes can also be mediated by a number of resiliency factors in the child. Factors also exist outside the child, as summarized by Hughes, Graham-Berman, and Gruber (95), such as at least one caring, consistent adult over time to provide support, less versus more IPV, parenting competence (69), maternal mental health (94), and caretaker social support (98). Although sufficient research exists to identify some of these factors associated with resilience, the framework has not been extensively applied. Issues such as cultural influences and the relative importance of internal competencies versus external context have not been documented, and almost none of the prospective studies needed to understand resilience have been conducted.

IMPLICATIONS FOR HEALTH CARE OF A STRENGTHS AND RESILIENCE APPROACH

General Prevention

The importance of changing public perceptions around IPV using a public education approach has been shown by Klein and associates (99) in their evaluation of the first national Family Violence Prevention Fund (FVPF) campaign on ending IPV. The current FVPF campaign, Coaching Boys Into Men (www.endabuse.org) is exciting because of its emphasis on bringing men into IPV prevention efforts and in its emphasis on positive characteristics in families and individuals, but it also needs evaluation. Other general prevention models that build on strengths include relationship-enhancement interventions, such as those in schools that emphasize teaching adolescents how to have healthy relationships (100).

Interventions for Women

Some interventions build on strengths, such as the survivor group model, developed by Campbell (101) and further used and tested by Dimmitt and Davila (51). The community advocacy intervention designed and tested by Sullivan and Bybee (102) has strengths- and choice-based orientation, as does the empowerment intervention developed by Dutton (103) and the brochure-driven intervention developed and tested by Parker and McFarlane (104). The Domestic Violence Survivor Assessment (DVSA) instrument (105) was developed to help healthcare professionals or advocates work with a woman in identifying where she is in the process of dealing with an abusive relationship and to base interventions on that assessment. An important part of all of these interventions is assessment of strengths and communication of those strengths to women, as well as to document her strengths as well as any problems.

INTERVENTIONS THAT SUPPORT BATTERED WOMEN'S PARENTING

Healthcare providers can help mothers understand their children's responses, behaviors, needs, and provide appropriate referrals, such as mental health counseling and other relevant community resources.

Pre-event risk/protective factors	→	Responses mediated by:	Outcomes
Demographics/Background • Age, socioeconomic status, gender, ethnicity • Religious participation • History of mental illness		**Resiliency Factors** • Positive child attributes • Family conflict • Social support for child	**Psychosocial Health** • Posttraumatic stress disorder • Depression
Family/Child-related Factors • Exposure to other trauma • Stressful family life events • Stressful child life events • Relationship to perpetrator • Child abuse	**IPV Against Mother (could also be child abuse)**	**Event-specific Factors** • Proximity/involvement • Degree of personal threat/injury • Perceptions of events • Self-blame/sense of responsibility	**Behavior Changes** • Behavior problems
		Coping Strategies • Effective child coping strategies • Effective family coping	**Academic Adjustment** • School attendance • School performance
		Caregiver Characteristics • Mental health problems • Social support	**Additional Violence** • Violence victimization • Violence perpetration

Figure 25.2 Conceptual model – resilience in children exposed to intimate partner violence.

Early identification and intervention in the lives of children is necessary to reduce the potential detrimental effects of witnessing IPV. When depression and/or PTSD are part of a woman's responses to the abuse, interventions to address these issues need to be part of a strengths-based approach. For instance, a maternal stress reduction intervention designed and tested by Meyer and colleagues (60) resulted in less maternal depression and better infant feeding in mothers of preterm infants. Therefore, similar interventions that help mothers cope with or reduce the stress, anxiety, and depressive symptoms they may be experiencing related to IPV also help mothers to redirect their energy into parenting their children.

Home Visit Interventions

Early home visitation (HV) historically has been an essential component of community health nursing practice to improve health outcomes for families (parents or children). Home visitation interventions have been demonstrated to reduce risks for poor pregnancy outcomes, improve parenting skills, and enhance infant development, especially nurse HV interventions that have been shown to be the one intervention with solid evidence for preventing child maltreatment (106). These programs usually target low-income "high-risk" single young mothers or families presumed to be at highest risk for poor physical and behavioral child outcomes. David Olds' Nurse Family Partnership (NFP) HV program is recognized as one of the most successful early HV program and as the most evidence-supported intervention to prevent family violence (105). The NFP program uses nurses only, and begins with prenatal visits through 2 years of age. It was found to significantly improve pregnancy outcomes and parenting, and decrease children's hospitalizations and emergency department visits. Long-term (4–15 years) evidence suggests that mothers visited by NFP nurses were less likely to be reported as child abusers (107). The model also was effective for poor families and families of color. However, it was found that child maltreatment was not prevented among families in which frequent IPV occurred, with the treatment effect decreasing as the level of IPV increased (108,109). Other outcomes, such as increased employment among mothers, were also attenuated by IPV. These findings suggest that HV programs need to be tailored specifically for the highest-risk families, such as those with frequent IPV. More frequent and structured systematic assessment for IPV is probably needed in the NFP program both pre- and postpartum, with a more comprehensive intervention than the referral process currently recommended. In two recent long-term (4- and 6-year) follow-ups of the NFP program, Olds and his colleagues (110) reported that even without systematic assessment and intervention, nurse home-visited families had significantly less IPV after 4 years; but even so, 15.8% reported such violence (compared to 23.7% of controls). In the Memphis follow-up, perhaps because of the extremely poor, inner-city nature of the sample, as well as the lack of systematic assessment and intervention, the regular NFP intervention was not able to achieve a significant decrease in IPV (111).

Sharps and Price (74) have pilot-tested the Passport to Health nurse HV program, specifically designed to reduce violence-related health disparities. Twelve women were enrolled in a 6-month HV intervention for women survivors of IPV who leave a residential shelter. At 6 months after leaving the shelter (end of HV protocol), of the 10 women who completed the protocol, eight reported no new abuse, two reported one incident of abuse, and all are in stable living situations, with no abuse of their children, and self-esteem and depressive symptoms scores have improved over baseline scores. Additionally, with the support of community health nurse HV, women were able to keep their children healthy, up-to-date on immunizations, and enrolled in schools. This pilot project presents empirical evidence that, with appropriate individualized interventions, battered women's parenting skills can be enhanced, and women can keep themselves and their children safe.

CONCLUSION

In summary, a strengths- and resilience-based approach to facilitating abused women in their quest to end the violence in their lives, address their health issues, and provide healthy parenting for their children requires a different examination and conduct of research and a different orientation to practice and policy. Substantive documentation of the strengths of abused women exists, as well as research demonstrating a normative process of dealing with the violence in their relationships that is important to understand and teach in order to be most effective in dealing with this issue. Resilience, as well as problems, has also been observed among the children of these women and has important implications for interventions.

IMPLICATIONS FOR POLICY, PRACTICE, AND RESEARCH

Policy

- Nurse HV can be an effective strategy for the amelioration of IPV, as well as the prevention of child abuse if there is a structured assessment for IPV with appropriate targeted interventions. Such nurse HV programs should be encouraged for at-risk families in every community.

- Prevention of IPV public education campaigns should be an annual part of state and national health promotion activities.
- Intimate partner violence against a parent should not be considered sufficient evidence of poor parenting on the part of the victim.

Practice

- Assessment of abused women and their children needs to include assessment of strengths as well as pathology, with documentation of those strengths.
- Interventions for abused women and their children are best based on an assessment of the stage in which a woman is in her process of dealing with the abuse.
- Interventions that facilitate strengths and encourage choices have been shown to be effective in helping women end the violence in their lives.
- Practice needs to take into account cultural norms and cultural influences on women's and children's responses.
- Culturally competent interventions need to be developed and tested, as well as culturally specific interventions in areas with high concentrations of particular racial and ethnic minority populations.

Research

- All studies of abused women and their children need to measure their strengths and resilience and other protective factors, as well as health and behavior problems. Important to include are such concepts as resilience, social support, and self-care agency (41,42), as well as where women are in their process of dealing with the abuse using measures such as the DVSA (105). More measures are also needed of relevant strengths—for instance: How do we measure courage?
- Researchers need to identify societal, community, and neighborhood, as well as individual, protective factors.
- More longitudinal studies of the women and especially their children are needed to find with more accuracy the predictors of resilience.
- In discussions of findings, as much attention must be given to strengths as is given to deficits and problems. Keywords related to resilience and strengths can be added to make sure that such studies can be found by others.
- Just as the Adverse Childhood Events study identified the long-term detrimental effects of childhood exposure to IPV, there needs to be a similar study of what factors protect children who have been exposed to adverse events.
- Research that identifies better services and supports to protect abused women and their children are also needed.
- Researchers need to do a better job of communicating the strengths of abused women and their children to advocates, healthcare professionals, and policy makers.

References

1. Abramson LY, Seligman MEB, Teasdale JD. Learned helplessness in humans: Critique and reformulation. *J Abnorm Psychol.* 1978;87:49–74.
2. Walker LE. The battered woman syndrome. New York: Springer, 1984.
3. Campbell JC. A test of two explanatory models of women's responses to battering. *Nurs Res.* 1989; 38:18–24.
4. Campbell JC, Cardwell MM, Belknap RA. Relationship status of battered women over time. *J Fam Violence.* 1994;9:99–111.
5. Campbell JC, Rose LE, Kub J, Nedd D. Voices of strength and resistance: A contextual and longitudinal analysis of women's responses to battering. *J Interpers Violence.* 1998;13:743–762.
6. Campbell JC, Lewandowski LA. Mental and physical health effects of intimate partner violence on women and children. *Psychiatr Clin North Am.* 1997;20(2):353–374.
7. Edleson JL. Children's witnessing of adult domestic violence. *J Interpers Violence.* 1999;14(8):839–870.
8. Edleson JL. The overlap between child maltreatment and woman battering. *Violence Women.* 1999;5(2):134–154.
9. Felitti VJ, Anda RF, Nordenberg D, et al. Relationship of childhood abuse and household dysfunction to many of the leading causes of death in adults: The Adverse Childhood Experiences (ACE) Study. *Am J Prev Med.* 1998;14(4):245–258.
10. Humphreys JC. Turnings and adaptations in resilient daughters of battered women. *J Nurs Scholarsh.* 2001;33(3):245–251.
11. Berman H, Hardesty JL, Humphreys JC. Children of abused women. In: Campbell JC, Humphreys JC, eds. *Family violence in nursing practice.* Philadelphia, PA: Lippincott, Williams, & Wilkins, 2003.
12. Luthar SS, Cicchetti D. The construct of resilience: Implications for interventions and social policies. *Dev Psychopathol.* 2000;12:857–885.

13. Garmezy N. Stressors of childhood. In: Garmezy N, ed. *Stress, coping, and development in children.* New York: McGraw-Hill;1983:43–84.

14. Werner EE. High risk children in young adulthood: A longitudinal study from birth to 32 years. *Am J Orthopsychiatrity.* 1987;59:72–81.

15. Kilpatrick KL, Williams, LM. Potential mediators of post-traumatic stress disorder in child witnesses to domestic violence. *Child Abuse Negl.* 1998;22: 319–330.

16. Neighbors B, Forehand R, McVicar D. Resilient adolescents and interparental conflict. *Am J Orthopsychiatry.* 1993;63:462–471.

17. Pynoos RS, Frederick C, Nader K, et al. Life threat and post-traumatic stress in school-age children. *Arch Gen Psychiatry.* 1987;44:1057–1063.

18. Hoff LA. *Battered women as survivors.* London: Routledge, 1990.

19. Gondolf EW. *Battered women as survivors.* Holmes Beach, FL: Learning Publications, 1990.

20. Kearney MH. Enduring love: A grounded formal theory of women's experience of domestic violence. *Res Nurs Health.* 2001;24(4):270–282.

21. Landenburger KM. A process of entrapment in and recovery from an abusive relationship. *Issues Ment Health Nurs.* 1989;10:209–227.

22. Lempert LB. Women's strategies for survival: Developing agency in abusive relationships. *J Fam Violence.* 1996;11:269–290.

23. Ulrich Y. What helped most in leaving spouse abuse: Implications for interventions. In: Campbell J, ed. *AWHONN'S clinical issues in perinatal and women's health nursing.* Philadelphia: Lippincott;1994: 385–390.

24. Belknap RA. Sense of self: Voices of separation and connection in women who have experienced abuse. *Can J Nurs Res.* 2002;33:139–153.

25. Draucker CB. Narrative therapy for women who have lived with violence. *Arch Psychiatr Nurs.* 2000;12:162–168.

26. Draucker CB, Madsen C. Women dwelling with violence. *Image J Nurs Sch.* 1999;31:327–332.

27. Ulrich Y, Torres S, Price-Lea P, et al. Postpartum mothers: Disclosure of abuse, role, and conflict. *Health Care Women Int.* 2006;27:1–20.

28. Landenburger KM. Exploration of women's identity: Clinical approaches with abused women. In: Campbell J, ed. *Empowering survivors of abuse: Health care for battered women and their children.* Thousand Oaks, CA: Sage Publications; 1998:61–69.

29. Merritt-Gray M, Wuest J. Counteracting abuse and breaking free: The process of leaving revealed through women's voices. *Health Care Women Int.* 1995;16: 399–412.

30. Campbell JC, Soeken, K. Women's response to battering over time: An analysis of change. *J Interpers Violence.* 1999;14(1):21–40.

31. Draucker CB. Impact of violence in the lives of women: Restriction and resolve. *Issues Ment Health Nurs.* 1997;18:559–586.

32. Wuest J, Merritt-Gray M. Not going back: Sustaining the separation in the process of leaving abusive relationships. *Violence Women.* 1999;5(2):110–133.

33. Langford DR. Developing a safety protocol in qualitative research involving battered women. *Qual Health Res.* 2000;10:133–142.

34. Bowker LH. *Beating wife-beating.* Lexington, MA: Lexington Books, 1983.

35. Ulrich Y. Women's reasons for leaving abusive spouses. *Women Health Care Int.* 1991;12:465–473.

36. Langford DR. Predicting unpredictability: A model of women's processes of predicting battering men's violence. *Schol Inq Nurs Pract.* 1996;10:371–385.

37. Belknap RA. Why did she do that? Issues of moral conflict in battered women's decision making. *Issues Ment Health Nurs.* 1999;20:387–404.

38. Mos VA, Pitula CR, Campbell JC, Halstead L. The experience of terminating an abusive relationship from an Anglo and African American perspective: A qualitative descriptive study. *Issues Ment Health Nurs.* 1997;18:433–454.

39. Wuest J, Merritt-Gray M. Beyond survival: Reclaiming self after leaving an abusive male partner. *Can J Nurs Res.* 2001;32(4):79–94.

40. Campbell JC, Miller P, Cardwell MM, Belknap RA. Relationship status of battered women over time. *J Fam Violence.* 1994;9:99–111.

41. Campbell JC, Soeken, K. Women's response to battering over time: An analysis of change. *J Interpers Violence.* 1999;14(1):21–40.

42. Campbell JC, Soeken K. Women's responses to battering: A test of the model. *Res Nurs Health.* 1999;22(1):49–58.

43. Campbell JC, O'Sullivan C, Roehl J, Webster DW. Intimate Partner Violence Risk Assessment Validation Study: The RAVE Study. Final Report to the National Institute of Justice. 2005. NCJ 209731–209732. At http://www.ncjrs.org/pdffiles1/nij/grants/209731.pdf. Accessed 11/04/2008.

44. Goodman L, Dutton MA, Vankos N, Weinfurt, K. Women's resources and use of strategies as risk and protective factors for reabuse over time. *Violence Women.* 2005;11(3):311–336.

45. Counts DA, Brown JK, Campbell JC. *To have and to hit: Cultural perspectives on wife beating.* Chicago, IL: University of Illinois Press, 1999.

46. Carrillo J, Tello J. *Family violence and men of color.* New York, NY: Springer, 1998.

47. Williams OJ. Developing an African American perspective to reduce spouse abuse: Considerations for community action. *Black Caucus: Journal of the National Association of Black Social Workers.* 1993;1:1–8.

48. Few A, Bell-Scott P. Grounding our feet and hearts: Black women's coping strategies in

psychologically abusive dating relationships. In: West CM, ed. *Violence in the lives of black women: Battered black and blue*. New York: Haworth Press; 2002:59–78.

49. Bent-Goodley T. Eradicating domestic violence in the African American community. *Trauma Violence Abuse*. 2001;2(4):316–330.

50. O'Campo P, McDonnell KA, Gielen AC, et al. Surviving physical and sexual abuse: What helps low-income women? *J Patient Educ Counsel*. 2002;46: 205–212.

51. Dimmitt J, Davila YR. Group psychotherapy for abused women: A survivor-group prototype. *Appl Nurs Res*. 1995;8(1):3–7.

52. Perilla JL. Domestic violence as a human rights issue: The case of immigrant Latinos. *Hispanic J Behavior Sci*. 1999;21:107–133.

53. Atkinson J. *Trauma trails recreating song lines: The transgenerational effects of trauma in indigenous Australia*. North Melbourne, Victoria: Spinifex Press, 2002.

54. Rose L, Campbell JC, Kub J. Role of social support & family relationships in women's response to battering. *Health Care Women Int*. 2000;21: 27–39.

55. Gielen AC, Fogarty L, O'Campo P, et al. Women living with HIV: Disclosure, violence, and social support. *J Urban Health*. 2000;77:480–490.

56. Golding JM. Intimate partner violence as a risk factor for mental disorders: A meta-analysis. *J Fam Violence*. 1999;14:99–132.

57. Essex M, Klein M, Cho E, Kalin N. Maternal stress beginning in infancy may sensitize children to later stress exposure: Effects on cortisol and behavior. *Biol Psychiatry*. 2002;52:773.

58. Ostberg M. Parental stress, psychosocial problems and responsiveness in help-seeking parents with small (2–45 months old) children. *Acta Paediatr*. 1998;87:69–76.

59. O'Connor TG, Heron J, Golding J, Beveridge M. Maternal antenatal anxiety and children's behavioural/emotional problems at 4 years: Report from the Avon Longitudinal Study of Parents and Children. *Br J Psychiatry*. 2002;180:502–508.

60. Meyer EC, Coll CT, Lester BM, et al. Family-based intervention improves maternal psychological well-being and feeding interaction of preterm infants. *Pediatrics*. 1994;93:241–246.

61. Anderson DK, Saunders DG, Yoshihama M, et al. Long-term trends in depression among women separated from abusive partners. *Violence Women*. 2003;9(7):807–838.

62. Campbell R, Sullivan CM, Davidson WS. Women who use domestic violence shelters: Changes in depression over time. *Psychol Women Q*. 1995; 19:237–255.

63. O'Campo P, Kub J, Woods A, et al. Depression, PTSD and co-morbidity related to intimate partner violence in civilian and military women. *Brief Treat Crisis Interv*. 2006;6:99–110.

64. Nixon R, Resick PA, Nishith P. An exploration of comorbid depression among female victims of intimate partner violence with posttraumatic stress disorder. *J Affect Disord*. 2004;82:315–320.

65. Woods AB, Page GG, O'Campo P, et al. The mediation effect of posttraumatic stress disorder symptoms on the relationship of intimate partner violence and IFN- levels. *Am J Community Psychol*. 2005;36(1/2):159–175.

66. Silva RR, Alpert M, Munoz DM, et al. Stress and vulnerability to posttraumatic stress disorder in children and adolescents. *Am J Psychiatry*. 2000;157: 1229–1235.

67. Sullivan CM, Nguyen H, Allen NE, et al. Beyond searching for deficits: Evidence that physically and emotional abused women are nurturing parents. *J Emotional Abuse*. 2000;2(1):51–70.

68. Casanueva C, Martin SL. *Mother-infant interaction among abused women*. Portsmouth, NH: International Family Violence Conference, 2003.

69. Levendosky AA, Graham-Bermann SA. Parenting in battered women: The effects of domestic violence on women and their children. *J Fam Violence*. 2001;16:171–192.

70. Salzinger S, Feldman RS, Ng-Mak DS, et al. Effects of partner violence and physical child abuse on child behavior: A study of abused and comparison children. *J Fam Violence*. 2002;17(1): 23–52.

71. Humphreys JC. The work of worrying: Battered women and their children. *Sch Inq Nurs Pract*. 1995;9(2):126–145.

72. Buchbinder E, Eisikovits Z. Reporting bad results: The ethical responsibility of presenting abused women's parenting practices in a negative light. *Child Fam Social Work*. 2004;9(4):359–367.

73. Berman H. Health in the aftermath of violence: A critical narrative study of children of war and children of battered women. *Can J Nurs Res*. 1999;31(3):89–109.

74. Sharps P, Price-Lea P. *Passport to health reducing violence related health disparities*. American Public Health Association Annual Meeting, 2004.

75. McFarlane J, Soeken K. Weight change of infants, age birth to 12 months, born to abused women. *J Pediatr Nurs*. 1999;25:19–23.

76. Schechter S, Edleson JL. *Effective intervention in domestic violence and child maltreatment cases: Guidelines for policy and practice*. Reno, Nevada: National Council of Juvenile and Family Court Judges, 1999.

77. Onyskiw, JE. Domestic violence and children's adjustment: A review of research. *J Emotional Abuse*. 2003;3(1/2):11–45.

78. Osofsky JD. Prevalence of children exposed to domestic violence and child maltreatment: Implications

for prevention and intervention. *Clin Child Fam Psychol Rev.* 2003;6:161–170.

79. Wolfe DA, Crooks C, Lee V, et al. The effect of children's exposure to domestic violence: A meta-analysis and critique. *Clin Child Fam Psychol Rev.* 2003;6:171–187.

80. Socolar RRS. Domestic violence and children: A review. *N C Med J.* 2000;61:279–283.

81. Koenen KC, Moffitt TE, Caspi A, et al. Domestic violence is associated with environmental suppression of IQ in young children. *Dev Psychopathol.* 2003;15:1–15.

82. Wright RJ, Mitchell H, Visness CM, et al. Community violence and asthma morbidity: The inner-city asthma study. *Am J Public Health.* 2004;94:625–632.

83. Cunningham S. The joint contribution of experiencing and witnessing violence during childhood on child abuse in the parent role. *J Emotional Abuse.* 2003;3:619–641.

84. Humphreys JC, Lee K, Neylan T, Marmar CR. Sleep patterns of sheltered battered women. *J Nurs Scholarsh.* 1999;31:139–143.

85. Whitfield CL, Anda RF, Dube SR, Felitti VJ. Violent childhood experiences and the risk of intimate partner violence in adults: Assessment in a large health maintenance organization. *J Interpers Violence.* 2003;18:166–185.

86. Solomon EP, Heide KM. The biology of trauma: Implications for treatment. *J Interpers Violence.* 2005;20(1):51–60.

87. Janssen PA, Nicholls TL, Kumar RA, et al. Of mice and men: Will the intersection of social science and genetics create new approaches for intimate partner violence? *J Interpers Violence.* 2005; 20(1):61–71.

88. Margolin G. Children's exposure to violence: Exploring developmental pathways to diverse outcomes. *J Interpers Violence.* 2005;20(1):72–81.

89. Mohr WR, Noone Lutz MJ, Fantuzzo JW, Perry MA. Children exposed to family violence: A review of empirical research from a developmental-ecological perspective. *Trauma Violence Abuse.* 2000; 1:264–283.

90. Finkelhor D, Wolak J. Reporting assaults against juveniles to the police: Barriers and catalysts. *J Interpers Violence.* 2003;18:103–128.

91. Kerig PK, Fedorowicz AE, Brown CA, et al. When warriors are worriers: Gender and children's coping with interparental violence. *J Emotional Abuse.* 1998;1:89–115.

92. Kernic MA, Wolf ME, Holt VL, et al. Behavioral problems among children whose mothers are abused by an intimate partner. *Child Abuse Negl.* 2003;27:1231–1246.

93. Margolin G., Gordis E., Medina, AM, Oliver P. Co-occurrence of husband-to-wife aggression, family-of-origin aggression, and child abuse potential in a community sample: Implications for parenting. *J Interpers Violence.* 2003;8(4): 413–440.

94. Hughes H, Luke DA. Heterogeneity in adjustment among children of battered women. In: Holden G, Geffner R, Jouriles E, eds. *Children exposed to family violence: Theory, research, and applied issues.* Washington, DC: American Psychological Association;1998;185–221.

95. Hughes HH, Graham-Bermann SA, Gruber G. Resilience in children exposed to domestic violence. In: Graham-Bermann S, Edleson JL, eds. *Domestic violence in the lives of children.* Washington, DC: American Psychological Association, 1990.

96. Nader K, Pynoos R, Fairbanks L, Frederick C. Children's PTSD reactions one year after a sniper attack at their school. *Am J Psychiatry.* 1990;147(11): 1526–1530.

97. Rossman BB, Bingham RD, Emde RN. Symptomatology and adaptive functioning for children exposed to normative stressors, dog attack, and parental violence. *Am Acad Child Adolesc Psychiatry.* 1997;36:1089–1097.

98. Graham-Bermann SA, Brescoll V. Gender, power, and violence: Assessing the family stereotypes of the children of batterers. *J Fam Psychol.* 2000; 14:600–612.

99. Klein E, Campbell JC, Soler E, Ghez M. *Ending domestic violence: Changing public perceptions.* Newbury Park, CA: Sage, 1997.

100. Yonas MA, Fredland N, Lary H, et al. An arts based initiative for the prevention of dating violence in African American adolescents: Theoretical foundation, program components and lessons learned. In: Jones L, Whitaker D, Shelley G, eds. *Centers for Disease Control and Prevention Monograph.* Atlanta, GA: CDC, 2007.

101. Campbell JC. A survivor group for battered women. *Adv Nurs Sci.* 1986;8(2):13–20.

102. Sullivan CM, Bybee DI. Reducing violence using community-based advocacy for women with abusive partners. *J Consult Clin Psychol.* 1999;67:43–53.

103. Dutton MA. *Empowering and healing the battered women.* New York: Springer, 1992.

104. Parker B, McFarlane J, Soeken K, et al. Testing an intervention to prevent further abuse to pregnant women. *Res Nurs Health.* 1999;22:59–66.

105. Dienemann JA, Campbell JC, Landenburger KM, Curry MA. The domestic violence survivor assessment: A tool for counseling women in intimate partner violence relationships. *J Emotional Abuse.* 2002;46:221–228.

106. Chalk R, King PA. *Violence in families: Assessing prevention and treatment programs.* Washington, DC: National Academy Press, 1998.

107. Olds DL, Hill P, Robinson J, et al. Update on home visiting for pregnant women and parents of young children. *Curr Probl Pediatr Adolesc Health Care.* 2000;30:107–141.

108. Cole R, Kitzman H, Olds D, Sidora K. Family context as a moderator of program effects in prenatal and early childhood home visitation. *Am J Community Psychol.* 1998;26(1):37–48.

109. Olds DL, Eckenrode J, Henderson CR, et al. Long-term effects of home visitation on maternal life course and child abuse and neglect: Fifteen-year follow-up of a randomized trial. *JAMA*. 1997;278:637–643.

110. Olds DL, Robinson J, Pettitt L, et al. Effects of home visits by paraprofessionals and by nurses: Age 4 follow-up results of a randomized trial. *Pediatrics*. 2004; 114:1560–1568.

111. Olds DL, Kitzman H, Cole R, et al. Effects of nurse home-visiting on maternal life course and child development: Age 6 follow-up results of a randomized trial. *Pediatrics*. 2004;114:1550–1559.

Chapter 26

Long-term Healthcare Intervention Models

Therese Zink and Karen Lloyd

KEY CONCEPTS

- Often intimate partner violence (IPV) is nonemergent, and care can be planned over time.
- Self-management by the patient should be encouraged, tailoring interventions to meet the unique needs of victims.
- Community partners must be engaged, and health systems should reach out to define how agencies and the health system can partner to care for victims of IPV.
- The health system's role is to make IPV a priority by setting policies and systems to identify and track IPV, train staff, and measure, monitor, and provide feedback on outcomes.
- New challenges and opportunities include learning to work with new partners, addressing ethical dilemmas, outlining evaluation and research plans, and sorting through the financial implications.

Although intimate partner violence (IPV) is sometimes emergent when the safety of the victim is a concern, it is often a chronic, recurrent, and usually escalating problem (1,2). Therefore, most care for victims is nonemergent. The patient is often not identified as a victim of IPV because of limited assessment and the fact that victims often choose not to disclose their abuse (3). Retrospective chart review demonstrated that approximately half of the women murdered through IPV made visits for general health or mental health problems during the year before they were killed (4). Intimate partner violence perpetrators and the exposed children also seek health care for health and behavioral issues (5–7).

Some researchers have begun to think about the management of both the abuser and the victim of IPV in a *stages of change model* (trans-theoretical model) (8–11). Many primary care clinicians are familiar with this model for helping patients make behavior changes. Most research with the model has been done with smoking cessation and substance abuse treatment (12–15). Five stages of change exist: pre-contemplation, contemplation, preparation, action, and maintenance. In attempting to change a behavior, an individual cycles through the stages, often moving back and forth between contemplation, action, and maintenance (16).

This chapter focuses on the victim. As opposed to smoking cessation or other behavior changes, the victim has no control over the actions of the abuser. Many factors shape the victim's process of managing the abuse. These factors include the victim's income and level of education; whether or not children are involved; whether mental health, physical health, or substance abuse problems are present for the victim and the severity of these problems; and what kind of support network the victim has. Given these factors, the victim does have some control over how she chooses to respond to the abuse. That might include asking for help from an IPV advocate or physician, seeking an order of protection, calling the police, or other strategies.

Guidelines for managing victims of IPV grew out of the emergency medicine literature (17,18). Generally, these recommend screening and identification, safety planning, and referral (19,20). These clinician interventions are generally targeted to victims who have disclosed the abuse and are seeking options to end the abuse, the contemplation stage in the stages of change model. However, many victims seeking health care are not at this stage. Some are unaware that their intimate relationships are abusive—the stage of precontemplation. Others may know that the abuse is a problem but are not ready to disclose the abuse to their healthcare providers (HCPs)—also the contemplation stage (11). The stage of contemplation can last quite long, even years, before the victim decides to take some action to stop the abuse and improve his safety. As a result, the management of IPV victims occurs over extended time. Care guidelines help structure the approach taken by care systems to health conditions, including IPV. Since individuals cycle through the stages of change, moving back and forth between contemplation, action, and maintenance, the use of a common set of guidelines assures that the victim gets appropriate care regardless of changes in personal readiness to change. Consistent approaches across levels of care and among health providers (primary care office, urgent care, emergency, or inpatient) help the victim of IPV have a coherent and additive healthcare experience over time. As discussed in other chapters, IPV victims have a variety of physical and mental health problems and often use healthcare resources frequently, so consistent use of a common set of guidelines and approaches can decrease confusion and support the patient in moving through the stages of change. Use of guidelines can also help HCPs avoid the misconception that behavior change is linear or sequential. "Meeting patients where they are" is foundational to effective health education and coaching. Use of guidelines can also help assure that evidence-based approaches are used with patients who are victims of IPV and that healthcare interventions are supportive, useful, and nonjudgmental.

We need to take action to adopt guidelines and supports to better help healthcare clinicians manage this chronic health issue within health systems and across healthcare organizations. Because of higher utilization, many opportunities may arise in which to plan care that assists both IPV victims and their families (21–23). In this effort, the Institute of Medicine report on family violence calls for the use of systems change models to move beyond education to behavior and practice change within health care (24).

The *planned care model* (PCM), formerly called the chronic care model, includes both evidence-based and best practice to reorganize the system of care to improve the management of chronic illnesses, improve patient outcomes, and reduce healthcare costs (25). Healthcare systems have used the PCM to address chronic illnesses such as congestive heart failure, diabetes, and asthma. Funding organizations have sponsored and continue to encourage research that uses the PCM to address clinical health problems (26–28). Although IPV is not a disease, the PCM may be useful for managing this chronic condition (29).

Figure 26.1 shows Wagner's chronic care model can be adapted for IPV (30). The health system partners with community agencies. Within the health system, clinicians, nonclinicians, and patients are involved in designing and organizing the appropriate system supports. Together the patient (IPV victim) and the practice team (clinicians, nonclinicians, and community agencies) work to better identify and manage IPV. Best practice guidelines address roles for each of the collaborating entities and help shape roles and expectations for referral, communication, and coordination of care.

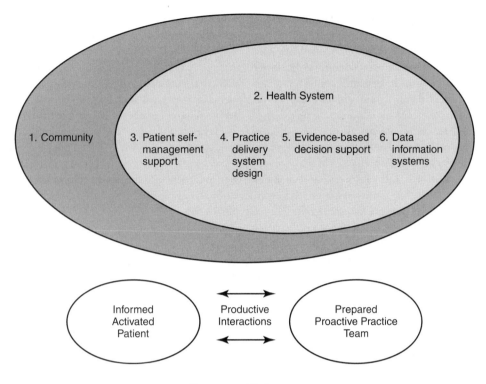

Figure 26.1 Overview of the chronic care model.
From Wager CC Model. Available at www.improvingchroniccare.org/change/model/components.html. Accessed 12/29/2005. *Source:* Zink T, Lloyd K, Isham G, et al. Applying the planned care model to intimate partner violence. *Manage Care.* 2007;16(3):54–61.

COMMUNITY PARTNERS

A number of community agencies provide crucial services for all members of the abusive family—victim, perpetrator, and exposed children—through IPV advocacy services for victims, treatment programs for perpetrators, and services for the exposed children. Clinicians make reports to child and adult protective services when abuse or neglect is a concern. Mental health agencies are often involved in providing care as well. Healthcare systems collaborate with all of these agencies.

Some domestic violence (DV) agencies already provide onsite services in emergency departments and clinics. Advocates from DV agencies are skilled at helping victims address their individual hurdles, have more practical experience, are less expensive, and have more time and interest in assisting IPV victims than clinicians and nurses. Some of these skills may

not be part of the proficiencies for existing healthcare staff, and it may not make sense to add new tasks to the roles of clinicians and nurses. A more efficient and effective approach may be for healthcare systems to cultivate referral and co-management arrangements with community DV agencies.

The health system's role is to make IPV a priority by setting policies and systems to identify and track IPV, train staff, and measure, monitor, and provide feedback on outcomes. Each of the components of PCM is discussed in light of IPV, but first let's discuss the role of the patient.

PATIENT SELF-MANAGEMENT

In PCM, the patient is empowered to participate in his care. For example, with congestive heart failure, the patient is asked to weigh himself daily and to dose diuretics based on the weight, checking in with the clinician if the weight is over a certain limit. Often nurse managers call the patient to monitor his progress. With asthma, an asthma action plan is developed in collaboration with the patient. This plan outlines how the patient doses his inhalers and medications according to his symptoms and when to seek help if symptoms are not improving. Healthcare providers and health systems each have roles in delivering ongoing heath education and coaching. This has become a standard part of health care for some conditions such as diabetes, asthma, or heart failure, and could become the standard for care for victims of IPV.

Historically, DV advocacy has honored the woman's timeline (31). Enhancing the patient's insight into the effect of IPV on health and then assisting the patient/victim in decision making in a way that honors her unique situation is important. This can be done in the healthcare setting, at the health plan level through case managers, at the advocacy agency, or at the worksite through employee assistance programs. Ideally, there should be support in each of these settings, so that the patient/victim has a number of opportunities to interact with knowledgeable others. The unique barriers for each patient, such as fear of losing the children, religious or cultural mores, or financial challenges should be identified (31). Victims have individual timelines and processes about how they want and are able to manage the abuse, given the realities of their abusers and their lives. Clinicians and case managers will need training about how to withhold judgment regarding the choices a patient/victim makes. Healthcare clinicians are notorious for trying to "fix" a problem, and often blame the victim for continuing to tolerate the abuse (32). Considering Prochaska's readiness to change behavior process may be a helpful approach (11). Scales for measuring a patient's activation have been developed (33). Standardized educational materials and resource guides should be assembled, but will need to be modified and interpreted for the unique challenges and needs of each victim/patient (e.g., education level, non-English speaking, gender). Managing IPV does not have a one-size-fits-all response.

Recent efforts have also focused on "harm reduction," helping the victim to define a set of practical strategies that reduce the negative consequences of the victim's survival and coping mechanisms (34). This approach avoids judging the victim's less helpful coping mechanisms, such as continued contact with the perpetrator, misusing alcohol, or survival sex. This creates a larger pool of options the victim can choose from, rather than narrowing them down through "paternalistic guidance" (34). "Harm reduction" is a philosophy first developed by people organizing against human immunodeficiency virus (HIV)/acquired immune deficiency syndrome (AIDS) crisis and other health issues among injection drug users. This approach acknowledged that drug use may not cease, but the development of certain practical strategies could reduce the negative consequences of drug use (35). Needle exchange programs are based on this philosophy.

PRACTICE DESIGN

Designing policies and systems within the healthcare system to support the planned and ongoing efforts of a healthcare team managing the patient is essential to PCM. Systems should be designed to identify IPV victims, stratify the victim's degree of risk (low/moderate/high), and coordinate care.

Screening should be encouraged in the setting of primary care clinics, urgent care, emergency department, hospital inpatient admissions, and behavioral health services. Validated questions and tools may be in verbal, written, or electronic formats. Adopting a policy that encourages adolescent or adult patients to be seen alone for some part of the visit will create the privacy needed for inquiring about IPV or other sensitive concerns. This saves the clinician the time of asking the parent, spouse, or friend to leave the room.

At present, less than 10% of clinicians routinely ask about IPV. Training, feedback, and system support does improve clinicians' identification rates (36,37). Efforts to improve and sustain clinician identification are important, but given the high prevalence of IPV, other methods of victim identification are important. Inserting validated screening tools at every opportunity will help to assess the extent of the problem, for example, by asking about IPV during intakes for phone support services such as pregnancy care or health risk assessments. Standardized screening of all patients in case and disease management programs, whether for chemical dependency, chronic pain, asthma, or high utilization should occur. Victims are usually high utilizers of healthcare resources and may already be targeted for medical management interventions. If IPV has not been identified, then an important factor contributing to the condition is not being addressed and health outcomes may not be maximized.

Risk stratification will characterize the unique risks of a victim and prioritize safety and care plans. Healthcare providers and healthcare systems use risk stratification to provide different levels or types of intervention based on the severity of the condition. This approach helps to both individualize treatment for the patient and to use resources, such as the HCP's time, efficiently. Some victims live with low-level verbal abuse that takes an emotional toll. Others are threatened with physical injury or weapons, and are at risk for serious injuries. Many victims minimize the abuse as a way of coping, which can make it difficult to assess the level of risk (38). Since readiness to change varies over time and is based on a series of decisions and experiences, having all parts of the health system prepared to be consistent, useful, and nonjudgmental in response to patients experiencing IPV can actually help move victims from the stage of contemplation toward taking more helpful actions for their own safety and well-being. Stratification based on level of need and level of risk systematizes the care system response to the individual patient's needs. The PCM approach may be unnecessary for some victims (29). Case management may be appropriate for patients who disclose abuse and want help. This might include victims with physical injuries and those who are high utilizers of healthcare resources.

Asking about abuse in itself is not harmful. The patient self-selects how she chooses to respond, but the management of the response is critical. The electronic medical record allows for a variety of algorithms that can walk clinicians through management options. Kaiser Permanente embarked on a collaborative process to develop "smart sets" of electronic prompts based on best practice guidelines for the identification and management of IPV (39). Standardized management referral tools such as these should be available at all points of care, primary care clinicians, inpatient hospitals, emergency and urgent care centers, and to behavioral HCPs. Services should be coordinated across clinical specialties, healthcare system divisions/departments, and with collaborative community agencies. For example, a patient identified as living with IPV in the urgent care area should be added to a confidential registry so that the patient's primary care clinician is aware of the IPV. The patient's participation in services, such as with a social worker, should also be documented in a way that preserves her confidentiality. If her children are seen by a pediatrician, then that physician should also be aware of the home situation.

EVIDENCE-BASED DECISION SUPPORT

Easy access to the expertise necessary to care for patients is essential to PCM. With IPV, validated screening questions, modes of assessment (computer versus verbal versus written tools), and guidelines for identification and referral have been developed (40–48). Despite their availability, only 10% of managed care plans have comprehensive systems for IPV, and only 28% have screening policies or guidelines (49). Research shows that on-site advocacy services in clinics and hospitals increase identification rates and referrals (50,51). Other educational interventions have resulted in a better process of care such as increased rates of provider inquiry, increased patient satisfaction with being asked, and increased case finding (36,37).

Making these decision supports available to clinicians in a systematic way, with ongoing feedback, has proven successful in other PCM approaches for smoking cessation and mammography screening (52). Health systems will need to identify appropriate evidence-based guidelines, develop performance standards, and provide ongoing assessment, feedback, and evaluation of what works and what does not.

Regarding interventions with victims, only a few studies demonstrate improved outcomes (53–55). Assisting victims with obtaining orders of protection decreased the occurrences of abusive incidents (56). Discussing safety behaviors with a nurse helped women to adopt more of these behaviors (57). Post shelter advocacy and counseling improved quality of life, social supports, and increased the depression and self-esteem scores for women, as well as elevated self-worth scores for children (58). Ongoing research will help to identify evidence-based approaches that can be incorporated.

DATA INFORMATION SYSTEMS

Clinical data systems that provide timely, useful data about individual patients and populations of patients are a critical component of PCM. With IPV, data systems should support a confidential patient registry and efforts to audit and provide feedback about identification, referral, communication, and collaboration efforts. Outcome measures and data for internal and external reports should be identified and planned from the outset, to plan for and build reportable data fields within electronic medical records and registries.

After case identification, developing and maintaining a patient registry in a confidential manner is needed for long-term follow-up. Therefore, the registry needs to be protected with the same layers of security that are currently in place to protect patients with HIV, mental health diagnoses, or sexual issues. Routine audits of those accessing the registry need to be extended to the IPV registry to assure that the health provider accessing the record has a "need to know" based on being one of the patient's treatment providers.

Feedback to clinicians might include rates of inquiry about IPV, missed screening opportunities (e.g., a patient with chronic headaches not asked about IPV), assessing the thoroughness of documentation about a patient's injuries or situation, the completeness of the safety assessment, and the patient's activation score and readiness to change. Tracking and comparing groups of patients on various clinicians' caseloads over time can identify those clinicians who are most helpful in supporting healthy behavior change. These clinicians then can be used as teachers and role models for others to help increase comfort and effectiveness among those clinicians who are less skillful in promoting health behavior change.

In addition to supporting communication and referral, electronic health records provide a variety of opportunities for monitoring identified IPV victims. These can contribute to ongoing evaluation efforts to measure what interventions work, and how utilization and costs are affected. External reports might include confidential communications with local advocacy agencies, oversight agencies, or employers. De-identified data can present financial and clinical benefits of the healthcare program for the employer's return on investment, through healthier employees, decreased absenteeism, and better performance. This employer-specific de-identified data can be compared with the developing body of research literature on IPV intervention outcomes to help estimate the positive impacts of IPV interventions on employer-related measures such as workplace productivity and work attendance.

As a result of these efforts, productive interactions should occur between the activated patient and the healthcare team. Employing a PCM approach to manage IPV broadens current approaches, which include clinician-focused screening and referral. This will require adopting guidelines, educating healthcare clinicians and staff, creating practice and documentation support systems, and fostering new partnerships. Since most patients with IPV present with chronic health problems, quality of care may be maximized by coordinating care across the health system and collaborating with local service agencies and worksites. This will stretch the limits of what is already done and present many challenges and opportunities. These include learning to work with new partners, addressing ethical dilemmas, outlining evaluation and research plans, and sorting through the financial implications.

NEW PARTNERS

It is imperative that healthcare systems reach out to their collaborative community partners, the advocacy agencies, and other services such as perpetrator treatment and support for the exposed children. Collaboration with healthcare systems may initially be threatening to some agency staff because of differences in education levels, levels of expertise and experience with IPV, and differing perspectives based on roles. Some advocacy agencies have a grassroots orientation and their advocates are former IPV victims. In addition, agencies keep minimal client records to avoid discovery in court. Discussions between agency staff and patients are not protected by doctor–patient privilege. Mutual data-sharing routines that preserve the patient's safety and confidentiality, but allow the health system to determine needs, outcomes, and quality of care provided will need to be defined. Some clinical settings use grant funding to support the work of advocates from local DV agencies with patients/victims. When funding ends, advocates are added to the clinical payroll because both victims and clinicians benefit from on-site services (59). Advocacy agencies are notoriously strapped for dollars and cannot be expected to fund an advocate within the health system without financial assistance.

Mandatory reporting issues will also need clarification. All states require healthcare professionals to report suspected child abuse or neglect and elder abuse or neglect, but the requirements differ for criminal DV (20,60,61). Teens who experience dating violence may be considered victims of DV or investigated as child abuse cases, and child exposure to IPV may be defined as child abuse or neglect. All of these statutes vary from state to state, so that understanding the local reporting obligations will require collaborative efforts between health care and protective services (62).

Finally, defining what services will be provided to victims, assuring consistency, and deciding how to measure the quality of the care will take work. Services may need to be tailored to the special needs of patients, as discussed in the section on patient self-management. These services may be delivered by advocates, social services, or mental health professionals, and all need to have support in using approaches that respect cultural and ethnic differences of victims of IPV while also applying best practice standards.

ETHICAL DILEMMAS

The PCM approach raises a spectrum of ethical issues that will need to be addressed. These include:

- How is confidentiality assured for the victim when the perpetrator is the financial guarantor through private or third-party payors?
- What are the mandated reporting obligations for IPV, the overlap between witnessing IPV and child abuse/neglect, and the uncertain boundaries between elder abuse/neglect or vulnerable adult and IPV?
- When the client refuses assistance, chooses to live with the abuse—especially if there are safety concerns for the victim or her children—what are a clinician's or healthcare system's obligations?
- What information should be shared, and how should information be communicated between advocacy organizations and the healthcare systems?

PRACTICAL DILEMMAS

For consistent messaging and expectations across systems of care, collaboration at the community level is required. A collaborative approach brings expertise from various fields and perspectives and can help build shared understanding and shared expectations.

Forming and maintaining a community collaborative is difficult and time consuming:

- Will partners rise to meet the challenge of working together to improve outcomes for victims of IPV?
- With limits on time and human and financial resources, community health focus areas need to be prioritized. How can IPV be added to the issues of interest among the community's health organizations?
- How will IPV as a topic fare when compared to other pressing community health needs like mental health, substance abuse, or teen pregnancy?
- How can models be developed and implemented to test the impact of shared evidence-based approaches, mutually agreed upon roles, and shared performance expectation?
- When found, how can effective models of collaboration to improve IPV outcomes be spread to other healthcare and community organizations?
- How can effective models, when found, be created to be adaptable enough to allow for varying state statutes, county-based policies, and judicial district interpretations and precedents, so that the model can be adoptable (with modifications) in nearly any locale?

EVALUATION AND RESEARCH PLANS

Because of the complexity of IPV and limited evidence about what interventions work for IPV (53–55), multifactorial and multilevel approaches that tackle the challenges of preserving confidentiality, safety, and ensuring follow-up are needed (29). Evaluation efforts will require outcomes measures that cross systems, with some data analysis based on aggregated group outcomes and other analysis based on longitudinal outcomes of individuals across systems. Lessons from using these outcomes will provide the opportunity to figure out what works and what does not, and can lead to adjustments with the ultimate goal of improved quality of care. This will require the creative planning and problem solving that has been necessary for constructing management programs for depression (63–66).

Measures based on management protocols might include the percent of patients screened for IPV in various settings, such as primary care, behavioral health, or urgent/emergency department care; or the percent of patients who receive a defined intervention such as the "Five A's,"—ask, assess, advise, assist, and arrange (67). Management and outcome measures must be tailored to individual patients. Leaving the abuser may not be an option or the current goal; nor does leaving mean that the abuse will stop. Outcomes might include the adoption of safety behaviors, securing an order of protection, decreased numbers of pain medications, improved scores on depression scales, increased stability as evidenced by fewer emergency department visits, decreased primary care visits, and decreased medical utilization. Setting goals (clinical and financial) based on the current state of knowledge is important. Ongoing evaluation can guide readjustment of strategies and goals as experience and knowledge grow.

Patient satisfaction about the system's efforts to identify and manage IPV should also be measured. Kaiser has done this for the last 2 years and reports that patients' satisfaction with their overall care is linked to efforts to assess for IPV (50,68).

Health employer data and information set (HEDIS) measures have driven healthcare system compliance in areas of immunizations, mammogram screening, and hemoglobin A1C measures for diabetics and depression management (69). In the future, HEDIS process of care measures for family violence may stimulate the efforts of healthcare systems to address violence and its burden on related healthcare conditions (69).

There will be many opportunities for research, such as determining the most effective curriculums and methods for training clinicians and staff in using consistent, useful, and nonjudgmental approaches that result in behavior change (i.e., assessing for IPV) (24); and determining the effectiveness of interventions for victims in terms of improved lifetime health status, health utilization, health costs, and the preservation of safety and security (2). The strategies to conduct this type of research will likely not be individual randomized control trials (70,71). Experts point out that sometimes randomization is not feasible or ethical in population-based research, and other study designs are necessary (70–72). Randomized trials are encouraged, where they can be done, and may answer specific interventional components, but the emphasis should be on the longitudinal evaluation of multifactorial and multilevel interventions that integrate care.

FINANCIAL IMPLICATIONS

Financial implications are largely uncharted, and return on investment (ROI) analysis must be innovative. Return on investment issues are important to employer groups and health insurers. Unlike PCM for diabetes, IPV needs to assess both direct (the direct cost of medical services covered by insurance) and indirect costs (the costs of employment productivity changes) and savings. These have been mapped with the treatment of depression and alcohol use disorders (63,73).

As with other initiatives, like breast cancer screening and smoking cessation, costs may initially increase because of pent-up demand and/or impeded access to care (74,75). However, it is also logical that care received after the initiation of the PCM would be "more appropriate" health care. For example, treating migraines without identifying IPV may result in less benefit to the overall health status; treating headaches and discussing safety is more comprehensive.

Since the literature shows IPV to adversely impact entire families, it might be useful to think of the family as the unit of analysis for ROI to evaluate the effectiveness of PCM for IPV (76,77). It is possible that aggregated health claims for current costs for the family may be impacted by an IPV PCM approach. Likewise, longitudinal analysis of the impact of early exposure to IPV on later healthcare costs may reveal that children exposed to IPV have different healthcare patterns or costs as adults.

The indirect costs and benefits of the program need to be quantified or estimated. The negative impact of IPV on work productivity, missed workdays or days of disability, job retention, career advancement, and educational achievement have been documented, but the degree to which these improve with a PCM approach needs to be assessed to fully evaluate the effectiveness of such a program (78–80). The HEDIS cost calculators, including one for depression, are based on research and include both direct and indirect savings that compare the impact of treating depression appropriately. An alcohol use disorders cost calculator has also been developed based on research findings (73).

Some of the services necessary for managing IPV are largely uncovered by medical dollars and are funded by the public sector (i.e., victims' advocacy, services, support groups, batterers' programs) or out of pocket. Health systems do not need to assume these costs, but will need to work with local agencies to assure that appropriate services are available for IPV victims and their families. Health systems do provide reimbursement for covered medical and behavioral health services, some of which may tend to be avoided by victims of IPV. However, these may be more acceptable when they are integrated into a comprehensive plan of care like PCM.

Despite the challenges of approaching IPV victims using PCM, quality of care may be greatly improved and resources better utilized with a care team approach across systems that involves both community agencies and worksite initiatives. It probably makes sense to start with a demonstration project in one department, make adjustments from the lessons learned, and then continue with a slow "roll out." Adapting PCM for IPV victims will require the sustained commitment of a few healthcare systems to work through the challenges. However, these efforts can move the field forward and provide improved quality of care, with better utilization of resources that tap the expertise of community partners in addressing this grave social problem.

IMPLICATIONS FOR POLICY, PRACTICE, AND RESEARCH

Policy

- It is imperative to determine how confidentiality is assured for the victim when private information is shared across departments, and between the health system and advocacy agencies.
- The mandated reporting obligations for IPV for clinicians, the overlap between witnessing IPV and child abuse/neglect, and the uncertain boundaries between elder abuse/neglect or vulnerable adult and IPV must be determined, as well as how advocacy agencies, child and adult protective services, and health systems work to define these obligations.

Practice

- When the client refuses assistance and chooses to live with the abuse, especially if there are safety concerns for the victim or her children, a clinician's or care system's obligations must be determined.

Research

- Process and outcome measures are needed to evaluate efforts across health system departments and between health systems and community agencies.
- The ROI for interventions must be defined and measured.

References

1. Chamberlain L. The USPSTF recommendations on intimate partner violence: What we can learn from it and what we can do about it. *Fam Violence Prev Health Pract.* 2005;1. At http://endabuse.org/health/ejournal/. Accessed 2/21/2008.
2. American Medical Association Council on Scientific Affairs. *Report 7 of the council on scientific affairs (A-05): Diagnosis and management of family violence.* June, 2005.
3. American Medical Association. AMA data on violence between intimates (I-00): CSA *report 7 at the 2000 AMA interim meeting. www.ama-assn. org/ama1/pub/upload/mm/443/csai-00.pdf+ama+ 2000+interim+meeeting&hl=en&ct=clnk&cd= 1&gl=us*
4. Campbell JC, Webster D, Koziol-McLain J, et al. Risk factors for femicide in abusive relationships: Results from a multisite case control study. *Am J Public Health.* 2003;93:1089–1096.
5. Sharps P, Koziol-McLain J, Campbell J, et al. Health care providers' missed opportunities for preventing femicide. *Prev Med.* 2001;33:373–380.
6. Onyskiw J. Health and use of health services of children exposed to violence in their families. *Can J Public Health.* 2002;93:416–420.
7. English D, Marshall D, Stewart A. Effects of family violence on child behavior and health during early childhood. *J Fam Violence.* 2003;18:43–57.
8. Burke J, Gielen A, McDonnell K, et al. The process of ending abuse in intimate relationships. *Violence Against Women.* 2001;7:1144–1163.
9. Frasier PY, Slatt L, Kowlowitz V, Glowa PT. Using the stages of change model to counsel victims of intimate partner violence. *Patient Educ Couns.* 2001;43:211–217.
10. Brown J. Working toward freedom from violence: The process of change in battered women. *Violence Against Women.* 1997;3:5–26.
11. Zink T, Elder N, Jacobson J. Medical management of intimate partner violence considering the stages of change: Precontemplation and contemplation. *Ann Fam Med.* 2004;2:231–239.
12. DiClemente CC. Changing addictive behaviors: A process perspective. *Curr Dir Psychol Sci.* 1993;2:101–106.

13. Prochaska JO, Velicer WF, Rossi JS, et al. Stages of change and decisional balance for 12 problem behaviors. *Health Psychol.* 1994;13:39–46.

14. Riemsma RP, Pattenden J, Bridle C, et al. Systematic review of the effectiveness of stage based interventions to promote smoking cessation. *BMJ.* 2003;326:1175–1177.

15. Brown VB, Melchior LA, Panter AT, et al. Women's steps of change and entry into drug abuse treatment: A multidimensional stages of change model. *J Subst Abuse.* 2000;18:231–240.

16. Prochaska JO, DiClemente CC, Norcross JC. In search of how people change: Applications to addictive behaviors. *Am Psychol.* 1992;47:1102–1114.

17. McLeer S, Anwar R. The role of the emergency physician in the prevention of domestic violence. *Ann Emerg Med.* 1987;16:1155–1161.

18. McLeer S, Anwar R. A study of battered women presenting in an emergency department. *Am J Public Health.* 1989;79:65–66.

19. Flitcraft A, Hadley S, Hendricks-Matthews M, et al. American medical association and treatment guidelines on domestic violence. *Arch Family Medicine.* 1992;1:39–47.

20. Family Violence Prevention Fund. National consensus guidelines on identifying and responding to domestic violence victimization in the health care setting. 2006. At http://store.yahoo.com/fvpfstore/healpractool.html. Accessed 1/20/2006.

21. Ulrich Y, Cain K, Sugg N, Rivara F, et al. Medical care utilization patterns in women with diagnosed domestic violence. *Am J Prev Med.* 2003;24:9–15.

22. Henning K, Klesges L. Utilization of counseling and supportive services by female victims of domestic abuse. *Violence Vict.* 2002;17:623–636.

23. Wisner C, Gilmer T, Saltzman L, Zink T. Intimate partner violence against women: Do victims cost health plans more? *J Fam Pract.* 1999;48:439–443.

24. Institute of Medicine. *Confronting chronic neglect: The education and training of health professionals on family violence.* Washington, DC: National Academy Press, 2002.

25. Bodenheimer T, Wagner EH, Grumbach K. Improving primary care for patients with chronic illness: The chronic care model, Part 2. *JAMA.* 2002;288:1909–1914.

26. Stanton MW, Dougherty D. *Chronic care for low-income children with asthma: Strategies for improvement.* (Issue 18. AHRQ Publication No. 05–0073). Rockville, MD: Agency for Healthcare Research and Quality, June 2005.

27. Institute for Health Care Improvement. Planned care. At http://www.ihi.org/IHI/Topics/OfficePractices/PlannedCare/. Accessed 12/29/2005.

28. Piepoli MF, Villani GQ, Aschieri D, et al. Multidisciplinary and multisetting team management program in heart failure patients affects hospitalization and costing. *Int J Cardiol.* 2006;111:377–385.

29. Nicolaidis C, Touhouliotis V. Addressing intimate partner violence in primary care: Lessons from chronic illness management. *Violence Vict.* 2006;21:101–115.

30. Zink TM, LLoyd K, Isham G, et al. Applying the planned care model to intimate partner violence. *Manag Care.* 2007;March:54–61.

31. Davies J, Lyon E, Monti-Catania D. *Safety planning with battered women.* Thousand Oaks CA: SAGE Publications, Inc., 1998.

32. Minsky-Kelly D, Hamberger KL, Pape DA, Wolff M. We've had training, now what? Qualitative analysis of barriers to domestic violence screening and referral in a health care setting. *J Interpers Violence.* 2005;20:1288–1309.

33. Hibbard J, Mahoney E, Stockard J, Tusler M. Development and testing of a short form of the patient activation measure. *Health Serv Res.* 2005;40:1918–1930.

34. Shlonsky A, Friend C, Lambert L. From culture clash to new possibilities: A harm reduction approach to family violence and child protection services. *Brief Treat Crisis Interv.* 2007;7:345–363.

35. Wikepedia, The free encyclopedia. Harm reduction. At http://en.wikipedia.org/wiki/Harm_reduction. Accessed 2/19/2008.

36. Waalen J, Goodwin M, Spitz A, et al. Screening for intimate partner violence by health care providers. *Am J Prev Med.* 2000;19:230–237.

37. Thompson R, Rivara F, Thompson D, et al. Identification and management of domestic violence: A randomized trial. *Am J Prev Med.* 2000;19:253–263.

38. Campbell JC. Helping women understand their risk in situations of intimate partner violence. *J Interpers Violence.* 2004;19:1464–1477.

39. KP HealthConnect: Patient Safety Work Group. *KP HealthConnect domestic violence SmartSet implementation guidebook.* Oakland CA: Kaiser Permanente Northern California, 2005.

40. Feldhaus K, Koziol-McLain J, Amsbury H, et al. Accuracy of 3 brief screening questions for detecting partner violence in the emergency department. *JAMA.* 1997;277:1357–1361.

41. Paranjape A, Liebschutz J. STaT: A three question screen for intimate partner violence. *J Womens Health.* 2003;12:233–240.

42. Peralta R, Fleming M. Screening for intimate partner violence in a primary care setting: The validity of "feeling safe at home" and prevalence results. *J Am Board Fam Pract.* 2003;16:525–532.

43. Sherin K, Sinacore J, Li X, et al. HITS: A short domestic violence screening tool for use in a family practice setting. *Fam Med.* 1998;30:508–512.

44. Smith PH, Earp JA, De Vellis R. Measuring battering: Development of the women's experience with battering (WEB) scale. *Womens Health: Research on Gender Behavior, and Policy.* 1995;1:273–288.

45. Brown J, Lent B, Schmidt G, Sas G. Application of the woman abuse screening tool (WAST) and WAST-short in the family practice setting. *J Fam Pract.* 2000;49:896–903.

46. Institute for Clinical Systems Improvement. Health care guideline: Domestic violence, 2006. At http://www.icsi.org/knowledge/detail. asp?catID=29&itemID=170. Accessed 1/20/2006.

47. Warshaw C, Ganley A. *Improving the health care response to domestic violence: A resource manual for health care providers,* 2nd ed. San Francisco CA: Family Violence Prevention Fund, 1996.

48. American Medical Association. American Medical Association diagnostic and treatment guidelines for domestic violence. *Arch Fam Med.* 1992;1:39–47.

49. The Family Violence Prevention Fund's National Health Resource Center on Domestic Violence. *National survey of managed care organizations.* San Francisco, CA. Family Violence Prevention Fund, August, 1999.

50. McCaw B, Bauer H, Berman W, et al. Women referred for on-site domestic violence services in a managed care organization. *Women Health.* 2002;35:23–40.

51. Short L, Hadley S, Bates B. Assessing the success of the WomanKind program: An integrated model of 24 hour health care response to domestic violence. *Women Health.* 2002;35:101–119.

52. Glasgow RE, Tracy CE, Wagner EH. Does the chronic care model serve also as template for improving prevention? *Milbank Q.* 2001;29: 579–612.

53. Nelson HD, Nygren P, McInerney Y, Klein J. Screening women and elderly adults for family and intimate partner violence: A review of the evidence for the US preventive services task force. *Ann Int Med.* 2004;140:382–386.

54. Wathen C, MacMillan H. Interventions for violence against women: Scientific review. *JAMA.* 2003;289:589–600, E1–E10.

55. Ramsay J, Richardson J, Carter Y, et al. Should health professionals screen women for domestic violence? Systematic review. *BMJ.* 2002;325:314–318.

56. Holt V, Kernic M, Wolf M, Rivara F. Do protection orders affect the likelihood of future partner violence and injury? *Am J Prev Med.* 2003;24:16–21.

57. McFarlane J, Malecha A, Gist J, et al. An intervention to increase safety behaviors of abused women: Results of a randomized clinical trail. *Nurs Res.* 2001;51:347–354.

58. Sullivan C, Bybee D. Reducing violence using community-based advocacy for women with abusive partners. *J Consult Clin Psychol.* 1999;67:43–53.

59. McKibben L, Hauf A, Must A, Roberts E. Role of victims' services in improving intimate partner violence screening by trained maternal and child health-care providers: Boston, Massachusetts, 1994–1995. *JAMA.* 2000;283:1559–1560.

60. Ramsey S, Abrams D. Child abuse and neglect. In: *Children and the law: In a nutshell.* St. Paul: West Group;2001:83–160.

61. Council on Scientific Affairs. Elder abuse and neglect. *JAMA.* 1987;257:966–971.

62. Zink T, Kamine D, Musk L, et al. What are physicians' reporting requirements for children who witness domestic violence (DV)? *Clin Pediatr.* 2004;43:449–460.

63. Rost K, Smity JL, Dickinson M. The effect of improving primary care depression management on employee absenteeism and productivity: A randomized trail. *Med Care.* 2004;42: 1202–1210.

64. Rost K, Nutting P, Smith J, et al. Improving depression outcomes in community primary care practice: A randomized trial of the QUEST intervention, quality enhancement by strategic teaming. *J Gen Intern Med.* 2001;16:143–149.

65. Nutting PA, Rost K, Dickinson M, et al. Barriers to initiating depression treatment in primary care practice. *J Gen Intern Med.* 2002;17: 103–111.

66. Katzelnick DJ, Simon GE, Pearson SD, et al. Randomized trial of a depression management program in high utilizers of medical care. *Arch Fam Med.* 2000;9:345–351.

67. US Public Health Service. Five major steps to intervention (the 5 A's). 2006. At http://www.surgeongeneral.gov/tobacco/5steps.htm. Accessed 1/22/2006.

68. McCaw B, Kotz K. Family violence prevention program: Another way to save a life. *The Permanente Journal.* 2005;9:65–68.

69. Sheehan D, Pesko L, Druss B. Does HEDIS affect compliance, length of therapy, or outcomes? *Manag Care.* 2003;12:13–19.

70. Lachs M. Screening for family violence: What's an evidence-based doctor to do? *Ann Intern Med.* 2004;140:399–400.

71. Zink T, Putnam F. Intimate partner violence research in the health care setting: What are appropriate and feasible methodological standards? *J Interpers Violence.* 2005;20(4):365–372.

72. Briss PA, Zaza S, Pappaioanou M, et al. Developing an evidence-based guide to community preventive services and methods. *Am J Prev Med.* 2000;18:35–43.

73. Ensuring Solutions to Alcohol Problems. Alcohol cost calculator. 2008. At http://www.alcoholcostcalculator.org/. Accessed 2/21/2008.

74. Thompson RS, Barlow WE, Taplin, SH, et al. A population-based case-cohort evaluation of the efficacy of mammographic screening for breast cancer. *Am J Epidemiol.* 1994;140: 889–901.

75. Wagner EH, Curry SJ, Grothaus L, et al. The impact of smoking and quitting on health care use. *Arch Intern Med.* 1995;155:1789–1795.

76. Kitzmann K, Gaylord N, Holt A, Kenny E. Child witness to domestic violence: A meta-analytic review. *J Consult Clin Psychol.* 2003;71:339–352.

77. Coben J, Friedman D. Violence: Recognition, management, and prevention. *J Emerg Med.* 2002;22:313–317.

78. EDK Associates for the Body Shop. *The many faces of domestic violence and its impact on the workplace.* New York: EDK Associates, 1997.

79. US General Accounting Office. Domestic violence prevalence and implications for employment among welfare recipients. Washington DC: Author, 1998:1–26.

80. Kramer FD. Screening and assessment for physical and mental health issues that impact TANF recipients' ability to work. *Welfare Information Network: Issue Notes.* 2001;5(3).

Chapter 27

Developing a Health System Response to Intimate Partner Violence

Brigid McCaw and Krista Kotz

KEY CONCEPTS

- The most successful strategies for improving intimate partner violence (IPV) services draw more on the strength and opportunities available in the healthcare setting as a "system" than on clinician training alone.
- The 2001 Institute of Medicine (IOM) report concluded that available evidence supports a multifaceted "systems change model" approach for IPV identification and management.
- Implementation challenges include coordination *within* the healthcare system, and *between* the healthcare system and community advocacy organizations.
- Quality improvement processes can be used to improve and sustain IPV services and ensure that these become an expected part of everyday care.

The high prevalence and cost of intimate partner violence (IPV), the associated health problems, and the impact on children, are compelling to both healthcare students and clinicians caring for patients. Since women access the health system throughout their lives, for preventive and routine care as well as for abuse-related visits, the healthcare setting can provide a safe and confidential setting for both outreach and early intervention (1–3). Clinical practice guidelines have been developed, and tools for IPV inquiry, assessment, and intervention are available. All this would suggest that an effective response to IPV should be present in most healthcare settings. Why is it, then, that inquiry and intervention for IPV in the healthcare setting is the exception and not the rule?

One reason is that most improvement efforts emphasize education of individual clinicians and overlook the powerful opportunities available in the healthcare environment surrounding clinicians and patients.

Although it is necessary to provide specialized training for clinicians to gain the awareness, knowledge, and skills to talk to patients about IPV, it is unlikely that this alone will yield significant and enduring change until the setting in which they provide patient care makes the clinician's role clear and easier to perform. This chapter describes an approach that draws upon the strength of health care as a system, rather than on clinician training alone.

This is not a new idea. The Institute of Medicine (IOM) report on The Education and Training of Health Care Professionals on Family Violence (4) supports a multifaceted, systems change approach to implementing IPV services, because this approach has the highest success rates (4). Several studies were cited that form the basis of the scientific evidence for using systems change models for improving healthcare services (5–11). Since the publication of the IOM report, additional studies have provided further evidence to support the use of systems change models in the delivery of IPV prevention and intervention services (12–19).

Although this chapter describes effective intervention models for practice settings in large multispecialty healthcare service delivery organizations (both public and private), smaller office-based practices may find the conceptual ideas applicable as well.

COMPONENTS OF A COMPREHENSIVE "SYSTEMS MODEL" APPROACH TO INTIMATE PARTNER VIOLENCE SERVICES

The key components of a health care "systems model" response to IPV are generally agreed upon as (4,20,21):
- *Supportive environment.* Using the entire healthcare setting to increase awareness of IPV, encourage disclosure to healthcare providers, and provide resource information that patients can access directly
- *Identification of IPV and appropriate referral.* Policies and protocols; specialized training; tools for inquiry, assessment, and intervention; and tools that assist the clinician in identifying IPV and referring patients to the appropriate services
- *Services within the healthcare setting.* Appropriate on-site resources provided by mental health or social work clinicians, or a dedicated IPV specialist who has received training and

can provide immediate advocacy services, including assistance with safety planning, danger assessment, and referral to appropriate community resources
- *Linkage to community resources.* Streamlined linkage from the healthcare system to community resources, including advocacy services, such as crisis hotline, shelter, support groups, legal advocacy, law enforcement, and job and career counseling
- *Leadership and oversight.* Management of the implementation and routine evaluation of the program and services, as well as obtaining committed institutional support to ensure program success and sustainability

One way of visualizing these key components is shown in Figure 27.1. This depiction shows how each component is interconnected and necessary for a coordinated healthcare response.

DESCRIPTION OF SELECT MODELS FOR INTIMATE PARTNER VIOLENCE SERVICES AND PREVENTION

In this chapter, four models for IPV prevention in the healthcare setting will be discussed. The models were chosen for discussion because they have been in place for at least 8 years and have some evaluation data.

WomanKind: An Integrated Model of 24-Hour Healthcare Response to Domestic Violence

WomanKind, the first program of its kind in the United States, was implemented in Minneapolis, Minnesota in 1986. This program has been operating successfully for more than 20 years, longer than any other comprehensive systems model for IPV services, education, and prevention. The program's mission is to provide (a) case management/advocacy services to victims of IPV in combination with (b) specialized education and consultation with healthcare providers. On-site resources are available 24 hours a day, 7 days a week and are provided by IPV specialists (mental health and social work clinicians with advanced IPV training). Policies and procedures help to ensure consistent response by health providers throughout the Fairview Health System, a not-for-profit organization serving over 2 million individuals per year. A vital aspect of the program services is the ongoing and follow-up contacts of the WomanKind

Systems Model for Intimate Partner Violence Prevention

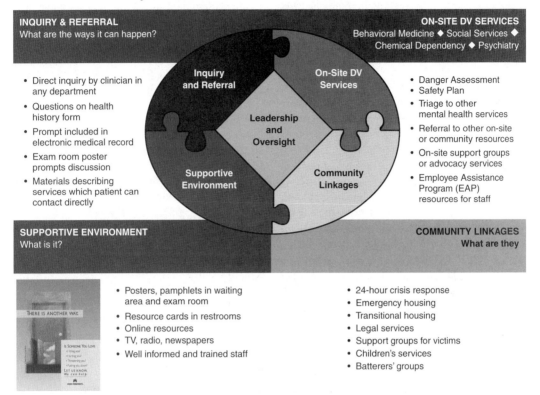

Figure 27.1 Kaiser Permanente "Systems Model" for intimate partner violence prevention.

staff with the patient/client. WomanKind facilitates the client's connection to the most appropriate community resource. Housed within the hospitals and clinics of the Fairview Health System in Minnesota, the vision of the WomanKind program has long been to integrate the issue of IPV into the total health care of each patient. The result is an overall system change in the medical system's response to victims of IPV, so that health providers treat not only the physical condition, but all also address the *underlying causes* of the medical or mental health problem (22–25). The evaluation of the WomanKind Program, conducted by the Centers for Disease Control and Prevention (CDC) in the late 1990s, showed that the "research results provide strong evidence that specialized provider training in combination with on-site client services have a significant, positive impact on the knowledge, attitudes, beliefs and behaviors (KABB) of health providers treating victims of domestic violence." The CDC concluded that the WomanKind program

is a useful model for both inpatient and outpatient healthcare settings (14,26). In a recent editorial in the publication *Contraception*, the Association for Reproductive Health Professionals affirmed the practices of WomanKind, stating "health care professionals can make a difference by screening all of their patients for past and current histories of abuse to effectively treat conditions arising from the violence, as well as conditions impacted by the abuse" (27).

Medical Advocacy Projects of the Pennsylvania Coalition Against Domestic Violence

Since 1993, domestic violence (DV) advocates working with the Pennsylvania Coalition Against Domestic Violence (PCADV) have been housed at many healthcare settings in the state. Medical advocacy is described as the identification of DV victims seeking health care and the provision of support, information, education, resources, and follow-up services within the healthcare setting. Medical advocacy also includes the development, refinement, and implementation of policies and procedures to enhance the healthcare response to victims of IPV, as well as ongoing training of healthcare personnel.

The PCADV provides funding and technical support to programs, which are collaborative efforts between a DV advocacy organization and a healthcare setting. The healthcare settings are predominantly hospitals, but also include community healthcare clinics. Thirty-four of these programs were evaluated using semi-structured interviews and the Delphi Instrument for Hospital-based Domestic Violence Programs (now called Family Violence Quality Assessment Tool, discussed in more detail below) (28). Program implementation was assessed at baseline, and 1 year later. The findings showed that all programs made progress in terms of implementation over 1 year, but that performance varied considerably (both overall and among the specific domains studied). Lessons learned from those most successful in implementation included the necessity of (a) an interdisciplinary IPV task force with the authority to influence hospital policy, (b) a formal training plan for hospital staff, (c) a valid method for screening, (d) a standardized, routinely used, victim safety assessment tool, and (e) standardized intervention checklists.

The PCADV model has also been implemented and evaluated in four rural counties in Pennsylvania. The authors concluded that the PCADV model can be successfully used in a rural setting, despite the access to care and advocacy resources issues that rural communities face (29).

Kaiser Permanente Family Violence Prevention Program, Northern California

Kaiser Permanente Northern California (KPNC) is a large nonprofit health plan serving over 3 million people. Kaiser Permanente provides a unique opportunity for comprehensive IPV services and prevention because the health plan is an integrated health delivery system, providing and coordinating the entire scope of care for its plan members, including outpatient, emergency, and inpatient care, with a strong commitment to prevention. In 1998, KPNC allocated funding to pilot an innovative, "systems model" approach to improving IPV services. This systems model approach consisted of five interrelated components described earlier in this chapter (see Figure 27.1): supportive environment, inquiry and referral, on-site services, community linkages, and leadership and oversight.

The initial goal of the pilot program was to increase clinicians' willingness to inquire about and identify IPV, then provide appropriate referral resources. It was designed to address the clinicians' concern "What do I do if the answer is 'yes?'" Another goal was to evaluate the effectiveness of the systems model approach by looking for evidence of change in clinician practice and change in patient experience.

A pilot program was developed, implemented, and tested at one facility (serving 70,000 members). A pre- and postimplementation evaluation demonstrated a dramatic and statistically significant increase in screening rates, identification, and referral to a mental health clinician. In addition, member satisfaction with the health plan improved, and the approach was well accepted by clinicians (12).

Over the next 3 years, the model was successfully transferred to six more KPNC facilities (serving approximately 350,000 members). Funding for a part-time physician director and project manager was made available to facilitate more efficient implementation across KPNC facilities, to coordinate dissemination of materials, identify best practices, provide consultation to facilities, and develop "infrastructure" tools designed to provide services to all the facilities (such as the appointment and advice call center, access to data systems for quality improvement, and online resources for clinicians) (see Sidebar 27.1). By 2004, implementation was well underway in all KPNC facilities, serving over 3 million members, and IPV identification and referral has continued to increase.

This program has shown continued improvements in identification of patients experiencing IPV from the program's inception in 2000 through 2007 (see Sidebar 27.2). Identification has steadily shifted to less acute settings, such as primary care and mental health, suggesting that patients are being identified earlier, before more potentially serious injury occurs (Figure 27.2) (30). Research associated with this program has also generated additional information on women who experience IPV, including demographics, perceived health status, and their reasons for accepting referrals for follow-up by mental health clinicians (31,32).

Sidebar 27.1: Steps for Implementation of the Kaiser Permanente Model

The first steps in implementation of the program in each facility are the selection of a local MD/ NP Champion and the development of a multidisciplinary IPV Implementation Team. This team develops an interdepartmental referral protocol designed to make referral to resources easy and straightforward for the front-line clinician.

Next, the IPV Implementation Team at each facility identifies local resources that can be used to carry out the key components of the "systems model."

- One example of *"on-site services"* that must be arranged are those for mental health. The mental health clinicians may belong to different departments or they may be part of social service or in psychiatry. The role of these specially trained mental health clinicians is to conduct the in-depth assessment and provide the needed support and information to the patient on the dynamics of IPV, and to guide patients in their decision-making.
- The *"community linkages"* component varies, and examples include a phone that patients can use to contact the National Domestic Violence Hotline, a local agency that can provide shelter or support groups, an emergency response team that can come to the facility and, in a few facilities, an on-site advocate.
- *"Inquiry and referral"* is performed using a variety of methods, such as the routine use of written questionnaires and exam room posters that prompt discussion or direct inquiry by various healthcare team members.

Sidebar 27.2: Quality Improvement Measures in the Kaiser Permanente Model

Two quantitative quality improvement measures are used to provide data to monitor performance over time and between facilities. These measures are also being used to demonstrate implementation of a behavioral health prevention guideline that shows coordination of care between primary care and mental health care to meet a NCQA standard. These are similar to those used to track quality improvement efforts for conditions such as depression:

- Percent of target population identified
- Percent of target population receiving appropriate referral

The measures utilize diagnosis codes from outpatient and emergency department medical visits, which are already entered into an automated database. The "target population" is based on a prevalence estimate of IPV (in the previous 12 months) among women members of the health plan aged 18–64. This estimate is drawn from a survey of health plan members and from published prevalence estimates.

Based on the successful adoption of the systems model approach in the Kaiser Permanente facilities in northern California, the remaining eight Kaiser Permanente Regions (8.7 million members) have been implementing the model since 2006. Electronic tools that facilitate inquiry, assessment, and documentation have been added to the electronic medical record to improve consistency of care. Similar patient education materials have been adopted by all the Regions as well.

Violence Intervention Program, Parkland Hospital, Texas

The Violence Invention Program (VIP) at Parkland Hospital in Dallas, Texas has been in place since 1999. The extensive Parkland Memorial Health and Hospitals System is a major healthcare provider in Dallas County, Texas, with 796 beds and over 40,000 admissions per year. Patients experiencing IPV are referred to the VIP, which then acts as an intermediary between medical providers and community agencies to help with acute needs and to facilitate referrals and follow-up visits. In addition, all rape patients in the county are seen at Parkland Hospital and, by extension, by the VIP team. The VIP Center, funded both publicly and privately, is characterized by the following components:

1. Rapid response by VIP caseworkers available 24 hours a day, 7 days a week. The rapid response includes:
   a. documentation of injuries and events associated with the abuse

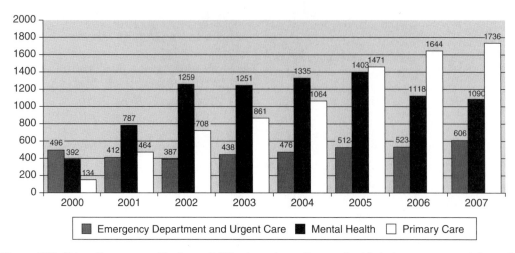

Figure 27.2 Kaiser Permanente Northern California patients diagnosed with intimate partner violence by year and department.

b. safety assessment and plan

c. assessment of need for immediate placement in a shelter, and need for legal intervention.

2. In-depth medical and mental health assessment and evaluation. As a follow-up to the rapid response, staff physicians complete a medical evaluation including a "well-woman" evaluation, crisis counseling intervention, and specific medical treatment and evaluation.

3. Case management and coordination of community services. A case manager with training specific to IPV coordinates outside referrals for services provided by community organizations. Pro bono legal aid is also provided, and victims are offered assistance with their legal cases as well as their medical and mental health problems.

4. Primary care placement. The VIP team works with the victim's primary care physician, or, if the patient does not have a primary care physician, a referral is made to one near the patient's home.

During a 1-year period in 1999–2000, VIP Center staff provided services during 1,274 patient/caseworker contacts and 359 patient/medical provider encounters (33). Emergency medical staff performance has been evaluated, and simple trainings, peer mentoring, and faculty modeling have resulted in sustained institutionalization of the VIP rapid-response referral system. In addition, focus groups have been conducted to evaluate patient preferences for services; the majority of patients consistently ranked having all services under one roof (medical, mental health, and legal) as an optimal arrangement (G.L. Larkin, VIP Medical Director, personal communication). Other ongoing VIP research has suggested that service needs differ by ethnicity, particularly for Hispanics (34).

ASSESSMENT OF HEALTHCARE ORGANIZATIONS' RESPONSE TO INTIMATE PARTNER VIOLENCE

One way to assess how a healthcare organization is responding to IPV from a "systems" perspective is by using a tool developed by the Agency for Healthcare Research and Quality (AHRQ) (21,35). This instrument can be used to assess whether a healthcare facility has in place many of the processes necessary for an effective systems' response to IPV. The categories of processes assessed include:

- Hospital policies and procedures
- Hospital physical environment
- Hospital cultural environment
- Training of providers
- Screening and safety assessment
- Documentation
- Intervention services
- Evaluation activities
- Collaboration

A component is given a weighted score, which can be combined to provide a total assessment of the facility's overall response or serve as benchmarks in tracking implementation or quality improvement efforts. Inter-rater reliability was very high (Kronbach's α ranging from 0.97 to 0.99 in the experienced coders and 0.96 to 0.99 in the inexperienced coders) (21). Guidelines, instructions for use, and interpretation of this tool can be accessed online through the AHRQ. Since its release in 2002, it has been used successfully in several healthcare settings in the United States and abroad, including in the evaluation of the PCADV model discussed earlier (29,36). In addition, the tool has been modified for use in primary care and tested in 32 medical practices (37).

IMPLEMENTATION CHALLENGES OF A "SYSTEMS MODEL" APPROACH

Incorporating new services, technologies, and therapies is a constant feature in health care. In addition to the usual challenges that accompany the introduction of something new, several aspects of implementing a coordinated approach to IPV pose unique challenges for most healthcare settings. These include the need for:

- Representation from and coordination between healthcare workers from multiple disciplines across multiple departments
- Establishing linkages and collaborating with community agencies
- Ongoing commitment and support of leadership within the healthcare institution
- Ongoing marketing of the program and of the importance of the healthcare response to IPV

According to the Family Violence Prevention Fund's manual on the healthcare response to IPV "a truly effective response requires an interdisciplinary approach involving physicians, nurses, social workers, health educators and other allied health personnel" (20). A variety of health specialties are needed to comprehensively address the health effects of IPV. Examples might include psychiatry to address co-existing depression or posttraumatic stress disorder; social services to link victims to safe housing, legal advocacy, and crisis counseling; orthopedics to address musculoskeletal injuries; and obstetrics to address prenatal safety and health. Institutionalizing a multidisciplinary approach ensures that clinicians know that it will be easy to access other members of the health team when a victim of IPV is identified and that, regardless of where a patient with IPV contacts the healthcare system, he/she will encounter an appropriate and welcoming response. This generally requires *representation from multiple departments* (e.g., emergency; mental health services; ambulatory, primary and specialty care; advice and appointment phone services; health education; labor and delivery) on the task force or team that oversees implementation. Representation is the first step toward developing *collaboration between* departments. This is particularly important *between mental and behavioral health clinicians* (such as social services, psychiatry, and chemical dependency services) who may be providing services in different venues with a different focus, perspective, and skill set.

Another challenge, unique to IPV, is *coordination between the healthcare setting and various community agencies and law enforcement.* As previously noted, a key component to the systems model approach is linkages to the community. This often requires a change in thinking by healthcare providers and by community agency staff, who frequently see the clinic or hospital as a self-contained entity. For an issue such as IPV, however, victims may need life-saving interventions (such as shelter and restraining orders), which are appropriately provided outside the healthcare setting and require the expertise of community advocates, law enforcement, and criminal justice. As noted previously, there are several models for effective partnerships. These include participation of the community agencies in the healthcare response implementation team, and/or making available advocates to provide services at the healthcare facility, and/or centers providing comprehensive services at one location (38–40).

Funding for most IPV programs in healthcare settings has been drawn from multiple sources, including grants from philanthropic organizations, and in-kind donations of space, office equipment, and personnel from nursing and social services. In some cases, the hospital may provide a stipend for a medical director. Programs that provide forensic exams may receive funding from law enforcement to provide this service. Those hospitals that have on-site advocacy services may have federal or state funding designated for that purpose (41).

Securing ongoing funding is frequently a challenge. An exception to this is the Kaiser Permanente model, in which institutional resources are allocated to support oversight and development, and coordination of consistent services across multiple facilities. This has facilitated the integration of IPV services into the usual systems of care in the outpatient and inpatient setting, quality improvement programs, Call Center protocols, and clinician training. Intimate partner violence services have been incorporated into the health plan's initiatives to improve efficiency and quality of service, and fulfill the organization's social mission.

As evidence mounts about the high prevalence and long-term healthcare costs associated with IPV (42,43), other health plans may be more inclined to provide consistent funding for IPV services.

In addition to financial resources, sustaining an IPV program beyond the initial enthusiasm requires *institutional support and the sponsorship of top leadership* within the healthcare organization. The importance of the healthcare role in IPV services and prevention must be communicated in an ongoing fashion to healthcare providers, employees, patients, and to community agency staff. To increase the likelihood of institutional support and continued growth of the program, the *successes of the program must be marketed* using quality improvement data and personal stories. This will demonstrate the benefit of IPV services to healthcare organizations, the patients they serve, the community, and healthcare purchasers (44).

USING QUALITY IMPROVEMENT PROCESSES TO SUSTAIN AND IMPROVE IPV PREVENTION SERVICES IN THE HEALTHCARE SETTING

The use of continuous quality improvement (CQI) and PDSA (plan, do study, act) are commonly used processes to improve clinical services, such as mammography screening, counseling for tobacco cessation, and blood pressure control (45). These methods can also serve as a valuable guide for improving IPV services. Some examples of process measures and quantitative measures for IPV are noted below (12,30,46–48):

- Examples of *process* measures include:
  - Agenda and notes from IPV taskforce meetings
  - Formal policies and protocols for IPV
  - Specialized training for clinicians
  - Availability of tools such as screening questionnaires, and intervention and referral protocols
  - Evidence of collaboration with community advocacy agencies
- Examples of *quantitative* measures include:
  - Percent of exam rooms containing patient information materials
  - Percent of patients identified as victims of IPV who have resources offered to them
  - Percent of patients with risk factors who are screened for IPV
  - Percent of charts of IPV victims with appropriate documentation
  - Percent of IPV victims who receive limited advocacy services by IPV specialist within healthcare setting
  - Percent of IPV victims who receive mental health services
  - Estimates of target population and identification rates

The AHRQ Family Violence Quality Assessment Tool described earlier can also be used as a formal assessment of a hospital or medical facility's performance in implementing a IPV program.

CONCLUSION

The systems model is an effective and sustainable method to improve IPV prevention services in the healthcare setting. Each component of the model is necessary: supportive environment, screening and referral, on-site services, community linkages, and leadership and oversight. How a particular healthcare setting chooses to accomplish these components may vary. Implementation challenges include coordination within the healthcare setting (between departments and between mental health disciplines) and coordination between the healthcare setting and community agencies. Quality improvement methods can be used to sustain IPV services and make inquiry and intervention for IPV in health care an expected part of every day care.

IMPLICATIONS FOR POLICY, PRACTICE, AND RESEARCH

Policy

- A systems-based approach supports and enhances individual clinicians and should be seriously considered by all major health organizations.
- Quality improvement measures for IPV monitor and document system and practitioner behavior change.
- Funders of community advocacy resources should encourage tighter linkages with hospitals and healthcare systems.

Practice

- Clinicians must advocate for system changes that facilitate identification and intervention and that benefit both patients and practitioners.
- Institutions can identify experts on their medical staff and provide start-up resources to develop a system response.

Research

- Research organizations should prioritize studies of the effectiveness of interventions in the healthcare setting, using outcomes such as safety, health status, quality-of-life measures, and healthcare utilization.
- Investigative models that compare models and outcomes across institutions would be valuable and could inform future healthcare practice and policy.
- The AHRQ Family Violence Quality Assessment Tool could be linked to outcome measures to determine which components of a health-based system response are most important in creating positive, long-term impact on victims of IPV.

References

1. WHO. *World report on violence and health.* Geneva: World Health Organization, 2002.
2. WHO. WHO *Multi-country study on women's health and domestic violence against women. Summary report.* Geneva: World Health Organization, 2005.
3. Black MC, Breiding MJ. Adverse health conditions and health risk behaviors associated with intimate partner violence: United States, 2005. *MMWR Morb Mortal Wkly Rep.* 2008;57(5):113–117.
4. Cohn F, Salmon M, Stobo J. *Confronting chronic neglect: The education and training of health professionals on family violence.* Washington, DC: Institute of Medicine, 2001.
5. Curry SJ, Kim EL. A public health perspective on addictive behavior change interventions: Conceptual frameworks and guiding principles. In: Tucker JA, Donovan DM, Donovan GA, eds. *Changing addictive behavior: Moving beyond therapy assisted change.* New York: Guilford, 1999.
6. DHHS. *Clinical practice guideline development: Methodology perspectives.* AHCPR Pub. No. 95–0009. Washington, DC: Department of Health and Human Services, Agency for Health Care Policy and Research, 1994.
7. Goodman NW. Who will challenge evidence-based medicine? *J R Coll Physicians Lond.* 1999;33(3): 249–251.
8. Green L, Kreuter M. *Application of PRECEDE/ PROCEED in community settings. Health promotion and planning: An educational and environmental approach.* Mountain View, CA: Mayfield, 1991.
9. Green L, Kreuter M. *Health promotion planning: An educational and ecological approach,* 3rd ed. Mountain View, CA: Mayfield, 1999.
10. Thompson RS. What have HMOs learned about clinical prevention services? An examination of the experience at Group Health Cooperative of Puget Sound. *Milbank Q.* 1996;74(4):469–509.
11. Walsh JM, McPhee SJ. A systems model of clinical preventive care: An analysis of factors influencing patient and physician. *Health Educ Q.* 1992;19(2):157–175.
12. McCaw B, Berman WH, Syme SL, Hunkeler EF. Beyond screening for domestic violence: A systems model approach in a managed care setting. *Am J Prev Med.* 2001;21(3):170–176.
13. Larkin GL, Rolniak S, Hyman KB, et al. Effect of an administrative intervention on rates of screening for domestic violence in an urban emergency department. *Am J Public Health.* 2000;90(9): 1444–1448.
14. Short LM, Hadley SM, Bates B. Assessing the success of the WomanKind program: An integrated model of 24-hour health care response to domestic violence. *Women Health.* 2002;35(2–3): 101–119.
15. Shye D, Feldman V, Hokanson CS, Mullooly JP. Secondary prevention of domestic violence in HMO primary care: Evaluation of alternative implementation strategies. *Am J Manag Care.* 2004;10(10): 706–716.
16. Thompson RS, Rivara FP, Thompson DC, et al. Identification and management of domestic violence: A randomized trial. *Am J Prev Med.* 2000; 19(4):253–263.
17. Campbell JC, Coben JH, McLoughlin E, et al. An evaluation of a system-change training model to

improve emergency department response to battered women. *Acad Emerg Med.* 2001;8(2):131–138.

18. Cole TB. Case management for domestic violence. *JAMA.* 1999;282(6):513–514.

19. McNutt LA, Carlson BE, Rose IM, Robinson DA. Partner violence intervention in the busy primary care environment. *Am J Prev Med.* 2002;22(2):84–91.

20. Warshaw C, Ganley AL. *Improving the health care response to domestic violence: A resource manual for health care providers,* 2nd ed. San Francisco, CA: Family Violence Prevention Fund, 1998.

21. Coben JH. Evaluating Domestic Violence Programs. September, 2002; At http://www.ahrq.gov/research/domesticviol/. Accessed 5/22/2005.

22. Randall T. Hospital-wide program identifies battered women, offers assistance. *JAMA.* 1991;266(9):1177–1179.

23. Hadley SM. Working with battered women in the emergency department: A model program. *J Emerg Nurs.* 1992;18(1):18–23.

24. Hadley SM, Short LM, Lezin N, Zook E. Woman-Kind: An innovative model of health care response to domestic abuse. *Womens Health Issues.* 1995;5(4):189–198.

25. Hadley SM. Linking the orthopaedic patient with community family violence resources. *Orthop Nurs.* 2002;21(5):19–23.

26. Reyes C, Rudman WJ, Hewitt CR. Domestic violence and health care: Policies and prevention. New York: Haworth Press, Inc.;2002:101–119.

27. Alam S, Hadley SM, Jordan B. The clinical implications of screening for violence against women. *Contraception.* 2007;76(4):259–262.

28. Coben JH, Fisher EJ. Evaluating the implementation of hospital-based domestic violence programs. *Fam Violence Prev Health Pract.* 2005;1(2):1–2.

29. Ulbrich PM, Stockdale J. Making family planning clinics an empowerment zone for rural battered women. *Women Health.* 2002;35(2–3):83–100.

30. McCaw B, Kotz K. Family Violence Prevention Program: Another way to save a life. *The Permanente Journal.* 2005;9(1):65–68.

31. McCaw B, Bauer HM, Berman WH, et al. Women referred for on-site domestic violence services in a managed care organization. *Women Health.* 2002;35(2–3):23–40.

32. McCaw B, Golding JM, Farley M, Minkoff JR. Domestic violence and abuse, health status, and social fuctioning. *Women Health.* 2007;45(2):1–23.

33. Taliaferro E, Smith D, Rogers J, Walker S. Violence intervention programs: The Parkland Domestic Violence Project. *Tex Dent J.* 2000;1 17(10):54–58.

34. Lipsky S, Caetano R, Field CA, Larkin GL. The role of intimate partner violence, race, and ethnicity in help-seeking behaviors. *Ethn Health.* 2006;11(1):81–100.

35. Coben JH. Measuring the quality of hospital-based domestic violence programs. *Acad Emerg Med.* 2002;9(11):1176–1183.

36. Kass-Bartelmes B. Women and domestic violence: programs and tools that improve care for victims. AHRQ Pub. No. 04–0055. *Research in Action.* 2004(15).

37. Zink T, Fisher BS. Family violence quality assessment tool for primary care offices. *Qual Manag Health Care.* 2007;16(3):265–279.

38. Guinn C. Dreaming big: Creating justice centers across America: Part 1. *Domestic Violence Report.* Oct/Nov 2004.

39. Guinn C. Dreaming big: Creating justice centers across America: Part 2. *Domestic Violence Report.* Dec/Jan 2005.

40. Hathaway JE. Listening to survivors' voices. *Violence Against Women.* 2002;8(6):687–719.

41. Mitchell C, Anglin D. Healthcare based models for IPV Intervention: An analysis of intervention strategies. *2002 National Conference on Health Care and Domestic Violence.* Atlanta, GA, 2002.

42. Rivara FP, Anderson ML, Fishman P, et al. Healthcare utilization and costs for women with a history of intimate partner violence. *Am J Prev Med.* 2007;32(2):89–96.

43. Thompson R, Bonomi A, Anderson M, et al. Intimate partner violence: Prevalence, types, and chronicity in adult women. *Am J Prev Med.* 2006;30(6):447–457.

44. Koss MP, Bailey JA, Yuan NP. Depression and PTSD in survivors of male violence: Research and training initiatives to facilitate recovery. *Psychol Women Q.* 2003;27:130–142.

45. Salber PR, McCaw B. Barriers to screening for intimate partner violence: Time to reframe the question. *Am J Prev Med.* 2000;19(4):276–278.

46. *National consensus guidelines on identifying and responding to domestic violence victimization in health care settings,* 2nd ed. Family Violence Prevention Fund, 2004.

47. ICSI. *Domestic violence.* Bloomington, MN: Institute for Clinical Systems Improvement, 2006.

48. Salber P, McCaw B. Preparing for an optimal response to intimate partner violence and abuse. In: Salber P, Taliaferro E, eds. *Physician's guide to intimate partner violence and abuse.* Volcano, CA: Volcano Press, 2006.

Chapter 28

Obstacles and Remedies for Criminal and Civil Justice for Victims of Intimate Partner Violence

Sara M. Buel and Eliza M. Hirst

KEY CONCEPTS

- Intimate partner violence (IPV) is one of the most rampant health problems in the United States.
- As a consequence of IPV, survivors often face significant physical, mental, economic, social, and legal obstacles.
- Victims do not always report incidents to practitioners or law enforcement because of the real or perceived risks of homelessness, removal of children, dual arrest policies, poverty, isolation, embarrassment, deportation (if undocumented), and/or unemployment.
- As part of safety planning, protection orders may be one of the most effective ways to help IPV victims.
- Healthcare practitioners may be asked to serve as experts in legal matters involving crimes, divorce, custody, torts, immigration petitions, and protective orders stemming from IPV.

Given the prevalence of intimate partner violence (IPV) in the United States, healthcare providers (HCPs) are highly likely to encounter abuse survivors in their practice. The Centers for Disease Control and Prevention (CDC) and the Department of Health and Human Services (HHS) have determined that IPV is one of the most critical national health epidemics (1). An estimated 5.3 million IPV incidents are reported annually, resulting in over 486,000 hospital emergency department visits and 18.5 million mental health counseling sessions each year (1). These numbers reflect massive underreporting because many IPV survivors do not report incidents of abuse to law enforcement authorities (2). Consequently, HCPs often play a unique role as the primary, and sometimes only, responders to acts of IPV (3). Therefore, they *must* integrate routine assessments for IPV into their medical practice. In doing so, they have an extraordinary opportunity to provide survivors with resources, social services, victims' advocates, and recourse through the legal system. By understanding the prevalence of IPV, the risks to victims, and the intersection between the medical and legal fields, HCPs will not only be equipped with powerful information that may ultimately serve as life-lines for their patients, but also help in the healing process.

The first section discusses the rates of IPV in the United States. The second part focuses on the reasons IPV survivors are reluctant to disclose their abuse to authorities. Finally, the third section provides information on the legal options available to victims and the role doctors can play in obtaining assistance.

CRIMINAL JUSTICE DATA AND TRACKING OF INTIMATE PARTNER VIOLENCE

Intimate Partner Homicides

Between 2001 and 2005, 30% of all female homicides resulted from IPV, with women ages 20–25 at greatest risk (4). In 2005 alone, 1,181 women and 329 men were killed by an intimate partner (4). These staggering numbers have led many states and cities to establish multidisciplinary IPV fatality review teams, which take a unique and comprehensive approach to examining each death. About 20 states have IPV fatality review teams established through statutes, executive orders, court panels, or volunteers (5,6). The teams often include forensic pathologists, medical examiners, attorneys, adult and child victims' advocates, and law enforcement (7). The intention of these teams is to promote prevention and track patterns of homicides (and suicides) resulting from IPV (6,8). These goals are achieved, in part, by carefully examining the chronology of events leading to a child or adult death in order to learn from past mistakes. Overall, death review committees are helpful because they identify IPV indicators and recommend reforms for all relevant professionals.

Fatality Review Committees: Warning Signs

Collectively, IPV fatality teams have discovered common warning signs among women who were murdered by their partners (9). Some important signs practitioners should be aware of include (10):

- A prior history of IPV and injuries
- Attempts to break away from the batterer (such as pending divorce, protective orders, moving out of the home)

- Relationship difficulties
- Stalking and threatening behavior
- Previous police calls
- History of drug and alcohol abuse (by the batterer and/or victim)
- History of mental illness

Danger assessment tools can also assist in assessing patient safety and are discussed in detail elsewhere in the text.

INTIMATE PARTNER VIOLENCE CRIMES

Although the homicide data offers a disturbing picture of IPV, the number of victims who suffer nonfatal attacks by intimate partners is significantly higher. The Bureau of Justice Statistics estimated that from 2001 to 2005, between 450,000 and 600,000 episodes of nonfatal incidents of IPV occurred, consisting primarily of assaults (e.g., hit, slapped, or knocked down) (4). The U.S. Department of Health and Social Services calculates that nonfatal IPV costs close to $8.3 billion annually in medical care, lost work time, and mental health treatment (1). Yet, no specific demographic indicators for IPV exist, as these incidents traverse all races and ethnicities (4). About two-thirds of reported nonfatal intimate partner victimizations occur at home (4). After the incident, fewer than one-fifth of victims reporting an injury obtain medical care, but females are more likely than their male counterparts to seek treatment at a hospital (4). The lack of reporting underscores the importance for doctors to identify IPV among their patients.

VICTIMS UNDERREPORT TO LAW ENFORCEMENT

Many survivors fail to report abuse to the police and their medical providers because of the range of adverse consequences. A recent study from the Bureau of Justice Statistics found the major reasons for non-reporting include a fear of reprisal (15%), a belief that the police do not or cannot help (6%), and a feeling that violence is a private matter (28%) (4,11). When incidents proceed to the courts, survivors feel prosecutors do not listen to them, judges often mete out light criminal sentences, and courts fail to enforce protective orders (10) (Figure 28.1).

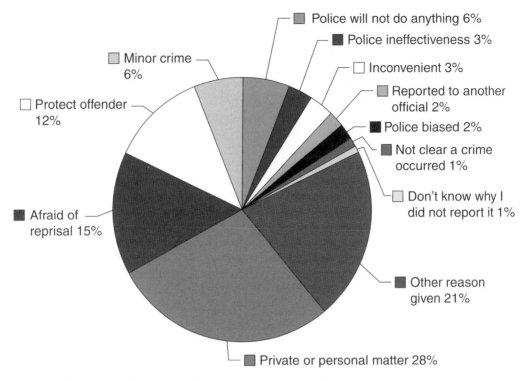

Figure 28.1 Why many victims/survivors do not report intimate partner violence.

The mistrust of the legal system for victims of IPV, unfortunately, extends to the health profession as well. Because of the real and perceived risks associated with divulging abuse to HCPs, studies also find that many survivors admit that they lie about the source of their injuries. Some survivors conceal abuse because of the shame or fear associated with reprisals for reporting (12). In many cases, abusers prevent victims from seeking medical treatment altogether (11). Compounding the problem, many survivors are loath to report abuse to their HCPs because of the risks to their financial circumstances, health, family integrity, or safety. Understanding these barriers will enable health professionals to provide more holistic care and resources for victims.

Increased Risk of Homelessness

Abusers often assert control by systematically destroying their partners' relationships with friends, family, and others (2), leaving them isolated with very few resources (13). Even when IPV victims are able to leave the violent environment, they may so lack

support networks that their only refuge is homeless shelters (2). In 2006, the United States Conference of Mayors' Report determined that IPV was the primary cause of homelessness in major cities including Los Angeles, San Francisco, and Seattle (14). In addition, this report found that, in a significant number of cities, IPV victims had no choice but to separate from their children in order to enter homeless shelters (13). For many survivors, disclosing their abuse to any professional is simply not an option when faced with the prospect of homelessness or family separation.

Children Exposed to Intimate Partner Violence

Children bear witness to incidents of IPV at an alarming rate. Between 2001 and 2005, children under the age of 12 were exposed to 38% of the incidents involving female victims and 21% of the incidents involving male victims (4). The short- and long-term consequences of witnessing violence are often more profound than the experience itself, as described in detail elsewhere in the text.

Still, many victims of IPV with children choose to remain silent because of the possible dual risks that child protective services will remove the children from the home and potential criminal charges for failure to protect (11). It is worth noting that in a recent class action brought in New York City, mothers who lost custody because their children were exposed to violence sued New York's Administration of Children's Services (ACS) (15). The New York Court ruled that the emotional harm to the child and the risk to family integrity outweighed the potential benefits of state removal, in part because battered mothers were being charged with "engaging in DV" (14).

Because implementation of court rulings and laws is often problematic, countless women still do not seek medical care or police protection for IPV-related injuries (11). They accurately fear child protective services and the potential criminal charges for failure to protect their children from violence (16). Therefore, when child protective services become involved in a family matter, doctors can play a profound role in preventing removal of their patients' children. Healthcare providers should document violence in medical records, and, when accurate, reassure social services that their patients are capable of parenting appropriately. Medical opinions and records in this arena may mean the difference between forcing a child into foster care for an extended period of time or maintaining family integrity.

Mandatory Arrests/Dual Arrests

In response to an IPV incident, many states mandate the arrest of the principal physical aggressor, while at the same time discouraging arrests for victim's acts of self-defense (17). When individuals do call the police, the officers must cull through differing accounts to determine who is the primary or "dominant aggressor." To arrest the offender, the police must develop probable cause that the individual committed a DV offense or violated a protection order (17). Too frequently, if a victim (or perpetrator) calls the police during a DV incident, the police will arrest *both* parties if they believe that mutual combat occurred (18).[1] Alternately, untrained police might arrest both the aggressor and the victim when the circumstances do

not provide a clear picture of the incident or when both sustain injuries (19).

With the looming threat of dual-arrest policies, doctors can be instrumental in helping both patients and the police. During an examination, when HCPs discover physical injuries resulting from IPV, they ought to encourage their patients to contact the police without delay. If the police respond during the exam, the victim can provide her statement without the batterer hovering. The police can also gather physical evidence on the spot (pictures, statements, and HCPs' assessments). Unlike responding to the crime scene, the police are less likely to arrest a victim in her practitioner's office because the incident will have already ended. At the same time, the presence of the practitioner may reassure and encourage the victim to reveal abuse to the police.

Becoming aware of the formidable obstacles victims of IPV face, HCPs may not only help their patients with medical care, but also with their long-term recovery.

PROTECTIVE ORDERS: WHAT ARE THEY AND DO THEY HELP VICTIMS ACHIEVE SAFETY?

Every state offers civil legal protection from abuse, usually called "protective orders," "restraining orders," or "protection from abuse orders."[2] The Violence

---

[1] Twenty states and Washington D.C. have mandatory arrest laws. See e.g., Alaska Stat. § 18.65.530 (2007), 42 U.S.C. § 3796hh, cal. Penal Code §13701 (West 2007).

[2] A list of state laws can be found in Interest of Amici Curiae, National Network to End Domestic Violence, 2004 U.S. Briefs 278, at 12, fn 14. n14 Ala. Code §§ 30–5-1 to -11, 30–5A-1 to -7, 30–5B-1 to -10 (1998 & Supp. 2004); Alaska Stat. §§ 18.66.100–.180 (Michie 2004); Ariz. Rev. Stat. Ann. § 13–3602 (West 2001 & Supp. 2004); Ark. Code Ann. §§ 9–15–201 to -216 (Michie 2002 & Supp. 2003); Cal. Fam. Code §§ 6200–6409 (Deering 1996 & Supp. 2005); Colo. Rev. Stat. §§ 13–14–101 to–104 (2004); Conn. Gen. Stat. §§ 46b-15 to -16 (2003), 46b-38c, amended by P.A. 03–202, 2003 Conn. Legis. Serv. § 5 (West); Del. Code Ann. tit. 10 §§ 1041–1053 (1999 & Supp. 2004); D.C. Code Ann. §§ 16–1001 to -1006, -1041 to -1048 (2001 & Supp. 2004); Fla. Stat. ch. 741.28- .315 (2004); Ga. Code Ann. §§ 19–13–3 to -6 (2004); Haw. Rev. Stat. §§ 586–1 to -11, -21 to -26 (1993 & Supp. 2003); Idaho Code §§ 39–6301 to—6316 (Michie 1998 & Supp. 2001); 725 Ill. Comp. Stat. 5/112A-1 to -31, 750 Ill. Comp. Stat. 60/101 to /104 (2002 & Supp. 2003); Ind. Code Ann. §§ 34–26–5-1 to -19 (Michie Supp. 2004); Iowa Code §§ 236.3–.11, .18–.19 (2003); Kan. Stat. Ann. §§ 60–3101 to-3112 (1994 & Supp. 2003); Ky. Rev. tat. Ann. §§ 403.720–.785 (LEXIS through 2004 Extraordinary Session); La. Rev.

Against Women Act (VAWA), makes protection orders enforceable across state lines and tribal nations under the U.S. Constitution's Full Faith and Credit Clause (20). Studies show that women who obtain permanent orders of protection experience an 80% drop in reported physical violence following their issuance (21).

Provisions of Protective Orders

A protective order's power is derived from provisions that limit contact and proscribe the batterer's future actions (21). The orders may include provisions that:

- Prohibit any abuse against the victim and any children in the home
- Maintain a 100-yard distance from the victim, her home, workplace, and any other appropriate location
- Refrain from contacting the victim in any way

- Determine who may stay in the residence (if the couple resides together)
- Pay compensation for damages the victim suffered as a result of abuse
- Award custody to the victim for any child in common with the batterer
- Require supervision for visitation, including the use of a visitation center
- Pay child support
- Pay spousal support
- Award possession of any personal property, like a car, a credit card or other items
- Prohibit any sale or disposal of property owned/leased by both parties
- Require appropriate counseling or treatment for the batterer
- Prohibit the purchase of a gun and require relinquishment of any guns during the duration of the order
- Provide any other relief that the court deems appropriate

In 1994, Congress amended the Federal Gun Control Act of 1968 to prohibit those subject to protective orders from possessing and purchasing a firearm or ammunition.[3] The protective order must either (a) contain a finding that the subject poses a credible threat to the victim's physical safety, or (b) explicitly prohibit the use, attempted use, or threatened use of physical force against the victim (22). Importantly, the federal firearm prohibition is effective regardless of relevant state law. Thus, the violation occurs when the court finds that the respondent possessed a firearm, even if he has not yet behaved in an overtly threatening manner.[4] Congress also codified it as a federal offense to sell or transfer a firearm or ammunition to a known subject of a qualifying protective order (22). Similarly, most states now permit judges to prohibit the possession and

---

Stat. Ann. §§ 46:2131–:2143 (West 1999 & Supp. 2005); Me. Rev. Stat. Ann. tit. 19-A, §§ 4001–4014 (West 1998 & Supp. 2004); Md. Code Ann., Cts. & Jud. Proc. §§ 3–1501 to -1509 (2002 & Supp. 2003); Md. Code Ann., Fam. Law §§ 4–501 to–511 (1999 & Supp. 2003); Mass. Gen. Laws ch. 209A §§ 1–10 (2002 & Supp. 2003); Mich. Comp. Laws Ann. §§ 600.2950–.2950m (West Supp. 2004); Minn. Stat. § 518B.01 (2002); Miss. Code Ann. §§ 93–21–1 to -29 (2004); Mo. Ann. Stat. §§ 455.005–.085 (West 2003 & Supp. 2004); Mont. Code Ann. §§ 40–15–101 to -408 (2003); Neb. Rev. Stat. §§ 42–901 to -940 (1998 & Supp. 2002, 2003); Nev. Rev. Stat. 33.017–.100 (2003); N.H. Rev. Stat. Ann. § 173-B:1–14 (2001 & Supp. 2004); N.J. Stat. Ann. § 2C:25–28 to -35 (West Supp. 2004); N.M. Stat. Ann. §§ 40–13–3 to -6 (McKinney 2005); N.Y. Fam. Ct. Act.§§ 841–842 (McKinney Supp. 2004); N.C. Gen. Stat.§§ 50B-1 to -7 (1999 & Supp. 2004); N.D. Cent. Code §§ 14–07.1–01 to -18 (2004); Ohio Rev. Code Ann. § 3113.31 (West 2000 & Supp. 2004); Okla. Stat. Ann. tit. 22, §§ 60–60.14 (West 2004 & Supp. 2005); Or. Rev. Stat. §§ 107.700 to -.732 (2003); 23 Pa. Cons. Stat. § 6108 (West 2001 & Supp. 2004); R.I. Gen. Laws §§ 8–8.1–1 to -8 (1997 & Supp. 2004); S.C. Code Ann. §§ 20–4-10 to -140 (Law. Co-op 1985 & Supp. 2004); S.D. Codified Laws§§ 25–10–1 to -13 (Michie 1999 & Supp. 2003); Tenn. Code Ann. §§ 36–3-601 to -622 (2001 & Supp. 2004); Tex. Fam. Code Ann. §§ 85.021–.026 (Vernon 2002); Utah Code Ann. §§ 30–6-1 to -15 (1998 & Supp. 2004); Vt. Stat. Ann. tit. 15, §§ 1101–1115 (2002); Va. Code Ann. § 16-1-279.1 (Michie 2003 & Supp. 2004); Wash. Rev. Code §§ 26.50.060–.120 (2004); W. Va. Code Ann. § 48–27–501 to -511 (Michie 2004); Wis. Stat. Ann. § 813.12 (West Supp. 2004); Wyo. Stat. Ann. §§ 35–21–103 to -111 (Michie 2003).

---

[3] 18 U.S.C.A. § 920 et. seq. §922 of this provision is part of the Violent Crime Control and Law Enforcement Act of 1994. It will be referred to hereafter as "the 1994 Amendment."

[4] U.S. v. Emerson, 270 F.3d 203, 213 (5th Cir. 2001) ("We likewise reject the argument that section 922(g)(8) requires that the predicate order contain an express judicial finding that the defendant poses a credible threat to the physical safety of his spouse or child.")

purchase of firearms by those persons subject to IPV protective orders.[5]

Types of Protective Orders

Protective orders can be filed on an emergency basis or for longer durations, with a few states providing permanent relief. Typically, emergency protective orders are heard *ex parte*, meaning that the victim is not required to give the batterer any notice of the hearing. This is considered an extraordinary option and only available if the survivor alleges she is in immediate danger. The judge will decide the merits solely from the victim's account and grant immediate temporary relief if finding that the accused poses a danger to the victim. For more lasting security, nonemergency protective orders require the batter to receive notice of the hearing and an opportunity to testify alongside the victim. Once awarded, the protective order lasts anywhere from 1 to 5 years, or is permanent, depending on the jurisdiction and the judge's order. (Protective orders can also be negotiated between the parties, which obviates the need for a hearing.)

The Enforceability of Protective Orders

Because the majority of states have central registries of protective orders,[6] when IPV victims call 911, the police should be notified immediately. Many states mandate that the batterer be arrested for violation of specific provisions of the protective order, such as those specifying no contact and refrain from abuse.[7] This mandate removes police discretion except to determine probable cause for violation of a protective order or other criminal offense. However, a recent Supreme Court case addressed the legal enforceability of protection orders (23).

In *Castle Rock v. Gonzales*, Mrs. Gonzales' sued the Castle Rock (Colorado) Police Department because her ex-husband violated her protection order and subsequently killed their three children. She alleged her husband was able to murder their daughters as a direct result of the repeated refusal of the police to take even minimal steps to locate the girls (24). She argued that she was deprived the right to property without due process of law because the police failed to enforce her protection order (in addition to physical property, "property" also includes legal entitlements or monetary damages). The U.S. Supreme Court ruled that Ms. Gonzales was not denied due process by the Castle Rock Police Department because the Court said that the protection order does not allow the recipient to demand an arrest or initiate contempt charges (23). Rather, a protection order only entitles a person to *request* that police investigate a reported violation of the order (23).

Steps to Obtain a Protective Order

Although *Castle Rock* poses some challenges for protective order enforcement, they are most often a comprehensive means to protect victims against repeated threats, stalking, and ongoing abuse. When safety planning with a victim of violence, it is important to refer the victim to a police victim's advocate or legal services organizations. Encourage them to get protection orders when possible. Most jurisdictions have protective order application forms that can be filled out without the assistance of an attorney. Before a patient who has experienced IPV leaves the clinical setting, HCPs may want to hand the patient the protection order form (most states have a downloadable form), and give the patient a safety plan brochure with local resource information. It is worth noting that when a victim obtains a protective order, the risk of aggravated violence may rise (23). Therefore, it is equally important for practitioners to safety plan with patients when recommending protective orders.

If a patient is an undocumented immigrant, however, the HCPs should encourage her to consult with an immigration attorney before recommending a protective order because of the potential implications to her legal status. Similarly, patients with a prior criminal record, or substance abuse and mental health challenges, should speak with an experienced advocate in deciding whether a protective order is a beneficial option. It is not that victims in any of these categories are statutorily prohibited from obtaining protective orders, but, rather, that court biases may deem other options more preferable.

---

[5] See, e.g., Tex. Fam. Code Ann. § 85.022(b)(6) ("In a protective order, the court may *prohibit* the person found to have committed family violence from . . . possessing a firearm . . .") (emphasis added).

[6] See Footnote 3.

[7] Ibid.

FIREARMS POSSESSION AND REGISTRY

In 1996, Congress passed the Lautenberg Amendment (also known as the Domestic Violence Gun-Offender Ban) making it a federal crime for a person convicted of a misdemeanor or felony DV crime to possess or purchase a firearm (25). The Lautenberg Amendment also includes a provision criminalizing the sale or transfer of a firearm or ammunition to a person convicted of an IPV offense (25). Because over two-thirds of intimate murders of spouses and ex-spouses involved firearms,[8] it is critical for medical providers to ask about weapons in the home. In 2002, for every female killed by a stranger, three women were killed by an intimate partner, two of whom used a firearm.[9] One study found that batterers with access to firearms are *five times more likely* to murder their intimate partners (26). Another study determined that there is a onefold increase in the chances of death occurring when IPV assaults involve firearms (27).

Additionally, firearms are often used to threaten and terrorize IPV victims (71.4% of firearm-associated assaults reported by the women involved such a threat) (28). Firearm-associated offenses may manifest in the batterer threatening to kill or shoot the victim, her children, himself, or beloved family pets.[10] Another effective form of threat occurs when the batterer deliberately cleans his gun in the midst of a dispute (29). Given the dangers posed by armed batterers,

safety planning must include direct questions about the previous or possible use of firearms against abused patients and their children.

THE COURTS: CRIMINAL AND CIVIL MATTERS

As important as it is to understand the barriers to survivors seeking help, legal remedies may hinge on the support of treating practitioners. Because many court cases rely heavily on experts, practitioners may be called upon to help victims obtain safety within the legal system. An overview of legal recourse available to IPV patients follows.

The legal system is divided into civil and criminal branches. The criminal side encompasses all crimes against the state, sentences, and violations of parole. Civil courts handle noncriminal matters between individuals or businesses, ranging from tort claims and contract disputes, to family and probate matters. Domestic violence cases are often an amalgam of criminal and civil matters. In the past, DV claims were often dismissed in family court proceedings as sheer manipulation (30). Over the last 20 years, however, specialized DV courts have emerged as a way to address the specific issues and problems inherent in these cases. There are various models of DV courts, but most divert DV cases into a more sensitive, private, and dedicated forum. This setting better protects victims because batterers may use repeated court proceedings as a way to continue their abuse (30).

Domestic Violence Courts

There are four types of DV courts (31). The first model channels pretrial conferences involving DV into a separate court calendar (31). Pretrial conferences are used to determine if the parties can reach a settlement or plea agreement. In this model, DV cases are guided into one court and heard on specific days of the week. Many of these courts have victim's advocates to help explain the system (31).

A second model limits DV courts to hearing nonevidentiary matters, and they make only legal decisions (31). Nonevidentiary issues are heard by a judge, with no jury, no trial, and no facts or evidence. Instead, only legal issues are presented to the court. A third type of court hears all criminal cases involving DV (31).

---

[8] Between 1990 and 2005, 68% of murders of women by their husbands involved firearms; 77% of murders of women by their ex-husbands involved firearms. Catalano, S., Ph.D., Bureau of Justice Statistics, Homicide Trends in the U.S.: Intimate Homicide, http://www.ojp.usdoj.gov/bjs/homicide/intimates.htm. Accessed February 13, 2008. In the same time period, 56% of murders of girlfriends involved firearms.

[9] In 2002, 1,112 females were murdered by a spouse, boyfriend, or girlfriend; 623 of these murders involved firearms. These numbers are compared to the relatively low number of 328 women killed by strangers. Durose, M, et al. U.S. Dept. of Justice, Family Violence Statistics: Including Statistics on Strangers and Acquaintances, 2005. Department of Justice Web Site. http://www.ojp.usdoj.gov/bjs/pub/pdf/fvs.pdf.

[10] Over two-thirds of victims living in a home where a gun is kept responded that the batterer used the gun to scare, threaten, or harm her. Sorenson, S Weibe, D Weapons in the lives of battered women. *Am J Pub Health*. 2004;94:1412.

Finally, a fourth iteration includes both criminal and civil DV cases, ranging from protective orders to assault charges (31). These courts are comprehensive because violations of civil orders can cross over into criminal sanctions. In addition, one court for all DV cases enables judges to follow-up with victims' safety issues and with defendants' attendance at batterer intervention programs (31). This model also creates coordination between the courts, the parties, and available services to better address IPV. Although this approach is praised as holistic, it may run afoul of a criminal defendant's right to remain silent if accused (31). This model may also allow defense attorneys to fish for statements from victims to be used in later criminal proceedings. Some courts have prohibited admissions of violence in the civil context (e.g., at protection order hearings) for use in future criminal proceedings (31). On the whole, however, diverting cases to a specialized court usually helps judges to become knowledgeable about the complexities of family violence.

Civil Suits by Victims

Most abuse victims are loath to use tort law as a remedy against batterers or professionals, even those who have caused them great injury (32). Tort law addresses civil wrongs. For a tort action, an individual must prove that she is owed a duty of care, and a wrong-doer has breached that duty. As a result, the individual suffers damage (emotional, physical or monetary), and then seeks a legal remedy (33). In the IPV context, tort cases include negligence of the batterer, the police, mental health/medical professionals, and others intervening with the victim or batterer. Given the polemics surrounding torts, it is helpful to note that the doctrines of corrective justice and compensation for harm (both intentional and negligent) make this option available to IPV victims. Because some abuse victims find the state and/or juries unwilling to treat their cases seriously, tort action may be their only alternative in seeking justice. Dropped at the doorstep of tort law, IPV victims face the prospect of too-brief statutes of limitations, confusing joinder mandates (which require adding parties or claims to a particular lawsuit), and difficulty in collecting judgments. It makes sense that criminal, family, and tort law be employed, as case facts warrant, in reforming policy and practice in DV cases.

Both during and after separation, batterers often tenaciously continue their pattern of abuse in whatever manner the court and police allow. If the court takes victim safety seriously and enforces protective orders, the batterer may resort to more covert tactics, such that he is still able to terrify the victim, but her pleas for help are viewed as exaggerated, neurotic, paranoid, or unwarranted (32). Batterers may stop direct violence, but continue harassment, psychological and economic coercion, and any other behavior designed to retain control of their victims. Judges, juries, police, doctors, and other professionals may minimize this ongoing psychological abuse if they are not adequately educated about compelling empirical data documenting the grievous harm it confers, whether or not there are evident physical manifestations (34). Likewise, batterers frequently sabotage victims' efforts to seek and maintain employment, causing tardiness, absenteeism, and harassment that may result in the women being fired (35,36). When they are able to work outside the home, victims are often denied access to their own earnings as well as those of their partners (35). Thus, separation and divorce may not solve the problem of abuse (37), but, in fact, could place the victim in greater danger. Because such nonviolent abuse may not constitute criminal offenses, tort litigation may be a victim's only recourse.

Generally, IPV victims only recover in tort for severe physical harm, and, even then for paltry amounts that they may never see. However, many victims report that at least some official recognition of their mistreatment can assist the healing process (38). Even when the initial judgment looks promising, victims are often forced to settle for much less. For example, a Virginia lawyer obtained a $50,000 judgment on behalf of a battered woman whose husband had pistol-whipped her. However, because there was no insurance, the batterer convinced the victim to settle for significantly less without consulting her lawyer.[11] Increasingly, albeit at a frustratingly sluggish pace, some victims are successfully suing their abusers as well as negligent third parties. In 2003, a Massachusetts superior court awarded $9 million to a battered woman left paralyzed by her former boyfriend (39).

Many regard tort litigation against police as the catalyst for much of the improved response with DV cases. However, several problematic doctrines remain.

---

[11] The case was heard in Chesapeake, Virginia circuit court, with Thomas Shuttleworth and Charles Hofheimer as co-counsel for the Plaintiff (Charles Hofheimer, esq., e-mail communication, February 17, 2004).

U.S. courts have also consistently imposed the premise that the police owe a duty to the whole community and, therefore, cannot be held responsible to one individual (40). Additionally, sovereign immunity (police departments and officers enjoy absolute protection unless they have acted with gross negligence; many states' tort claims acts do provide limited waiver of sovereign immunity based on good faith and reasonableness standards), qualified immunity (qualified immunity shields police officers from liability based on their discretionary functions), and the public duty doctrine make it quite difficult for IPV victims to bring suit against law enforcement.

A 14th Amendment equal protection claim can overcome qualified immunity if IPV victims can show that the police department discriminates against IPV victims because of gender bias. Extensive evidence collection is necessary, as was done successfully in *Thurman v. Torrington* (41). In *Thurman*, the federal district court found police liable because, "police protection was fully provided to persons abused by someone with whom the victim had no domestic relationship, but the police consistently afforded lesser protection when the victim was a woman abused or assaulted by a spouse or boyfriend, or when a child was abused by a father or stepfather" (41). The plaintiff, Tracy Thurman, who remains partially paralyzed and scarred from stab wounds inflicted by her husband, won a $2 million judgment against the City of Torrington. In response, Thurman is widely credited with Connecticut quickly enacting a mandatory arrest law. Often, IPV victims who bring suit against police departments or municipalities do not seek to recover monetary damages, but rather seek changes in police procedure.

Treating Professional's Duty to Warn

The 1974 case, *Tarasoff v. Regents of California*, held that therapists can be required to warn identifiable third parties when a patient has threatened harm (42), even absent a relationship with the third party (43). Since this decision, a majority of jurisdictions have adopted some form of the *Tarasoff* duty (44). Upon rehearing, which is known as *Tarasoff II*, the California Supreme Court expanded its previous ruling. Instead of merely a duty to warn the intended third-party victim, the health professional is now obligated "to use reasonable care to protect the intended victim against such danger" (45). According to the *Tarasoff*

decision, simply notifying law enforcement of the threat does not constitute reasonable care.

The Duty to Accurately Diagnosis

Given the frequency with which abuse victims seek healthcare treatment, the health profession has included routine screening for intimate partner abuse within the rubric of its standard of care (46–49).[12]

The premise is based on findings that, while many battered patients are too ashamed or afraid to self-disclose intentional harm to their physicians, directly asking a patient about abuse prompts some victims who might not otherwise do so to disclose the abuse (50,51). For example, Dr. Richard Jones III found that IPV victims rarely disclosed until he began routinely inquiring—that is, asking every patient if she had been hit or threatened at home—then victimization disclosures exponentially increased from an average of four or five per year to two to three per week. Just as with lawyers, social workers, pharmacists, and others held liable for failing to properly identify, treat, and warn, physicians, too, must adhere to a standard of care with IPV victims that prioritizes their safety or face liability (51).

In line with legal requirements to notify intended victims of threatened violence, courts are increasingly imposing the duty to warn on various professionals in contact with human immunodeficiency virus (HIV)-infected and acquired immune deficiency syndrome (AIDS) patients. In 1995, a California appellate court held that physicians have a duty to warn intimate partners of an AIDS patient's status (52). The court reasoned that although a professional has a special relationship with a patient or client, the duty to warn a third party takes precedence, "even if the third person is both unknown and unidentifiable"(52). Hospitals, too, may be required to warn in the context of HIV cases.

---

[12] AMA Council on Scientific Affairs, Policy H-515.965. Dec. 2000. AMA Web site. http://www.ama-assn.org/ama/pub/category/13577.html. Medical "curricula should include coverage of the diagnosis, treatment, and reporting of child maltreatment, intimate partner violence, and elder abuse and provide training on interviewing techniques, risk assessment, safety planning, and procedures for linking with resources to assist victims. The AMA supports the inclusion of questions on family violence issues on licensure and certification tests . . ." and the "AMA encourages physicians to: (a) Routinely inquire about the family violence histories of their patients as this knowledge is essential for effective diagnosis and care").

A Texas appellate court found that a hospital had a duty to warn its staff when they were treating an AIDS patient.[13] Similarly, in *Johnson v. West Virginia University Hospital*, a court ruled (a) that the hospital had a duty to notify a security guard that he was subduing an AIDS patient, and (b) that the officer could recover for emotional distress caused by his exposure to AIDS (53). Given the overlap with IPV and HIV/AIDS cases, HCPs should check with their legal counsel to become familiar with the legal obligations imposed in their state.

Problems with Family Courts

Custody Issues

Intimate partner violence is prevalent in custody, visitation, and divorce cases (54). In many family law matters, attorneys will employ medical experts for several reasons ranging from assessing the parties' abilities to parent to educating judges on the impact of family violence (55). An expert may be needed to counter the problem of an abusive parent being more likely to obtain child custody because he can present better in court than the victim (55). Survivors of IPV often suffer from depression, posttraumatic stress disorder, anxiety, or other mental health disorders (56), which may not bode well in court. Since custody and divorce battles often involve expert testimony, healthcare providers may play a crucial role in custody decisions. Because the impact on family law matters can be profound, health providers treating IPV victims should maintain detailed medical records and be extra attentive in visits.

NON-COURT REMEDIES FOR VICTIMS OF CRIME

Violence Against Women Act Legislation: What It Has Changed and What Protections It Offers

Protections for Immigrant Women

Those IPV survivors who are neither citizens nor lawful permanent residents (i.e., undocumented immigrants)

may elect to conceal their abuse because they risk being held in immigration detention, deportation, abandoning their children (especially if the children are U.S. citizens), or facing economic desperation (57). However, there are two main circumstances in which an undocumented immigrant can legally remain in the country if she reports IPV. The survivor may either apply for a VAWA self-petition or a U-Visa (the government grants up to 10,000 per year) (58). (The U.S. government also permits T-Visas for sex trafficking, but those visa requirements are exceedingly difficult to meet, and the government limits issuance of up to 5,000 per year [59]).

Enacted in 1994, VAWA includes provisions to combat the power abusers hold over battered immigrants, ranging from financial dependence and immigration status, to housing and medical care (58). The VAWA allows survivors of IPV to petition the U.S. Citizenship and Immigration Services for lawful permanent residency (60). To self-petition, an individual survivor of IPV must show (61,62):

- Her spouse is a U.S. citizen or a lawful permanent resident (i.e., green card holder).
- She is legally married to the abuser.
- Her spouse abused her and/or her children during the marriage.
  - Abuse includes threats of violence, physical injuries, emotional abuse at home or in public, forced sex, threats of deportation or kidnapping, controlling her actions.
- She currently lives with (or has lived in the past with) her spouse.
- She married her spouse in good faith (not to obtain immigration benefits).

The other legal option is a U-Visa, which developed from the Victims of Trafficking and Violence Protection Act (63). A U-Visa allows undocumented immigrants to petition for residence after witnessing/experiencing a crime and assisting law enforcement with prosecution. An individual immigrant applying for a U-Visa must meet five specific criteria (64):

- The applicant must be the victim of crime within the United States (such as DV, assault, kidnapping, false imprisonment, rape, or sexual assault).
- The applicant must have suffered substantial mental or physical abuse as a result of the criminal experience.

---

[13] A nurse contracted HIV after assisting a patient with AIDS; the hospital knew this was an AIDS patient but failed to notify the nurse.

- The applicant must be willing to assist law enforcement in the investigation of the crime. The type of assistance will vary depending on the crime, including statements to the police, descriptions of the perpetrator, and testifying at a trial.
- The applicant must also assist in the prosecution of the crime by cooperating with the police and the attorneys who try the case.
- Finally, the applicant must attach a signed certification from law enforcement indicating the victim cooperated with law enforcement in investigating the crime.

U-Visa status cannot exceed 4 years, but an applicant may apply for her spouse and children as well (64). After 3 years under a U-Visa, the survivor may then apply for Permanent Resident Status (64). Even with these legal protections, silence among immigrant survivors of IPV remains a serious problem. The requirements are cumbersome, and many immigrants do not know about their rights as victims of crime (64). Therefore, HCPs may assist their undocumented patients in two meaningful ways.

First, health providers should be aware that an undocumented patient may have a right to a visa under certain circumstances. Becoming familiar with nonprofit immigration agencies and immigration lawyers is a strong lifeline for many undocumented immigrants. Second, medical documentation of injuries and descriptions of abuse are equally important to help survivors flee dangerous situations. When undocumented immigrants apply for the U-Visa or a VAWA self-petition, they will need to submit "credible evidence" that they have suffered substantial physical or mental harm (65). Consequently, treating physicians are often asked to provide medical records or letters describing the physical or psychological injuries along with their patients' immigration applications. Working with an immigration attorney to determine how records and documentation should be submitted to the U.S. Citizenship and Immigration Services Administration is the most effective way to support immigrant patients in their quest to become legal residents and recover from the trauma they experienced.

VICTIMS OF CRIME RESOURCES

Every state and the federal government have crime victim compensation funds stemming from the Victims of Crime Act (66). The funds are generated from fines imposed on criminal defendants for acts of violence. Crime victims can apply for funds in their state (or for federal funds). Compensation from these funds can be used by victims for mental health treatment, medical or dental expenses, lost income, funeral expenses, relocation expenses, and financial support to care for the dependents of victims who died or became disabled (67). Some states, such as Florida and New York, have specific criteria to reimburse expenses stemming from IPV (68). Healthcare providers should become aware of these resources to assist victims who may need financial help to flee a dangerous situation.[14] The practitioner's state department of justice website will likely have information on the eligibility criteria for victims of crime. In addition, practitioners should provide their patients with medical records documenting the injuries. Reimbursement for crime victims may very well hinge on the proof and severity described in the medical records.

CONCLUSION

With all the obstacles and risks, it is not surprising that IPV victims often conceal the source of their injuries. Significant deterrents include fear of homelessness, loss of children, retaliation, and a dearth of accessible resources. The more health providers know about the personal consequences for survivors, the better able they will be to integrate the law and health care, thus decreasing the prevalence of IPV. Collectively, safety planning, learning of the resources in their patients' community,[15] and documenting all evidence of abuse are the most effective ways HCPs can enable victims to overcome the dangers and obstacles they face. Most significantly, becoming advocates for survivors of IPV will undoubtedly assist in the healing process.

---

[14] Health providers can access immediate guidance for themselves and assistance for patients 24/7 at the National Domestic Violence Hotline, 1–800–799-SAFE.

[15] Free information can be obtained from the National Coalition Against Domestic Violence (www.ncadv.org) and the American Bar Association's Commission on Domestic Violence (www.abanet.org/domviol).

IMPLICATIONS FOR POLICY, PRACTICE, AND RESEARCH

Policy

- Legal protective orders are an important option for patients to consider in an effort to prevent continued abuse, harassment, and stalking, and should be readily available on an emergency basis and easy to apply for on a nonemergent basis.
- Victims of IPV have complex health and safety needs, and victims of crime funding for both adult and child victims may be important to recovery.

Practice

- It is imperative for practitioners to be aware of legal protections and to act as advocates for more accessible resources for victims of IPV.
- Providers ought to be mindful of the types of documentation that help victims prove the necessity of a protective order. At the same time, practitioners should become knowledgeable about local resources, victim advocacy organizations, and assistance based on the needs of the patient.

Research

- Research is needed in regards to outcomes of civil or criminal remedies on the health and welfare of adult and child survivors of IPV.

Reference

1. Centers for Disease Control. Cost of intimate partner violence in the United States. Centers for Disease Control and Prevention Web Site. At http://www.cdc.gov/ncipc/pub-res/ipv_cost/03_incidence.htm.2003. Accessed 3/20/2008.
2. Buel S. Fifty Obstacles to leaving, A.K.A., Why abuse victims stay. *Colorado Law.* 1999;28:19–24.
3. U.S. Department of Justice, Office on Violence Against Women. A *National Protocol for Sexual Assault Medical Forensic Examinations: Adults/Adolescent.* 49NCJ206554. 1–141. Washington DC: Author, 2004.
4. Catalano, S., Ph.D., Bureau of Justice Statistics. Intimate Partner Violence in the United States Nonfatal violent victimization rate by victim/offender relationship and gender, 1993–2005, At http://www.ojp.

usdoj.gov/bjs/intimate/victims.htm. 2007. Accessed 2/13/2008.
6. Websdale N, et al. Reviewing domestic violence fatalities: summarizing national developments. Violence Against Women Online Resources Web site. At http://www.vaw.umn.edu/documents/fatality. Accessed 2/12/2008.
7. California penal code. §11163.3 (West 2007).
8. Delaware penal code. ANN. tit. 13, §2105 (2008).
9. Websdale N, Town M, Johnson B. Domestic violence fatality reviews: From a culture of blame to a culture of safety. *Juv Fam Court J.* 1999:61–74.
10. Campbell J, et al. Assessing risk factors for intimate partner homicide. *Natl Instit Justice J.* 2003;250:14–19.
11. Rodriguez MA, McLoughlin E, Nah G, Campbell JC. Mandatory reporting of domestic violence injuries to the police. *JAMA.* 2001;286:580–583.
12. Sullivan C, Hogan L. Survivors' opinions about mandatory reporting of domestic violence and sexual assault by medical professionals. *Affilia.* 2005;20(3):346–361.
13. The Mayo Clinic, Power and Control Wheel, At http://www.mayoclinic.com/health/domestic-violence/W000044. Accessed 10/12/2007. Domestic Abuse Prevention Project, Power and Control Wheel. National Center on Domestic and Sexual Violence Web site. At http://www.ncdsv.org/images/PowerControlwheelNOSHADING.pdf. Accessed 11/22/2007.
14. US Conference of Mayors, A Status Report on Hunger and Homelessness in America's Cities. 2006;75. U.S. Conference of Mayors Web site. At http://usmayors.org/uscm/hungersurvey/2006/report06.pdf. Accessed 10/12/2007.
15. *Nicholson v. Williams,* 203 F.Supp.2d 153 (E.D.N.Y. 2002).
16. Witcomb D. Prosecutors, kids and domestic violence cases. *Natl Instit Justice J.* 2002;248:2–9.
17. See e.g. Ala. Code §13–3601.B (2002), Cal. Penal Code §13701(b) (West 2007). Fla. Stat. Ann. §741.29(4)(b) (West 2007), Wash. Rev. Code §10.31.100(2)(c)(2008).
17. Ruttenberg M. A feminist critique of mandatory arrest: An analysis of race and gender in domestic violence policy. *Am Univ J Gend Soc Policy Law.* 1994;2:160–186.
18. Chestnut S. The practice of dual arrests in domestic violence situations: Does it accomplish anything? *Miss Law J.* 2001;70:971–981.
19. Mills L. Commentary: Killing her softly: Intimate abuse and the violence of state intervention. *Harv Law Rev.* 1999;113:550–613.
20. 18 U.S.C. §2266(5)(2007).
21. Holt V, Kernic MA, Lumley T, et al. Civil protection orders and risk of subsequent police-reported violence. *JAMA.* 2002;589–593.
22. 18 U.S.C.A. § 920 et. seq.
23. 545 U.S. 748 (2005).
24. 42 U.S.C. §1983 (2007).

25. 18 U.S.C.A.§ 921(a)(33).

26. Campbell J, Webster D, Koziol-McLain J, et al. Risk factors for femicide in abusive relationships: Results from a multisite case control study. *Am J Public Health*. 2003;93:1089–1092.

27. Saltzman L, Mercy JA, O'Carroll PW, et al. Weapon involvement and injury outcomes in family and intimate assaults. *JAMA*. 1992;267:3043.

28. Sorenson S, Weibe D. Weapons in the lives of battered women. *Am J Public Health*. 2004;94:1412.

29. Cukier W, Sidel V. The global gun epidemic: From Saturday night specials to AK-47s. *Praeger Security International*. 2006:21.

30. Freedman A. Symposium: Fact finding in civil domestic violence cases: Secondary traumatic stress and the need for compassionate witnessing. *Am Univ J Gend Soc Policy Law*. 2003;11:567–656.

31. Helling J. Specialized criminal domestic violence courts. Violence Against Women Online Resources Web site. At http://www.vaw.umn.edu/documents/helling/helling.pdf. Accessed 11/22/2007.

32. Buel S. Access to meaningful remedy: Overcoming doctrinal obstacles in tort litigation against domestic violence offenders. *Oregon Law Rev*. 2004;83: 945–1034.

33. Garner B, ed. *Black's law dictionary*. Eagan MN: West Group Publishing, 1996.

34. Perry B, Marcellus J. The Impact of Abuse and Neglect on the Developing Brain. Scholastic Web site. At http://teacher.scholastic.com/professional/bruceperry/abuse_neglect.htm. Accessed 1/22/2008.

35. Kinzel S. The effects of domestic violence on welfare reform: An assessment of the personal responsibility and work opportunity reconciliation act as applied to battered women. *Univ Kans Law Rev*. 2002;50: 591–627.

36. Raphael J. *Keeping women poor: How domestic violence prevents women from leaving welfare and entering the world of work*. In: Brandwein R, ed. Battered women, children, and welfare reform. Thousand Oaks, CA: Sage, 1999.

37. Buzawa E, et al. US *department of justice, response to domestic violence in a pro-active court setting: Final report*. Washington, DC: National Institute of Justice, 1999.

38. Herman J. *Trauma and recovery*. New York: Basic Books, 1992.

39. Domestic violence victim awarded $9 million dollars. Wmnbfm.com. December 14, 2003 At http://www.wmnbfm.com/news.php3?story_id=5197. Accessed 11/04/2008.

40. *Riss v. City of New York*, 22 N.Y.2d. 579, 585 (1968) (Keating, J., dissenting).

41. *Thurman v. Torrington*, 595 F. Supp. 1521 (D. Conn. 1984).

42. *Tarasoff v. Regents of the Univ. of Cal.*, 529 P.2d 553, 555 (Cal. 1974).

43. Hubbard A. Symposium: The future of "the duty to protect": Scientific and legal perspectives on Tarasoff's thirtieth anniversary, symposium introduction. *Univ Cincinnati Law Rev*. 2006;75:429–444.

44. Kachigian C, Felthous A. Court responses to Tarasoff statutes. *J Am Acad Psychiatry Law*. 2004; 32:263–273.

45. *Tarasoff v. Regents of the Univ. of Cal.*, 551 P.2d 334, 340 (Cal. 1976).

46. Draucker C. Domestic violence: The challenge for nurses. Online J Issues Nurs. 2002;7:1. At http://www.nursingworld.org/MainMenuCategories/ANAMarketplace/ANAPeriodicals/OJIN/Tableof Contents/Volume72002/Number1January31/Domestic ViolenceChallenge.aspx. Accessed 3/20/2008.

47. American Psychological Association. *Violence and the family: Report of the American Psychological Association Presidential Task Force on Violence and the Family*. Washington, DC: American Psychological Association, 1996.

48. American College of Obstetricians and Gynecologists. *The battered woman*. ACOG Bulletin 1989; No. 124. Washington, DC: Author.

49. Chambliss L. Domestic violence: A public health crisis. *Clin Obstet Gynecol*. 1997;40:630–638.

50. Jones R. Domestic violence: Let our voices be heard. *Obstet Gynocol*. 1993;81:1–4.

51. Buel S, Drew M. Do ask and do tell: Rethinking the lawyer's duty to warn in domestic violence case. *Univ Cincinnati Law Rev*. 2006;75:447–496.

52. *Reisner v. Regents of the Univ. of Cal.*, 37 Cal. Rptr. 2d 518 (Cal. Ct. App. 1995).

53. *Johnson v. W. Va. Univ. Hosps., Inc.*, 413 S.E.2d 889 (W. Va. 1991), abrogated in part on other grounds by *Helderth v. Marrs*, 425 S.E.2d 157, 160–61 (W.Va. 1991).

54. American Bar Association Commission on Domestic Violence. 10 Myths about Custody and Domestic Violence and How to Counter Them. 2006. ABA Web site. At http://www.abanet.org/domviol/custody_myths.pdf. Accessed 11/22/2007.

55. Aiken J, Meier J. Evidence: Litigation techniques and strategies in domestic violence cases: a Teleconference series. American Ban Association Commission on Domestic Violence, 2006. ABA Web site. At http://www.abanet.org/domviol/Evidence_outline.pdf. Accessed 11/22/2007.

56. AMA. Diagnostic and treatment guidelines on mental health effects of family violence. AMA Web site. At http://www.ama-assn.org. 1995 Accessed 1/13/2008.

57. Title IV of the Violent Crime Control and Law Enforcement Act of 1994. (Subtitle G). The Violence Against Women Act and Department of Justice Reauthorization Act of 2005, H.R. 3402 Title II Sec. 201.

58. Violence Against Women Act 2000 §1513 (a)(2) (B) Title VIII, Protection of Battered and Trafficked Immigrants of the Violence Against Women and Department of Justice Reauthorization Act of 2005, Pub. L. No 109–162, 119 Stat. 2960 (Jan. 5, 2006), amended by Violence Against Women and Department of Justice Reauthorization Act—Technical

Corrections, Pub. L. No. 109–271, 120 Stat. 750 (Aug. 12, 2006). 8 C.F.R. §204.1. (2007).

59. New Classification for Victims of Severe Forms of Trafficking in Persons; Eligibility for "T" Nonimmigrant Status. *Fed Reg.* 2002;67:4784.

60. Title IV of the Violence Crime Control Act and Law Enforcement Act of 1994. Subtitle G remedy for Self-petition.

61. Self Petition Visa Application, United State Citizen and Immigration Service website, At http://www. uscis.gov/portal/site/uscis. Accessed 11/10/2007.

62. HR3244 Title V Sec 1501–1513. T visa, victim of sex trafficking, U visa victims of crime.

63. 8 C.F.R. §102, 212, 214, 274(a), 299.

64. U Visa Application, United State Citizen and Immigration Service Web site. At http://www. uscis.gov/portal/site/uscis. Accessed 11/10/2007.

65. 8 C.F.R. § 214.14 (c)(4); 72 Fed. Reg. 53014 (Sept. 17, 2007).

66. 42 U.S.C. §10601 et. seq. (1984).

67. California Victim Compensation. California Office of Victim Services Web site. At http://ag.ca.gov/ victimservices/faq.php. Accessed 11/11/2007.

68. Florida Crime Victim Compensation Application. Florida Department of Justice Web site. At http://myfloridalegal.com/Compapp.pdf. Accessed 11/11/2007.

Chapter 29

Medical and Forensic Documentation

Sarah M. Buel and Eliza M. Hirst

<table>
<tr><td>

KEY CONCEPTS

- Documenting intimate partner violence (IPV) accurately (including injuries and statements made by patients) not only enhances patient care, but may also be a key evidentiary component to civil and criminal cases resulting from violence.
- When practitioners become aware of IPV, they must be knowledgeable of abuse reporting requirements in their jurisdiction, as well as how to help victims plan for safety (with local resources and strategies for survival).
- Practitioners may be required to undermine patient autonomy and informed consent to protect patient safety or comply with mandatory IPV reporting laws.
- The National Domestic Violence Hotline, 1-800-799-SAFE, is a useful resource for practitioners and survivors.

</td></tr>
</table>

Because victims of intimate partner violence (IPV) often face heightened risk of harm once they leave abusive situations, it is critical for healthcare providers (HCPs) to chronicle their patients' presenting problems, diagnoses, and statements in the medical records. Doctor–patient confidentiality, privacy protections, mandatory reporting requirements, and civil and criminal legal issues all influence medical documentation of IPV cases. Although medical records are helpful to maintain a history of patient treatment, forensic documentation is usually recorded with an eye toward the legal system. Whether used in a criminal prosecution for assault or a custody hearing to determine with which parent a child will reside, medical records provide uncontroverted, objective, and, thus, valuable information to the court. Meticulous documentation not only ensures compliance with continuity of care and treatment protocols, it also creates a record of forensic evidence that may prove crucial for an IPV victim ensnared in the legal system by a dangerous perpetrator.

MEDICAL DOCUMENTATION

Medical record keeping promotes continuity of care, demonstrates the competency of the health professional, avoids liability, and demonstrates a good faith effort to help the patient. Health professionals may be asked about the care of an IPV patient in civil or criminal proceedings, so detailed records can be helpful when elapsed time results in blurred or forgotten facts. The thorough history in the case of an IPV patient will include more detailed information about prior abuse, forms of abuse, and the nature of the acute event and threats of future injury. A thorough physical exam will note patient demeanor, mental status, sequelae of past injuries (scars, decreased range of motion), and detailed description of any current injuries using narrative, diagrammatic, and photographic documentation wherever possible.

Diagnosis

Intimate partner violence is a term preferred by the Centers for Disease Control (CDC) and *domestic violence* (DV) is both a lay term and used by the legal system. The diagnostic term described in the World Health Organization International Classification of Diseases is "adult maltreatment" (995.80) and includes specific codes for physical abuse, emotional abuse, sexual abuse, adult neglect, and other abuse. In version 10, a modifier code can be added to indicate whether the diagnosis is confirmed or suspected.

Risk of Malpractice Liability

A concern for many HCPs is that they barely have enough time to meet with patients, let alone address such a complex issue as IPV (1). Since the standards for patient care include accurate diagnosis of IPV, HCPs have a duty to their patients to incorporate identification and care of patients exposed to all forms of violence and abuse. Because not all patients will reveal IPV to their health practitioners, it is equally important for practitioners to document that they asked about partner violence in the patient's medical records, and document their concerns within a discussion of the differential diagnosis. Documentation of abuse (or the absence of it) demonstrates a good faith effort to diagnose accurately and provide for patient safety. However, breaching the appropriate standard of care to identify IPV creates two problems. First, by not identifying IPV, it may perpetuate the patient's risks of staying in an abusive relationship. Second, failing to identify IPV (and failing to report in some jurisdictions) exposes HCPs to criminal and civil liability, particularly in jurisdictions with mandatory reporting requirements. States with criminal statutes for failure to act (i.e., failure to report child abuse or IPV) often have corresponding statutes that provide immunity for reporters. At the same time, criminal liability creates the possibility for aggrieved individuals to file civil lawsuit for the practitioner's failure to act. Civil lawsuits have been filed on behalf of IPV patients who alleged that doctors and/or hospitals failed to accurately diagnose or demonstrated negligent care that resulted in further injury and harm (2).

Patient Statements, "Excited Utterances," Veracity

In legal proceedings, any *out of court* statement (verbal or written) offered for its truth is generally not admissible *in court*, as it is considered hearsay (3). One of the exceptions to the hearsay rule is an "excited utterance" (4), which allows some spontaneous, out of court statements to be admitted into evidence. The statement must be made under the stress or excitement related to a shocking event (4). An excited utterance is considered reliable because the declarant blurts out a statement during the moment of shock, without time to create a lie (5). The statement does not need to be made at the scene of the startling event, but the witness must relate it to the stress from the event (5). Statements upon regaining consciousness, when in shock from an injury, during a 911 phone call, or in the aftermath of an accident are usually considered inherently reliable.

In the context of medical treatment, when a patient exclaims that her partner harmed her or gives specific details about a physically or emotionally abusive incident, while still under the stress of the experience, the utterance is more likely to be admissible in court. However, to be useful in the legal system, the statement must be carefully (and legibly) recorded (6,7) noting the battered patient's demeanor and exact words. The following four steps are essential for accurate documentation (6):

1. The statement must be recorded exactly as it was uttered. Never write patient "alleges" or "claims." Instead, write patient "states," "reports," or "indicates . . ." Definitive statements have greater value in court.
2. The statement must concern the shocking incident (e.g., assault, threat, stalking, rape). It must either be specifically about the event or related to the event (e.g., a declarant's description of an injury and how she sustained it).
3. The provider should describe the condition of the patient at the time the statement was uttered (e.g., the patient was shaking, crying, distressed, hyperventilating, nervous, in shock, soiled, in her bloody clothes, etc.). If possible, the provider should also try to record the amount of time elapsed between the incident and the utterance (e.g., last night, early this morning, 1 hour ago.)
4. Importantly, the recorder should *not* draw conclusions such as "the patient is a victim of violence," "a battered woman," or "in a violent relationship" (6). Those are matters for a court to decide (6), and full, objective descriptions certainly make it easier for the judge or jury to do so.

Statements for the Purpose of Medical Diagnosis or Treatment

Another exception to the hearsay rule is a statement for the purpose of medical diagnosis or treatment (8). Any statement regarding medical assistance, past or present symptoms, pain, medical history, diagnosis, or treatment for a patient may be admissible under this exception (8). Consequently, this type of statement should be documented in a patient's medical records because it is considered reliable, based on the assumption that patients tend not to lie during medical examinations (5). As with excited utterances, HCPs should detail the conversation with the patient as accurately as possible. During investigations and legal proceedings, the records may be subpoenaed to corroborate, discredit, or supplant varying testimony about a specific incident (5).

Medical records may be particularly important in criminal IPV proceedings. The medical exception to live testimony can be vital to prosecuting cases

because a provider's statement may be the only admissible evidence against a perpetrator when a victim is too frightened to testify (9). The Sixth Amendment of the United States Constitution provides that a criminal defendant has the right to "be confronted with the witnesses against him." In *Crawford v. Washington* (10), the U.S. Supreme Court ruled when a declarant of a hearsay statement is unavailable, that statement is only admissible in court if the defendant has a prior opportunity to cross-examine the witness. However, some courts may make an exception to this evidentiary requirement if the defendant causes the witness to be unavailable, whether through threats, intimidation, bribes, violence, or spousal privilege (9). Since evidence may still be admissible through other sources, it is important for HCPs to elicit and record as much information about an incident as possible. Although *Crawford* has strong implications for IPV victims who cannot or will not testify, detailed medical records may be used later to help increase victim safety by prosecuting IPV perpetrators.

ETHICAL CONSIDERATIONS IN MEDICAL DOCUMENTATION OF INTIMATE PARTNER VIOLENCE

Autonomy and Informed Consent

The HCP–patient relationship is generally established through trust, communication, confidentiality, and informed consent (11).[1] Informed consent requires that a patient exercise free choice without force, fraud,

---

[1] According to the American Medical Association's Council on Ethical and Judicial Affairs patients should make their own decisions regarding their treatment; thus physicians have an obligation to: "present the medical facts accurately to the patient or to the individual responsible for the patient's care and to make recommendations for management in accordance with good medical practice. The physician has an ethical obligation to help the patient make choices from among the therapeutic alternatives consistent with good medical practice. Informed consent is a basic . . . policy *in both ethics and law that physicians must honor . . . unless* the patient is unconscious or otherwise incapable of consenting and harm from failure to treat is imminent." Council on Ethical and Judicial Affairs, *Informed Consent:* Opinion 2-I-06, E-8.08 *Amendment*, 15–23 (Updated June 2006). At http://www.ama-assn.org/ama1/pub/upload/mm/475/cej02i06.doc. Accessed11/02/08.

deceit, duress, or coercion (12). It also means that the HCP needs to explain the patient's diagnosis, type of treatment, risks and benefits, alternatives, and options (13). To give informed consent, a patient must have the capacity to understand the proposed course of action (14). Collectively, informed consent involves a thorough conversation between the HCP and the patient, in which the patient expresses her wishes, fully understands the information presented to her, and the practitioner is confident the patient has a meaningful appreciation of the medical treatment. (This is usually demonstrated by having the patient sign and date an authorization form to release information.) The American Medical Association (AMA) states that, absent a legal requirement to report the abuse, physicians should not act without patient consent (15). In the context of IPV, informed consent requires a frank discussion between HCP and patient of the possible risks patients may face when the police are notified as a result of mandatory reporting requirements (16). As challenging as open discussions may be in the realm of family violence, the HCP–patient relationship emphasizes respecting the rights and dignity of individual patients and keeping communication confidential (15).

Confidentiality

Generally, physicians, psychotherapists, and mental health providers have a duty to protect information disclosed during the course of medical treatment (17). However, when a patient expresses an intent to act in a manner that "presents a serious danger of violence" to herself or to another, doctors may be obligated to breach HCP–patient confidentiality (18). For example, in *Tarasoff v. Regents of University of California*, a patient, Prosenjit Poddar, told his therapist that he intended to kill a specific person (18). After learning of this threat, the therapist notified the police, but did not directly warn the victim before she was murdered.

Ultimately, the California Supreme Court determined that "once a therapist does in fact determine (or . . . reasonably should have determined), that a patient poses a serious danger of violence to others, he has a duty to exercise reasonable care to protect the foreseeable victim of that danger" (18). In most jurisdictions, HCPs are obligated to protect identifiable potential victims if their patients threaten imminent

harm. Since not all states follow *Tarasoff*, medical professionals must check with their legal counsel to determine what local obligations exist. For example, Texas does not follow *Tarasoff*, instead prioritizing confidentiality. In 1999, the Texas Supreme Court ruled, in *Thapar v. Zezulka* (19) that a patient's threat to kill an identifiable person did not impose a duty on a psychiatrist to warn the intended victim. In the context of IPV, however, practitioners may need to act with a heightened sensitivity to these obligations when treating both victims and batterers. The duty to warn is covered in detail elsewhere in this text.

STATUTORY HEALTH PRIVACY PROTECTION AND HEALTH INFORMATION PORTABILITY AND ACCOUNTABILITY ACT

The Health Information Portability and Accountability Act (HIPAA) provides federal guidelines to help protect and preserve health information (20). Under HIPAA, HCPs may not generally share confidential information or medical records without patient consent (20). At the same time, HIPAA sets a minimum standard and cannot override specific state and federal laws, including mandatory abuse reporting laws (20). When a mandatory reporting requirement exists, practitioners must report incidents of violence *even* when the disclosure would otherwise breach confidentiality (20).

Discretionary Disclosures Under HIPAA: Reporting Intimate Partner Violence to Police and Social Service Agencies

In the absence of mandatory reporting laws, medical entities covered by HIPAA *may* disclose an IPV victim's protected health information to appropriate governmental authorities or social services when they reasonably believe abuse has been perpetrated (20). Covered entities include health plans, HCPs, and healthcare clearinghouses. Covered entities may also release health information to law enforcement officials for crime victims or for medical emergencies *only* if state law requires or patients consent (20). When HCPs disclose IPV to law enforcement or social service agencies, they *must* inform their patients (either in writing or orally) that the report was or will be made (20). In fact, this disclosure to the patient is a critical part of safety planning. As discussed in the following section, HIPAA allows HCPs to forgo patient notification if the provider believes that it will place the patient in danger.

Discretionary Disclosures Under HIPAA: Assessing Patients for Serious Risk of Harm

Absent a state reporting requirement, a provider must obtain patient consent before reporting abuse; however, two exceptions exist. A doctor has discretion to withhold information when (a) she believes that notification will place the patient at "serious risk of harm" (20); (b) a patient is unable to consent; and (c) the doctor believes it would be dangerous to report to a patient's personal representative (if applicable) (20). A personal representative has the same rights and privileges to protected health information as an individual patient (20). Significantly, it is not uncommon for the personal representative to be the IPV perpetrator, because many abusive relationships are characterized by an acute power imbalance. Batterers may seek to control their partners' medical care (21) because, as personal representatives, they can access medical records, make treatment decisions, and be present for medical appointments (20).

The HIPAA anticipated the potential for coercion and, therefore, permits HCPs to disregard the personal representative's right to access such information when they suspect abuse (20). The test for an HCP to deny access to medical information is:

(a) The individual has been or may be subjected to domestic violence, abuse, or neglect (20), or
(b) treating such person as the personal representative could endanger the individual [patient]. In exercising professional judgment, providers decide that it is not in the best interest of the individual to treat the person as the individual's personal representative (20).

The discretion allowed by HIPAA has some important implications for the doctor–patient relationship when IPV is present. Although reporting abuse to the police may be one way to protect a battered patient, it may also prevent her from seeking future care. It may also lead to a confrontation with a patient's personal representative, particularly if the representative is controlling. In determining what course to pursue, HCPs ought to understand the consequences for all parties of electing to take specific actions. If a physician is unsure which strategy to use, it is wise to ask the patient what she needs and to contact a local IPV victim advocate to discuss realistic options.[2]

PROTECTIONS FOR MINORS AND VULNERABLE ADULTS

All states mandate that health providers report abuse of children (22) and vulnerable adults (23), because those populations may be unable to seek help on their own. These reporting statutes are intended to prevent abuse and neglect, and to prosecute perpetrators (24). Among mandated reporters, HCPs are likely to have greater contact with abused children and vulnerable adults than other professionals because violence often results in physical and mental injuries.[3] For example, one 2005 study found that allegations of child abuse affected an estimated 6 million children based on 3.3 million referrals to child protective services (8.1% of referrals came from medical professionals). A 2004 study found that, for all 50 states, adult protective services agencies received 565,000 reports of elder abuse (age 60+), with between 1.4% and 4.7% reported by medical professionals. In some instances, HCPs may be the primary or only responders to abuse-related injuries within these populations.[4]

Mandatory reporting laws are often controversial because many child and adult victims do not have the choice to self-report abuse, especially given that they may understand the implications of disclosure (25). Vulnerable adults may choose to keep abuse secret because of the diminished independence that might

---

[2] Open 24/7, the National Domestic Violence Hotline, 1–800–799-SAFE, can provide contact information for all U.S. shelters and advocacy organizations.

[3] Healthcare providers are listed as mandated reporters, due in part to their contact with children and vulnerable adults. See e.g., MINN. STAT. ANN. § 626.556 (West 2008), N.J. STAT. ANN. §9:6–8.8 (West 2002), FLA.STAT. ANN.§ 415.101 (West 2005).

[4] See e.g., DEL. CODE ANN. tit. 16, §903 (2007) (Healthcare providers are among a list of individuals who are required to report abuse).

result, or the increased danger to them if a report is made and the abuse becomes known (26). Children often understand the potential for family separation because of police or social service involvement (27). Children may also shy away from reporting violence because they are unable to escape dangerous circumstances and have no financial and external supports (28).

None of the mandatory reporting statutes require HCPs to obtain informed consent from children or vulnerable adults before reporting (29).[5] This is because these populations may not have the legal capacity to give consent (either due to age or functional limitations) (27). The policy implications for child and vulnerable adult abuse reporting are clear: family integrity and individual autonomy are secondary to the government's interest in preventing injuries, death, and the significant expenditures that result from family violence (29).

Mandatory Reporting of Intimate Partner Violence

Like the child and vulnerable adult abuse statutes, the prevalence of IPV has led many states to create a system of direct or indirect reporting of IPV incidents to law enforcement or social service agencies. Healthcare providers' obligations under the law and to IPV victims vary by state. California (30), Rhode Island (31), New Hampshire (32), Kentucky (33), Colorado (34), Ohio (35), and Pennsylvania specifically require HCPs to report IPV incidents to law enforcement or social service agencies. Currently, only a few states—New Hampshire (32), Pennsylvania,[6] and Tennessee (36)—condition physician reporting on patient consent.

In contrast, many states have general violence reporting requirements such as for life-threatening assaults, gun violence, or burn injuries. Only Alabama, New Mexico, Oklahoma, South Dakota, Washington, and Wyoming are silent on the need to report

violence to law enforcement authorities. At the same time, most states with mandatory reporting laws (of any form of violence) do not have corresponding requirements for safety plans and survival resources (37). Only Pennsylvania, Texas (38), New York (39), and North Dakota (40) require doctors to provide IPV patients with a written list of resources, such as referrals to family violence agencies, shelters, and other services.

Current Ethical Controversies of Mandatory Reporting Requirements

Many physicians believe laws mandating DV reporting violate medical ethics and are dangerous for victims (41). Absent well-planned assistance, victims may be more vulnerable and suffer increased injuries after they seek medical help or leave their batterers (42). Proponents of mandatory HCP reporting of adult IPV argue that the policy helps identify victims early on, making key information accessible regarding resources and safety planning. Victims can decide whether or not to utilize them, but at least they have some idea of the legal and social services available (43). In addition, recent studies indicate that the majority of IPV victims do not believe that mandatory reporting laws place them in greater danger and that such laws have not kept them from seeking medical care (44–46).

Opponents are concerned that abuse victims will not seek treatment if reporting is inevitable, thereby jeopardizing their safety, as well as violating the provider's confidentiality obligations (47). Studies indicate that many HCPs find mandatory reporting laws without patient consent objectionable for a variety of reasons. In a 1999 study, 59% of physicians reported that they might not comply with mandatory reporting laws if a patient objected (42). Of the physicians surveyed, primary care physicians were most reluctant to report IPV because of the "patient–provider relationship" (42). Physicians criticized mandatory reporting because (a) it overlooks patient choice and (b) the law violates confidentiality and autonomy (42). They were concerned that reporting requirements may inadvertently discourage patients from discussing abuse and, thus, deter patients from receiving referrals and support (42). Lastly, the physicians felt that reporting might trigger an increase in violence within intimate relationships (42). A 2000 study found that IPV incidents were

---

[5] Furthermore, when a child dies, healthcare providers do not need to obtain informed consent to disclose protected health information when the state is conducting a mortality investigation; see, e.g., DEL. CODE ANN. tit. 16, §1232 (d)(2007).

[6] Pennsylvania's law also permits doctors to make decisions together with their patients on whether or not to report 18 PA.CONS.STAT.ANN. § 5106 (West 2007).

underreported to police or were poorly documented in medical records (48).

Nonetheless, mandatory reporting laws, without patient consent, have the potential to place HCPs in an untenable position: they can either follow the law or uphold their duty to respect patient self-determination. The AMA Code of Ethics directs physicians to follow the law, while at the same time respecting their patients' privacy and autonomy (49). The AMA opposes mandatory reporting laws for competent adult IPV victims (49). Studies have found that due to the safety concern of their patients, physicians may omit documentation of injuries or suspected abuse as a way to protect patients or to circumvent compliance with reporting obligations (49). Although the goal of mandatory reporting is laudable, the requirements may trigger significant consequences, such as risk of increased violence, family disruption, loss of financial means, and home-lessness (50).

Mandatory IPV reporting may effectively create a "don't ask, don't tell policy" for many HCPs. Providers who object to mandatory reporting (or those who do not know how to routinely inquire about IPV) may simply fail to ask about the patient's safety or ignore signs/symptoms related to IPV (42). However, abuse cannot be ignored, and, as first responders (51), medical providers are well-placed to intervene. Although practitioners cannot subvert the laws of their state, they can help safety plan with patients, which is an invaluable tool to protect patients and prepare them for potential danger after reporting IPV. In addition, documenting violence can create an opening for HCPs to examine the reason behind chronic illnesses, and medical or mental health conditions that might result fromIPV. State reporting mandates vary (Figure 29.1). California delineates who must report, how, when, and the contents of the report. California healthprofessionals must report 24 different crimes related to violence and abuse and a state standardized one-page form is used. Although ethically patients should be informed of the limits of confidentiality prior to the health encounter, once IPV is suspected, then it is reported to law enforcement, with or without patient consent. In contrast, in Pennsylvania, reporting to law enforcement can occur only with patient consent, and practitioners are required to provide safety planning resources once DV is known or suspected.

FORENSIC DOCUMENTATION

As important as medical records are for quality patient care, forensic documentation is crucial to the legal system. Forensic evidence must be collected in a manner that protects IPV victims, while facilitating positive legal outcomes. California is the first state in the country to create a standardized form (CalEMA 2-502) for the medical forensic examination of victims of DV (Figures 29.2 through 29.4[52] are examples of sections of the 7 page form.)

Evidenced-based Prosecution

The outcome in legal proceedings may turn on the accuracy and presentation of forensic evidence. As rules change and vary, it is important to know the protocol within the practitioner's jurisdiction. For example, Nebraska and California have specific statutes addressing standardization of collecting sexual assault evidence (53,54). California also has added language in its Penal Code to establish a state supported medical forensic training center to develop and deliver standardized training on medical evidentiary examination, including child abuse, DV, elder abuse, and sexual assault. Other states and local jurisdictions may have uniform practices on evidence collection with which HCPs should become familiar.

In 2004, the U.S. Department of Justice developed a forensic medical examination protocol for sexual assault in order to coordinate resources between practitioners in health care and criminal justice (51). Healthcare providers play an important role in forensic evidence collection (51). When a victim initially enters a healthcare facility, the practitioner must conduct a medical assessment and examination, provide treatment, test for sexually transmitted disease and pregnancy, and make referrals for support services (51). Once the patient is stable, HCPs can move on to the forensic side, in which they obtain health history, collect evidence (such as DNA samples), take pictures, and document medical records (51).

Consent for Forensic Exams

Healthcare providers must get both verbal and written consent to administer a forensic exam (51). Intimate partner violence cases include both medical and forensic aspects, so medical professionals

California

(a) Any health practitioner employed in a health facility, clinic, physician's office, local or state public health department, or a clinic or other type of facility operated by a local or state public health department who, in his or her professional capacity or within the scope of his or her employment, provides medical services for a physical condition to a patient whom he or she knows or reasonably suspects is a person described as follows, shall immediately make a report in accordance with subdivision (b):

> **(1)** Any person suffering from any wound or other physical injury inflicted by his or her own act or inflicted by another where the injury is by means of a firearm.

> **(2)** Any person suffering from any wound or other physical injury inflicted upon the person where the injury is the result of assaultive or abusive conduct.

(b) Any health practitioner employed in a health facility, clinic, physician's office, local or state public health department, or a clinic or other type of facility operated by a local or state public health department shall make a report regarding persons described in subdivision (a) to a local law enforcement agency as follows:

> **(1)** A report by telephone shall be made immediately or as soon as practically possible.

> **(2)** A written report shall be prepared on the standard form developed in compliance with paragraph (4) of this subdivision, and Section 11160.2, and adopted by the agency or agencies designated by the Director of Finance pursuant to Section 13820, or on a form developed and adopted by another state agency that otherwise fulfills the requirements of the standard form. The completed form shall be sent to a local law enforcement agency within two working days of receiving the information regarding the person.

> **(3)** A local law enforcement agency shall be notified and a written report shall be prepared and sent pursuant to paragraphs (1) and (2) even if the person who suffered the wound, other injury, or assaultive or abusive conduct was a factor contributing to the death, and even if the evidence of the conduct of the perpetrator of the wound, other injury, or assaultive or abusive conduct was discovered during an autopsy.

> **(4)** The report shall include, but shall not be limited to, the following:

> > **(A)** The name of the injured person, if known.

> > **(B)** The injured person's whereabouts.

> > **(C)** The character and extent of the person's injuries.

> > **(D)** The identity of any person the injured person alleges.

(c) For the purpose of this section, "injury" shall not include any psychological or physical condition brought about solely through the voluntary administration of a narcotic or restricted dangerous drug.

Pennsylvania

Failure to report injuries by firearm or criminal act

(a) OFFENSE DEFINED. -- Except as set forth in subsection (a.1), a physician, intern or resident, or any person conducting, managing or in charge of any hospital or pharmacy, or in charge of an ward or part of a hospital, to whom shall come or be brought any person:

> **(1)** suffering from any wound or other injury inflicted by his own act or by the act of another which caused death or serious bodily injury, or inflicted by means of a deadly weapon as defined in section 2301 (relating to definitions); or

> **(2)** upon whom injuries have been inflicted in violation of any penal law of this Commonwealth; commits a summary offense if the reporting party fails to report such injuries immediately, both by telephone and in writing, to the chief of police or other head of the police department of the local government, or to the Pennsylvania State Police. The report shall state the name of the injured person, if known, the injured person's whereabouts and the character and extent of the person's injuries.

Figure 29.1 Examples of state statutes on mandating reporting of domestic violence.

(A.1) EXCEPTION. -- In cases of bodily injury as defined in section 2301 (relating to definitions), failure to report under subsection (a)(2) does not constitute an offense if all of the following apply:

(1) The victim is an adult and has suffered bodily injury.

(2) The injury was inflicted by an individual who:

    (i)   is the current or former spouse of the victim;

    (ii) is a current or former sexual or intimate partner of the victim;

    (iii) shares biological parenthood with the victim; or

    (iv) is or has been living as a spouse of the victim.

(3) The victim has been informed:

    (i)   of the duty to report under subsection (a)(2); and

    (ii) that the report under subsection (a)(2) cannot be made without the victim's consent.

(4) *The victim does not consent to the report under subsection (1)(2).*

(5) The victim has been provided with a referral to the appropriate victim service agency such as a domestic violence or sexual assault program.

(b) IMMUNITY GRANTED. -- No physician or other person shall be subject to civil or criminal liability by reason of complying with this section.

(c) PHYSICIAN-PATIENT PRIVILEGE UNAVAILABLE. -- In any judicial proceeding resulting from a report pursuant to this section, the physician-patient privilege shall not apply in respect to evidence regarding such injuries or the cause thereof. This subsection shall not apply where a report is not made pursuant to subsection (a.1).

(d) REPORTING OF CRIME ENCOURAGED. -- Nothing in this chapter precludes a victim from reporting the crime that resulted in injury.

(e) AVAILABILITY OF INFORMATION. -- A physician or other individual may make available information concerning domestic violence or sexual assault to any individual subject to the provisions in this chapter.

Figure 29.1 *Continued*

will need to obtain two stages of informed consent. The first addresses a patient's options to receive medical care and treatment (51). Possible pregnancy tests, sexually transmitted disease tests, medications, side effects, and the medical course of action should be discussed. The second level of consent concerns the patient's decision to undergo a forensic examination including:

- Notification to law enforcement or other authority (depending upon reporting requirements)
- Photographs, including colposcopic images
- The examination and evidence collection
- Toxicology screening
- Release of information and evidence to law enforcement
- Permission to recontact patients for reasons related to their criminal sexual assault case

- Patient notification in case of DNA match or additional victims (51)

Without a forensic exam, law enforcement may lack evidence to prosecute criminal acts.

The cost of the exam should not be a deterrent for patients who need medical and forensic documentation. The Violence Against Women Act (VAWA) provides grants to health practitioners for medical care and forensic exams resulting from IPV (51,55). Under VAWA, the STOP program covers the "full out of pocket costs" for these examinations through federal grants (56). Other expenses may be covered by the Crime Victims Compensation Fund, a state-administered resource designed to assist victims of violent crime with costs directly related to the offense. The invasiveness of medical and forensic examination after an incident

7. Methods employed by assailant(s) and circumstances

              No Yes If yes:

Weapons   ☐ ☐ ☐ Firearm ☐ Knife ☐ Blunt object ☐ Other _____

Threatened?   ☐ ☐ Describe: _____

Displayed?   ☐ ☐ Describe: _____

Used?   ☐ ☐ Describe: _____

Injuries?   ☐ ☐ Describe: _____

Physical blows ☐ by hands ☐ by feet ☐ by head ☐ Other, describe: _____

    ☐ Grabbing ☐ Holding ☐ Pinching ☐ Slapping ☐ Punching ☐ Other, describe: _____

Hair pulling? ☐ No ☐ Yes ☐ If yes, describe: _____

Physical restraints ☐ No ☐ Yes ☐ If yes, describe: _____

Strangulation

	One Hand	Two Hands	Forearm	☐ Ligature, describe:
	Frontal Assault	Frontal Assault	Frontal Assault	_____
	Rear Assault	Rear Assault	Rear Assault	_____

Bites ☐ No ☐ Yes, describe: _____

Burns ☐ Thermal ☐ Chemical ☐ Other_____

Threat(s) of harm ☐ No ☐ Yes   If yes, target of threat: ☐ Patient ☐ Children ☐ Pet(s) ☐ Property ☐ Other, describe: _____

    Describe what was said or done: _____

Sexual relations with assailant as part of this assault?   ☐ No ☐ Unsure ☐ Yes If yes: ☐ Forced ☐ Coerced

Involuntary use of alcohol/drugs   ☐ No ☐ Yes If yes: ☐ Forced ☐ Coerced ☐ Suspected

    If yes: ☐ Alcohol ☐ Drugs Describe: _____

Figure 29.2 Details of the assault from California Forensic Medical Report: Domestic Violence Examination (CalEMA 2-502).

4. Describe condition of clothing upon arrival. Collect outer and under clothing if applicable.   ☐ Not Applicable

5. Examine the face, head, ears, hair, scalp, neck, and mouth for injury. Document findings using photographs, diagrams, legend, and consecutive numbering system.

6. Collect dried and moist secretions, stains and foreign materials from the scalp, head and neck.

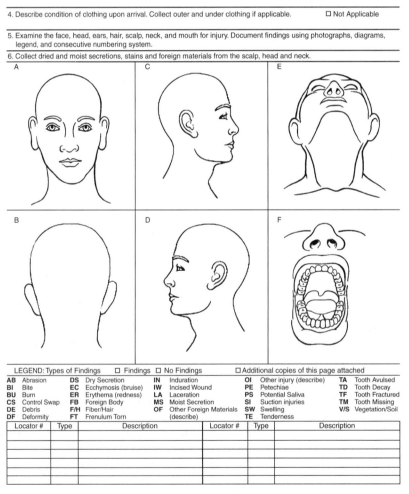

LEGEND: Types of Findings   ☐ Findings ☐ No Findings   ☐ Additional copies of this page attached

AB	Abrasion	**DS**	Dry Secretion	**IN**	Induration	**OI**	Other injury (describe)	**TA** Tooth Avulsed
BI	Bite	**EC**	Ecchymosis (bruise)	**IW**	Incised Wound	**PE**	Petechiae	**TD** Tooth Decay
BU	Burn	**ER**	Erythema (redness)	**LA**	Laceration	**PS**	Potential Saliva	**TF** Tooth Fractured
CS	Control Swab	**FB**	Foreign Body	**MS**	Moist Secretion	**SI**	Suction injuries	**TM** Tooth Missing
DE	Debris	**F/H**	Fiber/Hair	**OF**	Other Foreign Materials	**SW**	Swelling	**V/S** Vegetation/Soil
DF	Deformity	**FT**	Frenulum Torn		(describe)	**TE**	Tenderness	

Locator #	Type	Description	Locator #	Type	Description

Figure 29.3 Face diagrams for California Forensic Medical Report: Domestic Violence Examination (CalEMA 2-502)

L. EVIDENCE COLLECTED AND SUBMITTED TO CRIME LAB		
1. Clothing Collected ☐ No ☐ Yes	**Clothing Placed in Evidence Kit**	**Clothing Placed in Paper Bag**
Bra ☐		
Dress/skirt ☐		
Jacket/sweater ☐		
Nylons ☐		
Pants/shorts ☐		
Shirt/top ☐		
Shoes (1 or 2) ☐		
Socks (1 or 2) ☐		
Underwear ☐		
Undershirt ☐		
Other ☐		

2. Foreign Materials Collected

	N/A	No	Yes	Collected by:
Swabs/suspected blood	☐	☐	☐	_____
Dried secretions		☐	☐	☐	_____
Fiber/loose hairs		☐	☐	☐	_____
Soil/debris/vegetation	☐	☐	☐	_____
Swabs/suspected saliva	☐	☐	☐	_____
Foreign body		☐	☐	☐	_____
Fingernail scrapings		☐	☐	☐	_____
Control swabs		☐	☐	☐	_____

Other, describe:_____

Figure 29.4 Additional physical evidence from California Forensic Medical Report: Domestic Violence Examination (CalEMA 2-502).

of IPV demands that the examiner act with compassion and thoroughness. These exams are not only used for the legal system, but also may improve the victim's ability to heal physically and emotionally.

Training and Expertise

When conducting a forensic exam, HCPs should be mindful of the precision with which evidence must be collected and maintained. Time constraints play a major role in collecting and preserving accurate evidence. It is also essential for the examiner to remain objective (51). Providers must ensure that evidence is properly labeled, kept in a "chain of custody" (meaning its placements and storage can be easily identified and have not been corrupted) (51). Importantly, evidence should not be handled by extraneous staff, in order to preserve the integrity of possession since damaged evidence is useless in criminal investigations and prosecutions (51). If damaged, the potential to reconstruct or retest is virtually impossible. Because forensic evidence demands cooperation between

HCPs and attorneys, they must learn to work together. California, for example, trains court personnel, criminal investigators, and health professionals on how to conduct a forensic exam (57). This type of crossover between the medical and legal fields enables both sides to collaborate in the criminal prosecution of batters and to enhance the safety of IPV victims. Other states can replicate California's legislative mandate (Penal Code 13823.93) for a medical forensic training center as a means of improving practice.

Expert Witnesses

After forensic evidence is captured, it will be used primarily for the investigation and prosecution of criminal acts (51). Tangible evidence often provides the necessary proof to convict a guilty perpetrator, when witness testimony will not be enough. Forensic evidence may even allow prosecutors to avoid placing the victim on the witness stand in certain circumstances. Instead, the attorney can rely on medical evidence and the testimony of medical responders when an IPV victim is too frightened or refuses to testify (9). Practitioners should be mindful that they might be called to testify either to explain the forensic examination, or to discuss medical diagnosis and treatment. If not immediately apparent when subpoenaed to testify, HCPs may want to contact the prosecutor or victim advocate to find out what to bring to court, how to prepare for the direct and cross-examination, and what information will support the patient. (Bear in mind, the attorneys cannot coach the practitioner about what to say in court.)

JOINT COMMISSION ON ACCREDITATION OF HEALTH CARE ORGANIZATIONS AND HOSPITAL REGULATIONS

As a result of the laws and regulations regarding family violence, the Joint Commission on Accreditation of Health Care Organizations (JCAHO) requires doctors to evaluate and document IPV for every patient (58). This body is highly influential in determining a facility's compliance with medical care standards. By highlighting routine screenings, JCAHO reinforces the important role medical providers play in identifying and treating IPV victims.

Many hospitals also have their own policies to universally identify and report IPV. These policies often stem from the duty owed to patients while under medical care. For example, in 2008, an Indiana Court of Appeals determined that an IPV victim's estate could sue the hospital for negligence and breach of a mandatory reporting statute (59).(The decision also left open the possibility for future malpractice lawsuits against doctors for failure to screen for IPV.) After she was discharged, the victim's husband killed her on their way home from the hospital. The court found the hospital had (a) a statutory duty to report suspected abuse of an endangered adult (60), and (b) a general duty to exercise reasonable care in protecting patients from harm (especially the danger of discharge to a suspected abuser) (59). The court found that, based on the batterer's suspicious conduct while accompanying the injured patient in the hospital, the risk of releasing the battered woman into his custody was reasonably foreseeable.

Specifically relevant in the context of IPV, the court stated: "We believe a hospital's duty of reasonable care

requires consideration of evidence [that] its patient is a victim of domestic abuse . . ." Here, it was uncontroverted that the injured patient had received a general anesthetic for the surgery, a relaxant, various opiates for pain relief, and then was told by hospital staff not to make key decisions. For her to subsequently be released to the very person whom hospital staff suspected had caused the injuries rendered negligence liability (59). Both JCAHO and hospital requirements underscore the importance of routinely inquiring for and properly treating IPV. When HCPs fail to incorporate IPV routine inquiry into their practice, they may not only be at risk of losing accreditations and licenses, but also subject to negligence lawsuits.

CONCLUSION

Good medical documentation helps patients obtain quality medical care, improves the preservation of evidence, and provides information for criminal and civil legal matters. Healthcare providers play an instrumental role in gathering evidence and convincing the court of victims' injuries (both physical and emotional). Without solid documentation, perpetrators may be set free, victims may not receive compensation to pay for their injuries or time lost recovering from IPV, and police may choose not to investigate egregious IPV cases. The stakes are high because, at the intersection of medicine and justice, HCPs can become the greatest advocates for their IPV patients.

IMPLICATIONS FOR POLICY, PRACTICE, AND RESEARCH

Policy

- Health professionals should advocate for resources to study the harms and benefits of mandatory reporting and, in the meantime, advocate for voluntary IPV reporting requirements in states that either have mandatory or no reporting requirements.
- Health professionals should standardize how they determine whether a patient has the capacity to give informed consent.
- Check with the hospital or medical practice policy on the HIPAA standard to

determine whether disclosure of protected health information is appropriate under certain circumstances.

Practice

- Quality improvement efforts should be directed toward the accurate diagnosis of IPV-exposed patients and documentation that services to address patient safety were provided.
- Intimate partner violence patients should routinely be informed of their additional protections under HIPAA and assisted in their patient safety needs.

Research

- Research is needed on the costs and benefits of mandatory reporting to law enforcement.
- It is essential to determine if these laws result in improved health outcomes for IPV patients.
- It must be determined if standardized approaches to forensic exams result in higher prosecution and conviction rates.
- Research is needed to determine if the effect of time and care during the forensic exam impact the development of posttraumatic stress disorder in IPV survivors.

References

1. Johnson R. Rural health response to domestic violence: Policy and practice issues, emerging public policy issues and best practices. The US Department of Health and Human Services Health Resources and Services Administration website. At http://ruralhealth.hrsa.gov/pub/domviol.htm. 2000. Accessed 2/19/2008.
2. *Kringen v. Boslough and Saint Vincent Hospital*: A new trend for healthcare professionals who treat victims of domestic violence? [Electronic version.] *Journal of Health Law*, 33 (4), p.629. *McSwane v. Bloomington Hospital and Health Care System*, No. 53A04–0705-CV-243, (Ind. Ct. App. decided March 14, 2008.)
3. Federal Rules of Evidence, Rule 801, 28 U.S.C.A. 1997.
4. Federal Rule of Evidence, Rule 803(2), 28 U.S.C.A. 1997.
5. Bocchino A, Sonenshein DA. *A practical guide to federal evidence*, 6th ed. Notre Dame, IN: National Institute for Trial Advocacy, 2003.
6. Isaacs N, Enos P. Documenting domestic violence: How health care providers can help victims. National Institute of Justice Research in Brief. 2001.

National Criminal Justice Service website. At http://www.ncjrs.gov/pdffiles1/nij/188564.pdf. Accessed 2/12/2008.
7. Around the school, researchers look at the role of medical records in domestic violence legal Cases. Harvard School of Public Health. August 11, 2000. Harvard School of Public Health website. At http://www.hsph.harvard.edu/ats/Aug11/. Accessed 2/12/2008.
8. Federal Rules of Evidence: 803(4) 28 U.S.C.A (1997).
9. Leventhal J, Aldrich L. The admission of evidence in domestic violence cases after *Crawford v. Washington*: A national survey. *Berkeley Journal of Criminology and Law*. 2006;11:77–100.
10. 541 U.S. 36 (2004).
11. Appelbaum P. Assessment of patients' competence to consent to treatment. *N Engl J Med*. 2007; 357(18):1834–1840.
12. N.Y. PUB. HEALTH § 2441 (McKinney 2001).
13. AMA. Resources/Standards E-10.01: Fundamental elements of the patient-physician relationship. AMA website. At http://www.ama-assn.org/ama/pub/category/4608.html. Accessed 3/24/2008.
14. DEL. CODE. ANN. tit. 16, §1230 (2006).
15. AMA. Abuse of Spouses, Children, Elderly Persons, and Others at Risk, E-2.02 AMA website. At http://www.ama-assn.org/apps/pf_new/pf_online? f_n=browse&doc=policyfiles/HnE/E-2.02.HTM&&s_t =&st_p=&nth=1&prev_pol=policyfiles/HnE/E-1.02. HTM&nxt_pol=policyfiles/HnE/E-2.01.HTM&. (2006). Accessed 11/2/2007.
16. Council on Ethical and Judicial Affairs, Informed Consent: Opinion 2-I-06, E-8.08 Amendment, 2006;15–23. American Medical Association website. At http://www.ama-assn.org/ama1/pub/upload/mm/475/cej02i06.doc. Last Updated June 2006. Accessed 11/2/2007.
17. AMA. Principles of Medical Ethics of the American Medical Association, Confidentiality, E-505. American Medical Association website.2004. At http://www.ama-assn.org/ama/pub/category/8353.html. Accessed 11/3/2007.
18. *Tarasoff v. Regents of University of California*, 551 P.2d 334 (Cal. 1976).
19. 994 S.W.2d 635 (Tex. 1999).
20. Health Information Portability and Accountability Act (HIPAA) 45 C.F.R. §160 et. seq. (2002).
21. Mayo Clinic. Women's health: Domestic violence towards women: Recognize the patterns and seek help. Mayo Clinic website. May 23, 2007. At http://www.mayoclinic.com/health/domestic-violence/W000044. Accessed 3/24/2008.
22. See e.g., Alaska Stat. §§ 47.17.020 (2008), Alaska Stat. §47.17.050 (2008), Alaska Stat. §47.17.068 (2008); 23 Pa. Cons. Stat. §§ 6311 (2008) (mandatory reporters, protection from retaliatory discharge), 6313 (procedure), 6318 (immunity), 6319 (penalty); N.J. State. Ann. §§ 9:6–8.10 (2002) (mandatory reporters, procedure), 9:6–8.13 (immunity), 9:6–8. 14 (penalty), Vt. Stat. Ann. tit. 33, §§ 4913 (2007)

(mandatory reporters, voluntary reporters, confidentiality, immunity, penalty), 4914 (procedure), 4920 (retaliatory discharge prohibited). See e.g. Child Abuse Treatment and Prevention Act, 42 U.S.C. §5101 et. seq. (2003).

23. See, e.g., Alaska Stat. §§ 47.24.900 2008 (definition of vulnerable adult), 47.24.010 (mandatory reporters, procedure, penalty), 12.55.035 (fine for class B misdemeanor), 47.24.120 (immunity), Maine Rev. Stat. tit. 22, §§ 3477 (West 2003) (mandatory reporters, procedure), 3479-A (immunity) 2003, 3475 2003 (penalty); Ohio Rev. Code Ann §§ 5101.61 (West 2008) (mandatory reporters, procedure, immunity), 5101.99 (penalty).

24. See e.g., Del. code ann. tit. 16, §90 (2007), Child Abuse and Neglect Reporting Act. Cal. Penal Code § 11164 (West 2007), Ga. Code Ann., § 19–7-5, I.C. 2006), § 39–5301A (2006).

25. Moskowitz S. Saving granny from the wolf: Elder abuse and neglect-the legal framework. *Conn Law Rev.* 1998;31:77–204.

26. AMA. E-2.02 Abuse of spouses, children, elderly persons, and others at risk. AMA website. At http:// www.ama-assn.org/apps/pf_new/pf_online?f_n= resultLink&doc=policyfiles/HnE/E-2.02.HTM &s_t=consent&catg=AMA/HnE&catg=AMA/BnGnC &catg=AMA/DIR&&st_p=60&nth=1&. Accessed 11/2/2007.

27. AMA. E-2.02 Abuse of spouses, children, elderly persons, and others at risk. American Medical Association website. At http://www.ama-assn.org/apps/ pf_new/pf_online?f_n=resultLink&doc=policyfiles/ HnE/E-2.02.HTM&s_t=consent&catg=AMA/ HnE&catg=AMA/BnGnC&catg=AMA/DIR&&st_ p=60&nth=1&. Accessed 11/2/2007.

28. Freedman A. Symposium: Fact finding in civil domestic violence cases: Secondary traumatic stress and the need for compassionate witnessing. *Am Univ J Gend Soc Policy Law.* 2003;11:567–656.

29. Child Abuse Treatment and Prevention Act, 42 U.S.C. §5101 et.seq. (2003). At http://www.acf. dhhs.gov/programs/cb/laws_policies/cblaws/capta03/ index.htm. See e.g., Ala. C. §38–9-3 (2007), protection from abuse and exploitation, Fla. Stat. § 415.101 (2005), Tenn. Code Ann. § 71–6-101 (2007).

30. Cal. Penal Code. §11160 (18) (West 2007).

31. R.I. Gen. Laws § 12–29–9 (2007) also requires a report be documented in a patient's file.

32. N.H. Rev. Stat. Ann. §631:6 (2008) Failure to Report Injuries (c).

33. Ky. Rev. Stat. Ann. § 209A.030 (Michie. 2007).

34. Col. Rev. stat. §12–36–135 (West 2003).

35. Ohio Rev. Code Ann. §2921.22 (West 2008).

36. Tenn. Code Ann. §36–3-621 (2007).

37. American Academy of Orthopedic Surgeons. Family Violence State Statutes. American Academy of Orthopedic Surgeons. At http://www.aaos.org/about/ abuse/ststatut.asp. Accessed 11/3/2007.

38. Tex. Fam. Code Ann. § 91.003 (Vernon 2002).

39. N.Y. Pub Health Law § 2803-p (McKinney 2007).

40. N.D. Cent. Code §43–17–41 (2007).

41. Rodriguez M, McLoughlin E, Nah G, Campbell JC. Mandatory reporting of domestic violence injuries to the police. *JAMA.* 2001;285(5):580–583.

42. Rodriguez M, Bauer HM, McLoughlin E, Grumbach K. Screening and intervention for intimate partner abuse, practices and attitudes of primary care physicians. *JAMA.* 1999;282:468–474.

43. Fritsch TA, Frederich KW. Mandatory reporting of domestic violence and coordination with child protective services. *Domestic Violence Report.* 1998;3:4:51–52.

44. Houry D, Feldhaus K, Thorson A, Abbott J. Mandatory reporting laws do not deter patients from seeking medical care. *Ann Emerg Med.* 1999;34:336–341.

45. Sachs C, Campbell J, Chu L, Gomberg L. Intimate partner violence victims' attitude toward mandatory reporting. *Acad Emerg Med.* 1999;6:46–566.

46. Smith A. It's my decision, isn't it? A research note on battered women's perceptions of mandatory intervention laws. *Violence Against Women.* 2000;6: 12:1384–1402.

47. Rodriguez M. Mandatory reporting of domestic violence: What do patients and physicians think? In 1997 wellness lectures, the California Wellness Foundation and the University of California. Oakland, CA: California Wellness Foundation, 1997.

48. Biroscak B, Smith P. Intimate partner violence: Findings from emergency department surveillance 1999–2000. Michigan Department of Community Health. Justice Research and Statistics Association website. August 2003. At http://www.jrsa.org/ dvsa-drc/michigan/1999–2000EDIPVreport. pdf#xml. Accessed 2/19/2008.

49. AMA. Family and intimate partner violence policy. H-515.965. AMA website. At http://www.ama-assn. org/apps/pf_new/pf_online?f_n=browse&doc= policyfiles/HnE/H-515.965.HTM. Accessed 3/24/2008.

50. CDC, Intimate Partner Violence Overview. CDC website. At http://www.cdc.gov/ncipc/dvp/IPV/ default.htm. 2005. Accessed 1/16/2008.

51. US Department of Justice. A National Protocol for Sexual Assault Medical Forensic Examinations: Adults/Adolescent. 49NCJ206554. 1–141. Washington DC: US Department of Justice, Office on Violence Against Women, 2004.

52. State of California, California Emergency Management Agency. Forensic Medical Report: Domestic Violence Examination. www.ccfmtc.org/forensic.asp (accessed 3/10/09).

53. Neb. Rev. Stat. § 29–4306 (2007).

54. Cal. Penal Code 13823 (West 2007).

55. Violence Against Women Act 42 U.S.C. § 10607 1994, 28 C.F.R. § 90.2 (2008), 28 C.F.R. § 90.14 (2008).

56. 28 C.F.R. § 90.14(a) (2008).

57. California Office of Emergency Services. Forensic examinations. Cal. Office of Emergency Services website. www.oes.ca.gov. Accessed 4/12/2008.

58. Joint Commission on Accreditation of Healthcare Organizations. Standards for victims of abuse P.C. 3.10. The Family Violence Prevention Fund website. At http://www.endabuse.org/programs/display.php3?DocID=266. Accessed 2/12/2008.

59. *McSwane v. Bloomington Hospital and Health Care System*, No. 53A04–0705-CV-243, (Ind. Ct. App. decided March 14, 2008.)

60. Ind. Code Ann. § 35–47–7-1 (West 2004), Ind. Code Ann. § 35–46–1-13 (West 2004).

Chapter 30

Treatment Approaches for Men Who Batter Their Partners

L. Kevin Hamberger, Jeffrey M. Lohr, Lisa M. Parker, and Tricia Witte

KEY CONCEPTS

- A number of models have evolved to help male batterers end intimate partner violence (IPV).
- Research has shown that treatment to end IPV has a beneficial but weak impact.
- Research has only recently begun to compare the effectiveness of different batterer treatment models.
- Matching type of batterer with type of treatment approach may improve treatment effectiveness.

TRANSACTIONAL CONTEXT OF PARTNER VIOLENCE

Intimate partner violence (IPV) is a transaction between perpetrator and victim. It is defined not only by the perpetration of violence and abuse, but by the fact that it occurs in an interpersonal relationship in which both parties participate. As such, the violence perpetrated is construed in more psychological terms than violence perpetrated upon strangers or on victims in other social roles, such as co-workers. There is little doubt that it represents a serious "relational problem." However, it is difficult to construe IPV as a psychiatric disorder in need of diagnostic criteria and formal classification.

Psychological Dysfunction Versus Diagnosis

Although IPV may not be a classifiable diagnosis, it certainly fits the definition of "mental disorder" as a harmful dysfunction (1). That is, it is a pattern of behavior that: (a) reflects a value term based on social norms and (b) is a failure of a natural function having evolutionary significance or function. Moreover, research has revealed perpetrator typologies (2,3) that clearly indicate a substantial proportion of domestic violence (DV) perpetrators show serious forms of psychopathology, some of which conform to diagnostic characterization, such as antisocial and borderline personality disorders (2,4). However, to develop effective and relevant treatments for IPV perpetrators, it is necessary to develop a working definition of the problem. Such a definition helps to frame the parameters of treatment targets and provides a basis for evaluating treatment effectiveness.

INTIMATE PARTNER VIOLENCE: DESCRIPTION AND DEFINITION

Battery and Violence

Earlier conceptualizations emphasized physical violence and assault. Barnett, Miller-Perrin, and Perrin (5) state "when people talk about marital violence, they are talking about slaps, assaults, rapes, and murders between intimate partners" (p. 186). There is no universal agreement about what, exactly, constitutes partner violence. In fact, Pagelow (6) states that the disagreement over definitions of partner violence is "fundamental" (p 27). For example, some researchers take a primarily psychological approach (7), a social structural approach (8), or a socio-political approach (8). Barnett and colleagues (5) further review the distinctions that a number of researchers make between the terms "abuse," "battering," and "violence."

Number of violent attacks contributes to the definition of some workers. For example, Pagelow (6) differentiates *primary battering*, the first incident of violence in a relationship, from *secondary battering*—subsequent, repeated violent attacks. Other early conceptualizations of partner violence emphasized the degree of injury to the victim (9,10), as well as frequency of physical assault (11). Some researchers (12,13) define violence as a continuum of acts ranging from relatively mild (e.g., push or shove) to severe and likely to cause injury (e.g., assault with or without a weapon). Barnett and Wilshire (14) developed a type of frequency × severity algorithm whereby a person is classified as a batterer if he or she admits to frequent episodes of less severe violence (e.g., pushing, restraining, slapping), or one or more episodes of severe violence (e.g., punching, multiple blows, using a weapon).

Abuse More Broadly Defined

Other scholars, such as Pagelow (6) define violence within the family more broadly than the commission of specific acts and their frequency. Rather, Pagelow

defines violence as the misuse of force or power to deny the rights and freedom of choice of another. More broadly defined as such, IPV or abuse can include not only acts of physical violence but any type of act that interferes with the development and growth of another, or deprives them of the right to make their own choices or to exercise their human rights.

Partner violence also has been defined in terms of intentionality, or purpose. For example, Flynn (15) defined partner violence in terms of physically aggressive acts designed to inflict bodily harm. Saunders (16) referred to violence as "the intentional use of physical force or threatened use of physical force to harm another" (p. 16). Saunders (17) further differentiates "abuse" from "battery" or "physical aggression." Specifically, Saunders considers "abuse" to have political connotations that include both intended physical and psychological harm, whereas battery and physical aggression refer to actual physical acts intended to cause harm. Hamberger and Lohr (18) argue that the intentionality of the violence contributes to functional significance of violent and coercive behaviors to perpetrators, as well as to victims. For the perpetrator, violent and abusive behaviors function to control the victim through their consequences (e.g., "winning" arguments, ending unpleasant internal arousal states, acquisition of goods, such as money, or services, such as sex). For the victim, violence and abusive behaviors acquire highly negative meaning, both direct and symbolic, leading to fear, terror, and behavioral attempts to limit such aversive states. Hamberger and Lohr (18) provide a detailed analysis of the manner in which violent and abusive behavior acquire controlling functionality in abusive relationships.

Barnett and colleagues (5), as well as Pagelow (6), further discuss the function of such behaviors to control or exercise dominance by one partner over the other through fear induction. Adams (19) also addresses the function of battering by defining violence as any type of act that causes a victim to do something they do not want to do, or causes the victim to be afraid. He applies this definition primarily to male-to-female violence from a feminist perspective and, similarly to Saunders (17), discusses that partner violence has political meaning beyond the actual assault that affects the balance of power in the relationship. Pence (20) focuses on the coercive, controlling functions of male violence toward female partners, as well as the interconnections between physical and sexual violence and other tactics of control and domination, such as minimization and denial, intimidation and threats, economic control, using children as tools of coercion, and asserting male dominance and privilege. A number of other clinicians and researchers have also included nonphysical or psychological forms of abuse and aggression in their working definitions of partner violence (21–23). Ganley (21) further differentiates between psychological battering and psychological abuse. She notes that, although the two sets of behavior look identical topographically, psychological battery occurs in the context of a history of actual physical violence in the relationship. Thus, such acts, when they occur, portend the possibility of further physical violence. In relationships without such a violent context or history, such acts are hurtful and damaging, but do not elicit fear or terror that violence is imminent. Ganley (21) and Yllo (8) also identify the function of violence as control through fear induction.

Defining partner violence has an important role in clarifying the effectiveness of batterer intervention programs. In particular, not only is it important in evaluating the effectiveness of batterer treatment to consider its impact on continued physical violence, but also to consider the coercive, fear-inducing nature of IPV. That is, treatment outcome studies need to measure the impact of treatment on the batterer's use of psychologically abusive and terroristic tactics. Further, victim fear and safety should also be included in batterer treatment program evaluations.

PREDOMINANT TREATMENT MODELS OF BATTERER INTERVENTION

Discussion of treatment modalities concerns the format or the manner in which batterer treatment is conducted. Discussion of treatment models focuses on the primary theoretical reasons treatment is conducted, as well as the specific intervention targets. There are a number of different models, or approaches to conceptualizing treatment of batterers. Primarily, specific treatment models reflect the source of their primary development. For example, feminist-based, socio-political models tend to have emerged from battered women's programs and feminist-based men's programs. Cognitive-behavioral and psychodynamic models tend to have emerged from mental health systems and programs. The predominant models are described herein. Following description of the

predominant models of treating men who batter their partners, we will turn our attention to what is known about their effectiveness.

Feminist-based Models

Feminist-based models view battering as part and parcel of broader societal norms and practices that subordinate and oppress women within institutions and individual relationships. Within this model, battering is a *socio-political* problem, and not an individual problem. Men learn, through male socialization processes, to oppress women through any means necessary, including violence. Psychological problems are not viewed as importantly related to battering. In fact, from a feminist-based approach, batterers are viewed as essentially not different from nonviolent men. All men benefit from the oppression of women, and all men must be part of the solution to ending violence and oppression of women. Ending men's violence and oppression of women requires changing community and societal institutions and values in ways that both acknowledge and support the social and economic equality of women, and support the rights of women to live free from violence and oppression. As such, community systems are accountable to battered women for making appropriate changes. As part of the overall community response to IPV, batterer treatment programs are also accountable to battered women to work with batterers in ways that lead to safety and freedom from oppression for the women. Intervention with batterers is primarily educational, to increase awareness of oppressive, sexist attitudes and behaviors that function to dominate and control their partners, and women in general. Following awareness, nonoppressive, egalitarian behaviors and attitudes are introduced and practiced. Intervention also emphasizes batterer accountability to his partner and his community for both his oppressive behavior and for making and maintaining appropriate changes. Hence, within treatment sessions, the client receives regular confrontation and feedback for both undesirable and desirable behaviors. Consistent with the socio-political emphasis on changing communities, male clients of batterer treatment programs are also encouraged to get involved and participate in community efforts to end violence against women, such as speaking at antiviolence rallies, volunteering for projects that aim to enhance equality for women, and so on. The Duluth program (24) and the Emerge program (19) are classic examples of feminist batter treatment models.

Cognitive-Behavioral Model

Within the cognitive-behavioral perspective, battering behavior is a complex combination of thought and attitudinal processes and overt behaviors that serve particular functions for the batterer. In particular, through direct or indirect, vicarious experience, batterers learn that certain behaviors lead to positive outcomes for them. For example, thoughts and actions that lead to sex are likely to be used again in future similar situations. Other behaviors lead to the ending of negative situations. For example, thoughts and actions that lead to ending a difficult argument are reinforced and likely to be used again in similar future situations. With respect to batterers, the behaviors and thought processes are viewed as deficient. That is, batterers are believed to possess rigid or limited problem-solving skills and limited, sexist attitudes and beliefs that set them up for oppressive and abusive behaviors (25,26). In addition, the actual battering behavior is conceptualized as constituting deficient behavioral skills for coping with interpersonal conflict and/or expression of personal needs, expectations, and vulnerabilities (27). Hence, responsibility for perpetrating violent and abusive behaviors, and for ending it, is placed with the perpetrator. His beliefs and actions lead to abuse and oppression. Therefore, he, alone, needs to change to end his abusiveness. Cognitive-behavioral treatment focuses on identification of deficient thought patterns and abusive behaviors, and their modification to nonabusive, noncontrolling skills. Treatment consists of in-session role-modeling, practice of appropriate skills, and feedback for the adequacy of the client's efforts and progress. Cognitive-behavioral treatments frequently include feminist-based analysis of how particular attitudes and behaviors support violence, abuse, and oppression. Hamberger (28) provides a detailed description of a cognitive-behavioral model for treatment that incorporates pro-feminist principles.

Psychodynamic/Trauma-based Model

A model that is experiencing a renaissance posits that IPV is related to unresolved physical and emotional trauma to which batterers were exposed as children. Because the emotional pain related to trauma has not yet been resolved, batterers have learned a number of survival tactics to avoid facing their bad feelings, including high-risk behaviors such as substance abuse, violence, and controlling behaviors (29,30).

Other complications of early trauma and deficient parent–child bonding include the development of attachment disorders (31), particularly an anxious, preoccupied attachment style. Such an attachment style is manifest in the batterer having a relationship model in which he is consistently less worthy than his partner. In addition, compared to nonviolent men, batterers report higher rates of having witnessed abuse (32), which in turn has been shown to adversely affect children in a number of psychosocial and relational factors in predicable ways along a developmental continuum (33). Further, compared to nonviolent men, batterers report having experienced parental rejection as children (34), which combines with a number of other factors to shape disordered personality styles, particularly borderline and narcissistic personality disorders (35). All of these different variations of psychodynamic theory have common themes. First, adult IPV is functionally related to early, negative, and pervasive childhood experiences. Second, the early traumatic and rejection experiences set the child on a developmental trajectory that leads to personal and relationship problems that can include IPV. The goal of psychodynamic/trauma-based treatment is to end violence by helping men to face their pain and its associated shame, and resolve it, leading to new ways of experiencing relationships and relating to intimate partners. Early phases of treatment work on helping clients to develop trust and safety within the treatment context (29). Once safety and trust are achieved, the men are assisted to identify and name the traumatic events of their childhood. Such uncovering leads to giving and receiving support and empathy. Other therapeutic themes include processing and examining how men's alienation from themselves can lead to repetition of alienation from their families and from each other, and learning how to use the therapeutic process to overcome the alienation. Therapeutic approaches that aim to heal attachment disorders by creating a safe place for men to face and examine their feelings and related behavior problems are also utilized (36). Once the trauma has been resolved, violent and abusive behavior will no longer have the function of "covering" or avoiding the bad feelings. Hence, the abusive behavior will end and be replaced by nonviolent, noncontrolling modes of relating to others. Cogan and Porcerelli (37) have described a treatment approach that uses a psychodynamic perspective, whereas Sonkin and Dutton (36) have described treatment approaches with batterers that focus on attachment disorders.

Conjoint Treatment Models

Although the predominant format for treating abusive men and battered women has been to work with them in gender-specific, gender-segregated treatment formats, such as male perpetrator's groups and female victim's groups, models that have advocated working with couples who struggle with IPV have existed for a long time within the history of the DV movement. Some of the earliest descriptions of conjoint treatment to end IPV were published in the mid-1980s (38,39). Since that time, a number of programs have emerged that treat the abusive man and his partner together and that combine a cognitive-behavioral theoretical model (22,40). Other conjoint treatment models are based on a family systems theory of relationships and aggression escalation (41). In general, conjoint approaches to end IPV are viewed as different from standard marital therapy (40). The abuser is held completely responsible for his use of violent and abusive behavior and for ending it. In contrast to gender-specific abuse abatement programs, however, conjoint treatment formats do acknowledge that abuse victims contribute to conflicts and escalation processes that can lead to aggression. As pointed out in the chapter entitled "Risk Factors for Intimate Partner Violence Perpetration" in this text, Murphy and O'Leary (42) found in their longitudinal study that verbal aggression predicted the onset of physical aggression in relatively new marriages. Further, as pointed out by O'Leary (40), most IPV emerges out of interpersonal conflict and not "out of the blue." Hence, as pointed out by Geffner and colleagues (22), if the couple wishes to remain together, the couple, as a unit, needs help to end the violence.

Conjoint approaches are controversial and not well supported by mainstream DV workers or batterer treatment program proponents. Primary objections to conjoint approaches center around safety concerns and messages communicated about causes and responsibility for violence and for ending it. Regarding safety, the primary concern is that the therapy setting may support the idea that both partners are equally safe to express themselves and discuss any relationship material deemed relevant to the treatment process. Thus, victims may be encouraged and convinced that they can safely bring up certain issues that could cause significant discomfort to the abuser. Although such discussion may appear to be dealt with in the session, the victim may be punished for her disclosures by further abuse and intimidation following the session. Conversely, if the victim perceives danger to herself for disclosing certain information in the counseling session, she may be labeled as uncooperative by the therapist for resisting attempts to get her to open up and honestly disclose sensitive information, when all the while, her reluctance is caused and controlled by her abusive partner's intimidation.

The second objection to conjoint treatment approaches concerns the messages that are communicated about the causes and responsibility to end the violence. In particular, conjoint approaches may communicate the subtle message that ending the violence is the responsibility of both parties, not only the perpetrator. Moreover, focusing on what victims can do to reduce conflict that leads to violence may communicate the message that she is partially responsible for causing her own victimization in the first place. Further, the presence of both partners at treatment could suggest that both partners share equal power in the relationship, despite the fact that one partner is abused and the other is the abuser.

Proponents of conjoint treatment approaches argue that they do not dilute responsibility for the violence and for ending it, but instead place such responsibility squarely on the male abuser (22,40). In addition, conjoint treatment programs typically contain detailed steps for assessing victim safety on a session-by-session basis (22). Further, O'Leary, Heyman, and Neidig (43) reported that women in conjoint treatment did not feel less safe than women in gender-specific treatment programs, and the men in conjoint treatment programs and gender-specific programs did not differ in the degree to which they took responsibility for their violence. Heyman and Schlee (44) and Vivian and Heyman (45) present in-depth analysis of the rationale and method for conducting conjoint treatment for IPV.

INTIMATE PARTNER VIOLENCE PROGRAM EVALUATIONS

Gender-specific Treatment Outcome

Each of the models just reviewed has strong philosophical, theoretical, and even empirical bases. Each model focuses on different treatment targets thought to be necessary to end men's violence against female intimate partners. Two questions emerge from this review.

First, how well do these programs work? Second, do certain approaches to treatment work better than others? The first question has begun to receive a considerable amount of research attention. Regarding the second question, comparative studies in the field of batterer treatment are few, making it difficult, and in many cases, impossible, to develop empirically based conclusions.

Babcock, Green, and Robie (46) conducted a meta-analysis of IPV treatment outcome reports to quantitatively summarize the measured effects of batterer treatment programs. Sixty-eight empirical studies were identified and classified according to methodology: experimental (k = 5), quasi-experimental (k = 17), and uncontrolled pre-/post-treatment assessments (k = 48). The uncontrolled pre-/post-assessments were excluded from the analysis because a tendency of such studies to overestimate effect size (47). Comprehensive reviews of such studies have been previously published (48–50).

The experimental studies evaluated by Babcock and colleagues (51) randomly assigned participants to treatment or to no-treatment conditions. Quasi-experiments compare participants who complete treatment to matched participants who did not receive treatment or who dropped out of treatment. The treatment conditions evaluated by Babcock and colleagues included the pro-feminist Duluth Model, cognitive-behavioral treatment, or other types of intervention. Criterion variables included subsequent violence recidivism based on police records or partner report. The effect size was calculated with the d statistic, which is represented in standard deviation units. An effect size of .50 reflects improvement of one-half of a standard deviation as compared to no treatment. An effect size of .20 or less is considered "small," .50 is considered medium, and an effect size of .80 is considered large (52).

Overall, Babcock and colleagues (51) found that the effect size of treatment is within the "small" range. Further, effect sizes for method of reporting were equivalent (police report $d = .18$; partner report $d = .18$). In addition, there was no statistically significant difference in effect size among the Duluth model and cognitive-behavioral programs for either police records or victim report of recidivism. Moreover, there was no statistically significant difference in effect size among quasi-experimental and experimental design studies. Thus, the results indicate that regardless of the reporting method, type of treatment, and methodological

procedure, the effect size on recidivism is small in comparison to psychotherapy outcome studies in general (53). Given the apparently small statistical effect, it may be instructive to examine the randomized controlled trials in greater detail.

Conjoint Treatment Outcome Studies

Because the meta-analysis reviewed above did not include conjoint treatment approaches, this section will review the small but growing literature that has evaluated them. Such studies have typically compared conjoint counseling with gender-specific treatment approaches (43,54,55). Dunford (55) also included a no-treatment, intensive supervision control condition. Further, in addition to assessing impact of treatment on violent and abusive behavior, research in this area has also investigated victim perception of safety, as well as other variables, such as the perpetrator's sense of responsibility, as reviewed earlier (43).

Overall, studies examining the effect of conjoint treatment versus gender-specific treatment have reported few differences between the two approaches, including reductions of violence (43,54,55), victim safety (43,54,55), and responsibility for the violence and for ending it (43). Brannen and Rubin (54) reported that abusive men with alcohol problems showed more violence reduction from conjoint treatment than from gender-specific treatment. Controlling for alcohol abuse, no differences were observed between treatment approaches on measures of communication or marital satisfaction. O'Leary and co-workers (43) also found no differences in levels and changes in marital satisfaction over treatment. Further, follow-up of 6 months (54) and 1 year (43) revealed no differential rates of recidivism between conjoint and gender-specific treatment.

Although these reviews suggest that conjoint treatment approaches have promise for helping some abusers end their violence, there are limitations in the research in this area that bear mention. First, the studies by Brannen and Rubin (54) and O'Leary and co-workers (43) worked with intact couples who wanted to stay together. Moreover, although Brannen and Rubin utilized couples who were involved with the courts, O'Leary and co-workers studied couples who were not. Further, O'Leary's group reported that the level of violence assessed in their samples was mild compared to that frequently observed among court-involved abusers. Hence, as pointed out by

O'Leary (40), conjoint approaches for IPV are not indicated for all couples or abusive men and require careful pretreatment assessment and different methodology than would be used in marital therapy.

EXPERIMENTAL CONTROL VERSUS QUASI-EXPERIMENTAL EVALUATION: DEBATE AND ISSUES

The Case for Experimental Designs

Debate has emerged within the field of batterer treatment program evaluation as to how such programs would best be evaluated to determine efficacy. One side of the argument is that experimental analysis, which includes random assignment to treatment and no-treatment groups to control for placebo and other effects is the only way to truly determine program success (56). Dunford asserts that conclusions drawn from nonexperimental evaluations may lead to erroneous conclusions, because rates of violence reduction and recidivism from treatment conditions are not compared against some no-treatment standard. Thus, it is impossible to conclude that observed changes in violence and recidivism from such evaluations are (a) due to treatment and (b) better than what could be achieved from no treatment. Dunford showed, using data from the San Diego Navy Study (55), that when the no-treatment control condition was eliminated from analysis, the other three, randomly assigned treatments (gender-specific, conjoint, and rigorous monitoring) showed significant reductions in violence and recidivism across a 1-year follow-up. Further, the three interventions were roughly equivalent. When the no-treatment control group was included in the analysis, Dunford reports no significant differences between the three intervention conditions and the control condition, leading to the conclusion that treatment did not significantly reduce continued violence against wives in the Navy.

Other support for Dunford's thesis regarding the importance of experimental control is noted in other studies that have utilized experimental designs. Davis, Taylor, and Maxwell (57) randomly assigned batterers to one of three conditions: a 26-week psycho-educational group, a brief 8-week psycho-educational group, or community service. Group assignment was random except when a judge ordered reassignment from the community service condition to psycho-educational treatment. Recidivism, based on police records at 12-month follow-up, was lower in the 26-week educational condition compared to the 8-week educational or community service conditions. There was no difference in recidivism between the 8-week condition and community service condition. However, when victim report of violence was used as the dependent variable, neither treatment condition was different from the community service condition.

Feder and Forde (58) randomly assigned male batterers to either no treatment probation or feminist cognitive-behavior group treatment that was administered once per week for 26 weeks. Dependent variables included recidivism based on police report and victim report. Statistical analyses showed no significant differences between the two groups on any outcome variable. As the attrition rate in the treatment condition was high (60%), post hoc analyses were conducted on treatment completers, which showed a statistically significant reduction in both measures of recidivism.

The cumulative findings of the controlled experimental trials of treatment efficacy are informative in several ways. It is clear from the findings of Dunford (55) that serious consideration needs to be given to designing outcome studies that include control conditions that assess and provide control for possible treatment artifacts and inappropriate conclusions about treatment efficacy. Although legitimate reasons exist to question the feasibility and ethics of such controls (59,60), their inclusion increases confidence in the effect of treatment. Indeed, Dunford (56) has observed that without the inclusion of a no-treatment control group (55), he would have concluded that treatment had a beneficial effect when there was none.

The Case for Quasi-experimental Designs

The other side of the debate is that "real world" evaluations of batterer treatment programs are sufficiently complex as to preclude meaningful randomization into treatment and no-treatment conditions. Gondolf (61) has described the difficulties with actually implementing random assignment in community-based batterer treatment evaluations. For example, he noted that in the Davis, Taylor, and Maxwell (57) study, judges changed almost 30% of randomized assignments, leading to questions of selection/assignment bias and problems with interpretation. Gondolf noted that the study by Feder and Forde (58), another experimental study, suffered from data collection problems, including a response rate of victims of only 21% at 1-year follow-up. Such a low follow-up rate leads to concerns about selection bias, generalizability problems, and problems of interpretation of the data. The validity of other outcome measures, such as probation violence and post-treatment arrest record is also questionable.

Gondolf (60) therefore argues that quasi-experimental designs that employ a public health–type of analytic approach may be the most appropriate for conducting real-world batterer treatment outcome research.

In a large, multisite treatment outcome study using a quasi-experimental design, Gondolf (60,62,63) evaluated the effect of batterer treatment with four model programs from different geographical areas in the United States, representing different treatment lengths, levels of comprehensiveness of services, and levels of connection to court processes. Program length ranged from 3 to 9 months. Some programs focused exclusively on DV abatement, whereas the most comprehensive program offered in-house substance abuse and mental health treatment, and case management, in addition to abuse abatement treatment. Some programs also provided gender-specific women victim's groups, and others did not.

Initial results, over a 15-month follow-up from initial program intake, showed no significant difference between treatment groups of differing length and comprehensiveness for any reassault. Between 27% and 35% of men in all four programs reassaulted within the 15-month follow-up period. Longer, more comprehensive programs did, however, show significantly lower reassault rates for severe violence, although subsequent logistic regression analyses that controlled for a number of potential confounding factors showed only a weak program effect. Gondolf (60) refers to the use of logistic regression analysis to determine program effect as a naïve analysis, because it does not take into account program contextual influences, and further, does not account for the fact that dropouts received some treatment, albeit a lower dose. Specifically, dropouts from treatment receive a smaller dose of the intervention, but within the context of logistic regression analysis, a case is classified as either a dropout or a completer. To address this limitation of statistical analysis, Gondolf has applied instrumental variable analysis, a methodology used more frequently in public health research. Gondolf reports that, depending on the specifications used

for instrumental variable analysis, program completion reduced the likelihood of reassault by 44%–64% (60,61). Gondolf argues that such analyses are appropriate substitutes for experimental designs in situations in which the rigorous control required by such designs is impossible due to practical and logistical difficulties (60), and provides a more "real-world" look at batterer treatment program effectiveness (61, p. 693).

The debate about the relative benefits of experimental designs or quasi-experimental designs that utilize sophisticated public health analytic techniques to determine batterer treatment effectiveness cannot be conclusively answered, either by the present exposition or by the present state of the art and knowledge. More work needs to be done to determine the most appropriate and effective ways to both treat abusive men and to measure the effectiveness of such treatment. Another emerging strategy to conduct treatment effectiveness studies is to compare different models of batterer treatment against each other.

The Potential of Treatment Matching

The findings of the controlled outcome studies also suggest that the content of the treatment could be matched to the psychological and behavioral characteristics of the perpetrator. As we know from the extant research, perpetrators are a heterogeneous group of men in terms of generality of violence, severity of violence, and psychopathology (2,3). Whereas treatment outcome studies in other areas of psychotherapy typically use stringent inclusion and exclusion criteria to target on particular disorder (64), batterer treatment studies typically include all batterers without reference to potentially important psychological characteristics. Therefore, the small effect sizes reported for batterer intervention studies (51) may be partially explained by the inclusion of a heterogeneous group of men in the treatment conditions.

As reviewed in the chapter on batterer characteristics earlier in the text, researchers have cluster-analyzed personality and psychopathological characteristics of large samples of adjudicated batterers and typically have found three or four subtypes. Holtzworth-Monroe and Stuart (3) theorized three identifiable subtypes. Hamberger, Lohr, Bonge, and Tolin (2) subsequently conducted large sample cluster analysis of adjudicated batterers and confirmed the prediction of: (a) generally violent antisocial, (b) passive-aggressive dependent, and (c) nonpathological, family-only.

If the typology can be generalized to previous treatment outcome research, it is reasonable to infer that all of these subtypes have received the same content of treatment in randomized, quasi-randomized, and uncontrolled studies. If the content of treatment could be matched to batterer subtype, treatment outcome (such as effect size) might be enhanced (65).

Saunders (29) conducted a study that incorporated psychological characteristics as predictors of treatment outcome. He found that perpetrators with antisocial traits showed better outcome with the feminist cognitive-behavioral treatment, whereas those with dependent personality traits showed better outcome with psychodynamic treatment. It is important to note, however, that several methodological limitations threaten the internal validity of the study: absence of a wait-list control condition, absence of fidelity assessment, and use of dependent variables with unknown reliability and validity. More important, the psychological variables that determine batterer subtype were not matched beforehand to different content of treatment.

Batterer typologies may be useful in the conduct of future research on treatment matching. White and Gondolf (66) suggest that batterers who fit the antisocial subtype described by Hamberger and colleagues (2) would best respond to direct therapeutic challenge in group therapy. The therapist should enforce limits on behavior and frame the goal of treatment as a more pro-social means by which to attain desired goals. Compliance with treatment process and goals should be framed as enlightened self-interest. The development of team-oriented group cohesion might reduce the tendency of such individuals to try to take over the group. The objective of treatment would be the containment and abatement of violent and abusive behavior, rather than modifying personality characteristics.

White and Gondolf (66) suggest that the passive-aggressive dependent perpetrator may benefit most from treatment that is aimed at modifying interpersonal skills that may reduce fear of negative evaluation (interpersonal judgment). A nonjudgmental and collaborative context might facilitate the development of more adaptive interpersonal relationships. The use of imitation, role-play rehearsal, and positive social feedback could be used for social skill development. Cognitive-behavioral procedures could be applied to improving affect regulation, anger control, and modification of cognitive distortions that occur in the context of partner conflict. For the non-pathological (family-only) subtype, the more familiar

feminist cognitive-behavioral strategy (24) might be most effective. The content of treatment focuses on violence and abuse as an instrumental means by which to assert power and control over the female partner. Treatment procedures include exposure to prototypic violence scenarios as exemplars that are analyzed for such control functions. The purpose is to improve the male abuser's ability to self-monitor and self-regulate such behaviors and to initiate alternative, egalitarian, adaptive means by which emotions are expressed and interpersonal influence is exercised.

IMPLICATIONS FOR POLICY, PRACTICE, AND RESEARCH

Policy

- Although batterer treatment programming has thus far proven to have a weak impact on ending IPV, it nevertheless remains an appropriate vehicle, as one component of a broader societal response, for holding perpetrators accountable for committing and ending IPV.
- Support must continue for development of innovative, effective treatments to end IPV. Such support would take the form of adequate funding to develop and evaluate different treatment approaches.
- Information on batterer treatment effectiveness will be enhanced by requiring programs to gather and report annual outcome statistics. This will facilitate natural studies to determine what types of treatments work best with which types of perpetrators, under which specific circumstances.

Practice

- Although very little research to date has targeted IPV perpetrators in the healthcare setting, recent studies have shown increasing interest in male batterers.
- Such research is at a very foundational stage, focusing primarily on the question of whether men who use IPV will even respond to survey requests to estimate prevalence of such men in healthcare settings. Oriel and Fleming (67) studied prevalence of partner-violent men in primary care settings. They reported a participation rate of 85% and violence perpetration rates of 13%. Phelan and associates (68) also

found high response rates (85%) among men seeking emergency services who were asked to participate in a survey about their use of IPV. The 85% response rate reported for both studies does suggest that male patients are open to answering questions about the role of partner violence in their lives.

- It appears that the identification of individual exemplars of batterer clusters can be accomplished reliably and accurately by clinicians familiar with the psychological assessment procedures (e.g., MCMI interpretation) and background information on psychological predictor variables. The clinician may be able to use such information to provide informed recommendations as to the feasibility of different types of treatment and informed expectations of treatment efficacy.

- In this way, clinical judgment would be based more on extant evidence rather than intuition.

- Little evidence argues against the use of the conjoint treatment modality in certain cases, but more work needs to be done to determine appropriate indications for its use. In particular, most of the research to date supporting the effectiveness of conjoint treatment for IPV has utilized couples willing to participate in such a treatment, and who used lower levels of violence.

- The various findings reviewed suggest that HCPs are in an important position to ask their male patients about IPV and, when they become aware of IPV, to make informed referrals.

- For referral to a batterer treatment program to be informed, the clinician must know whether batterer intervention programs exist in his community. Over 40 states presently require batterer intervention programs or providers to be certified, demonstrating that they meet minimum require ments of program content and provider training (69).

- Healthcare providers must be aware of the certification requirements in their state and community and refer male patients only to such programs.

- Given the controversy surrounding conjoint treatment for partner violence, despite emerging research supporting its effectiveness with certain intact couples, it is important for HCPs to exercise caution in referring batterers to couples counseling. In particular, conjoint treatment has been used primarily with intact couples who: (a) wish to stay together, (b) *both* agree to participate, and (c) exhibit low levels of violence. Further, clinicians who provide conjoint treatment for IPV must demonstrate that they are conducting specialized abuse abatement counseling, as opposed to regular marital therapy (40).

- HCPs understand that research to date has fallen short of providing stellar endorsement of batterer treatments, regardless of theoretical model. On the other hand, batterer treatment does appear to have a positive effect on reducing and ending IPV (61–63). Thus, HCPs can make referrals to qualified providers with appropriate cautions that such treatment is not a panacea, and no guarantee that it will result in violence cessation.

Research

- Methodological refinement of efficacy on batterer treatment is necessary (51). Despite logistical and ethical challenges (60), experimental research methods must be applied to determine which treatments are efficacious, the nature of essential content and components, and whether some content is more effective with some types of perpetrators than others. Accomplishing this goal requires control conditions for nonspecific factors of treatment in general, and component control conditions to identify "active ingredients" (70) .

- Proponents of rigorous experimental designs are challenged to overcome many of the problems posed by attempting such research in community settings, where the researcher has precious little actual control. It may be necessary to further develop and refine methodological and analytic strategies that are more consistent with public health approaches to research.

- More research is needed to examine whether matching perpetrator type to treatment content reveals differential effectiveness of the many models of treatment that have evolved. One strategy would be to identify a priori batters based on typology and then randomly assign them to either a wait-list control condition or active treatments as described. Magnitude of change within each treatment condition could be assessed for each perpetrator type. If the results of such a study indicated a differential response to treatment, then subsequent studies providing for a priori matching of batterer type to treatment content could be conducted to identify optimal treatment responsiveness, if any.

References

1. Wakefield JC. The concept of mental disorder: On the boundary between biological facts and social values. *Am Psychol.* 1992;47:373–388.
2. Hamberger LK, Lohr JM, Bonge D, Tolin DF. A large sample empirical typology of male spouse abusers and its relationship to dimensions of abuse. *Violence Vict.* 1996;11:277–292.
3. Holtzworth-Munroe A, Stuart GL. Typologies of male batterers: Three subtypes and the differences among them. *Psychol Bull.* 1994;116:476–497.
4. Dutton DG, Saunders K, Starzomski A, Bartholomew K. Intimacy anger and insecure attachments as precursors of abuse in intimate relationships. *J Appl Soc Psychol.* 1994;24:1367–1386.
5. Barnett OW, Miller-Perrin CL, Perrin RD. *Family violence across the lifespan: An introduction.* Thousand Oaks, CA: Sage, 1997.
6. Pagelow MD. *Family violence.* New York: Praeger, 1984.
7. O'Leary KD. Through a psychological lens: Personality traits, personality disorders, and levels of violence. In: Gelles RJ, Loseke DR, eds. *Current controversies on family violence.* Thousand Oaks, CA: Sage Publications;1993:7–30.
8. Yllo KA. Through a feminist lens: Gender, power, and violence. In: Gelles RJ, Loseke DR, eds. *Current controversies on family violence.* Thousand Oaks: Sage Publications;1993:47–62.
9. Stewart MA, deBlois CS. Wife abuse among families attending a child psychiatry clinic. *J Am Acad Child Psychiatry.* 1981;20:845–862.
10. Rounsaville BJ, Weisman MM. Battered women: A medical problem requiring detection. *Int J Psychiatry Med.* 1978;8:191–202.
11. Parker B, Schumaker DN. The battered wife syndrome and violence in the nuclear family of origin: A controlled pilot study. *Am J Public Health.* 1977;67:760–761.
12. Straus MA. Wife-beating: How common and why? *Victimology: An International Journal.* 1977;2:412–418.
13. Gelles RJ, Straus MA. Determinants of violence in the family: Toward a theoretical integration. In: Burr WR, Hill R, Nye FI, Reiss IL, eds. *Contemporary theories about the family,* Vol. 1. New York: Free Press;1979:549–581.
14. Barnett OW, Wilshire TW. Forms and frequencies of wife abuse. *Third National Family Violence Research Conference.* Durham, NH, 1987.
15. Flynn JP. Recent findings related to wife abuse. *Soc Casework.* 1997;58:13–20.
16. Saunders DG. Counseling the violent husband. In: Keller PA, Ritt LG, eds. *Innovations in clinical practice: A source book,* Vol. 1. Sarasota, FL: Professional Resource Exchange;1982:16–29.
17. Saunders DG. Cognitive and behavioral interventions with men who batter: Application and outcome. In: Caesar PL, Hamberger LK, eds. *Treating men who batter: Theory, practice, and programs.* New York: Springer;1989:77–100.
18. Hamberger LK, Lohr JM. Proximal causes of spouse abuse: A theoretical analysis for cognitive-behavioral interventions. In: Caesar PL, Hamberger LK, eds. *Treating men who batter: Theory, practice, and programs.* New York: Springer;1989:53–76.
19. Adams D. Feminist-based interventions for battering men. In: Caesar PL, Hamberger LK, eds. *Treating men who batter: Theory, practice, and programs.* New York: Springer;1989:3–23.
20. Pence E. Batterer programs: Shifting from community collusion to community confrontation. In: Caesar PL, Hamberger LK, eds. *Treating men who batter: Theory, practice, and programs.* New York: Springer;1989:24–50.
21. Ganley AL. Integrating feminist and social learning analyses of aggression: Creating multiple models for intervention with men who batter. In: Caesar PL, Hamberger LK, eds. *Treating men who batter: Theory, practice, and programs.* New York: Springer;1989:196–235.
22. Geffner R, Mantooth C, Franks D, Rao L. A psychoeducational, conjoint therapy approach to reducing family violence In: Caesar PL, Hamberger LK, eds. *Treating men who batter: Theory, practice, and programs.* New York: Springer;1989:103–133.
23. Rosenbaum A, Maiuro R. Eclectic approaches in working with men who batter. In: Caesar PL, Hamberger LK, eds. *Treating men who batter: Theory, practice, and programs.* New York: Springer;1989:165–195.
24. Pence E, Paymar M. *Education groups for men who batter: The Duluth Model.* New York: Springer, 1993.
25. Barnett OW, Hamberger LK. The assessment of maritally violent men on the California Psychological Inventory. *Violence Vict.* 1992;7:15–28.
26. Holtzworth-Munroe A, Hutchenson G. Attributing negative intent to wife behavior: The attributions of martially violent men versus nonviolent men. *J Abnorm Psychol.* 1993;102:206–211.
27. Holtzworth-Munroe A, Anglin K. The competency of responses given by maritally violent men to problematic marital situations. *Violence Vict.* 1991;6:257–269.
28. Hamberger LK. The Men's Group Program: A community-based, cognitive, behavioral, profeminist intervention program. In: Aldarondo E, Mederos F, eds. *Batterer intervention programs: A handbook for clinicians, practitioners, and advocates.* Kingston, NJ: Civic Research Institute, 2002.
29. Saunders D. Feminist-cognitive-behavioral and process-psychodynamic treatment for men who

batter: Interaction of abuser traits and treatment model. *Violence Vict.* 1996;11:393–414.

30. Stonsy S. Treating attachment abuse: The compassion workshop. In: Aldarondo E, Mederos F, eds. *Programs for men who batter: Intervention and prevention strategies for a diverse society.* Kingston, NJ: Civic Research Institute;2002:9–17.

31. Dutton DG, Starzomski AJ. Psychological differences between court-referred and self-referred wife assaulters. *Crim Justice Behav.* 1994;21:203–222.

32. Hamberger LK, Hastings JE. Personality correlates of men who batter and nonviolent men: Some continuities and discontinuities. *J Fam Violence.* 1991;6:131–137.

33. Edleson J. Children's witnessing of adult domestic violence. *J Interpers Violence.* 2000;14:839–870.

34. Dutton DG. *The abusive personality.* New York: Guilford, 1998.

35. Coleman V. Treating the lesbian batterer: Theoretical and clinical considerations: A contemporary psychoanalytic perspective. *Journal of Aggression, Maltreatment, and Trauma.* 2003;7:159–206.

36. Sonkin DJ, Dutton D. Treating assaultive men from an attachment perspective. In: Dutton D, Sonkin DJ, eds. *Intimate violence: Contemporary treatment innovations.* Binghampton, NY: The Haworth Maltreatment and Trauma Press;2003:105–134.

37. Cogan R, Porcerelli JH. Psychoanalytic psychotherapy with people in abusive relationships: Treatment outcomes. In: Dutton D, Sonkin DJ, eds. *Intimate violence: Contemporary treatment innovations.* Binghampton, NY: The Haworth Maltreatment and Trauma Press, 2003.

38. Geller JA, Wasserstrom J. Conjoint therapy for the treatment of domestic violence. In: Roberts AR, ed. *Battered women and their families: Intervention strategies and treatment programs.* New York: Plemum Press;1984:457–481.

39. Neidig PH, Friedman DH. *Spouse abuse: A treatment program for couples.* Champaign, IL: Research Press, 1984.

40. O'Leary KD. Conjoint therapy for partners who engage in physically aggressive behavior: Rationale and research. *Journal of Aggression, Maltreatment, and Trauma.* 2001;5:145–164.

41. Lane G, Russell T. Second-order systemic work with violent couples. In: Caesar PL, Hamberger LK, eds. *Treating men who batter: Theory, practice, and programs.* New York: Springer;1989: 134–162.

42. Murphy CM, O'Leary KD. Psychological aggression predicts physical aggression in early marriage. *J Consult Clin Psychol.* 1989;57:570–582.

43. O'Leary KD, Heyman RE, Neidig PH. Treatment of wife abuse: A comparison of gender-specific and couples approaches. *Behav Ther.* 1999;30: 475–505.

44. Heyman RE, Schlee K. Stopping wife abuse via physical aggression couples treatment. In: Dutton D,

Sonkin DJ, eds. *Intimate violence: Contemporary treatment innovations.* Binghampton, NY: The Haworth Maltreatment and Trauma Press;2003:135–157.

45. Vivian D, Heyman RE. Is there a place for conjoint treatment of marital violence? *In Session.* 1996;2:25–48.

46. Babcock J, Green CE, Webb SA, Graham KH. A second failure to replicate the Gottman, et al. (1995) typology of men who abuse intimate partners, and the possible reasons why. *J Fam Psychol.* 2004;18:396–400.

47. Lipsey MW, Wilson DB. The efficacy of psychological, educational, and behavioral treatment: Confirmation from meta-analysis. *Am Psychol.* 1993;48:1181–1209.

48. Davis RC, Taylor BG. Does batterer treatment reduce violence: A synthesis of the literature. *Women Crim Justice.* 1999;10:69–93.

49. Hamberger LK, Hastings J. Court mandated treatment of men who assault their partners: Issues, controversies, and outcomes. In: Hilton NZ, ed. *Legal responses to wife assault.* Newbury Park CA: Sage Publications;1993:188–229.

50. Rosenfield DB. Court ordered treatment of spouse abuse. *Clin Psychol Rev.* 1992;12:205–226.

51. Babcock JC, Green CE, Robie C. Does batterers' treatment work? A meta-analysis. *Clin Psychol Rev.* 2004;23:1023–1053.

52. Cohen J. *Statistical power analysis of the behavioral sciences.* Hillsdale, NJ: Lawrence Erlbaum, 1988.

53. Smith ML, Glass GV, Miller T. *The benefits of psychotherapy.* Baltimore, MD: Johns Hopkins University Press, 1980.

54. Brannen SJ, Rubin A. Comparing the effectiveness of gender specific and couples groups in a court mandated spouse abuse treatment program. *Res Soc Work Pract.* 1996;6:405–424.

55. Dunford FW. The San Diego Navy experiment: An assessment of interventions for men who assault their wives. *J Consult Clin Psychol.* 2000;68:468–476.

56. Dunford FW. Determining program success: The importance of employing experimental research designs. *Crime Delinq.* 2000;46:425–434.

57. Davis RC, Taylor BG, Maxwell C. Does batterers' treatment reduce violence: A randomized experiment in Brooklyn. *Justice Q.* 1998;18:171–201.

58. Feder L, Forde D. *A test of efficacy of court-mandated counseling for domestic violence offenders: The Broward experiment.* Washington, DC: National Institute of Justice, 2000.

59. Dutton DG, Bodnarchuk M, Kropp R, Hart SD. Wife assault treatment and criminal recidivism. *Int J Offender Ther Comp Criminol.* 1997;41:9–23.

60. Gondolf EW. Limitations of experimental evaluation of batterer programs. *Trauma Violence Abuse.* 2001;2:79–88.

61. Gondolf EW, Jones AS. The program effect of batterer programs in three cities. *Violence Vict.* 2001;16:693–704.

62. Gondolf EW. Patterns of reassault in batterer programs. *Violence Vict.* 1997;12:373–387.

63. Gondolf EW. A comparison of four batterer intervention systems: Do court referral, program length, and services matter? *J Interpers Violence.* 1999;14:41–61.

64. Hsu LM. Random sampling, randomization, and equivalence of contrasted groups in psychotherapy research. In: Kazdin AE, ed. *Methodological issues and strategies in clinical research.* Washington, DC: American Psychological Association;1992: 119–133.

65. Beutler LE, Clarkin J. *Systematic treatment selection: Toward targeted therapeutic interventions.* New York: Brunner/Mazel, 1990.

66. White RJ, Gondolf EW. Implications of personality profiles for batterer treatment. *J Interpers Violence.* 2000;15:467–488.

67. Oriel KA, Fleming MF. Screening men for partner violence in a primary care setting: A new strategy for detecting domestic violence. *J Fam Pract.* 1998;46:493–498.

68. Phelan, M.B., Hamberger, L.K., Guse, C.E., Edwards, S., Walczak, S., & Zosel, A. Domestic violence among male and female patients seeking emergency medical services. *Violence Vic.* 2005:20: 187–206.

69. Austin JB, Dankwort J. Standards for batterer programs: A review and analysis. *J Interpers Violence.* 1999;14:152–168.

70. Lohr JM, DeMaio C, McGlynn FD. Specific and nonspecific factors in the experimental analysis of behavioral treatment efficacy. *Behav Modif.* 2003;27:322–368.

Chapter 31

Stalking Victimization: The Management of Its Consequences

Keith E. Davis and Mindy B. Mechanic

KEY CONCEPTS

- Stalking is a series of behaviors directed at another individual, including repeated unwanted approaches, communication, harassment, and threats or implied threats, that would make a reasonable person afraid.
- Females are more likely to be victims of stalking than males.
- Stalkers differ in their motives, the nature of the prior relationship between the stalker and their victim, the degree of reality contact of the stalker, and the degree of dangerousness of the stalker.
- The crime of stalking is unique for its serial and chronic nature. The resultant degree of fear is attributable to the omnipresent yet unpredictable potential for violence.
- Stalking results in numerous adverse physical and mental health consequences.
- Because of its serial and chronic nature, stalking results in symptoms due to ongoing traumatic stress, and is not a response to prior stress, or posttraumatic stress disorder (PTSD).
- Stalking is a significant predictor of lethal risk in victims of intimate partner violence (IPV).
- Current management approaches for victims of stalking focus on victim safety and treatment of psychological distress.

In this chapter, we shall (a) delineate the development of stalking as a crime, (b) identify prevalence estimates, (c) distinguish among types of stalkers, (d) describe the characteristic features of stalking victimization, and (e) identify the physical and mental health consequences of being stalked. Furthermore, we shall address the issue of safety planning and the management of the high levels of fear associated with this crime. We strongly suggest that viewing the treatment of victims of ongoing stalking through the lens of effective treatments of posttraumatic stress is mistaken in crucial ways. Finally, we end with recommendations for education and prevention efforts.

Only 15 years ago, the word stalking had the connotation of avid pursuit of particular kinds of species, such as deer, moose, butterflies, or even of special delicacies—the wild asparagus. Now, the first image that comes to mind is the stalking of celebrity figures, with potentially lethal results. We will show, however, that stalking is in fact a more common occurrence—not at all limited to celebrity or power figures—but a far-too-typical part of relationship pursuit, of some ongoing intimate relationships, and of separation or breakup (1). The transition in our conception of persistent, obsessive expressions of love from an extreme but recognizable part of love madness into unacceptable harassment or psychological rape is illustrative of the social construction of a problem (2,3). The transition in conceptualization was accomplished by the spirited social action of individuals who had suffered the harmful consequences of stalking—physical attacks, persistent intrusions into privacy, and long-term distress—joined with mental health advocates, district attorneys, judges, and other members of the criminal justice community to insist that state legislatures pass antistalking statues.

From the perspective of legislators, stalking presents some difficulties for the creation of effective criminal statues. First, stalking is an activity description. By this, we mean that to say that George[1] stalked Susan does not commit one either (a) to an inference about George's intent, nor (b) to the specific forms of behavior that George has engaged in, but legally it does commit one to both of the following: (c) the victim's judgment that her privacy is being unreasonably invaded and (d) that she has reason to be concerned for her safety and that of relatives, friends, pets, or other significant property. Although the perpetrator's intent may be benign—establishing a relationship—it is the victim's construal that matters. Most states followed the recommendations of the uniform antistalking statues proposed by the National Criminal Justice Association (4) as a course of conduct directed at a specific person that involves repeated visual or physical proximity, nonconsensual communication, or verbal, written, or implied threats, or a combination thereof, that would cause a reasonable person fear (pp. 43–44). The course of

action engaged in by the perpetrator must be persistent, which at the minimum requires at least two actions: it must be of the sort that a reasonable person would take to be invasive, threatening, or harassing. And the victim must have a high level of fear for her own safety or that of family and friends. The elements of the typical antistalking statue—both in the 50 United States, and in Australia, Canada, England, and Wales—require more than mere annoyance on the victim's part. Practically, a burden of proof is placed on the victim to document the form and persistence of the courses of action, to make the case for these actions being a threat to her safety, and to establish that she has reasonable grounds for distress (to avoid coming off as a hysterical woman).

In general, prosecutors prefer to make cases that are not dependent upon the victim's reaction. Thus, the police and district attorneys treat rape and stalking as harder cases to successfully prosecute than battery, harassment, or property damage (5). Victims are loath to report stalking cases for some of the same reasons that they are reluctant to report rape and sexual molestation victimization.

PREVALENCE ESTIMATES

National Violence Against Women Survey Estimates (with Different Criteria)

The National Violence Against Women Survey (NVAW), conducted in 1995, was a major joint undertaking of the National Institute of Justice and the Center for Disease Control (CDC) designed (1) to survey 8,000 men and 8,000 women about their experiences with four major types of violence: (a) physical abuse, (b) psychological abuse, (c) sexual abuse, and (d) stalking—and to document a broad range of health, mental health, and substance abuse problems plausibly related to such experiences.

Three different criteria have been used to calculate prevalence rates from this sample. The most conservative of these is Tjaden and Thoennes (1), which require both multiple occurrences and that the victim was very afraid. It yielded an estimate that 8.1% of U.S. women between the ages of 18 and 85 (not residing on college campuses, residential treatment centers, or correctional facilities) had been stalked, with a corresponding estimate of 2.2% for men. In that same sample, 12.1% of the women (and 6.2% of men)

---

[1] Throughout, we shall refer to the stalker as male and the victim as female both for ease of communication and because this is the statistically most common gender pattern. In fact, men are often victims and women stalk both men and, sometimes, other women·

answered the question, *Have you ever been stalked?* affirmatively. When Davis, Coker, and Sanderson (6) excluded those participants over 65 and relaxed the criteria from being very afraid to merely being afraid, 14.3% of the women and 4.3% of men were classified as having been stalked.

College Samples

Routine activity theory (7) suggests that we should expect higher rates of stalking among younger samples who lived among strangers and socialized together in clubs. The data are consistent with this expectation. Fisher (8) found that 13.7% of a representative sample college women self-reported being stalked enough to be afraid in the previous 7 months. Many convenience samples on college campuses find rates of self-reported victimization of 15%–30%, with small to nonsignificant gender differences in reported victimization. One of the most consistent findings in this arena is that victims and perpetrators have different perspectives on what counts as harassment or illegal stalking (9).

MULTIDIMENSIONAL ANALYSIS OF STALKER TYPES AND THEIR RELATION TO INTIMATE PARTNER VIOLENCE

Those who have encountered stalkers in the criminal justice and mental health systems quickly became aware that several types of stalkers exist (10,11). In our view, the two best published studies of the variety of stalkers have been done in Australia (12) and in Great Britain (13). But useful information about variations in stalker types and their management can be found in Meloy (10,14) and in Zona, Palarea, and Lane (15). Because the independent results of the two major classifications are so similar, we have drawn on them extensively for this section. When the descriptions of their types are compared, they agree in finding four distinctions essential to their sorting of types: (a) The motives of the stalker, (b) the nature of the prior relationship between stalker and victim, (c) the degree of reality contact of the stalker, and (d) the degree of dangerousness of the stalker (16).

Almost all research groups have noted three categories of motives: (a) desire for revenge for perceived mistreatment or rejection—which includes trying to leave a partner, (b) pursuit of an unrequited love, or (c) desire to degrade the victim (where the victim has not mistreated the stalker). The primary variation in *relationship history* is whether the perpetrator had an intimate enough relationship so that perceived *betrayal* was a possible motive versus being merely a stranger or acquaintance. Perceived betrayal is possible in both romantic and nonromantic relationships. In the former, having been sexually intimate prior to a breakup dramatically increases the risk of violence (14). In the case of co-workers and friends, evidence from case studies suggests that whenever the persons are interdependent enough so that one person can harm the other's reputation or standing in an important community, then perceived betrayal or humiliation can lead to stalking and violence (17–19).

The issue of *reality contact* can best be summed up by the answer to the question: Are crucial beliefs (e.g., that he and the victim have had an intimate relationship or that he is being persecuted by the victim) of the stalker delusional or not? Psychiatrists have long been interested in the variety of delusions and obsessions that their patients have, and patient stalkers have been no exception, but thus far, no type of delusion other than persecutory has not been linked to risk of violence (11,12). Finally, stalkers vary greatly in how likely they are to be engaged in physically *dangerous behavior* toward their victims, including property damage as well as personal harm or death. Many stalkers want merely to be in their beloved's world and have no desire to inflict physical harm. Yet, out of their insistence on being part of that world, they become a major violator of their victim's privacy and engage in harassing and stalking behaviors, such as persistent unwanted telephone calls or e-mails. They show up at the victim's home, school, or workplace uninvited and at inappropriate times. They presume a relationship with the victim that does not exist, and although this may not technically be dangerous, the inappropriateness of the stalker's behavior strikes fear in the heart of the object of his attention. It is worth noting that stalking episodes often go on over extended periods of time, with the median time being between 18 and 27 months (1). To have an unwanted suitor in one's life for such a period of time is highly distressing. Furthermore, in most cases, nothing seems to work to dissuade the stalker. Initially, many victims try the polite "No, I am not interested in a relationship," only to find that such statements may increase the intensity of stalking. Some stalkers take this polite rejection as a test of their intentions and respond with redoubled effort. The plight of the victim takes on even more stressful aspects to the degree that the stalker makes verbal threats, damages property, and/or gains access to private information about the victim (9,17). Unfortunately, no good longitudinal study allows an estimate of the probability of dangerous behavior by stalkers as a function of time, specific types of events, or stalker characteristics. By extrapolating from extensive research on intimate partner violence (IPV), some useful guidelines can be offered (20). The best predictor of future behavior is past behavior; thus any evidence that the stalker has been violent previously toward the victim or toward others immediately indicates higher risk. Threats by the stalker to harm himself or the victim again must be given some weight—although these are often ploys to force the victim to take the stalker seriously and thus to continue interacting with him.

Stranger stalking brings in a different set of concerns, one of which is the likelihood of initially innocent stalking developing into dangerous obsessive pursuit. The NVAW data provide one of the best opportunities to examine the associations of stalking with physical violence, psychological abuse (coercion and control), and forced sexual acts. Both the Australian (12) and British (13) data affirm that a subset of stalkers are sexual predators who use stalking as means of gaining enough information to romance the victim before subjecting her to sexual degradation.

CHARACTERISTICS OF STALKING VICTIMIZATION: ITS DURATION AND DEGREE OF FEAR

Stalking victimization, in contrast to many other time-limited forms of victimization, is unique for its serial and chronic nature (1). In the NVAW survey, Tjaden and Thoennes (1) found that stalking episodes lasted on average 1.8 years, with lengthier periods of stalking found for women experiencing concurrent forms of IPV (2.2 years on average). In contrast, college populations tend to report much briefer episodes of stalking. Fisher (2001), in her national sample of college women, reported that stalking episodes lasted an average of 2 months.

Although most incidents of stalking do not erupt in physical violence or injuries (21), the menacing nature of stalking is attributable to the omnipresent yet *unpredictable* potential for violation that looms on the horizon, generating severe fear, distress, and a range of lifestyle disruptions (1,12,22,23).

Consequently, the stalking experience as described by victims is one of becoming a psychological hostage to a relentless pursuer who intrudes into every crevice of life, leaving no inner space sacrosanct and no physical place immune from the potential for violation. It is no surprise then, that stalking victims, particularly those with co-occurring forms of IPV, report high levels of psychological distress and symptomatology (24).

STALKING AND PHYSICAL HEALTH SEQUELAE

The National Violence Against Women Survey

Stalking victims reported worsening of preexisting physical conditions and the development of new somatic complaints. Victims acknowledged general deterioration in their physical health as a result of stalking. These findings have been replicated in several studies. The specific diseases and disorders most frequently reported in Pathe and Mullen (25), of a sample of 100 volunteers were (a) digestive disturbances (23%–30%), (b) headaches (47%), (c) appetite and weight fluctuations (45%–48%), and (d) excessive tiredness and weaknesses (55%).

A major innovation of the Davis, Coker, and Sanderson (6) analysis of the NVAW data was the use of the temporal information on each incident of violence and stalking and each starting point for illness symptoms to construct a dataset in which only those health ill effects occurring after the first instance of stalking are included in the analysis. Thus, in their analysis, they have constructed a time-controlled dataset that makes it more plausible that they were dealing with effects, not merely with correlations. The results of Davis, Coker, and Sanderson (6) were summarized:

> In comparison with persons who did not report being stalked and adjusting for age, race, health insurance, childhood physical or sexual abuse, and partner violence, those who were stalked and were very afraid of the stalker were significantly more likely to report poor current health status (aRR = 1.7 for women and aRR = 3.7 for men), to develop a chronic disease (aRR = 1.5 for women), and to become injured (aRR = 2.2 for women) and this association held among women for injuries to the neck (aRR = 2.2; 95% CI = 1.1, 4.2) and back

injuries (aRR = 2.5, 95% CI 1.5, 4.2) . . . Being stalked independent of the level of fear was associated with current depression for both women and men. Fearful stalking was significantly associated with developing a chronic mental illness among women (aRR = 3.4) and with current antidepressant use (aRR = 2.2). Being stalked independent of the level of fear was associated with current use of tranquilizers and recreational drugs for women and men. In general, among women, the associations between mental and physical health outcomes and stalking were stronger for those reporting being very afraid of the stalker. (p. 437)

Other Research

One statewide study of stalking among female residents of Louisiana documented a 32% injury rate among women reporting lifetime stalking victimization and who perceived their stalking to be somewhat dangerous or life threatening (26). These injuries, resulting from assaults committed by the stalker, included swelling, cuts, scratches, bruises, strains/sprains, burns, bites, broken teeth, and knife or gunshot wounds. Injury rates were four times higher among women stalked by current or former intimate partners than by other types of stalkers.

Among a sample of battered women, stalking in combination with psychological abuse contributed unique variance to the prediction of severe injuries, both when entered first into the regression model, and again after controlling for physical violence (27). These data highlight the importance of nonphysical forms of IPV as risk factors for severe injuries among women who are battered by their intimate partners.

FEAR AND PHYSICAL HEALTH CONSEQUENCES OF STALKING

Long-term fear and arousal system activation contribute not only to psychological distress, but are also tied to decrements in long-term physical health functioning through a variety of possible mechanisms, including suppressed immune function secondary to hormonal activation, as well as behavioral responses to trauma, including poor self-care and increased health-risk behaviors (28–30). Physical and psychological forms of relationship abuse have both been

documented to result in chronic health problems, as have a variety of other traumatic stressors (31–33).

Interestingly, Sutherland, Bybee, and Sullivan (33) found that the detrimental (non–injury based) physical health effects of intimate partner abuse were mediated by symptoms of anxiety and depression, and these effects continued to persist over time even in the absence of continued abuse. Thus, their study underscores the point that mental health consequences of intimate partner abuse appear to provide critical links between experiences of intimate partner abuse and resulting decrements in functioning, at least in terms of physical health outcomes. It is thus important to consider the role of fear, distress, and psychological symptomatology in potentially mediating the negative physical health consequences of stalking victimization as it occurs with and without concurrent IPV (29).

Coercive Control

When stalking occurs in the context of current or dissolving romantic or intimate partnerships, stalking functions as a coercive control tactic that may manifest in a variety of additional abusive behaviors that include emotional or psychological abuse, physical violence, and sexual coercion (1,23). The exercise of coercive control through the use of abusive behavior functions to instill fear and uncertainty, thus increasing the probability that the victim will engage in compliant behavior or other behavior organized around reducing the risks associated with the potential but unpredictable threat posed by the perpetrator. Although the possibility of harm posed by an unknown stalker is undoubtedly associated with significant fear, stalking transacted in the context of previous relationship violence is menacing precisely because the victim knows the perpetrator to be capable of, and willing to use, physical violence to achieve domination and control. In a recent study of battered women, stalking significantly predicted women's fears that their partners would commit future violence against them and predicted their fears of lethal harm, even after controlling for the effects of physical violence (23). A study of 187 women stalked by former intimate partners (34) reported that both power and control dynamics previously established during the abusive relationship were evidenced during stalking, as partners attempted to reestablish waning control over their intimate partners.

Loss of Control and Schema Disruptions

Schema disruptions or shattered assumptions are classic responses to a range of traumatic events, particularly traumas that are interpersonal in nature (in contrast to a natural disaster). It is precisely the loss of control engendered by trauma that wreaks havoc with a victim's sense of control and predictability about the world. Traumatic events, such as stalking, pose a challenge to one's views about personal control. Moreover, victimization disrupts a victim's sense of personal control and power—often leading to a variety of efforts to regain a sense of control over her world.

Disrupted schemas have been observed among victims of various forms of interpersonal victimization, including sexual assault, sexual abuse, and domestic violence (24,35,36). Traumatic events challenge core beliefs about the both the predictability and meaning of the world as well as the trustworthiness of oneself and others—at times resulting in attempts to restore schematic structures by disavowing the traumatic event, or by holding oneself accountable for the victimization through self-blame (36,37). Schema disruptions related to themes of safety, trust, control/power, and esteem have been documented among survivors of interpersonal trauma (35,37).

Cognitive schemas play an important role in information processing because they function as filters for organizing information and integrating a traumatic experience into existing cognitive structures. When a traumatic event and a schematic structure are in conflict, the result can be failed information processing, resulting in traumatic stress symptoms (38). Moreover, disruptions in schemas about trust and safety can result in massive curtailment of life activities, including interpersonal relationships, due to fear that others are likely to cause harm or betrayal. Treatment with survivors of trauma often involves working with disruptions in cognitive schemas to integrate the traumatic experience with world views and restore functional capacities (38,39). Unfortunately, little research has addressed the impact of stalking on cognitive schemas, although it is expected that the nature of stalking victimization would be likely to impair the victim's sense of trust and control.

Other Efforts to Reestablish Control

Apart from schematic disruptions, victims of stalking may attempt to regain a sense of control over their worlds by engaging in a variety of safety-related and lifestyle changing behaviors. For example, some stalking victims have attempted to reestablish their sense of control by securing a firearm (1,26). Although securing a firearm might create the illusion of increased safety, easy access to a weapon may actually increase the risk of violent victimization against the stalking victim (40). Medical and mental health professionals might consider working with stalking victims to manage heightened levels of fear and anxiety and increase a sense of empowerment through other means (e.g., stress management approaches), and to conduct a comprehensive risk assessment that might incorporate the potential added danger associated with the purchase of a weapon. Risk assessment approaches, traditionally employed only with offender populations, have recently been used with battered women with some success to predict the likelihood of reabuse (40,41).

Paradigm Shift

As discussed earlier, stalking is a serial event that tends to persist for lengthy periods of time in a victim's life. When stalking co-occurs with other forms of IPV, the picture is complicated by both realistic threats of violence, as well as continued harassment, stalking, and reassault even after separation from an abusive partner (23,42,43). In a small sample of battered women ($N = 75$) followed over a 6-month period, Mechanic, Marelich, and Resick (42) found that, whereas battered women who remained with abusive partners were more likely to be physically and sexually reassaulted by those partners, stalking was unrelated to relationship status. That is, 25% of the sample reported stalking over a 6-month period, whether they were separated or still with their abusive partners. Women in this sample reported very high rates of depression and postraumatic stress disorder (PTSD), suggesting a pattern of chronic symptomatic adaptation to the stalking and violence in their lives. Anecdotally, these women described enormous frustration with having taken all the right steps—by seeking help, separating from their abusive partners, etc.—and yet they continued to be stalked and harassed over lengthy periods of time. The limits of victim-only interventions are underscored by these cases. Clearly, efforts to develop more responsive criminal justice, legal system, and mental health interventions with stalking populations are crucial. For victims, even doing all the "right things," does not necessarily end the reign of terror endured under stalking.

MENTAL HEALTH CONSEQUENCES OF STALKING VICTIMIZATION

Surprising little research has systematically explored the mental health consequences of stalking victimization. Research on stalking victimization has been descriptive or anecdotal, lacking standardized assessments of clinical constructs, such as depression and PTSD. General distress, anxiety, and fear are among the most frequently described responses to stalking victimization (25). Fear and general distress are among the most frequently reported victim reactions to stalking (25,44,45). In a re-analysis of the NVAW study, Davis and colleagues (6) found that fear was 13 times more likely among female than male stalking victims in data collected from the NVAWS. Behavioral changes and lifestyle disruptions are also commonly reported by stalking victims (1,22,46,47). Behavioral strategies made in response to stalking victimization include changing residence and telephone numbers, varying daily routines and travel patterns, and increased attention to personal security.

Psychological responses to traumatic events commonly include PTSD, depression, and substance abuse problems, as well as alterations in schemas about the self, the world, and other people, as discussed earlier. Carlson and Dalenberg (48) identified three features of an event that are necessary in order for that event to be experienced as traumatic: suddenness, uncontrollability, and perception of the event as negative. Many cases of stalking victimization are likely to be consistent with the three defining features of a traumatic event. Although an event may be experienced as traumatic, many factors influence whether or not a particular individual will experience symptoms sufficiently severe to warrant a diagnosis of a psychological disorder.

Depression

Depression is another very common response to victimization. Research assessing depression in the wake of stalking has generally not systematically evaluated depression using standardized assessment tools, thus limiting the conclusions that can be offered about clinical levels of depression. Using data from the NVAWS, Davis and colleagues (6) reported that nearly 20% of stalked individuals reported current depression. Stalking was associated with increased rates of depression for both male and female stalking victims. Pathe and Mullen (25) reported suicidal ideation among nearly one-quarter of the stalking victims studied. Depression at the clinically significant level was documented to occur at high rates among the battered and stalked women studied by Mechanic and her colleagues (24). Levels of depressive symptoms were higher among college students reporting stalking, compared to those who were victims of harassment and to comparison participants experiencing neither stalking nor harassment (45). Like PTSD, future research on the impact of stalking victimization would benefit from evaluation of depression using standardized measures of symptomatology, such as the Beck Depression Inventory.

Posttraumatic Stress Disorder

Posttraumatic stress disorder is comprised of a triad of symptom clusters: reexperiencing, avoidance, and hyperarousal. Although formally a minimum number of symptoms from each cluster are required to fulfill the diagnostic criteria for PTSD, research has found that even subsyndromal forms of PTSD that fall short of the required number of symptoms can result in clinically significant distress and functional impairment (49). Moreover, even a client presenting with the full panoply of PTSD symptoms is ineligible for the diagnosis if the traumatic event to which they were exposed failed to pose a threat of physical harm and concomitant fear, distress, and horror (criterion A). Research on stalking victims suggests that, although they may experience significant fear and distress, threats to the physical integrity of oneself or others (as required for a diagnosis of PTSD) may not be present. Pathe and Mullen (25) reported that 18% of stalking victims fulfilled symptom criteria for PTSD, but were not eligible for the diagnosis because of the absence of threatened harm.

Because not all individuals exposed to a traumatic event will develop PTSD, research has begun to delineate factors that increase the odds of symptomatic responding in the context of traumatic event exposure. Risk factors for developing PTSD following exposure to a traumatic event include female gender (50), prior history of traumatic event exposure (51), physical injury and/or perceived life threat during the traumatic event (39), repeat victimization (52), and interpersonal victimization, particularly physical and sexual assault (50). Given that many of these risk factors are also features of stalking victimization or co-occur with it, it can be argued that stalking carries a high risk of PTSD liability. This is particularly true when stalking co-occurs with physical and sexual violence. Unfortunately, very few studies have assessed PTSD in relation to stalking victimization. Rates of PTSD in the context of stalking without concomitant physical violence are difficult to obtain, as stalking has not been included in most epidemiological studies of traumatic event exposure and resultant PTSD. However, PTSD symptomatology was assessed with the Posttraumatic Stress Diagnostic Scale (53) in two studies with very different populations—one comprised of harassed and stalked college students (45) and the other composed of infrequently and relentlessly stalked battered women (43). Westrup and colleagues (45) reported significantly higher PTSD scores among stalked women ($M = 16.84$; $SD = 14.17$) compared to harassed women ($M = 7.00$; $SD = 6.63$) and control subjects ($M = 5.79$; $SD = 8.47$). Among the battered women, those reporting relentless stalking ($M = 49.6$; $SD = 10.4$) reported more severe PTSD than those who experienced less frequent stalking ($M = 44.0$; $SD = 9.3$). The less severely stalked battered women reported PTSD symptoms that were 2.6 times higher than the stalked college women, and 6.3 times higher than the harassed college students. Similarly, the relentlessly stalked battered women had PTSD scores that were nearly three times higher than the college stalked women and about seven times higher than the college harassed women. These differences suggest the obvious—more severe stalking and associated violence results in greater psychological symptomatology. These comparisons also caution us about generalizing from findings on symptom indices obtained on college populations to clinical populations of stalking victims. Nonetheless, even at the lower levels of stalking, female victims report clinically significant symptoms of traumatic stress reactions.

Finally, because stalking often co-occurs with a number of other forms of IPV, it is reasonable to question the extent to which stalking victimization contributes uniquely to posttraumatic symptomatology, after controlling for the effects of physical and sexual violence. Two recent studies (24,54) using multivariate models both found that stalking victimization contributes uniquely to the prediction of PTSD symptoms, even after controlling for other more violent forms of IPV.

Substance Use

In the face of high levels of psychological symptomatology and distress, some victims of traumatic events cope with their distress through the use of alcohol and/or drugs as a self-medicating strategy to cope with distressing psychological symptoms (55,56). Elevated rates of substance abuse, compared to general-population samples of women, have been documented among battered women (57,58) and among stalked men and women (6). Although substance use may, in part be motivated by a self-medication strategy to attenuate disturbing symptoms of PTSD and depression, it is also possible that in the context of exposure to serial forms of victimization (i.e., stalking and partner abuse), substance use is a maladaptive strategy to cope with the uncontrollable, unpredictable threat of looming potential violence. Unfortunately, although the use of substances may have short-term beneficial effects by temporarily reducing emotional distress, the long-terms complications include the development of secondary substance abuse disorders that further hinder recovery from trauma and may impede the deployment of more effective strategic and coping responses to ongoing threats of harm.

STALKING AND LETHAL VIOLENCE

Of paramount concern is the potential eruption of stalking into acts of violence that may increase the risk of lethal or near lethal outcomes. Stalking has been identified as a significant risk factor for lethal and near-lethal assaults on battered women (59–61). In an interesting case control study of 821 women in 10 different U.S. cites, McFarlane, Campbell, and Watson (61) compared a sample of 437 women who were killed or nearly killed by their intimate partners with a control sample of 384 abused women residing in the community. A set of potential risk factors was assessed to determine their relative ability to predict femicide (i.e., homicide of a woman by her intimate partner) or near femicide (i.e., cases that could have but did not result in death for the victim). Stalking emerged as a significant predictor of lethal risk. Specifically, a substantially higher proportion of the killed/nearly killed women had histories of stalking (79%) in their abusive relationships compared to the control group of abused women (49%). Although there was a link between physical abuse, stalking, and acts of lethal or near-lethal violence, it is notable that in 15% of the cases of femicide/attempted femicide, there was a history of stalking alone without a concomitant history of relationship abuse. These findings underscore the importance of stalking, either alone or in conjunction with other forms of IPV, as a significant risk factor for lethal and near-lethal violence.

McFarlane and her colleagues sought to identify specific risk factors for lethality. After controlling for the influence of demographic factors, in multivariate analyses the authors found being followed or spied on by the abuser in the 12-months prior to the lethal or near-lethal incident resulted in a nearly 2.5-fold risk. More detailed analyses focused on the risk associated with specific threatening behaviors. Again, multivariate analyses controlling for demographic variables identified five threat factors that were associated with increased odds of becoming a femicide/attempted femicide victim: (a) threatened to harm children if the woman left (aOR = 8.99); (b) frightened the woman with a weapon prior to the incident (aOR = 5.89); (c) left scary notes on the woman's car prior to the incident (aOR = 4.37); (d) threatened to kill the woman (aOR = 3.02); and (e) frightened or threatened the woman's family prior to the incident (aOR = 2.31). (Note: aOR = increased risk of femicide/near femicide when this risk factor was present, after controlling for other relevant factors.) Clearly, practitioners working with abused women should incorporate assessment of these factors in their risk assessments with clients.

THE PROBLEM OF POSTTRAUMATIC STRESS DISORDER

Previous sections concluded that PTSD and depression are the most likely symptomatic responses to trauma and victimization and are thus likely to be the target of intervention in mental health settings. As described elsewhere (42), it can be argued that the PTSD conceptualization is problematic when applied to cases of serial forms of victimization, such as stalking and IPV. Specifically, the construct of *post*-traumatic stress disorder is predicated on the idea that a person experienced a traumatic event that occurred in the past (1 month minimum) but, although the traumatic event has ceased, the individual continues to respond as though danger still exists, resulting in a range of intrusive, avoidant, and hyperarousal symptoms. That these symptoms constitute a disorder codified in the

Diagnostic and Statistical Manual of Mental Disorders (DSM-IV) (62) underscores the point that when a person who is no longer in danger responds as though the danger still persists, she is manifesting a pathological overreaction—that is, she is behaving as though the trauma is ongoing and that danger persists when indeed, threatened danger has passed and objectively she is now safe. Herein lies the problem. For women experiencing IPV and stalking, harassment and continued threats are perpetrated even after exiting the abusive relationships (23,43). Further, women experience the same intrusive, avoidant, and hyperarousal symptoms (43) when the objective threat to their well-being poses a present and future danger of unknown magnitude and duration, although the reactions are clearly not post event. To reframe the meaning of these symptoms—in the face of threatened harm to oneself or loved ones, hyperarousal symptoms are no longer *symptomatic reactions* experienced by a fearful, but otherwise safe individual, but rather, they may be conceptualized as reasonable responses to actual/threatened harm. Therefore, in the face of actual or threatened danger, *hyperarousal reactions* are just that—survival-based fear *reactions* rather than (pathological) symptomatic responses to conditioned cues experienced in the context of objectively safe but previously dangerous conditions. By extension, because trauma-based treatments for PTSD adopt the conceptualization of PTSD as a pathological reaction to one or more *past* events, their goals are to extinguish the maladaptive fear/hyperarousal response to threat cues. Such approaches are clearly contraindicated in the case of ongoing stalking with or without concurrent forms of IPV.

Finally, with respect to diagnostic conceptualization and classification of traumatic stress responses, future efforts should attempt to either redefine the PTSD construct to account for peritraumatic conditions, or additional categories ought to be developed that adequately capture the nature of responses to traumatic events that pose ongoing threats of danger and violence.

CLINICAL AND THREAT MANAGEMENT APPROACHES WITH VICTIMS

This section, outlining clinical and threat management approaches, draws heavily on the work of Mechanic (63) in describing a variety of approaches to managing victim safety and psychological distress. Progress has been made in the development and empirical evaluation of treatment approaches for both of these disorders. Empirically validated approaches have been developed for treating PTSD resulting from a variety of traumatic stressors, including sexual assault, combat, childhood sexual abuse, and natural disasters (64,65). Recently, the International Society for Traumatic Stress Studies (ISTSS) published guidelines to assist practitioners in choosing empirically validated approaches for treating PTSD (64). Interestingly, the guidelines intentionally omitted offering treatment recommendations for "peritraumatic" events posing a continued risk of danger—this would include stalking and other forms of partner abuse. Reasons offered for this omission were the multitude of ethical, forensic, and clinical complications faced by individuals exposed to ongoing relationship violence. Thus, whereas practice guidelines for the treatment of PTSD do exist, they are unfortunately not applicable to the majority of stalking and relationship violence victims because of the continued risk of violence exposure. Consequently, stalking victims facing active stalking at the time they seek treatment are not candidates for active trauma therapies.

Nonetheless, some issues can be the focus of clinical intervention in cases characterized by ongoing stalking. These include documentation of stalking incidents, safety planning, risk assessment, and crisis management to deal with symptoms of distress, fear, anxiety, depression, and traumatic stress. Developing a paper trail can be useful, even if a victim has not decided whether to pursue criminal justice system remedies. Obtaining records from caller ID output, logs of phone calls, copies of threatening letters, and pictures of injuries or of the stalker sitting outside the home, are examples of evidence that may help build a case if a victim decides to seek criminal justice system assistance. When stalking occurs absent threatened or actual violence, law enforcement personnel may not pursue the matter vigorously. Similarly, stalking transacted in the context of other forms of domestic abuse may be ignored by law enforcement (66). Although victims frequently do not feel empowered within the criminal justice system, it may be helpful to remind them of their rights and to suggest that they contact a supervisor or a prosecuting attorney if the reporting officer does not take their stalking complaints seriously.

Although controversial (12), a restraining or protective order may be an option to consider—although it is critical to recognize that restraining orders do not always prevent stalking from escalating into violence and sometimes may contribute to the escalation of stalking and its eruption into acts of violence (10). Irrespective of the decision about a protective order, it is important to develop a safety plan. One component of a safety plan is creating a network of informed individuals, including relatives, friends, neighbors, and co-workers who are apprised of the situation and can assist in developing an effective response system. The workplace is another venue that might warrant attention in designing a safety plan. For example, it might be useful to leave a photo of the stalker with security personnel at the victim's workplace. Additional strategies for increasing the safety and security of a stalking victim in the workplace environment can be developed by working with managerial, security, and human resources staff at the workplace. Although the shame and self-blame associated with stalking (and other forms of victimization) might result in social isolation and secrecy, mobilizing the support and involvement of other people is important for enhancing physical safety and for securing needed emotional support and validation.

In the case of telephone harassment, one potentially useful strategy is to obtain an unlisted phone number for private use, and to install another answering machine to accept calls made to the published phone number. In the event that a victim has to make a quick exit, securing easy access to a reserved set of valuables would facilitate the process. This list of items includes money, credit cards, medication, important papers, keys, and other valuables. The value of advance planning cannot be underestimated—suggest that the victim anticipate and identify a safe place to go in an emergency, and rehearse (using imaginary or in vivo procedures) going to that location, so that the behaviors become automatic. Another useful suggestion is to keep a small business card–sized list with helpful telephone numbers, such as victim assistance agencies, in case a crisis suddenly erupts. Alternatively, cellular telephones can be easily programmed with important emergency contact phone numbers and speed-dial procedures. Other safety suggestions include varying the routes taken to and from work and other places, and trying to travel with others present. Victim assistance agencies are excellent sources of support and provide detailed information about safety planning. Safety planning materials can also be obtained via several helpful stalking and victim assistance websites.

Although risk assessment methods have primarily been utilized with offenders, such tools may be useful in working with victims of stalking to evaluate the potential risk of harm in her particular situation. Earlier in this chapter, risk factors for the escalation of stalking into physical violence were reviewed. If stalking co-occurs in the context of relationship violence, these factors should figure into an appraisal of risk, including risk of lethal violence. Specific safety plans should be devised around planned separation or service of a restraining/protective order. Victim assistance, criminal justice, or mental health professionals can work with stalking victims in an effort to appraise risk and develop appropriate safety planning strategies that are tailored to the case-specific assessment of risk.

Although active trauma treatment may not be appropriate for most stalking victims, supportive treatments aimed at reducing psychological distress, reducing self-blame, and increasing self-efficacy may be helpful. Supportive treatment approaches include the following components: (a) education about trauma and traumatic responses, (b) emotional support and validation, (c) tools for managing stress and anxiety symptoms, and (d) skills training to enhance strategic responding and increase feelings of self-efficacy. Psychoeducational interventions provide basic information about the intrusive, avoidance, and arousal symptoms of PTSD. Information about trauma symptoms is often experienced as "normalizing," because many PTSD symptoms result in the feeling that one is going crazy. This is particularly evident for symptoms such as flashbacks and other unbidden memories that may or may not include sensory elements. Psychoeducational programs emphasize that PTSD symptoms are normal reactions to abnormal events involving powerlessness, loss of control, perceived threat to life, fear, helplessness, or horror (see ref. 69, for a self-help book on PTSD). One particularly important aspect of PTSD education aims to prevent or reduce the use of maladaptive coping behavior, such as avoidance or substance use, to alleviate emotional distress. One aim of this intervention is to help the victim understand the link between the deployment of avoidance behaviors, including suppression of thoughts and feelings or use of alcohol or drugs to numb feelings, and the subsequent development of chronic PTSD and secondary comorbid conditions, including depression, suicidality, panic, and substance use disorders. Clients are encouraged to minimize their use of avoidance behaviors to cope with distress from unbidden memories and heightened arousal and to engage in more active coping efforts that include talking about their feelings and managing symptomatic distress through relaxation or other methods. Other effects of trauma, including somatic reactions and behavioral changes, are also explored. Finally, clients can be provided with information about how trauma can affect basic schemas or beliefs about the world that may contribute to self-blame and to disruptions in beliefs about safety, trust, intimacy, esteem, and control (see ref. 67, for a client workbook on these themes).

Informal peer and family support, in addition to the validation provided through professional counselors and support groups, can be of assistance in coping with stalking victimization. Rosenbloom and Williams (67) provide guidelines for family and friends to support their efforts in caring for a trauma survivor. Suggestions include listening to the survivor instead of trying to fix the problem, and helping the survivor access other formal and informal sources of support in the community. Professional and personal support providers should avoid asking questions or making statements that might subtly suggest that the victim is responsible for the stalking that is targeted towards her ("why" questions, which suggest personal responsibility/blame should generally be avoided when providing a victim with support). More information and helpful hints for family and friends and other aspects of PTSD can be obtained from the National Center for PTSD (http://www.ncptsd.org) and the PTSD Alliance (1–800–877–507-PTSD or http://www.PTSDAlliance.org).

A number of stress management approaches can be used to assist with anxiety and other forms of emotional distress. Relaxation procedures (67–69) and breathing retraining approaches (70) are effective for reducing emotional distress and managing panic symptoms. These techniques can be used alone as self-help tools or can be effective adjuncts to professional individual or group therapies. Pharmacologic intervention has also been used with some success to manage anxiety and traumatic stress symptoms. Friedman and colleagues (2000) reviewed the empirical evidence supporting pharmacological intervention with PTSD. They concluded that selective serotonin reuptake inhibitors (SSRIs) are the first-line drugs for treating PTSD. Monoamine oxidase inhibitors (MAOIs) were reported to be moderately effective, and tricyclic antidepressant drugs were found to be mildly effective, but with adverse side effects for both classes of drugs. No evidence yet exists to support the use of antiadrenergic or anticonvulsant agents because of a lack of randomized clinical trials with these medications. Friedman and colleagues (46) caution against the use of benzodiazepines for treating the intrusive and avoidant symptoms of PTSD.

Stress inoculation training (SIT) (71) is a cognitive-behavioral approach that combines education about stress, coping skills for managing distress, and opportunities to practice those skills; SIT has been found to be effective in managing PTSD symptoms with sexual assault survivors (72). Enhanced coping skills that replace avoidant coping behaviors with more proactive engaging behaviors are likely to be effective at reducing some of the symptoms of PTSD, as well as in gaining access to needed resources from community and criminal justice agencies. Moreover, the acquisition of problem-solving skills and other active coping behaviors can help a victim regain some sense of self-efficacy and control in the aftermath of victimization, which tends to induce a sense of helplessness and loss of control.

For nonacute stalking cases, clinical service providers might consider adapting any one of the available cognitive-behavioral therapies for treating PTSD. These therapies include prolonged exposure, cognitive therapy, cognitive processing therapy, and systematic desensitization. Empirical support for each of these therapeutic modalities, both alone and in combined approaches, can be found in a review by Rothbaum and co-workers (72). A systematic exposition of these therapies is beyond the scope of the present chapter.

EDUCATION ABOUT STALKING AND PREVENTION OF STALKING VICTIMIZATION

Given the serious health and mental health consequences of stalking victimization, it is imperative that education about its reality be included in programs designed to alert young men and women to its genuine risks. It is a potentially fatal error to treat persistent unwanted attention as merely a nuisance that will cure itself over time. It is important that victims do not unthinkingly blame themselves but rather, if polite but firm refusals do not work, treat the state of affairs as one requiring profess-

ional advice and perhaps intervention by criminal justice authorities. Second, it is essential that educational campaigns make explicit the strong empirical linkages between stalking and other forms of coercive control and relationship violence. Just as some of the recent efforts to change campus climates of tolerance for rape have utilized the education of men (73), it may well be that creating a climate of male intolerance for persistent pursuit will help to prevent some stalking and even more of its negative consequences.

IMPLICATIONS FOR POLICY, PRACTICE, AND RESEARCH

Policy

- Comprehensive, multisystemic responses to stalking victimization are essential, yet practically nonexistent. Without mobilizing the efforts of law enforcement and criminal justice systems to respond appropriately to stalking offenders, no amount of state-of-the-art intervention will be successful in addressing victim distress and symptomatology. Victims will continue to live in heightened states of fear and distress (leading to longer-term physical and mental health complaints) as long as stalking continues to be a real or potentially continued course of action.
- Education and training of criminal justice and law enforcement personnel on the serious psychological and physical consequences of stalking victimization may improve practices related to the arrest, detention, and treatment of stalking offenders.
- Enforceable policies and practices that provide serious penalties for stalking victimization are also a critical link in the chain.
- The development of intervention strategies for stalking victims goes hand in hand with reconceptualization of traumatic stress responses and peritraumatic (instead of posttraumatic) events, for those individuals exposed to stalking, which tends to be serial and chronic.
- Future efforts should attempt to either redefine the PTSD construct to account for peritraumatic conditions, or add additional categories that adequately capture the nature of responses to traumatic events that pose ongoing threats of danger and violence.

Practice

- To date, criminal justice responses to stalking have been marred by high dismissal rates (74) and failure to charge and prosecute stalking behavior as stalking (i.e., charges bargained down to less severe offenses) (1,66). Law enforcement and criminal justice responses need to be augmented by the development and implementation of effective intervention strategies that target treatment of problems relating to stalker psychopathology and motivation for engaging in unwanted pursuit-oriented acts.

- Because stalking perpetration is heterogeneous in terms of motivation for engaging in stalking behavior and the specific type of stalker psychopathology, it is imperative that new stalking interventions be developed and appropriately tailored to address the specific motivation and form of psychopathology of the stalking offender (16).

- Although arrest and incarceration of the offender represent two critical steps in the process of addressing the complexities of stalking, the engagement of mental health professionals armed with successful (i.e., empirically supported) stalker-specific intervention strategies that address both stalking motives and relevant psychopathology are essential.

- When stalking and battering are co-occurring, victims' needs often extend beyond the realm of traditional mental health services. Specifically, comprehensive advocacy services that assist women to find resources to meet economic, housing, childcare, healthcare, and other material and personal needs are required (75,76).

- Finally, although we advocate for the development of appropriate interventions to respond to the distress produced by stalking victimization, without more effective law enforcement, criminal justice, and mental health responses to stalking perpetration, such interventions will be of limited utility. Thus, by more effective means of incapacitating and rehabilitating stalking offenders, the needs of stalking victims are served.

Research

- Although stalking may appear relatively innocuous on its surface, the research reviewed here underscores the variety of deleterious physical and mental health consequences arising from stalking victimization. Victims report high levels of fear and distress, in addition to symptoms of psychological disorders, such as anxiety, depression, and posttraumatic stress. A variety of behavioral and lifestyle changes and a host of long- and short-term physical health sequelae are documented to occur as a consequence of stalking victimization. Further health surveillance data as to the magnitude of the problem and impact on health are needed.

- We are in need of further research to increase our knowledge about how to predict which stalkers will become dangerous.

- Although much effort has been devoted toward the development and evaluation of batterer intervention programs, parallel research to develop and systematically evaluate stalker-specific interventions has been almost nonexistent, with the one possible exception of the promising work of Rosenfeld and his colleagues (77), who are in the process of empirically evaluating a treatment model they developed based on dialectical behavior therapy to target specific forms of behavior disruption and psychopathology evidenced among stalking offenders. Rosenfeld's approach is on the cutting edge of new and promising directions in clinical research that may provide another crucial link in what must be a multisystemic response to the problem of stalking victimization.

- Although the field of traumatic stress has made great advances in developing and testing interventions that can be used in most victim populations, most if not all of these treatments are contraindicated for use among victims with ongoing threats of violence or potential violence. Clinical research attention to the development of intervention strategies and practice guidelines that can be effectively used to enhance the physical and emotional well-being of stalking victims is needed.

References

1. Tjaden P, Thoennes N. *Stalking in America: Findings from the National Violence Against Women Survey.* NCJ 169592. Washington, DC: National

Institute of Justice and Center for Disease Control and Prevention;1998.

2. Lowney KS, Best J. Stalking strangers and lovers: Changing media typifications of a new crime problem. In: Best J, ed. *Images of issues: Typifying contemporary social problems.* New York: Aldine De Gruyter;1995:33–57.

3. White J, Kowalski RM, Lyndon A, Valentine S. An integrative contextual model of male stalking. In: Davis KE, Frieze IH, Maiuro RD, eds. *Stalking: Perspectives on victims and perpetrators.* New York: Springer Publishing Company;2001:163–185.

4. National Criminal Justice Association. Project to develop a model anti-stalking code for states. Washington, DC: Author,1993.

5. Tjaden P, Thoennes N. *Extent, nature, and consequences of intimate partner violence.* NJC 169592 Washington, DC: US Department of Justice, 2000.

6. Davis KE, Coker A, Sanderson M. Physical and mental health effects of being stalked for men and women. *Violence Vict.* 2002;17:429–443.

7. Mustaine EE, Tewksbury R. A routine activity theory explanation of women's stalking victimization. *Violence Against Women.* 1999;5:43–62.

8. Fisher BS. Being pursued and pursuing during the college years: The extent, nature, and impact of stalking on college campuses. In: Davis JA, ed. *Stalking crimes and victim protection: Prevention, intervention, threat assessment, and case management.* Boca Raton, FL: CRC Press;2001:207–238.

9. Davis KE, Frieze IH. Research on stalking: What do we know and where do we go? In: Davis KE, Frieze IH, Maiuro RD, eds. *Stalking: Perspectives on victims and perpetrators.* New York: Springer Publishing Company;2002:353–375.

10. Meloy JR. The clinical risk management of stalking: "Someone is watching over me . . ." *Am J Psychother.* 1997;51:174–184.

11. Zona MA, Sharma KK, Lane J. A comparative study of erotomanic and obsessional subjects in a forensic sample. *J Forensic Sci.* 1993;38:894–903.

12. Mullen P, Pathe M, Purcell R. *Stalkers and their victims.* New York: Cambridge University Press, 2000.

13. Sheridan L, Boon J. Stalker typologies: Implications for law enforcement. In: Boon J, Sheridan L, eds. *Stalking and psychosexual obsession.* London: John Wiley and Sons, 2002:63–82.

14. Meloy JR. Stalking and violence. In: Boon J, Sheridan L, eds. *Stalking and psychosexual obsession.* London: Wiley;2002:105–124.

15. Zona MA, Palarea RE, Lane JC. Psychiatric diagnosis and the offender-victim typology of stalking. In: Meloy JR, ed. *The psychology of stalking: Clinical and forensic perspectives.* New York: Academic Press, 1998; 69–84.

16. Davis KE. Stalkers and their worlds. In: Davis KE, Bergner RM, eds. *Advances in descriptive psychology,* Vol. 8. Ann Arbor, MI: Descriptive Psychology Press;2006:326–347.

17. DeBecker G. *The gift of fear.* New York: Bantam/Dell Publishing Co., 1997.

18. Kienlen KK. Developmental and social antecedents of stalking In: Meloy JR, ed. *The psychology of stalking: Clinical and forensic perspectives.* London: Academic Press;1998:52–69.

19. Meloy JR. Stalking (obsessional following): A review of some preliminary studies. *Aggression and Violent Behavior.* 1996;1:147–162.

20. Walker LE, Meloy JR. Stalking and domestic violence. In: Meloy JR, ed. *The psychology of stalking: Clinical and forensic perspectives.* San Diego: Academic Press;1998:140–159.

21. Spitzberg BH. The tactical topography of stalking victimization and management. *Trauma Violence Abuse.* 2002;3:261–288.

22. Bjerregaard B. An empirical study of stalking victimization. *Violence Vict.* 2000;15:389–406.

23. Mechanic MB, Weaver TL, Resick PA. Intimate partner violence and stalking behavior: Exploration of patterns correlates in a sample of acutely battered women. In: Davis KE, Frieze IH, Maiuro RD, eds. *Stalking: Perspectives on victims and perpetrators.* New York: Springer Publishing Company; 2002: 62–88.

24. Mechanic MB, Weaver TL, Resick PA. Mental health consequences of intimate partner abuse: A multidimensional assessment of four different forms of abuse. *Violence Against Women.* 2008; 14: 634–654.

25. Pathe M, Mullen P. The impact of stalkers on their victims. *Br J Psychiatry.* 1997;170:12–17.

26. Centers for Disease Control. Prevalence and health consequences of stalking: Louisiana 1998–1999. *MMWR Morb Mortal Wkly Rep.* 2000; 49: 653–655.

27. Mechanic MB, Weaver TL, Resick PA. Risk factors for physical injury among help-seeking battered women: An exploration of multiple abuse dimensions. *Violence Against Women.* 2008; 14:1148–1165.

28. Resnick HS, Acierno R, Kilpatrick DG. Health impact of interpersonal violence 2: Medical and mental health outcomes. *Behav Med.* 1997;23:65–78.

29. Schnurr PP, Green BL. An integrative model and its implications for research, practice, and policy. In: Schnurr PP, Green BL, eds. *Trauma and health: Physical health consequences of exposure to extreme stress.* Washington, DC: American Psychological Association;2004:247–275.

30. Weaver TL, Resnick H. Toward developing complex multivariate models for examining the intimate partner-physical health relationship: Commentary on Plichta. *J Interpers Violence.* 2004;19:1342–1349.

31. Coker AL, Smith PH, Bethea L, et al. Physical health consequences of physical and psychological intimate partner violence. *Arch Fam Med.* 2000;9:451–457.

32. Plichta SB. Intimate partner violence and physical health consequences: Policy and practice implications. *J Interpers Violence.* 2004;19:1296–1323.

33. Sutherland CA, Bybee DI, Sullivan CM. The long-term effects of battering on women's health. *Womens Health.* 1998;4:41–70.

34. Brewster MP. Power and control dynamics in stalking and prestalking situations. *J Fam Violence.* 2003;18:207–217.

35. Dutton MA, Burghardt KJ, Perrin SG, et al. Battered women's cognitive schemata. *J Trauma Stress.* 1994;7:237–255.

36. Janoff-Bulman R. Victims of violence. In: Everly G, Lating J, eds. *Psychotraumatology: Key papers and core concepts in posttraumatic stress.* New York: Plenum Press;1995:73–86.

37. Mechanic MB, Resick PA. The personal beliefs and reactions scale. Unpublished manuscript. 2002.

38. Resick PA, Schnicke MK. *Cognitive processing therapy for rape victims: A treatment manual.* Newbury Park, CA: Sage Publications, 1993.

39. Resnick HS, Kilpatrick KG, Dansky BS, et al. Prevalence of civilian trauma and posttraumatic stress disorder in a preresentative sample national sample of women. *J Consult Clin Psychol.* 1993;61:984–991.

40. Campbell JC. The danger assessment scale: Research validation from the 12-city femicide study. Paper presented at American Society of Criminology, 2001, Atlanta, GA.

41. Goodman LA, Dutton MA, Bennett L. Predicting repeat abuse among arrested batterers: Use of the danger assessment scale in the criminal justice system. *J Interpers Violence.* 2000;15:64–74.

42. Mechanic MB, Marelich W, Resick PA. Assessment of stalking as a risk factor for escalated violence among battered women. Paper presented at Symposium presented to American Psychology Law Society, 2004, Scottsdale, AZ.

43. Mechanic MB, Uhlmansiek MH, Weaver TL, Resick PA. The impact of severe stalking experienced by acutely battered women: An examination of violence, psychological symptoms, and strategic responding. *Violence Vict.* 2000; 15:443–458.

44. Hall DM. The victims of stalking. In: Meloy JR, ed. *The psychology of stalking.* San Diego, CA: Academic Press;1998:115–136.

45. Westrup D, Fremouw WJ, Thompson RN, Lewis SF. The psychological impact of stalking on female undergraduates. *J Forensic Sci.* 1999;44:554–557.

46. Friedman MJ, Davidson JR, Mellman TA, Southwick SM. Treatment guidelines: Pharmacotherapy. In: Foa EB, Keane TM, Friedman MJ, eds. *Effective treatments for PTSD: Practice guidelines from the international society for traumatic stress studies.* New York: Guilford Press, 2000.

47. Fremouv B, Westrup D, Pennypacker J. Stalking on campus: The prevalence and strategies for coping with stalking. *J Forensic Sci.* 1997;42:666–669.

48. Carlson EB, Dalenberg CJ. A conceptual framework for the impact of traumatic experiences. *Trauma Violence Abuse.* 2000;1:4–28.

49. Stein M, Walker JR, Hazen A, Forde D. Full and partial posttraumatic stress disorder: Findings from a community survey. *Am J Psychiatry.* 1997;154:1114–1119.

50. Kessler RC, Sonnega A, Bromet E, et al. Posttraumatic stress disorder in the National Comorbidity Survey. *Arch Gen Psychiatry.* 1995;52:1048–1060.

51. Nishith P, Mechanic MB, Resick PA. Prior interpersonal trauma: The contribution to current PTSD symptoms in female rape victims. *J Abnorm Psychol.* 2000;109:20–25.

52. Norris FH, Kaniasty K. Psychological distress following criminal victimization in the general population: Cross-sectional, longitudinal, and prospective analyses. *J Consult Clin Psychol.* 1994;16:665–685.

53. Foa EB, Cashman L, Jaycox L, Perry K. The validation of a self-report measure of posttraumatic stress disorder: The posttraumatic diagnostic scale. *Psychol Assess.* 1997;9:445–451.

54. Basile KC, Arias I, Desai S, Thompson MP. The differential association of partner physical, sexual, psychological, and stalking violence and posttraumatic stress symptoms in a nationally representative sample of women. *J Trauma Stress.* 2004; 17:413–421.

55. Chilcoat HD, Breslau N. Investigations of causal pathways between PTSD and drug use. *Addict Behav.* 1998;23:827–840.

56. Stewart SH, Pihl RO, Conrod PJ, Dongier M. Functional associations among trauma, PTSD, and substance-related disorders. *Addict Behav.* 1998; 23: 797–812.

57. Golding JM. Intimate partner violence as a risk factor for mental disorders: A meta-analysis. *J Fam Violence.* 1999;14:99–132.

58. Mechanic MB, Griffin MG, Resick PA. The effects of intimate partner abuse on women's psychological adjustment to a major disaster. Unpublished manuscript. 2002.

59. Block CR. *Chicago women's health risk study of serious injury or death in intimate violence: A collaborative research project.* Illinois Criminal Justice Authority; Revised report, June 6, 2000.

60. McFarlane JM, Campbell JC, Wilt S, et al. Stalking and the intimate partner femicide. *Homicide Studies.* 1999;3:300–316.

61. McFarlane JM, Campbell JC, Watson K. Intimate partner stalking and femicide: Urgent implications for women's safety. *Behav Sci Law.* 2002;20:51–68.

62. American Psychiatric Association. *Diagnostic and statistical manual of mental disorders,* 4th ed. Washington, DC: American Psychiatric Press, 1994.

63. Mechanic MB. Stalking victimization: Clinical implications for assessment and intervention. In: Davis KE, Frieze IH, Maiuro RD, eds. *Stalking and obsessive behavior: Perspectives on victims and perpetrators.* New York: Springer Publications, 2001;31–61.

64. Foa EB, Keane TM, Friedman MJ. *Effective treatments for PTSD: Practice guidelines from the*

international society for traumatic stress studies. New York: Guilford Press, 2000.

65. Follette VM, Ruzek JI, Abueg FR. *Cognitive behavioral therapies for trauma.* New York: Guilford Press, 1998.

66. Tjaden P, Thoennes N. The role of stalking in domestic violence crime reports generated by the Colorado Springs police department. *Violence Vict.* 2000b;15:427–442.

67. Rosenbloom D, Williams MB. *Life after trauma: A workbook for healing.* New York: Guilford Press, 1999.

68. Davis M, Eshelman ER, McKay M. *The relaxation and stress reduction workbook,* 4th ed. Oakland, CA: New Harbinger Press, 1995.

69. Schiraldi GR. *The posttraumatic stress disorder sourcebook: A guide to healing, recovery, and growth.* Los Angeles, CA: Lowell House, 2000.

70. Barlow DH, Craske MG. *Mastery of your anxiety and panic.* Albany, NY: Graywind, 1989.

71. Meichenbaum D. Stress inoculation training: A twenty-year update. In: Woolfolk RL, Lehrer PM, eds. *Principles and practices of stress management.* New York: Guilford Press, 1993.

72. Rothbaum BO, Meadows EA, Resick PA, Foy DW. Cognitive behavioral therapy. In: Foa EB, Keane TM, Friedman MJ, eds. *Effective treatments for PTSD: Practice guidelines from the international society for traumatic stress studies.* New York: Guilford, 2000.

73. Berkowitz AD. Fostering men's responsibility for preventing sexual assault. In: Scheur PA, ed. *Preventing violence in relationships: Interventions across the life span.* Washington, DC: American Psychological Association;2002:163–196.

74. Jordan CE, Logan TK, Walker R, Nigoff A. Stalking: An examination of the criminal justice response. *J Interpers Violence.* 2003;18:148–165.

75. Allen N, Bybee DI, Sullivan CM. Battered women's multitude of needs: Evidence supporting the need for comprehensive advocacy. *Violence Against Women.* 2004;10:1015–1035.

76. Riger S, Raja S, Camacho J. The radiating impact of intimate partner violence. *J Interpers Violence.* 2002;17:184–205.

77. Rosenfield DB. Court ordered treatment of spouse abuse. *Clin Psychol Rev.* 1992;12:205–226.

Chapter 32

Weapons and Intimate Partner Violence

Susan B. Sorenson

KEY CONCEPTS

- A woman is more than twice as likely to be shot and killed by her male intimate than killed in any other way by a stranger. Handguns account for most of these gun deaths.
- Focusing solely on the homicide of an intimate partner underestimates the full scope of fatal outcomes associated with intimate partner violence (IPV).
- Guns can be used to intimidate and coerce, as well as to harm, an intimate partner.
- Persons under a restraining order and those convicted of misdemeanor domestic violence (DV) are prohibited from purchasing and possessing a firearm.
- Future considerations in IPV and firearms include personalized weapons, contacting the spouse when application is made to purchase a gun, seizing weapons at the scene of DV, how to increase the mandated

relinquishment of firearms by batterers, and the risks and benefits of battered women arming themselves.

Weapons figure prominently in intimate partner violence (IPV). The most commonly used weapons are what law enforcement call "personal weapons," that is, hands, fists, and feet. Although it is possible to inflict substantial injury with personal weapons, assaults are made more efficient through the use of external weapons. External objects are used with great frequency in IPV. Sometimes the weapon is a gun or knife; it typically is a nearby household object that is seized in haste and rage.

This chapter focuses on external weapons, primarily firearms, in IPV. The emphasis on firearms is indicated because they are highly lethal and because they are already identified as an intervention point (i.e., some limits are placed on the possession of firearms by certain persons). Data and policies from the

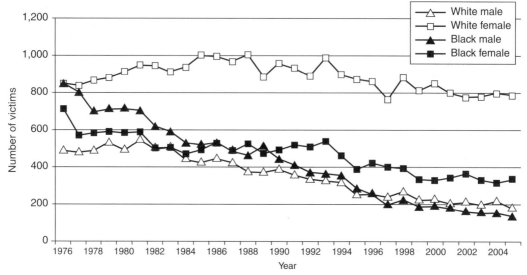

Figure 32.1 Intimate partner homicide victims in the United States, by race and gender, 1976–2005. *Source:* Department of Justice, Bureau of Justice Statistics, 1976–2005. At http://www.ojp.usdoj.gov/bjs/homicide/intimates.htm. Accessed 10/20/2007.

United States will be reviewed, largely because firearms in general and handguns in particular are more available to civilians in the United States than in most other developed countries. In addition, unless otherwise specified, the focus is on intimate partner relationships, that is, on relationships with a current or former spouse or a current or former boyfriend or girlfriend. Grouping married and unmarried persons together is indicated because violence against an intimate is not limited to legally recognized relationships.

EPIDEMIOLOGY OF WEAPON USE IN INTIMATE PARTNER VIOLENCE

Fatal Intimate Partner Violence

Fatal IPV has decreased in recent years. As shown in data from law enforcement agencies across the nation (Figure 32.1), the decline has not been consistent across population groups. The homicide of men at the hands of an intimate partner has dropped farther and faster than the homicide of women. In the past decade, among 20- to 44-year olds, rates of intimate partner homicide have been highest for girlfriends (1).

Firearms predominate in intimate partner homicides (IPH). Firearms account for about half of the IPHs of men and about three-fifths of the IPHs of women (Figures 32.2 and 32.3). The proportion of IPHs that are committed with a firearm is about one-fifth lower than the proportion of overall homicides that are committed with a firearm (2). The same pattern holds for homicides committed with a handgun: about 42.2% of IPHs and 51.7% of all homicides are committed with a handgun.

National data from the 1980s suggested that women were at particular risk from an intimate with a firearm (3). Updating these data to 2005, the most recent year for which national homicide data are available, indicates that risk is particularly high for fatal assaults by intimates with handguns. As shown in Figure 32.4, women were nearly 2.3 times as likely to be shot and killed by an intimate as to be shot, stabbed, strangled, beaten, or killed in any other way by a stranger. This finding is driven largely by handguns: women were nearly 1.7 times as likely to be killed by a handgun-wielding intimate as to be shot, stabbed, strangled, beaten, or killed in any other way by a stranger.

Research documenting that keeping a firearm in the home increases risk of homicide in that home has gotten widespread attention (4). Less well

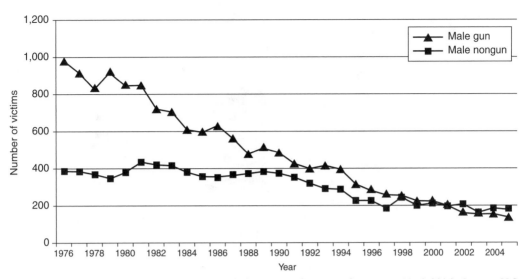

Figure 32.2 Intimate partner homicide, U.S. male victims, by type of weapon, 1976–2005. *Source:* U.S. Department of Justice, Bureau of Justice Statistics, 1976–2005. At http://www.ojp.usdoj.gov/bjs/homicide/intimates.htm. Accessed 12/8/2007.

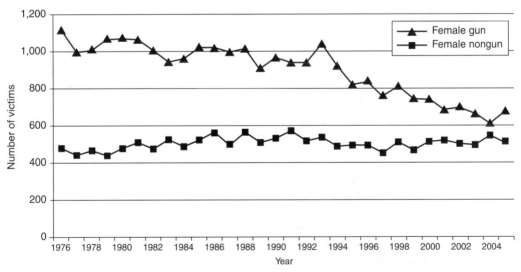

Figure 32.3 Intimate partner homicide, U.S. female victims, by type of weapon, 1976–2005. *Source:* U.S. Department of Justice, Bureau of Justice Statistics, 1976–2005. At http://www.ojp.usdoj.gov/bjs/homicide/intimates.htm. Accessed 12/8/2007.

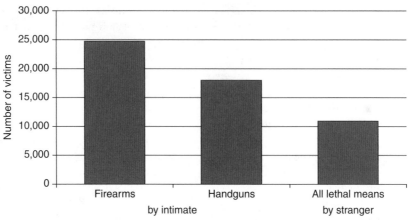

Figure 32.4 Homicide of women, U.S., by intimates with firearms versus strangers using all methods, 1976–2005. *Source:* Unweighted data compiled from Uniform Crime Reports [United States], Supplementary Homicide Reports, 1976–1999, Part 1: Victim Data. At http://webapp.icpsr.umich.edu/cocoon/NACJD-SDA/03180.xml, accessed 10/28/2007 and using computer files for 2000–2005 data from U.S. Dept. of Justice, Federal Bureau of Investigation. Uniform Crime Reporting Program Data [United States]: Supplementary Homicide Reports. Compiled by the U.S. Dept. of Justice, Federal Bureau of Investigation. ICPSR ed. Ann Arbor, MI: Inter-university Consortium for Political and Social Research.

known is that the study also found that violence in the home is an independent risk factor for homicide in the home. Subsequent research focusing solely on women indicates that prior domestic violence (DV) and having one or more guns in the home substantially increases the risk of homicide at the hands of a spouse, intimate acquaintance, or close relative (OR = 14.6 and 7.2, respectively) (5).

The homicide of an intimate partner is not the only fatal outcome. Violent partners sometimes kill the children, other family members, or friends of their partners. A study of IPHs in Massachusetts found that 38% of the perpetrators killed more than one person (6). In addition, sometimes the intimate partner is not the one who is killed at all; another—a child, a current partner, a family member—is killed as a way to punish the intimate partner.

Suicide is another outcome. About 40% of the homicides of intimate partners are immediately followed by the suicide of the perpetrator (7). And, in a topic that has received scant attention, suicide is the choice of some battered women (5,8,9). Firearms are the primary weapon of choice in each of these lethal acts.

In war, unintended harm to civilians is labeled "collateral damage" and, if fatal, included in the body count of total lives lost. The murder of members of

the victim's family, her friends, her current partner, or her co-workers can be viewed as collateral damage in that they are not the primary target. Given that "collateral damage" in fatal intimate homicides—that is, fatalities that are "side effects" of the IPV itself—is not included in the official counts of the problem, the full scope of IPH has yet to be realized. In terms of the present chapter, it is important to note that regardless of whether it is a homicide of an intimate partner or her family or friends or whether it is a suicide by a perpetrator or victim, the most common weapon used is a firearm.

Nonfatal Intimate Partner Violence

In the 1970s and 1980s, family sociologists studied assault and aggression toward spouses and children in two national community-based surveys (10). They concluded that women and men were equally likely to engage in assaultive behaviors in intimate relationships, and that women sometimes were more likely to engage in certain behaviors. Practitioners, by contrast, typically focus on injury outcomes. Given general size and strength differentials, physical damage will be more likely to result when a man hits a woman with a closed fist than vice versa.

Recent national research confirms clinical experience—women are more likely than men to incur injury as a result of IPV (11).

Weapon-related findings, however, have received less attention from researchers, advocates, and practitioners. Family sociologists found that about two in 1,000 U.S. women and men reported that they had used a knife or gun against an intimate partner (10). Recent research on IPV indicates that women are more likely than men to be threatened with a knife (2.8% versus 1.6%) or gun (3.5% versus 0.4%) and to have a knife or gun used against them (0.9% versus 0.8% for knife and 0.7% versus 0.1% for gun) (11). Thus, the use of knives and guns is relatively rare in IPV, yet troubling to realize that 16 in every 1,000 U.S. women have been threatened with a gun and 7 in 1,000 have had a gun used against them by an intimate partner.

Men are more likely than women to be shot, but women are more likely than men to be shot by an intimate partner. National hospital discharge data indicate that men are eight times more likely than women to be treated for a gunshot wound (12). These same national hospital discharge data indicate that women are 3.6 times more likely than men to be shot by a current or former spouse than by a stranger (13).

The emergency department is the main healthcare delivery setting that has focused on identifying IPV. It also is the location where practitioners are beginning to assess firearm ownership and access in the context of IPV. Relatively little research has been published on the topic to date. In a South Carolina emergency department in which over half of the female patients had ever experienced IPV, when demographic characteristics were taken into account, whether there was a firearm in the household was not associated with IPV (14). These findings were replicated in a multistate survey (15). Recent findings from a multisite study indicate, however, that the assailant's access to a firearm and him threatening her with it increases the risk of her being killed by him (16). The researchers also found that, compared to other methods, the risk of homicide was higher for women when the male intimate used a gun.

The most common calls for assistance from law enforcement are DV calls (17). About two-thirds of these calls involve weapons. Although DV calls were widely believed to be the most dangerous calls for police, armed robberies in progress are the most

dangerous for officers (18). When an officer is killed at the scene of a family quarrel, it almost always is with a gun (19).

Surveys of victims and perpetrators of IPV document the widespread presence of and use of firearms. In a statewide survey of residents of battered women's shelters, 36.7% of the women reported that there was a gun in the home during their most recent relationship (20). This compares to 15.7% of women in the general population of that same state who report that there is a gun in the home (21). When there was a gun in the home, nearly two-thirds of the women reported that her partner used it to scare, threaten, or harm her (20). When the gun was used in the relationship, it was used to threaten to shoot/kill her (71.4%) or to actually shoot at her (5.1%), as well as to threaten to kill himself (4.1%) or the children (3.1%).

And batterers themselves acknowledge their use of firearms against their intimate partners. In a review of the records of 8,529 men enrolled in Massachusetts-based batterers' intervention programs, 7% reported owning a gun during the previous 3 years (22). Nearly 12% of these gun-owning batterers report that they had used the gun to scare or threaten their intimate partner, and 4.3% reported that they had shot the gun during an argument with their partner. Far fewer had used a knife against their partner.

In sum, firearms are used to intimidate, coerce, injure, and kill intimate partners.

INTERVENTION POINTS

This section of the chapter focuses on policies designed to keep firearms out of the hands of persons deemed to be a risk to their intimate partners. Persons convicted of aggravated assault, which is a felony, are prohibited from purchasing or possessing a firearm. The prohibition applies regardless of the relationship of the assailant to the victim. Federal legislation in the 1990s added two categories of persons to the list of prohibited purchasers and possessors—those under a DV order of protection and those convicted of misdemeanor DV.

Orders of Protection

With the Violence Against Women Act (VAWA) of 1994, the U.S. Congress amended the Gun Control

Act to prohibit firearm purchase and possession by a person who is subject to a DV protection order (Title 18 U.S.C. § 922(g)(8) and (d)(8)). The federal restriction applies to orders of protection in which the alleged abuser was given notice and the opportunity to appear at a hearing. To be consistent with federal laws, states needed to pass similar legislation. Moreover, how the information was to be collected and reported was left to individual states. Some states already had similar restrictions in place, but many did not.

Orders of protection, also known as restraining orders or stay-away orders, are a legal intervention in which one person is deemed to be a threat to another and ordered to stay a specified distance from the person to be protected. All 50 states have stay-away orders, but the criteria for obtaining them, the length of time for which they are issued, and other conditions vary. The orders can be issued through criminal courts or through civil procedures, the latter of which typically are victim initiated.

Each year, more than 1 million people in the United States obtain restraining orders for intimate partner assault, rape, or stalking (11). About one in five women who experience these forms of violence seek and are granted a restraining order. Given that different types of restraining orders are issued for varying lengths of time, many more restraining orders are in effect than are issued during 1 year. For example, on any given day in California, nearly a quarter of a million restraining orders are in effect—about the same number of restraining orders as there are marriages recorded in 1 year (23). Thus, each year, persons under a restraining order are the single largest class of persons who are added to the roll of those prohibited from purchasing and possessing a firearm.

The National Instant Criminal Background Check System (NICS), however, often does not identify and prevent such individuals from purchasing a firearm (24). More than a decade after the legislation was enacted, the system remains compromised because many states do not provide information about DV restraining orders to NICS (24,25). Intimate partner homicide rates of women are 7% lower in states that do (versus do not) have restraining order and firearms laws in place (25).

Even in states where firearm prohibitions related to restraining orders have been in place before the federal law was changed, problems remain. For example, a recent review in California identified multiple problem practices, including the observations that some courts are not issuing restraining orders although required by law to do so, some jurisdictions are not entering restraining orders into the database against which applications to purchase firearms are checked, and some judges cross out the firearms prohibitions language on the restraining order form or use another form thinking that it will not be entered into the database (26). Obviously, state legislation must be enacted and procedures established and followed for the federal law to have its intended effect.

Moreover, restraining orders must be perceived as an available option for those who are being abused. Recent research suggests that only about 1 in 10 women who are killed by an intimate partner had ever been under the protection of a restraining order (27).

Domestic Violence Misdemeanors

In 1996, the U.S. Congress amended the Gun Control Act with what is widely known as the Lautenberg Amendment (Title 18 U.S.C. § 922(g)(9) and (d)(9)). The amendment prohibited firearm purchase and possession by persons who are convicted of a DV misdemeanor. Persons convicted of felony assault on an intimate partner were already barred from purchasing or possessing a firearm. This action was hailed by advocates, who testified that assaults on intimate partners often are tried as misdemeanors.

For this provision to be effective, states must provide detailed information on DV misdemeanants to the federal NICS database used in background checks on gun buyers. Because no consistent definition of DV exists across the states, in May 2001, NICS was modified to include a "flag" to indicate that a record was related to DV. More than 2 years later, only 19 states participated in the flagging system (28).

Despite the problems in implementing the federal laws prohibiting persons with a DV restraining order or with a DV misdemeanor conviction from purchasing or possessing a firearm, the laws may be having an impact. In 2005, the most recent year for which data are available, about 15% of the persons applying to purchase a firearm from a federally licensed firearm dealer were denied the ability to do so on the basis of a DV misdemeanor conviction or a DV restraining order (29).

Personalized Weapons

Personalized firearms, currently in the prototype stage of development, are engineered so that only an authorized user can fire the gun. Hailed as a way to reduce a wide range of ills—shootings of law enforcement officers by a suspect who is able to wrest away the officer's service weapon, adolescent suicide (in fact, suicide by anyone other than the authorized user), and residential burglaries (cash and guns are the usual items targeted)—an unintended consequence may be the heightened threat value of personalized weapons in intimate relationships.

If a batterer has a personalized firearm, he could more thoroughly intimidate and coerce his partner—even if she was able to access the weapon, it would be useless in her hands. A recent survey of residents of battered women's shelters indicates that most would be against the introduction of such weapons (20). It is possible, however, that personalized weapons, which would be more expensive than conventional nonpersonalized guns, would reduce the number of homes with guns and, by extension, reduce the risk of IPH. Given that it is not possible to fully predict their impact, it would be wise if discussions about personalized weapons would include considerations of their implications in IPV.

Spousal Query Upon Application to Purchase a Firearm

In some locales, intimate partners are taken into account when a gun is purchased. For example, in New Jersey, when someone wants to purchase a handgun, the opinion of the spouse or partner (as well as others) is sought and taken into account in the decision whether to issue a purchase permit.

Three-fourths of battered women residing in shelters thought it would be good to require that the spouse or partner be contacted when a gun is purchased (20). Regardless of their perspective on the advisability of such a policy, nearly all (91.8% of 417 women

surveyed) said that if their opinion were sought in such a circumstance, they would say that it would not be a good idea for their partner to get a gun.

Seizing Weapons at the Scene of Domestic Violence

Some states allow or require law enforcement officers to seize firearms at the scene of a DV incident (30). The circumstances surrounding such allowed seizures vary, for example, when the gun is in plain sight or when the victim and suspect agree to a voluntary search of the premises. The limits placed on firearm seizures at the scene of a DV incident generally are more restrictive than those placed on firearm seizures at the scenes of a drug bust, where weapons are confiscated and held as evidence regardless of whether they were used in the incident.

Relinquishment of Firearms by Batterers

Federal law prohibits the purchase and possession of a firearm by a batterer who is under a restraining order or convicted of misdemeanor DV. Prohibiting purchase is relatively easy if restraining orders are entered into an electronic database and if potential purchasers are checked against the database. Prohibiting possession of a firearm by a batterer is far more difficult.

Persons subject to a restraining order can be ordered to relinquish their firearm(s) within a specified time period (e.g., 24 hours, 48 hours). Written proof is to be provided that the guns have been sold, transferred to another person, or turned in to a law enforcement agency. In reality, firearm relinquishment rarely occurs, in no small part, because of the lack of adequate administrative records. Substantial bureaucratic procedures go into effect when a vehicle is sold or transferred; the buyer and seller complete paperwork that includes the unique vehicle identification number, and it is forwarded to the responsible agency in the state in which the transaction occurred. The states that do maintain gun purchase records could determine that an individual purchased a gun at one point, but not provide accurate, current information about the firearm. This is largely because procedures by which to track the sale and transfer of firearms among individuals are not as clearly specified, not as closely monitored as sales by dealers, largely not enforced, or some combination of the aforementioned. Thus, when told to relinquish a firearm, a person under a restraining order could falsely say "I don't have one," and there often is no way to ascertain otherwise, aside from having law enforcement conduct a search of the individual and his residence. Precluding a substantial infusion of resources into law enforcement across the country for the express purpose of conducting searches for firearms of these two classes of persons, individuals under a DV restraining order or convicted of misdemeanor DV are not likely to relinquish their firearms.

Another part of the problem with the firearm possession prohibition is that law enforcement agencies are, at best, ambivalent about implementing the law. Agencies are, perhaps understandably, not eager to deal with substantial numbers of gun-carrying individuals who were very recently ordered to give up their guns because they harmed or threatened to harm someone. In addition, limited storage space presents a problem. Lockers used to store crime scene evidence are sometimes in short supply, and priority is given to their use for this purpose. The storage problem likely is some combination of real and perceived: if law enforcement agencies can establish procedures by which to store impounded vehicles, they likely can figure out how to store firearms that are relinquished by batterers.

Risks and Benefits of Battered Women Arming Themselves

Advocates for battered women have been largely silent on the questions of whether a battered woman should arm herself. There is, to my knowledge, no research reporting the proportion of battered women who arm themselves or estimating the risks incurred and the benefits accrued by such action.

The available evidence, from research based on the general population, indicates that women who purchase a gun to protect themselves may unwittingly place themselves at higher risk of homicide and suicide. A sophisticated study comparing mortality among those who did and did not purchase a gun found a particularly strong effect among women (31). In the first year following handgun purchase, suicide attributed to firearms accounted for 51.2% of all deaths of 21- to 44-year-old women. The risk of homicide by a firearm also was elevated among women. The elevated risk of homicide and suicide following handgun purchase

by women was maintained during the entire 6-year follow-up period.

CONCLUSION

Firearms pose a particular risk in IPV. Knowledge about the use of firearms in IPV is limited largely to fatalities. Recent research on emergency department visits expands our understanding to include some of the nonfatal physical assaults. A more thorough understanding of the use of firearms in IPV may help elucidate intervention points. Specifically, more research is needed about the use of firearms to threaten and coerce an intimate partner and the mental health outcomes of such experiences. Given that psychological intimidation is a substantial component of battering, and the relatively common use of guns for this purpose, (at least as reported by residents of battered women's shelters), healthcare professionals would be wise to ask about and to take into account gun threats and gun use when treating a woman injured by a partner.

Although firearm injury inflicted by another often is considered an urban problem, the importance of guns in IPV should not be overlooked in rural areas, where gun ownership is high and guns often are easily at hand. Firearm-related deaths are highest for women in states where guns are more prevalent, a finding that remains even when poverty and urbanization are taken into account (32).

Well-intended laws to keep guns out of the hands of batterers lack adequate implementation; more resources and increased political will are needed before federal policies can fulfill their intended effects. Advocates are increasingly focusing on how to reduce batterers' access to firearms (see, for example, the 2003 report *Disarming Domestic Violence Abusers* issued by the Brady Campaign to Prevent Gun Violence [28] and the 2005 report *The Impact of Guns on Women's Lives* published by Amnesty International, the International Action Network on Small Arms

IMPLICATIONS FOR POLICY, PRACTICE, AND RESEARCH

Policy

- Well-intended laws to keep guns out of the hands of batterers lack adequate implementation.

- More resources and increased political will are needed before federal policies can fulfill their intended effects.

Practice

- Healthcare professionals would be wise to ask about and to take into account gun threats and gun use when treating a woman injured by a partner.

Research

- Whether gun ownership or keeping a gun in the home is associated with IPV, the costs and benefits of battered women arming themselves, and other key considerations regarding IPV and weapons merit investigation.

[IANSA], and Oxfam International [33]). Support from various quarters, including medical personnel, may help policy makers understand the importance of fully implementing existing laws.

References

1. Fox J, Zawitz M. *Homicide trends in the United States, Intimate Homicide.* US Department of Justice, Bureau of Justice Statistics; 2005. At http://www.ojp.usdoj.gov/abstract/fvs.htm.Accessed 7/12/2005.
2. Durose M, Harlow C, Langan P, et al. *Family violence statistics.* Washington DC: US Department of Justice; 2005. At http://www.ojp.usdoj.gov/bjs/abstract/fvs.htm. Accessed 7/11/2005.
3. Kellermann A, Mercy J. Men, women, and murder: Gender-specific differences in rates of fatal violence and victimization. *J Trauma.* 1992;33:1–5.
4. Kellermann A, Rivara F, Rushforth N, et al. Gun ownership as a risk factor for homicide in the home. *N Engl J Med.* 1993;329:1084–1091.
5. Bailey J, Kellermann A, Somes G, et al. Risk factors for violent death of women in the home. *Arch Intern Med.* 1997;157:777–782.
6. Langford L, Issac N, Kabat S. Homicides related to intimate partner violence in Massachusetts. *Homicide Studies.* 1998;2:353–377.
7. Lund L, Smorodinsky S. Violent death among intimate partners: A comparison of homicide and homicide followed by suicide in California. *Suicide Life Threat Behav.* 2001;31:451–459.
8. Kaslow N, Thompson M, Jacobs DML, et al. Factors that mediate and moderate the link between partner abuse and suicidal behavior in African American women. *J Consult Clin Psychol.* 1998; 66:533–540.
9. Olson L, Huyler F, Lynch A. Guns, alcohol, and intimate partner violence: The epidemiology of female suicide in New Mexico. *Crisis.* 1999;20:121–126.
10. Straus M, Gelles R. Societal change and change in family violence from 1975 to 1985 as revealed by two national surveys. *J Marriage Fam.* 1986;48:465–479.
11. Tjaden P, Thoennes N. *Extent, nature, and consequences of intimate partner violence.* Washington, DC: US Department of Justice, 2000.
12. Gotsch K, Annest J, Mercy J, Ryan G. Surveillance for fatal and non-fatal firearm-related injuries: United States, 1993–1998. *MMWR Morbid Mortal Wkly Rep.* April 13 2001;50(No. SS-2).
13. Wiebe D. Sex differences in the perpetrator-victim relationship among emergency department patients presenting with non-fatal firearm injuries. *Ann Emerg Med.* 2003;42:405–412.
14. Coker A, Smith P, McKeown R, King M. Frequency and correlates of intimate partner violence by type: Physical, sexual, and psychological battering. *Am J Public Health.* 2000;90:533–539.
15. Vest J, Catlin T, Chen J, Brownson R. Multistate analysis of factors associated with intimate partner violence. *Am J Prev Med.* 2002;22:156–164.
16. Campbell J, Webster D, Koziol-McLain J, et al. Risk factors for femicide in abusive relationships: Results from a multistate case control study. *Am J Public Health.* 2003;93:1089–1097.
17. California Attorney General's Office. *Domestic violence-related calls for assistance, 1993–2003.* Sacramento, CA: Criminal Justice Statistics Center. At http://caag.state.ca.us/cjsc/publications/misc/dvsr/rpt.pfd. Accessed 4/4/2005.
18. Garner J, Clemmer E. *Danger to the police from domestic disturbances: A new look.* NCJ 102634. Rockville, MD: National Institute of Justice, 1986.
19. Federal Bureau of Investigation. *Law enforcement officers killed & assaulted, 2003.* Washington, DC: US Department of Justice, 2004. At http://www.fbi.gov/ucr/killed/leoka03.pdf. Accessed 7/19/2005.
20. Sorenson S, Wiebe D. Weapons in the lives of battered women. *Am J Public Health.* 2004;94:1412–1417.
21. California Health Interview Survey. At http://www.chis.ucla.edu. Accessed 7/7/2005.
22. Rothman E, Hemenway D, Miller M, Azrael D. Batterers' use of guns to threaten intimate partners. *J Am Med Womens Assoc.* 2005;60:62–68.
23. Sorenson S, Shen H. Restraining orders in California: A look at statewide data. *Violence Against Women.* 2005;11:912–933.
24. Kessler J, Kimbrough L. *Broken records: How America's faulty background check system allows criminals to get guns.* Washington, DC: Americans for Gun Safety Foundation, January 2002.
25. Vigdor E, Mercy J. Do laws restricting access to firearms prevent intimate partner homicide? *Eval Rev.* 2006;30:313–346.

26. California Department of Justice. *Keeping the promise, victim safety and batterer accountability*. Sacramento, CA: California Department of Justice, 2005. At http://safestate.org/documents/DV_Report_AG.pdf. Accessed 12/7/2007.

27. Vittes K, Sorenson S. Restraining orders among victims of intimate partner homicide. *Injury Prev.* 2008;14:191–195.

28. Jose J. Disarming domestic violence abusers: States should close legislative loopholes that enable domestic abusers to purchase and possess firearms. At http://endabuse.org/programs/publicpolicy/files/BradyReport.pdf. Accessed 2/13/2005.

29. Bowling M, Lauver G, Hickman M, Adams D. *Background checks for firearms transfers, 2005.* NCJ 214256. Washington, DC: US Department of Justice, November 2006.

30. Frattaroli S, Vernick J. Separating guns and batterers: A review and analysis of gun removal laws in 50 US states. *Eval Rev.* 30:296–312.

31. Wintemute G, Parham C, Beaumont J, et al. Mortality among recent purchasers of handguns. *N Engl J Med.* 1999;341:1583–1589.

32. Miller M, Azrael D, Hemenway D. Firearm availability and suicide, homicide, and unintentional firearm deaths among women. *J Urban Health.* 2002;79:26–38.

33. Amnesty International the International Action Network on Small Arms (IANSA) and Oxfam International. *The impact of guns on women's lives.* Oxford, UK: Oxfam, 2005. At http://www.controlarms.org/downloads.indes.htm. Accessed 5/2/2005.

Chapter 33

The Impact of Intimate
Partner Violence on Children

Cynthia L. Kuelbs

KEY CONCEPTS

- Children are overrepresented in violent homes.
- Living in a violent home constitutes witnessing violence.
- Abuse to pregnant women may cause direct trauma or harm to the fetus through the effects of stress, inadequate prenatal care, smoking, alcohol and drug use, and poor nutrition.
- The chronic stress from living in violent homes, by directly affecting brain growth, synapse formation, myelination, and neurotransmitters, may explain the behavioral, mental health, and academic problems seen in exposed children. Not all children exposed to intimate partner violence (IPV) will have significant problems however.
- Identifying children exposed to IPV requires a high index of suspicion.
- The presence of IPV may be a predictor of other forms of child abuse. All children exposed to IPV should be assessed for other forms of abuse, safety, and need for mental health treatment.

We are guilty of many errors and many faults but our worst crime is abandoning the children, neglecting the fountain of life. Many things we need can wait. The child cannot. Now is the time his bones are being formed, his blood is being made, his mind is being developed. To him we cannot answer 'Tomorrow.' His name is 'Today.'

Gabriela Mistral

The Institute of Medicine, in the report "Children's Health, the Nation's Wealth: Assessing and Improving Child Health" (1), recognized the societal importance of healthy children and recommended that child health be defined as: "the extent to which an individual child or groups of children are able or enabled to develop and realize their potential, satisfy their needs, and develop the capacities that allow them to interact successfully with their biological, physical, and social environments." Three specific health domains were defined: health conditions, functioning, and health potential. Recognizing that health influences are multifactorial, the report outlines a model that highlights the impact of social, behavioral, biological, and physical environmental factors on child health. Exposure to intimate partner violence (IPV) can impact child health through influences in each of these areas. This chapter addresses the ways in which this occurs.

PREVALENCE

To mediate these health effects, it is important to identify those children affected. Although it is clear that IPV is an important public health problem, it is not known exactly how many children are affected each year. Some knowledge of prevalence is necessary in order to change attitudes, educate practitioners and patients, improve identification, and drive practice guidelines.

Living in a violent home likely constitutes witnessing violence. Witnessing may not mean direct observation of the violence; rather, children may hear violence, witness the aftermath, or sense tension between adults. Battered women have reported their children were aware of most of the marital arguments (2). In a police survey study conducted at domestic violence (DV) scenes, 85% of children had witnessed the assault (3). In another police study, half of the women who called police for an assault stated that the children had witnessed the event. In about two-thirds of the cases, children had witnessed arrival of the police (4).

Children are overrepresented in violent homes. Using data from the National Crime Victimization Survey, the Bureau of Justice Statistics reported that children under 12 lived in 43% of homes where IPV occurred. By contrast, only 27% of households in general in the United States had children younger than 12 years (5). Data from the Sexual Assault Replication Program also revealed that homes with IPV not only more frequently had children present, but also had a greater proportion of children younger than 5 years of age compared with census data. The younger children were exposed to more incidents of IPV compared to older children. In addition to being present in the homes where the violence occurred, the children were

also involved in the abuse in many ways; they called the police in about 10% of the cases, were themselves physically abused in 6%–7%, and were a factor in the dispute leading to the abuse in almost 20% (6).

Commonly cited estimates are that 3.3–10 million children witness IPV each year (7,8). The 3.3 million child estimate is derived from data that exclude divorced and separated families and those families with children under 3 years of age. The 10 million child estimate, from the National Family Violence Survey, is based on recall data from adults asked about exposure during teenage years to IPV between their parents (9). A more recent study estimates that 15.5 million children live in dual-parent homes where at least one episode of physical violence occurred between the parents in the past year; 7 million of those children lived in homes where severe IPV had taken place (10). This study derived data from a sample of 1,625 randomly selected heterosexual couples, each partner of which was interviewed independently in the home. Partner violence occurred in almost 22% of the couples, and 59% of these couples had children. Such estimates, although necessary for policy development, are not useful for the practicing clinician. Of more benefit are studies that give estimates about how frequently a condition occurs in a given population.

Many small clinical studies have addressed this issue. If the presence of IPV in the home equates to witnessing IPV, the prevalence of assaults on mothers estimates the exposure rate of children. Clinical studies reveal prevalence of current exposure to IPV, defined as that occurring in the preceding 2 years, to range from 2% to 16%. Higher prevalence numbers result if women are asked about past violence. The following selected studies reveal strikingly similar prevalence data in a variety of clinical settings reflecting varying socioeconomic statuses.

Using a child safety questionnaire with questions on IPV in an academic primary care pediatric practice, 2% of children ages 0–18 years were currently exposed to IPV, and 13% of children had been exposed to violence at some time in the past (11). In a private pediatric practice, when mothers of children ages 1 month to 10 years of age were questioned for IPV during well-child visits, 2.5% disclosed current relationship violence and 14.7% disclosed past violence (12). In an inner-city, resident-run pediatric clinic, the prevalence rate for assault by an intimate partner to mothers in the past 12 months was 3.7% (13). A community suburban pediatric setting noted much higher rates of adult assault: 31% of women screened at well-child visits had been physically assaulted by an intimate partner as adults, 16% in the past 2 years. Although the children ranged in age from 0–18 years, the average age was young, just under 2 years (14). Ten percent of mothers of children under 3 years of age seen in a pediatric emergency department reported physical abuse by an intimate partner in the preceding year (15). The prevalence of past-year IPV in female caregivers of children reported to child protective services was 29% (16).

These studies were done on women of different races, in different settings, and from different socioeconomic groups. What is unclear in some of these studies is whether the assault predated the birth of the child. What is also unclear is where the children were when the assault occurred, and whether the children were directly involved. What is clear, however, is that a healthcare provider seeing children can expect to see children who have been exposed to IPV, regardless of race or socioeconomic status. A growing body of knowledge addresses how this exposure may impact children.

PHYSICAL HARM

The Institute of Medicine Report recognizes that children in violent homes are at increased risk of physical harm through a variety of mechanisms, including physical abuse and neglect. The presence of IPV in the home may, in fact, be a predictor of other forms of child abuse. The physical harm to children from IPV can actually begin prior to birth.

Harm During Pregnancy

Prenatal harm may occur through direct trauma to the developing fetus when a pregnant mother is assaulted; more commonly, the harm is from secondary effects of abuse, such as tobacco, alcohol, and illicit substance use, poor nutrition, and poor prenatal care. Prenatal trauma may have significant consequences for the baby, directly resulting in fetal death, fetal injuries, or preterm labor. Blunt abdominal trauma during pregnancy leads to fetal death most commonly through placental abruption (17). This occurs when the relatively elastic uterus deforms, separating from the more rigid placenta. At the same time, the increase in intra-amniotic pressure causes further shearing of the placenta away from the uterus (18). Interestingly,

pregnant women assaulted by intimate partners were more likely to have peripartum complications, including premature rupture of membranes, preterm labor, and placental abruption compared with women suffering abdominal trauma from other causes (19).

Actual fetal injuries are rare after assault on the mother due to the relative protection the pregnant abdomen and uterus provide. The literature provides few clinical studies on fetal injuries. One series described 20 stillborn infants with unexplained intraventricular and subdural hemorrhages. The authors speculated on maternal assault as the cause of the unexplained hemorrhaging, arguing that maternal trauma is the "best documented cause" of both intraventricular and subdural bleeding prior to birth (20). More compelling are case reports involving live births of battered infants (21,22).

Abdominal trauma may lead to preterm labor, delivery, and fetal death, even in the absence of placental abruption or fetal injuries. Blunt abdominal trauma in a pregnant woman releases arachidonic acid, precipitating uterine contractions and leading to preterm labor. Controlling for confounding variables for preterm labor, battered women were more likely to have preterm *labor* than those who were not battered, but had no increase in preterm *delivery* perhaps because these women had good prenatal care (23). More recent work has contradicted this, noting an association between violence and preterm delivery (24,25). Interestingly, women reporting injury due to abuse within the past year were much more likely to have preterm births, although the injuries may have occurred prior to the pregnancy (26). Finally, women physically assaulted during pregnancy had higher rates of antepartum hemorrhage, intrauterine growth retardation, and perinatal death (27).

In addition to the physical harm suffered from maternal assault, IPV may cause fetal harm through associated comorbidities seen in battered women. These include elevated stress, inadequate prenatal care, smoking, alcohol and drug use, and poor nutrition. Abused women are more likely to have unplanned pregnancies and to enter prenatal care after 20 weeks (28,29). Abused women are more likely to smoke, drink alcohol, and use illicit drugs during pregnancy than are nonabused women (28,30,31). All these factors contribute to the increased risk of low-birth-weight infants seen in battered pregnant women (24,26,32). They also are factors contributing to poorer pregnancy outcomes.

Caught in the Crossfire

After birth, the physical environment of children exposed to IPV continues to be dangerous. Children in violent homes are at increased risk of physical harm due to direct abuse, to being caught in an assault between intimate partners, and to neglect resulting in inappropriate supervision and oversight. How frequently physical harm occurs is unknown but it is likely underreported.

Children may be injured when caught in the middle of an assault on an adult. However, children are not likely to be identified as having been harmed if they do not have clear evidence of physical injury (6). If the injuries to the child are minor, health care may not be sought. When health care is sought for these children, parents may be reluctant to tell healthcare providers how the injuries occurred due to concern that they may be reported to child welfare and the children taken into protective custody. The batterer may not allow the nonbattering parent to state what occurred. A false or partial history is then given, so that the children present with injuries that are not explained by the history provided.

The one study in which children were evaluated by healthcare professionals for injuries sustained during IPV found injuries to be minor. Adolescents were harmed while trying to intervene, and younger children were harmed as they were held during the assault (33).

Physical Abuse

Children in violent homes are clearly at increased risk of physical harm through physical abuse. The co-occurrence of childhood physical abuse and adult IPV is estimated to be at least 30%–60% (34). It is essential that all children in violent homes be assessed for physical abuse. This may be done through careful history and physical examination, including a developmental assessment. The physical abuse is often by the battering adult (9,35,36).

Sadly, though, these children are also at greater risk of physical abuse by the nonbattering parent (9). Battered women are more likely to hit their children, leaving a mark, than those who do not report abuse (37). Theories on why the battered parent abuses are varied. They may overdiscipline to control children's behavior, thus protecting children from abusive discipline by the batterer; the victim may view his/herself as more in control of anger and punishment than a violent partner; or the victim may take out anger on the children.

Children in violent homes may be at increased risk of death due to abuse. The role that IPV plays in childhood deaths is poorly studied. Limited data reveal that IPV was present in many homes where children died from abuse or neglect. The role that IPV played in these deaths, however, is unclear. Child welfare data from three states illustrate the connection (38). In Oregon, IPV was present in 43% of families in which child abuse and neglect contributed to critical injuries. In Massachusetts, 43% of mothers of children dying from abuse or neglect were themselves victims. And in New York City, 55.6% of families with child homicides had documented IPV in the 4 years preceding the homicide.

Home visitation data provide another view into the co-occurrence of IPV and child physical abuse. Intimate partner violence noted in the first 6 months of child-rearing was a significant predictor of child physical abuse; when present, there was a threefold increase of child physical abuse in the first 5 years of the child's life compared to families without IPV (39). Important for the healthcare provider is that IPV preceded the child abuse in 78% of the cases in which both were present.

SEXUAL ABUSE

Child sexual abuse may impact child health by influencing the social, behavioral, biological, and physical environment of the child, and must be considered in children living in violent homes. Although child sexual abuse shares the secrecy and control dynamics seen in IPV, the overlap between the two is just now being realized. And although sexual abuse may be declining, it is still a prevalent problem for children (40). Twenty percent of adult women and 5%–10% of adult men describe sexual abuse as children in recall studies (41). Recent studies shed some light on how often sexual abuse of children co-occurs in the home with adult IPV. In an adverse childhood experiences survey of over 8,000 adults, 2.3% of men and 3.9% of women were physically and sexually abused as children and also witnessed the abuse of their mothers (42). In child sexual abuse evaluation clinics, IPV was present in slightly more than half of the homes (43,44). Fifty-eight percent of the child sexual abuse perpetrators were also perpetrators of adult intimate partner abuse; in three-fourths of the cases, the sexual abuse and adult abuse occurred during the same time period. Quite compelling was that when adult violence was present, more children delayed in disclosing the sexual abuse because of fear of the perpetrator (44). Healthcare providers for children must inquire about child sexual abuse in children living in violent homes.

NEGLECT

Child neglect may be defined as a failure to meet basic needs of a child. Neglect may influence child health again through influences in social, biological, behavioral, and physical environments. This can include lack of supervision, adequate food, clothing, and shelter, and failure to meet medical, emotional, and educational needs. Emotional neglect may include exposure to IPV. Neglect is the most common form of child maltreatment, comprising more than 60% of confirmed cases nationally (45). Neglect has been associated with maternal depression, parental substance and alcohol abuse, and parental mental health problems (46). Intimate partner violence noted in the first 6 months of life has also been found to be a significant predictor of child neglect (39).

The comorbid substance and alcohol abuse and maternal depression often present in battered women are also risk factors for child neglect and may manifest as general neglect of the child. Depressed women may be emotionally unavailable and unable to care for the children adequately. Self-identified depressed women are more likely to have been physically abused as adults (47). In a study comparing neglect-only families to families where both neglect and IPV were present, differences were seen between the two groups. The IPV and neglect group had more mothers with a history of alcohol and drug use and mental health problems (48).

MENTAL HEALTH IMPACT OF EXPOSURE TO INTIMATE PARTNER VIOLENCE

Neurobiology

Exposure to IPV affects the child's biologic environment, with the potential to cause social, behavioral, and physical health problems. Although the physical health effects of IPV on children are sobering, perhaps even more concerning are the possible long-term mental health effects of chronic exposure to IPV on the developing brain. No longer recognized as a purely psychological problem, the stress resulting from the exposure may cause permanent neurobiological effects. This has implications for practice, intervention, and prevention. To discuss this, a brief review of developmental neurobiology is in order.

The most primitive portion of the brain controlling autonomic functions develops first—the brainstem and midbrain. This is followed by development of the limbic system, which controls emotions. Last, the cortex is formed, allowing for cognition, abstract thoughts, and higher-order functioning. As the brain develops, the cortex moderates the more reactive parts of the brain. Chronic stress can cause the emotional, more primitive parts of the brain, to become too active or reactive.

The fetal brain has two to three times the number of adult neurons. About half of these die prior to birth. New neuron formation ends at birth, with few exceptions. Brain growth occurs from birth to 5 years of age due to myelination and arborization; in fact, the brain will triple in mass during this time period. At birth, although billions of neurons are present, there are relatively few synapses. Those synaptic connections present control vital functions, so that babies can eat, breath, sleep, and eliminate. With stimulation, new synaptic connections expand after birth. Synaptic connections are pruned constantly, as those that are not used are discarded. Neural pathways are developed as these connections form, allowing the baby to gain new skills.

Babies' brains are often thought of as *plastic* or able to adapt to many situations by creating and discarding synapses. Stimulation, positive or negative, is required for this learning. Repeated stimulation is needed to strengthen these pathways, or the pathways will be discarded. The pathways can be physical, cognitive, or emotional. Children exposed to violence are exposed to chronic stress. Stress can be positive, preparing children to cope. Chronic stress, however, can be detrimental to child development. A cascade model that outlines the neurobiological alterations caused by extreme stress has been described and is useful in understanding why children exposed to violence may have physical, behavioral, social, and mental health problems (49). A brief review of this model is in order prior to outlining these problems.

First, the model emphasizes that exposure to stress activates stress response systems. These include the hypothalamic-pituitary-adrenal (HPA) axis, the noradrenergic and adrenergic system, and the vasopressin-oxytocin system. The HPA axis, along with the hippocampus, forms a system that utilizes cortisol. When activated, cortisol is released, which mobilizes energy stores, potentiates the release of adrenaline, increases cardiovascular tone, and inhibits growth, immune, and inflammatory responses. Increased stress also affects myelination and synaptogenesis. The noradrenergic-adrenergic system is comprised of the amygdala, locus coeruleus, adrenal gland, and sympathetic nervous system. Together, they respond to stress by affecting blood flow and increasing awareness, creating the fight or flight response. Little is known about the vasopressin-oxytocin arm of the stress response system, but it causes adrenocorticotropin hormone to be released from the pituitary. Early stress emphasizes these response systems and primes humans to be more fearful.

Second, stress hormones, particularly cortisol, affect the developing brain. Brain weight, myelination, neural morphogenesis, and neural and synaptic formation are affected. The effects are likely not due to cortisol alone but rather to the activation of all the stress response systems together.

Third, some portions of the brain are more vulnerable to stress than others. The reticular activating system is a network of arousal-related neural systems that is involved in arousal, anxiety, and modulation of limbic and cortical functioning. The locus coeruleus consists of norepinephrine-containing neurons. It originates in the pons and sends axons to almost all regions of the brain, functioning as a regulator of noradrenergic tone and activity. Its major role is in determining the value of incoming sensory information. It increases in activity if information is new or threatening; fear increases its activity.

The hippocampus is involved in memory storage and retrieval, as well as learning. It links with the reticular activating system and has a central role in the fear response. The hippocampus grows slowly, and is unusual in that it continues to form new neurons after birth. It has a high density of cortisol receptors, so is exquisitely sensitive to stress. It is crucial in inhibiting behavior and arresting inappropriate behavior. Repeated, chronic stress may inhibit development of neurons and pathways in the hippocampus, resulting in problems with learning, memory, and behavior.

The amygdala processes, interprets, and integrates emotions, weighing the emotional value of sensory input. It is sensitive to kindling, whereby intermittent stimulation increases neuronal excitability. It has a role in fear conditioning and in controlling aggressive behaviors. Stress decreases the density of γ-aminobutyric acid (GABA; an inhibitory neurotransmitter) receptors.

The cortical hemispheres and corpus callosum are vulnerable to stress. Since stress may affect myelin formation, it impacts myelinated areas such as the corpus callosum. This may affect hemispheric integration of memory. The prefrontal cortex continues to develop well into adulthood. It is rich in glucocorticoid receptors, making it sensitive to stress, yet plays an inhibitory role in the stress response system through a negative feedback role in the HPA axis. Stress also inhibits development of the left hemisphere, which is important in language and logic.

The cerebellum has recently become important to consider in children exposed to trauma, as it seems to play a role in mental health maintenance. Like the hippocampus, it grows slowly after birth, continues neurogenesis, and has a high density of glucocorticoid receptors, making it sensitive to stress. The cerebellum has a role in moderating limbic irritability and is involved in attention, language, affect, and thinking.

Although the stress response system is designed to allow humans to fight or flee, and so favors hyperarousal, infants and young children are not able to flee. These young children may then activate a dissociative pathway. In this pathway, in addition to activation of stress hormones and epinephrine, vagal tone is increased. This leads to decreased blood pressure and heart rate. Dopaminergic systems, and perhaps opioids, seem to play an important role in these pathways in animals (50).

Understanding this neurobiology makes sense of the social, behavioral, and physical health problems seen in so many children exposed to violence. When children are exposed to chronic stress, their focus is on survival, and the brain develops to meet that goal. The effects of stress include more excitable neurons, decreased development of the left side of the brain, decreased size of the corpus callosum, and blunted activity in the cerebellum.

IMPACT OF INTIMATE PARTNER VIOLENCE EXPOSURE

The end result of these neurobiological changes is a myriad of functional problems for children. Stress may affect the ability of a child to attach to others, to learn empathy, to be aware of his or her relation to others. The well-developed fight or flight response results in aggressive and impulsive behavior. The overdeveloped limbic system allows for more emotional rather than cognitive responses to problems. The lack of empathy may manifest as antisocial behavior.

Early studies were descriptive, without comparison groups, and many were done on children living in battered women's shelters. More recently, using the Child Behavior Checklist, children exposed to violence have been found to have both externalizing or aggressive behaviors, internalizing or fearful behaviors, and total behavioral problems as compared to nonexposed controls (51,52). These behaviors are explained by the neurobiologic changes that occur when children are exposed to stress.

Further, school-aged children exposed to IPV are at risk of academic problems. They may have a hard time attending to tasks and processing information if in a chronic state of arousal. They are more likely to be suspended for disruptive behavior. They are more likely to be absent from school. They more often have school nurse visits for social or emotional problems, and the nurse visits often result in children being sent home (53). Maternal depression coexisting with violence exposure may exacerbate these academic challenges. Kindergarten children exposed to both violence and maternal depression scored more poorly on mathematics, reading, and general knowledge tests than did those exposed to either one alone (54).

Children exposed to violence with symptoms of traumatic stress have been shown to have higher rates of health problems including asthma, allergies, gastrointestinal problems, and headaches (55). Compounding this, they may be less likely to have a medical home and receive recommended well-child visits (56). Interestingly, children whose mothers were abused had higher healthcare utilization and costs for primary care, mental health, specialty care, and pharmacy services compared with those of nonabused mothers. This held true even if the IPV stopped prior to the birth of the child (57).

Adverse childhood experiences data link witnessing IPV as a child to alcoholism, illicit drug use, and depression in adulthood (58). These adult behaviors, problematic for healthcare providers, may be solutions for patients, making them feel better as they struggle with the hard-wired neurobiological consequences of their early childhood exposure to stress.

It is important to remember that not all children exposed to IPV will have significant problems. Several factors may mediate the effect of the exposure. These include the severity of the violence, the amount of exposure to the violence, whether other forms of child abuse were present, the length of time since last exposure, and the presence of other stressors such as alcohol or substance abuse and mental health issues in the parents.

IDENTIFICATION OF INTIMATE PARTNER VIOLENCE-EXPOSED CHILDREN

An American Academy of Pediatrics (AAP) policy statement notes that "intervening on behalf of battered women is an active form of child abuse prevention," and that pediatricians should attempt to recognize IPV (59). Identifying these children can be challenging and requires a high index of suspicion. The U.S. Preventive Services Task Force found insufficient evidence to recommend *for* or *against* screening for IPV, as no study has directly addressed the effectiveness of screening in reducing harm and preventing premature death and disability. Additionally, optimal interventions are not clearly established or widely available (60).

That said, healthcare providers for children have opportunities to identify these children. Anticipatory guidance is geared toward prevention and early detection. Pediatricians form longitudinal relationships with families, having opportunities to meet with families frequently, at scheduled intervals. Six visits are recommended by the AAP in the first year of life. Pediatricians establish rapport with parents, as well as children, so that parents may feel comfortable discussing sensitive and confidential topics with them. Pediatricians are often viewed as nonthreatening to parents.

Women abused postpartum are likely to be injured yet unlikely to seek medical care for the injuries. These women do bring their children for well-child care, offering healthcare providers for children an opportunity to identify intimate partner abuse (61). Although healthcare providers for children are in a unique position to ask about IPV, few do so (62,63). In a community-based practice, pediatricians identified IPV in 0.3% of patients, while 4.2% of parents self-reported IPV. Reasons given for not inquiring about IPV include lack of education, protocols, time, and adequate staff. Other barriers include concern of offending patients' mothers and a belief that IPV is not a problem within the physician's patient population (63). Women are likely to disclose IPV to pediatricians when asked (14,15). Including questions about IPV in a psychosocial screening tool identified some abused women, but had limited sensitivity compared with the Conflict Tactics Scale (64).

RESPONDING TO INTIMATE PARTNER VIOLENCE-EXPOSED CHILDREN

Tension has existed between child advocates and battered women's advocates on how to approach the issue of children exposed to IPV. Some child advocates and child welfare agencies have favored reporting child exposure as child emotional abuse or child neglect, with some states specifically mandating reporting IPV exposure to child welfare agencies. Unfortunately, resources do not always exist to support families who are reported for exposure to IPV. When Minnesota required reporting DV exposure as child abuse, agencies experienced a 50%–100% increase in reports, without additional resources, and the legislature repealed the law (65).

Battered women's advocates argue that reporting penalizes women caught in the cycle of DV who may actually be staying with a batterer because it truly is the safest place for her children, as threats may have been made about the children should she leave. Additional arguments against reporting include that the varying needs of children may not be considered in the child welfare response, removal of the child is punitive to the mother and may be detrimental to the child, and removal takes away a mother's autonomy to do what she feels is best. Pediatricians may not believe that child welfare intervention will help their patient; in fact, past experience with child welfare may make the pediatrician less likely to report (66).

Safety of the child is surely linked to the safety of adults. A risk model is required that, based on need, allows for appropriate interventions for IPV-exposed children. Until an assessment of the child is done, it is difficult to know the level of risk. It is important that healthcare providers for children define who can be responsible for that assessment, as well as a safety assessment of the child, keeping in mind the potentially devastating long-term consequences of chronic exposure to violence. If a healthcare provider for children has concerns about a child's safety, however, a report must be made to child welfare services.

If IPV is identified, a careful evaluation for child physical and sexual abuse and neglect should be done. In addition to a history and physical examination, careful attention should be paid to child development and school functioning, as well as emotional and behavioral concerns. Height, weight, and head circumference should be plotted against norms to evaluate nutritional status and brain growth. Skeletal imaging should be considered to evaluate for occult fractures in nonambulating children in whom a concern of physical abuse is raised.

Perhaps most important for these children is mental health treatment. Understanding the neurobiology mandates that these children have a careful mental health evaluation by a professional with expertise in childhood trauma. In most states, children exposed to IPV qualify for victim-of-crime funding to help underwrite unreimbursed medical and mental health care interventions. Ongoing treatment should also be done by professionals with experience and knowledge in this area. A growing body of literature addresses this issue.

The multidisciplinary team approach to child maltreatment is well established. Given that exposure to IPV can affect the social, behavioral, biological, and physical environments of the child, these children deserve a multidisciplinary team response as well. Healthcare providers for children should form connections to professionals with expertise in mental health treatment, battered women's services, educational support services, family support services, public health nursing, parenting education, and child abuse, in order to provide appropriately for these children.

CONCLUSION

Children exposed to IPV may be exposed to chronic stress resulting in physical, neurobiological, emotional, and social problems. By identifying these children early and intervening to ensure safety and provide needed treatment, these vulnerable members of our society might be allowed to reach their full potential. The time for each individual child is now.

IMPLICATIONS FOR POLICY, PRACTICE, AND RESEARCH

Policy

- Public policy should reflect the significant risk IPV-exposed children have for mental health problems and allow for effective and accessible mental health treatment.
- Child protection and DV agencies should collaborate to create a coordinated system response to meet the needs of all victims in a violent home.

Practice

- All healthcare providers for children must be prepared to identify, appropriately assess, and appropriately refer IPV-exposed children.
- Exposure to IPV should be considered in all children also being assessed for physical or sexual abuse or neglect.

Research

- Research is needed to determine optimal methods of identification and intervention for children exposed to IPV, as well as why some children are affected more than others.
- Effective prevention strategies must be developed and disseminated, as exposure to IPV in the family of origin appears to be one of the biggest risk factors for either victimization or perpetration of IPV as an adult.

References

1. National Research Council, Institute of Medicine. Children's Health, the Nation's Wealth: Assessing and Improving Child Health. Committee on Evaluation of Children's Health. Board on Children, Youth, and Families, Division of Behavioral and Social Sciences and Education. Washington, DC: The National Academies Press, 2004.
2. Holden G, Ritchie K. Linking extreme marital discord, child rearing, and child behavior problems: Evidence from battered women. *Child Dev.* 1991;62(2):311–327.
3. Brookoff D, O'Brien KK, Cook CS, et al. Characteristics of participants in domestic violence. Assessment at the scene of domestic assault. *JAMA.* 1997;277(17):1369–1373.
4. Hutchison I, Hirschel J. The effects of children's presence on woman abuse. *Violence Vict.* 2001;16(1):3–17.
5. Rennison C, Welchans S. *Bureau of Justice statistics special report: Intimate partner violence.* Washington DC: US Department of Justice, Office of Justice Programs, 2002.
6. Fantuzzo J, Boruch R, Beriama A, et al. Domestic violence and children: prevalence and risk in five major US cities. *J Am Acad Child Adolesc Psychiatry.* 1997;36(1):116–122.
7. Straus MA. *Children as witnesses to marital violence: A risk factor for lifelong problems among a nationally representative sample of American men and women.* Columbus, OH: Ross Laboratories, 1992.
8. Carlson BE. Children's observations of interparental violence. In: Roberts AR, ed. *Battered women and their families.* New York: Springer;1984:147–167.
9. Straus MA, Gelles RJ. *Physical violence in American families.* New Brunswick, NJ: Transaction Publishers, 1990.
10. McDonald R, Jouriles E, Ramisettu-Mikler S, et al. Estimating the number of American children living in partner-violent families. *J Fam Psychol.* 2006;20(1):137–142.
11. Wahl R, Sisk D, Ball T. Clinic-based screening for domestic violence: Use of a child safety questionnaire. *BMC Med.* 2004;2(1):25.
12. Parkinson GW, Adams RC, Emerling FG. Maternal domestic violence screening in an office-based pediatric practice. *Pediatrics.* 2001;108(3):e43.
13. Holtrop TG, Fischer H, Gray SM, et al. Screening for domestic violence in a general pediatric clinic: Be prepared! *Pediatrics.* 2004;114(5):1253–1257.
14. Siegel RM, Hill TD, Henderson VA, et al. Screening for domestic violence in the community pediatric setting. *Pediatrics.* 1999;104(4):874–877.
15. Duffy SJ, McGrath ME, Becker BM, Linakis JG. Mothers with histories of domestic violence in a pediatric emergency department. *Pediatrics.* 1999;103(5):1007–1013.
16. Hazen AL, Connelly CD, Kelleher K, et al. Intimate partner violence among female caregivers of children reported for child maltreatment. *Child Abuse Negl.* 2004;28(3):301–319.
17. Ribe J, Teggatz J, Harvey C. Blows to the maternal abdomen causing fetal demise: Report of three cases and a review of the literature. *J Forensic Sci.* 1993;38(5):1092–1096.
18. Pearlman M, Tintinalli J, Lorenz R. Blunt trauma during pregnancy. *N Engl J Med.* 1990;323(23):1609–1613.
19. Pak L, Reece E, Chan L. Is adverse pregnancy outcome predictable after blunt abdominal trauma? *Am J Obstet Gynecol.* 1998;179(5):1140–1144.
20. Gunn T, Becroft D. Unexplained intracranial haemorrhage in utero: The battered fetus? *Aust N Z J Obstet Gynaecol.* 1984;24:17–22.

21. Stephens RP, Richardson AC, Lewin JS. Bilateral subdural hematomas in a newborn infant. *Pediatrics.* 1997;99(4):619.

22. Akduman E, Luisiri A, Launius G. Fetal abuse: A cause of fetal ascites. *AJR Am J Roentgenol.* 1997;169(4):1035–1036.

23. Berenson A, Wiemann C, Wilkinson G, et al. Perinatal morbidity associated with violence experience by pregnant women. *Am J Obstet Gynecol.* 1994;170(6):1760–1766.

24. Coker AL, Sanderson M, Dong B. Partner violence during pregnancy and risk of adverse pregnancy outcomes. *Paediatr Perinat Epidemiol.* 2004;18(4):260–269.

25. Covington D, Hage M, Hall T, Mathis M. Preterm delivery and the severity of violence during pregnancy. *J Reprod Med.* 2001;46:1031–1039.

26. Neggers Y, Goldenberg R, Cliver S, Hauth J. Effects of domestic violence on preterm birth and low birth weight. *Acta Obstet Gynecol Scand.* 2004; 83(5):455–460.

27. Janssen PA, Holt VL, Sugg NK, et al. Intimate partner violence and adverse pregnancy outcomes: A population-based study. *Am J Obstet Gynecol.* 2003;188(5):1341–1347.

28. Curry M, Perrin N, Wall E. Effects of abuse on maternal complications and birth weight in adult and adolescent women. *Obstet Gynecol.* 1998;92(4):530–534.

29. Parker B, McFarlane J, Soeken K. Abuse during pregnancy: Effects on maternal complications and birth weight in adult and teenage women. *Obstet Gynecol.* 1994;84(3):323–328.

30. Grimstad H, Backe B, Jacobsen G, Schei B. Abuse history and health risk behaviors in pregnancy. *Act Obst Gynecol Scand.* 1998;77(9):893–897.

31. Perham-Hester K, Gessner B. Correlates of drinking during the third trimester of pregnancy in Alaska. *Matern Child Health J.* 1997;1:165–172.

32. Murphy CC, Schei B, Myhr TL, Mont JD. Abuse: A risk factor for low birth weight? A systematic review and meta-analysis. *CMAJ.* 2001;164(11): 1567–1572.

33. Christian CW, Scribano P, Seidl T, ePinto-Martin JA. Pediatric injury resulting from family violence. *Pediatrics.* 1997;99(2):e8.

34. Edleson J. Children's witnessing of adult domestic violence. *J Interpersonal Violence.* 1999;14(8): 839–870.

35. Ross S. Risk of physical abuse to children of spouse abusing parents. *Child Abuse Negl.* 1996;20(7): 589–598.

36. Tajima EA. The relative importance of wife abuse as a risk factor for violence against children. *Child Abuse Negl.* 2000;24(11):1383–1398.

37. Kerker BD, Horwitz SM, Leventhal JM, et al. Identification of violence in the home: Pediatric and parental reports. *Arch Pediatr Adolesc Med.* 2000;154(5):457–462.

38. Spears L. *Building bridges between domestic violence organizations and Child Protective Services.* National Resource Center on Domestic Violence, 2000.

39. McGuigan WM, Pratt CC. The predictive impact of domestic violence on three types of child maltreatment. *Child Abuse Negl.* 2001;25(7):869–883.

40. Finkelhor D. Improving research, policy, and practice to understand child sexual abuse. *JAMA.* 1998;280(21):1864–1865.

41. Finkelhor D. Current information on the scope and nature of child sexual abuse. *Future Child.* 1994;4(2):31–53.

42. Edwards VJ, Holden GW, Felitti VJ, Anda RF. Relationship between multiple forms of childhood maltreatment and adult mental health in community respondents: Results from the Adverse Childhood Experiences Study. *Am J Psychiatry.* 2003;160(8):1453–1460.

43. Bowen K, Aldous MB. Medical evaluation of sexual abuse in children without disclosed or witnessed abuse [see comments]. *Arch Pediatr Adolesc Med.* 1999;153(11):1160–1164.

44. Kellogg ND, Menard SW. Violence among family members of children and adolescents evaluated for sexual abuse. *Child Abuse Negl.* 2003;27(12): 1367–1376.

45. *Child Maltreatment 2003.* Washington, DC: US Department of Health and Human Services, Administration on Children, Youth and Families, 2005.

46. Kelleher K, Chaffin M, Hollenber J, Fischer E. Alcohol and drug disorders among physically abusive and neglectful parents in a community-based sample. *Am J Public Health.* 1994;84(10): 1586–1590.

47. Scholle S, Rose K, Golding J. Physical abuse among depressed women. *J Gen Int Med.* 1998;13(9): 607–613.

48. Hartley CC. The co-occurrence of child maltreatment and domestic violence: Examining both neglect and child physical abuse. *Child Maltreat.* 2002;7(4):349–358.

49. Teicher MH, Andersen SL, Polcari A, et al. Developmental neurobiology of childhood stress and trauma. *Psychiatr Clin North Am.* 2002;25(2): 397–426.

50. Perry BD. The neurodevelopmental impact of violence in childhood. In: Schetky D, Benedek E, eds. *Textbook of child and adolescent forensic psychiatry.* Washington, DC: American Psychiatric Press, Inc.;2001:221–238.

51. McFarlane JM, Groff JY, O'Brien JA, Watson K. Behaviors of children who are exposed and not exposed to intimate partner violence: An analysis of 330 black, white, and Hispanic children. *Pediatrics.* 2003;112(3):E202–E207.

52. Kernic MA, Wolf ME, Holt VL, et al. Behavioral problems among children whose mothers are

abused by an intimate partner. *Child Abuse Negl.* 2003;27(11):1231–1246.

53. Kernic MA, Holt VL, Wolf ME, et al. Academic and school health issues among children exposed to maternal intimate partner abuse. *Arch Pediatr Adolesc Med.* 2002;156(6):549–555.

54. Silverstein M, Augustyn M, Cabral H, Zuckerman B. Maternal depression and violence exposure: Double jeopardy for child school functioning. *Pediatrics.* 2006;118(3):E792–E800.

55. Graham-Bermann SA, Seng J. Violence exposure and traumatic stress symptoms as additional predictors of health problems in high-risk children. *J Pediatr.* 2005;146(3):349–354.

56. Bair-Merritt MH, Crowne SS, Burrell L, et al. Impact of intimate partner violence on children's well-child care and medical home. *Pediatrics.* 2008;121(3):E473–E480.

57. Rivara FP, Anderson ML, Fishman P, et al. Intimate partner violence and health care costs and utilization for children living in the home. *Pediatrics.* 2007;120(6):1270–1277.

58. Dube S, Anda R, Felitti VJ, et al. Exposure to abuse, neglect, and household dysfunction among adults who witnessed intimate partner violence as children: Implications for health and social services. *Violence Vict.* 2002;17(1):3–17.

59. Committee on Child Abuse and Neglect. The role of the pediatrician in recognizing and intervening on behalf of abused women. *Pediatrics.* 1998;101(6):1091–1092.

60. Nygren P, Nelson, HD, Klein J. *Screening children for family violence:* A review of the evidence for the US Preventive Services Task Force. March 2004. *Ann Fam Med.* 2004;2:161–169.

61. Martin SL, Mackie L, Kupper LL, et al. Physical abuse of women before, during, and after pregnancy. *JAMA.* 2001;285(12):1581–1584.

62. Erickson MJ, Hill TD, Siegel RM. Barriers to domestic violence screening in the pediatric setting. *Pediatrics.* 2001;108(1):98–102.

63. Lapidus G, Cooke MB, Gelven E, et al. A statewide survey of domestic violence screening behaviors among pediatricians and family physicians. *Arch Pediatr Adolesc Med.* 2002;156(4):332–336.

64. Dubowitz H, Prescott L, Feigelman S, et al. Screening for intimate partner violence in a pediatric primary care clinic. *Pediatrics.* 2008;121(1):E85–E91.

65. Edleson J. Should childhood exposure to adult domestic violence be defined as child maltreatment under the law? In: Jaffe PG, Baker, LL, Cunningham A, eds. *Protecting children from domestic violence: Strategies for community intervention.* New York, NY: Guilford Press, 2004.

66. Flaherty EG, Sege R, Binns HJ, et al. Health care providers' experience reporting child abuse in the primary care setting. *Arch Pediatr Adolesc Med.* 2000;154(5):489–493.

Chapter 34

Adolescent Relationship Violence

Lyndee Knox, Carmela Lomonaco, and Elaine Alpert

KEY CONCEPTS

- In national and state level surveys, between 10% and 20% of girls and boys report experiencing intimate partner violence (IPV) or relationship violence (RV), with higher rates among vulnerable populations such as homeless youth, minority youth, pregnant and parenting teens, and also youth from rural communities. These figures likely underestimate the problem.
- Adolescent RV is underreported by public health systems, and its relationship to other forms of youth violence, such as school violence, is not understood and often not recognized.
- Although rates of victimization and perpetration reported by girls and boys are similar, significant differences exist between the genders in the type and severity of the violence and reasons for use of violence in an intimate relationship.
- Characteristics common to the adolescent stage of development can increase young people's vulnerability to RV; in turn, experiencing RV during adolescence can interrupt critical developmental processes and have life-long effects.
- Adolescent and adult RV share many features in common. However substantial differences also exist between the two phenomena that have important implications for policy and practice.
- Prevention and intervention services for adolescent RV are scarce. Funds for youth violence prevention have been directed mainly to gang intervention/prevention programs and to programs for other forms of peer-on-peer violence. Depending on state statutes, adolescents may not be able to access traditional intimate partner violence (IPV) or RV services.
- Healthcare professionals are uniquely situated to assist in the primary, secondary, and tertiary

> prevention of adolescent RV. However, most providers do not incorporate routine inquiry, counseling, and referral activities for RV into their practice despite recommendations from professional associations and others.

Dating violence among adolescents tends to come to the public's attention in rare and extreme cases, such as assault, homicide, and suicide. A growing body of research shows that adolescent relationship violence (RV) is not limited to tragic events. Less extreme but still harmful episodes of dating violence are common among teenagers and take a serious toll on the health and well-being of a sizable percentage of young persons in the United States. For the purpose of this chapter, adolescent RV can be defined as a pattern of assaultive and coercive behaviors adolescents (age 12-19) use against dating or intimate partners.

Adolescent RV can occur as early in a relationship as the first date. It may exhibit itself as a single act of coercive violation such as date rape, or present as a chronic pattern of physical, sexual, or emotional abuse. Adolescent RV includes physical violence, sexual violence, threat of physical or sexual violence, and psychological or emotional abuse (1) and is a concern for both heterosexual and same-sex couples (2).

Adolescent RV should be understood and addressed by the healthcare professional as part of a larger continuum of violence. In discussing the different forms of violence in our society, such as intimate partner violence (IPV), child abuse, and elder abuse, researchers have fragmented violence into artificially distinct categories. Although necessary to some degree in order to address the unique aspects of each type of violence, such compartmentilization also obscures the relationships among them. In fact, the different forms of violence are, more often than not, interconnected . Early victimization or witnessing of violence in the home places children at risk for victimization or perpetration as they grown older, thus increasing risk for involvement in RV or community violence and other forms of violence later in life. Without an understanding of these interconnections, health professionals who may be prepared to respond to one type of violence may fail to consider other forms of violence that may also be impacting their patients, such as the teen victim of RV who witnessed violence between her parents at home, or the teen perpetrator who is at the same time a victim of abuse at the hands of a caregiver. Conversely, the provider may be prepared to respond to one individual affected by violence, but fail to consider the potential impact on others in the family system. For example, an emergency physician or nurse who has received training in working with a teen victim of RV may overlook the needs of the victim's child, who may have witnessed the violence. To be effective in any area of violence prevention, health professionals must be aware and willing to develop the knowledge and skills necessary to identify and address the continuum of violence as it occurs within a family and within a community (3).

PREVALENCE OF ADOLESCENT RELATIONSHIP VIOLENCE

The true prevalence of adolescent RV in the United States is difficult to establish. Estimates vary widely depending on the sample used (national, regional, or local), whether the estimate is based on lifetime exposure or experiences in the preceding year, whether the definition of RV is limited to physical abuse or expanded to include emotional and verbal abuse, reluctance of teens to disclose victimization, and the methods used for data collection (e.g., in-depth interviews, surveys, crime reports).

In studies of RV conducted specifically with adolescents, anywhere from 9% to 30% of young people report experiencing violent victimization or perpetration in the context of a dating relationship. On the 2005 Youth Risk Behavior Survey System (YRBSS) conducted by the Centers for Disease Control and Prevention (CDC), 9.2% of male and female high school students reported being victims of dating violence in the preceding year (4). This trend has remained constant since 1999 (5). Analyzing YRBSS and additional data collected in Massachusetts, Silverman and colleagues determined that 18%–20% of adolescent girls reported ever having experienced physical and/or sexual coercion at the hands of a dating partner (6). Twelve percent of adolescents from South Carolina reported being victimized or perpetrating severe dating violence in the preceding year on the YRBSS (7). On the 1998 Minnesota Student Survey administered to 81,247 9th and 12th graders, primarily Anglo students, 9% of girls and 6% of boys reported ever being the victim of violence on a date, and 4% of the girls and 3% of the boys reported ever having been the victims of date rape (8). Seventeen percent of girls and 9% of boys reported experiencing dating violence on the Commonwealth Fund Survey of the Health of Adolescent Boys and Girls administered to a nationally representative sample of 9th through 12th graders (9). Finally, 32% of a nationally representative sample of 7,500 adolescents who responded to the National Longitudinal Study of Adolescent Health reported experiencing some form of victimization (psychological, physical, or any) in an opposite-sex relationship over the past 18 months. Twelve percent reported experiencing physical violence (10).

An even higher prevalence of RV has been found in targeted surveys of special populations. Higher rates of RV have also been found among adolescents from lower socioeconomic backgrounds (9), and among youth living in rural communities compared to urban and suburban communities (11). In one survey of 719 high school students living in low-income communities, 39.3% reported perpetrating physical dating violence and reported being physically victimized in a dating context in the past 5 years (12). In another study of 689 girls aged 14–23 years seeking care from an urban healthcare facility, 30% reported having an unwanted sexual experience in the past year, and 25% reported having experienced verbal sexual coercion or rape/attempted rape by a date or acquaintance in the past year (13). Finally, 18% (N = 522) of Black girls who received care from a single family medicine clinic reported a history of dating violence (14). In surveys of homeless youth, foster children and other especially vulnerable groups, as many as 68% report having experienced date rape or severe dating violence at some point in the past (15,16). Although international estimates focused specifically on adolescent RV are not available, the World Health Organization's Study on Women's Health and Domestic Violence found that between 35% and 76% of women age 15 and older in 13 sampled countries had been victims of sexual assault, with a majority of these assaults coming from an intimate partner (17,18).

Differences in prevalence have also been found among different ethnic and racial groups. On the 2005 YRBSS, Black teenagers (12%) were the most likely to report being victims of adolescent RV, followed by Hispanic (10%) and White (7%)

youth (19). Other studies, however, have not demonstrated ethnic and racial differences when socioeconomic status (20) and exposure to other forms of violence are controlled (12).

An alarming proportion of pregnant adolescents and teen mothers experience RV. Prevalence studies of RV during pregnancy range from 3.9% to 8.3% (21). In one study of 724 pregnant adolescents on a postpartum unit, 11.9% reported being physically assaulted by the fathers of their babies during the preceding 12 months (22). Of these, 40% also reported experiencing violence at the hands of a family member or relative in the preceding year. Although the incidence of RV declined over the follow-up period (21% at 3 months and 13% at 24 months), the percentage of abused mothers who reported experiencing severe RV increased from 40% to 62%. Also, the majority (78%) of young women who reported being abused by their partner in the first 3 months postpartum had not reported RV before delivery, suggesting that both pregnancy and the early postpartum period represent high-risk times for the onset of adolescent RV (23). Chang and colleagues found that one of the risk factors associated with homicide for pregnant women included age (under 20), suggesting that the younger the mother, the higher prevalence of severe violence against women (24).

Even with these multiple sources of data on RV, it is likely that they underestimate the true prevalence of adolescent RV in the United States. As is true with self-reports of other problems, youth may underreport their RV experiences on self-report surveys. In addition, official statistics on adolescent RV are of limited utility. Some states classify adolescent RV as child abuse rather than IPV, a practice that leads to consistent underreporting. In addition, adolescent RV that occurs in the context of other forms of youth violence is often unrecognized and unreported. The role adolescent RV may have played in U.S. school shootings over the past decade is a case in point. In her recent review of the dating violence literature, Sousa (25) points out that gender-based motives have been factors in many recent school shootings. Sousa points out that the perpetrators of these tragic events have almost all been male, that their victims have been overwhelmingly female, and that forensic reviews of the shooters themselves often later report that gender-based motives, such as anger about a refused date, played a role in their actions.

GENDER DIFFERENCE IN ADOLESCENT RELATIONSHIP VIOLENCE

Although similar numbers of girls and boys report experiencing RV, substantial differences exist between genders in the nature, severity, and purpose of the violence. Girls are substantially more likely than boys to report experiencing severe violence such as being strangled, burned, punched, beaten, raped, or threatened with a weapon. They are also substantially more likely than boys to experience physical injuries that require medical attention and to report sexual violence as a part of dating violence. Boys, on the other hand, are more likely to report experiencing less severe acts such as being pinched, slapped, scratched, or kicked (26–29). Where boys most frequently reported laughing at the experiences of a physical altercation (50%) or ignoring it (33%), girls more often reported having fought back, having tried to talk to their partner, or having obeyed their partner, after experiencing violence (30). Where boys report being relatively unconcerned about RV, girls as young as 8 to 12 years old describe RV as a serious worry (31).

This same research finds that girls are more likely than boys to report perpetrating RV against a dating partner (12). Twenty-eight percent of girls and 11% of boys in a longitudinal study of middle school students in North Carolina reported ever behaving violently toward a dating partner (32). However, again, substantial differences exist between genders, both in the severity of the violence each inflicts as well as the reasons for its use (27,28,33).

Girls are more likely to report perpetrating less serious forms of violence such as slapping, pushing, kicking, and biting; they are also more likely to report that they engaged in physical violence as a means of self-defense (26,34,35). In contrast, boys are more likely to report committing more severe acts of violence such as threatening a partner with a gun or knife, sexually assaulting a partner, using physical violence likely to cause injury, and using physical violence or threats of violence to terrify and control a partner (26,27,34–37).

ADOLESCENT DEVELOPMENT AND RELATIONSHIP VIOLENCE

Adolescence is a unique stage in human development, one that creates unique vulnerabilities for victimization within the context of an interpersonal relationship. Adolescence is formally defined as a prolonged period between childhood and adulthood that prepares a young person for occupation, marriage, and mature social roles (38). During this period, young people experience rapid changes in anatomy, physiology, and psychological development. They enter puberty, modify their body images, and grapple with emerging sexuality. Changes in the brain foster the capacity for abstract, planful thought but, at the same time, adolescents typically are imbued with a sense of invulnerability. The belief that "it can't happen to me" is a hallmark of the stage.

During adolescence, young people typically begin a process of separation from their parents or primary caregivers and seek to establish a sense of independent personal identity. Questions such as "Who am I? Am I normal? Am I competent?" and "Am I lovable and loving?" are central concerns of normally developing adolescents. Narcissism and the strong desire to fit in with peers are also hallmarks of the stage. The great risk of this period is that a young person will fail to establish a sense of self that is coherent, and in which the young person experiences him or herself as competent and capable both alone and in relationship to others. The myriad and exciting changes that take place in adolescence pave the way for a young person to transition into mature adulthood, but these same changes also increase a young person's vulnerability to RV. In turn, the experience of RV can impair a young person's ability to accomplish many of the critical developmental tasks of adolescence.

By age 15, 61% of adolescent females and 66% of adolescent males report dating (39), and 50% of adolescents aged 14–18 years report having had sexual intercourse (40). By age 18, almost all (89%) adolescents are or have been involved in a dating relationship (41). Adolescents experiment with romantic relationships in the context of limited life experience. Their models for romantic relationships most usually are drawn from their families, their peers, and the media. In the absence of effective working models, particularly when they have observed violence in their own homes or communities, adolescents may emulate or accept the abusive and violent behavior they have observed as the norm.

Because of their relative lack of life experience, teenagers are also more likely to endorse stereotyped gender roles that hold that the male should be dominant and sexually aggressive, and the female should be submissive and supportive—a set of beliefs that has been found to predict sexual victimization in girls and violent victimization among boys (42). Adolescents can also be vulnerable to confusing control with devotion and see violence in a relationship as acceptable. In a study of adolescent RV victims, 35% interpreted their partners' violent acts as signs of devotion and love, and 60% indicated that the violent behavior was of so little importance that it had no effect on the relationship (43,44).

The experience of violence in an early romantic relationship can profoundly damage an adolescent's sense of self in intimate relationships and the young person's emerging sexuality. Instead of developing a feeling of competence in negotiating intimacy, a young person who experiences violence in an intimate relationship may come to view him or herself as unsafe and unlovable, and the world and others as unsupportive and unfair. In the narcissism of adolescence, a young person may blame him or herself for the abuse and translate this into a sense of self as flawed or broken. The patterns of violence and submission learned and then practiced in adolescence may then be carried into adulthood, and become the foundation for intimate relationships in adulthood.

Relationship violence may disrupt critical nonromantic socialization processes of adolescence. The young victim's ability to socialize with peers may be interrupted by a jealous partner who seeks to limit his or her partners' exposure to others, and his or her freedom to participate in school activities, to study, and to make forays into early work environments.

The normal distancing that occurs between teenagers and their parents/caregivers during the individuation process of adolescence may prevent a young person from sharing concerns he or she has about a romantic relationship. Finally, adolescents may be reluctant to disclose abuse to their peers as they may fear being out-of-step with their classmates, or even rejected by them, especially if the abuser is socially popular (45). If a young person's friends accept abusive behavior as a normal part of romantic relationships, the young person may decide that his or her concerns are abnormal and simply accept the abuse as being an unavoidable and expected consequence of the desire to belong. In fact, most adolescent victims and perpetrators of RV do not disclose the abuse. In a study conducted by Ashley and Foshee (46) of 225 adolescent victims and 140 adolescent perpetrators, fewer than 40% of victims and 21% of perpetrators

sought help. When help was sought, the adolescents were most likely to turn to a close friend or a family member over a professional.

For certain groups of adolescents, such as lesbian, gay, bisexual, and transgender (LGBT) teenagers; those already experiencing abuse in their homes; and pregnant and parenting teens, the developmental challenges of adolescence are often even more complex and the risks associated with RV further heightened. For example, LGBT adolescents tend to be even more hesitant than other teens to seek help, as they must also contend with fear of being outed; ostracized by family, friends, community, and faith; assaulted; or even killed (2). Teenagers from abusive homes may not trust adults to turn to for help and may fear abuse, by or among family members, if they disclose RV. Similarly, pregnant teens and young mothers may be hesitant to come forward out of fear that their pregnancy will be discovered or because they have already encountered criticism from family, community, teachers, and peers for becoming pregnant outside of marriage. In instances in which the adolescent is younger than the abuser, the abuser may use age as a tool of control, for example, by threatening to turn tthe dating partner in to child protective services as a runaway if the abuse is disclosed to anyone (45). Table 34.1 contains an outline of the unique developmental characteristics of adolescence and possible vulnerabilities for RV.

RISK FACTORS FOR ADOLESCENT RELATIONSHIP VIOLENCE

Like other forms of youth violence, adolescent RV appears to be the result of the interaction of multiple factors. Riggs and Houry et al (47) hypothesize that violence emerges between adolescent partners due to a combination of contextual (observing family violence, beliefs that support use of violence in relationship) and situational (alcohol use, conflict in relationship, economic stress) factors. Similarly, social-ecological models of human development locate risk factors for adolescent RV in the individual, family, and broader social environment, as well as in the interactions among these various systems.

At the individual level, risk factors for adolescent RV include low self-esteem, poor problem-solving and conflict resolution skills, low social responsibility, and personal beliefs regarding the acceptability of

Table 34.1 Developmental Characteristics of Adolescence and Vulnerability to Relationship Violence (RV)

Developmental Characteristics	Vulnerability to RV
Individuation and separation from parents and adult caregivers	May be reticent to approach caregivers with concerns about RV out of fear of "being wrong" or losing independence
Drive to form intimate attachments and practice adult roles in the context of limited life experience	Desire to have a romantic partner may outweigh concerns about abuse; may accept abuse in order to not "fail" at romantic relationship; looks to media, family, and cultural stereotypes that may support RV to determine how to behave in intimate relationships
Strong peer orientation; desire to "fit in" with peers	May stay in abusive relationship in order to "fit-in" with peers; may be influenced by peers who view abusive behavior as normal/acceptable

aggressive behavior in dating relationships (15,42,48). Some studies have found a link between depression and sexual victimization among girls, and between depression and perpetration of RV (49). Substance use has also been shown to be a factor in adolescent RV (49) and is one of the strongest predictors of sexual aggression within the context of a date (50,51). One study found that as many as 38% of boys who report perpetrating physical abuse against an intimate partner also report being intoxicated at the time of the violence (30). In date rape victimization, forced use of drugs such as Rohypnol or "roofies" and γ-hydroxybutyric acid (GHB) are also factors that must be considered (15).

The family environment also contributes to risk for RV. The National Institute of Justice's (NIJ) longitudinal study of abused and neglected children links early exposure to abuse or neglect to an increased likelihood of arrest as a juvenile by 59%, and as an adult by 28% (52). In studies examining the link between early violence exposure and later health problems, exposure to physical or sexual abuse as a child, or the witnessing of violence in the home, doubles a

person's risk for involvement in RV later in life (53). Divorce and less than optimal parental support have been associated with perpetration (54). For example, low maternal education was found to be associated with sexual victimization in a dating relationship for females (42). Although family variables are a source of risk for both girls and boys, some studies suggest that their effects vary by a child's gender. For example, a study of 1,317 primarily White high school students (55) found that for boys, a childhood history of maltreatment was significantly correlated with dating violence and attitudes justifying dating violence, and that trauma symptoms were associated with perpetration of emotional abuse in the following year. For girls, a childhood history of maltreatment predicted deficits in empathy and self-efficacy, and was less strongly related to dating violence or attitudes justifying dating violence compared to boys. O'Hearn and colleagues (56) found that boys (but again not girls) who witness serious conflict between their parents are more likely to believe that aggression is permissible in a romantic relationship. In addition to violence exposure in the home, other factors such as low parental supervision and monitoring have been found to be associated with increased risk for RV victimization (51,57). The exact nature of how risk exposures impact girls and boys differently, and how these same variables may affect future likelihood of victimization and perpetration, are not yet well understood.

In addition to family, a young person's peers are another important source of risk. Male adolescents who have sexually aggressive peers are more likely to engage in sexual violence against a partner (58). Teenage girls and boys who have a friend who is a victim of dating violence or who are involved in coercive relationships are more likely to be involved in similar relationships themselves (32,42), and to view coercion, violence, and extreme jealousy as an acceptable part of dating, even interpreting it as a sign of their partner's devotion (59).

At the community-level, poverty and related factors such as overcrowding, low social capital, stress and frustration, and weak sanctions against RV have all been linked to increased risk for RV perpetration (60,61), as have low school attachment and neighborhood monitoring (54). Malik and colleagues (12) found that exposure to weapons and violent injury in the community, and cultural values and characteristics also influence the occurrence of adolescent RV. In her classic study of culture and RV, Campbell

Table 34.2 Risk Factors for Serious Adolescent Relationship Violence (RV)		
	Victim	Perpetrator
Individual	Depression Low self-esteem Poor problem-solving Attitudes accepting of violence in dating relationship Alcohol use	Low social responsibility Poor problem-solving Attitudes justifying dating violence Substance use
Family	Hit by an adult History of sexual victimization by non-date Mother education Witnessing serious violence between parents Low parental supervision	Childhood history of maltreatment (boys) Witnessing serious violence between parents (boys) Divorce Low parental supervision Low social support
Peer group	Friend victim of dating violence Physical fights with peers	Having sexually aggressive peers Having a friend who condones or uses violence in dating relationship
Community/society	Community or societal norms that accept and normalize use of violence against females or in intimate relationships Poverty Overcrowding Low social capital	Community or societal norms that encourages male aggression and a male role of "disciplining" female or intimate partner Low school attachment Low neighborhood monitoring Poverty Overcrowding Low social capital Norms supporting use of violence in intimate relationships

observes that most perpetrators of RV come from cultures in which the male is encouraged to be aggressive, believes his role includes disciplining his partner, and views himself as owning his female partner (60–62). Table 34.2 provides an overview of risk factors for adolescent RV victimization and perpetration.

DIFFERENCES BETWEEN ADOLESCENT AND ADULT RELATIONSHIP VIOLENCE

Adolescent and adult RV share similar dynamics of jealousy, power, and control, and the use of physical, sexual, and emotional forms of coercion. However, substantial differences also exist between adolescent and adult RV that merit viewing adolescent RV as a phenomenon distinct from adult RV, and that have important implications for practice.

Unlike adult victims of RV, adolescent RV victims most often live with their parents, not their abusers, and generally do not have children in common with their abusers. Except in cases in which an adolescent is involved in a relationship with an older partner, the young person is not economically bound to their abuser, and does not depend on the abuser for necessities of living such as food, shelter, or clothing.

While at first glance these differences would appear to simplify the logistics of leaving violent relationships for adolescents, a closer examination suggests that this is not the case. It may be difficult or impossible for an adolescent living at home to obtain geographic distance from an abuser; this may be difficult if not impossible to achieve if parents and family members are unable or unwilling to move to another community. Teenage intimate partners often are enrolled in the same school and may even attend the same classes. To separate from an abusive partner, the teenager may be required to change schools, or at the very least, alter classes and schedules. If the abuser is popular, the young victim may be ostracized by classmates and have to cope not only with the loss of an important love relationship, but also with rejection and blame by peers (63). In instances in which the victim or abuser is involved in gangs, retaliation by gang members can be a significant concern.

Compared to adult RV, adolescent RV may not be taken seriously by adults (25). Police may view the involved teenagers as just "kids being kids." Parents and primary caregivers may not recognize the importance their teenagers give to the dating relationship, and expect them to get over it quickly or to grow out of it. Schools, preoccupied with other pressures, may be impatient with young people whose academic achievement is slipping.

Like adults, teenage victims may be hesitant to disclose RV to others in their lives, but their reasons for this often differ. In addition to concerns about loss of confidentiality, retaliation by the abuser, and beliefs that they are at fault for the abuse, teenagers may also fear losing hard-won independence that they have only recently achieved during adolescence. Runaways may fear being reported to police and returned to what may be equally or even more abusive family situations. Young mothers may fear that, because of their age, they will be seen as unfit mothers and lose custody of their children; LGBT youth may fear being outed. Undocumented youth may fear deportation.

The many obstacles to disclosure, adolescents' natural affinity for peers, and efforts to separate from caregivers, make other young people, not adults or members of the professional community, the likely first responders to disclosure of adolescent RV. Molidor and Tolman found that among 8th and 9th grade victims of RV, fewer than 3% reported violent incidents to authority figures (e.g., police, social workers, counselors, or teachers);, only 6% of physically or sexually abused adolescents reported their abuse to a family member (30). Of those who did tell someone about their victimization, 61% stated they told a friend. This unique characteristic of adolescent RV has important implications for intervention and underscores the importance of ecological approaches to preventing adolescent RV that engage not only young people and their families, but also peers.

Heise and García-Moreno describe two primary patterns that occur in adult RV (17)—escalating violence that includes multiple and severe forms of abuse, terrorization and threats, and increasingly controlling and possessive behavior; and a less severe form called *common couple violence*, in which anger and frustration occasionally erupt into physical aggression between the two partners. Less is known about the patterns of interaction that underlie adolescent RV or its

Table 34.3 Similarities and Differences Between Adolescent and Adult Relationship Violence (RV)	
Adolescent RV	Adult RV
Most often does not live with abuser	Often lives with abuser
Generally, no children w/ abuser	Children may be involved
Not usually economically bound to abuser	Often economically dependent on abuser
Often not taken seriously by adults and professional community; seen as a "phase"	Taken seriously by professional community— mandated reporting, special police units, etc.
Peers are first responders	Professional community or family are first responders
Both partners may behave violently	Victim and perpetrator roles are more clearly defined
Geographic separation is difficult and sometimes impossible if victim and abuser attend same school; or if parents unable or unwilling to move; shelters are usually unavailable	Geographic separation is possible; shelters many times are available in community
Legal protections may or may not be available to teenager depending on laws in state and statues defining RV; may require consent or involvement of parent or guardian	Legal protections usually available; able to pursue without involvement of family/others

longitudinal course. Understanding how normative interactions between adolescents and their partners progress toward violence will be important in designing effective prevention and intervention programs, and more research is needed in this area (64). Some research suggests that mutual violence, in which both partners engage in abusive and violent behavior, may be more common among adolescents than adults (65,66). Gray and Foshee reported in 1997 that the majority of the youth in their sample were involved in mutual violence (66%) and that violence in these relationships was more severe and injuries were more common than in relationships in which violent behavior was one-sided (26).

The reasons why adolescents are more likely than adults to experience mutual violence are not clear, but one possible explanation is that it may reflect defensive responses on the part of the victim. Molidor and Tolman (1998) report that 36% of the girls in their study who were victims of RV reported using violence against an intimate partner in self-defense (30). Similarly, Watson and colleagues found that fighting back was the most common way high school students respon to experiences of RV, followed by informal help-seeking, breaking up, doing nothing, and crying (67).

Studies that have examined relational patterns leading to adolescent RV suggest that interactions progress from minor coercive and aggressive behaviors, such as the teasing and pseudo-bullying often used by adolescents to signal romantic interest, RV-type features including physical and sexual violence emerging during mid-adolescence (66). Table 34.3 provides a comparison of the characteristics of adult and adolescent RV.

HEALTH EFFECTS OF ADOLESCENT RELATIONSHIP VIOLENCE

Relationship violence has serious health effects for adults and adolescents, and research has demonstrated a connection between RV and eight of the 10 Leading Health Indicators (LHIs) of Healthy People 2010 (Family Violence Protection Fund [FVPF], accessed online December 20, 2007). Although literature on physical injuries associated with adolescent RV is sparse, there is a large body of literature on physical injuries and adult RV or IPV. Women in abusive relationships may present to healthcare settings (clinics, urgent care settings, and emergency departments) with a wide variety of medical complaints and physical injuries. The head, face, neck, and areas usually covered by clothing are the most common sites of IPV-related injuries. Injuries to multiple parts of the body, injuries in various stages of healing, and explanations that do not fit the nature of the injuries may all be suggestive of trauma sustained through partner violence. However, in many instances, women experiencing IPV will not present to the healthcare setting with direct trauma or injuries, but with medical complaints related to stress such as anxiety, depression, sleep and appetite disturbances, fatigue, and gastrointestinal complaints.

Adolescents experiencing RV may present in the clinical setting with obstetrical and gynecologic issues. The connection between teen exposure to sexually transmitted infections (STIs) and RV is strong enough that it should raise a clinical red flag for providers when a teen presents for testing. Adolescents experiencing RV frequently feel powerless to refuse sexual requests by their partner or require use of a condom. In a study of African-American adolescent girls, those with a history of RV were three times more likely to have contracted an STI, three times more likely to report being with a nonmonogamous male partner, and half as likely to use a condom. In yet another study of young mothers receiving public assistance, more than half reported that their dating partner sabotaged their birth control. Adolescent victims of RV are significantly more likely to delay prenatal care until the third trimester, and are also at heightened risk for physical violence during and immediately after pregnancy.

Adolescent victims of RV may present without overt injuries or medical conditions such as an STI, but rather with psychiatric symptoms such as anxiety or depression, or may suffer from an eating disorder or substance abuse. Adolescents involved in RV are more likely to engage in a variety of health-risk behaviors including smoking, substance abuse, and unprotected sex. In one study, 53% of high school students who reported severe dating violence reported smoking compared to 34% of students who did not report dating violence; and 34% admitted use of illegal drugs (excluding marijuana) compared to 18% of students reporting no dating violence. Finally, in a survey of RV victims and perpetrators attending California high schools, both were more likely to have carried a gun or other weapon to school, as well as to have been threatened or injured by a weapon at school, compared to their non-RV involved peers.

It is important but not surprising to note that, in addition to the negative health effects outlined here, teens involved in RV are also significantly less likely than their nonabused peers to engage in health-promoting behaviors such as using seat belts, not driving while drinking or riding with a driver who is drinking, using safe sexual practices, and obtaining recommended dental care (6,9,14,68–86).

Sadly, involvement in RV in the adolescent years can set a young person up for a lifetime of violent victimization or perpetration. In a longitudinal survey of 1,569 college students, Smith, White, and Holland (87) found that women who experience physical violence in a dating relationship during adolescence are three times more likely than their nonabused peers to be victimized in a dating relationship during college. Similarly, Foshee (89) found that adolescents who experienced mild forms of dating violence in the preceding year were 2.4 times more likely than non-victimized peers to experience severe dating violence (violence likely to lead to injury) and 1.3 times more likely report being sexually assaulted by their partners in the following year.

PREVENTING ADOLESCENT RELATIONSHIP VIOLENCE

Although many interventions and resources are available for adult victims of RV, including legal remedies, treatment groups, emergency shelters, and community outreach groups (61), far fewer are available for adolescents. The majority of resources for youth violence prevention have been directed toward gang and bullying prevention efforts, with less attention paid to RV. In addition, adolescent RV victims, because of their legal status as minors, are frequently ineligible for or excluded from RV services that do exist—the majority of which are focused on serving adult populations. Although emergency shelters are available to adult female RV victims, many if not most of these shelters refuse to accept adolescent RV victims out of concern that the young person may break the rules, divulge the location of the shelter, or otherwise fail to fit into the shelter services (63). Male adolescent RV victims are essentially ineligible for emergency shelter.

In states where IPV services are tied to a minimum age limit or require current or prior cohabitation, characteristics that are common to adult relationships but less so in adolescent ones, civil remedies such as restraining orders may not be available to adolescent RV victims. Even if civil remedies are available, the young person may lack the knowledge, skills, experience, and basic resources such as transportation to negotiate the court system successfully. In many instances, the teenager may need his or her parent or guardian to file the court papers or to give consent, actions which the teenager may not want to request, especially if he or she is also experiencing abuse in the home. Finally, even if a young person prevails in obtaining a protective order, it can be difficult to enforce if victim and abuser legitimately frequent the same places, for example, if the victim and perpetrator both attend the same school (88).

Although child protective services systems should ostensibly provide an alternative to these adult-oriented systems, in general they also fail to meet the needs of the adolescent victim of RV. These typically overburdened systems are designed to respond to reports of suspected abuse of a child by someone within the home or family, and generally are not prepared to address abuse that is taking place outside the home and between peers. Similarly, they are more likely to give priority to abuse reports involving young children, not adolescents (63).

On a more positive note, services for the primary prevention of adolescent RV are more available. A number of school- and community-based programs have been developed over the last decade specifically for adolescents; some have demonstrated beneficial short- and longer-term effects. Most of these programs incorporate cognitive behavioral approaches and seek to educate both girls and boys about the problem of dating violence and to change attitudes and behaviors thought to increase risk for RV victimization or perpetration. Safe Dates is a well-researched example of a school-based prevention program. Designed for middle and high school students between the ages of 12 and 18 years, the program targets both potential victims and perpetrators, and uses both primary and secondary prevention strategies. It includes nine 50-minute educational sessions, a 45-minute play that students perform, and a poster contest. Early studies of the intervention without follow-up or booster sessions, demonstrated positive effects on participants at 1-month follow-up; however, only attitude changes were maintained at 1-year follow-up. After booster sessions were added to the interventions, attitude and behavior chan were sustained at 4-year follow-up, with participants significantly less likely to be perpetrators or victims of RV at 4-year follow-up than controls (51,89,90).

Another approach to preventing RV among adolescents seeks to change local norms and culture that either tacitly or directly support violence against girls and women. These programs are based on a bystander model of violence prevention and seek to involve otherwise uninvolved bystanders, often young men in the community or on a sports team, as allies in discouraging acts of violence against girls and young women. The Mentors in Violence Prevention Program (MVP) is an example of this type of program. Founded in 1993 by Northeastern University's Center for the Study of Sport in Society, MVP raises participants' awareness of the extent to which men physically, verbally, emotionally, and sexually abuse women; creates an environment in which men can talk about dating violence without feeling defensive or guilty; and inspires leadership by showing how men can teach fellow students and others in their community that dating violence is unacceptable (91,92).

National awareness campaigns also exist that aim to increase young persons' and parent/caregivers' awareness of RV and ways to prevent it. Liz Claiborne Inc.'s Love Is Not Abuse Initiative is an example of a national awareness and educational campaign that spotlights relationship abuse. The campaign includes educational brochures for girls, boys, and their parents, as well as public service announcements about adolescent RV (93,94).

Very limited information is available on RV prevention interventions conducted in the healthcare setting. Although RV interventions for adults in the healthcare setting have demonstrated some positive effects in improving women's help-seeking and self-protection in relation to RV (95,96), studies of healthcare-based interventions for adolescent RV are not yet available. However, findings from a recent study examining the effects of a healthcare-based screen and referral intervention for more general incidents of aggression hint at the promise healthcare-based prevention efforts may hold for various types of youth violence. In this study, universal screening of 7- to 15-year-olds for psychosocial and emotional problems is conducted in the waiting rooms of primary care clinics; based on the results, parents were referred to a telephone-based parent training and counseling resource. Compared to young people in the care-as-usual control group, those in the intervention group showed significant reductions in aggressive behavior, delinquent behavior, and attention problems on the Child Behavior Checklist; lower rates of parent-reported bullying, physical fighting, and fight-related injuries requiring medical care; and child-reported bullying victimization (97).

Despite existing school-, community-, and healthcare-based efforts, serious gaps in services for adolescent RV exist. School-based prevention and intervention programs do not reach the vulnerable groups of youth who have already dropped out of school, fewer services are available in lower-income communities, and the usefulness of programs with minority populations in some cases is not known. In addition, with scarce resources available for such prevention efforts, some

groups recommend that particular focus be placed on those groups at highest risk for RV. In 2002, the FVPF released a report on adolescent RV that recommends that future prevention efforts be directed toward four specific subgroups of adolescents: teenage mothers, adolescents transitioning from foster care and juvenile detention, serious offenders, and young adolescents aged 10–15 years (45). Finally, prevention programs that target perpetrators of adolescent RV are almost non-existent. The expansion of services and research in this area is a clear priority, given that the behavior of young perpetrators may be more malleable than that of older perpetrators, and as such, it may be possible to alter patterns of violent behavior and prevent RV in future relationships.

HEALTHCARE PROVIDERS AND ADOLESCENT RELATIONSHIP VIOLENCE

Many professional healthcare associations have in some way recognized youth violence and/or family violence, including teen dating violence, as serious threats to the health of the public. A 1998 position statement by the American Academy of Pediatrics (AAP) advised its members to attempt to recognize evidence of RV and to intervene in a sensitive and skillful manner. This effort, although stopping short of a guideline, is an important first step in the healthcare response to violence in adolescent relationships.

Clinical experts and professional associations such as the American Medical Association (AMA) and American Association of Family Practitioners (AAFP) recommend that health professionals begin anticipatory guidance regarding interpersonal violence at age 11, just before patients are ready to begin dating relationships (98). The AMA's Guidelines for Adolescent Preventive Services (GAPS) recommends that providers begin to screen for emotional, physical, and sexual abuse beginning in early adolescence (11–14 years) and continue to late adolescence (18–21 years) (99). The Maternal and Child Health Bureau, Health Resources and Services Administration of the United States Department of Health and Human Services' *Bright Futures*, another resource intended to support preventive health care for children and adolescents, also recommends screening for abuse and assault in adolescents starting at age 11. Preventive counseling for caregivers is also recommended (100) to increase their awareness of factors that increase a child's risk for RV and of effective prevention strategies. Bright Futures provides a fact sheet that healthcare providers can use to educate parents on the warning signs of adolescent RV and supportive resources (100).

During these early preventive counseling sessions, health professionals can describe healthy and unhealthy dating behaviors; describe and label violent, aggressive, and controlling behaviors as unacceptable within the context of dating; model skills for preventing abusive behavior in dating relationships; and provide instructions on where to go for assistance if unacceptable behaviors do occur (98).

ASSESSMENT FOR ADOLESCENT RELATIONSHIP VIOLENCE

Although many major healthcare organizations in the United States recommend routine inquiry for one or more aspects of family violence, including adolescent RV, few providers inquire about adolescent RV. A recent study of 204 pediatric residents found that, whereas most reported being knowledgeable about the prevalence of adolescent RV, 91% do not routinely inquire about RV among their adolescent patients (101).

Reasons providers give for low compliance with recommendations for routine inquiry include lack of time, discomfort, fear of causing harm, lack of places to refer patients for further assistance, and lack of training in dealing with family violence issues (102–105). The relatively low base rate of RV and the infrequency of a positive response can also reduce provider motivation to ask about RV and its perceived usefulness. Some point to a lack of evidence that routine inquiry is helpful to patients, and voice concerns that it may produce harm rather than good, especially when discussing universal inquiry vs symptom- or presentation-based inquiry (e.g., evidence of physical harm) (106,107). As recently as 2004, the U.S. Preventive Services Task Force (USPSTF), which provides clinical guidelines and recommendations to clinicians, found insufficient evidence to recommend *for* or *against* routine screening of women for IPV. This recommendation has stimulated vigorous debate in the field; a comprehensive analysis and criticism of the USPSTF recommendation can be found on the Family Violence Prevention Fund's website at www.endabuse.org. This is discussed in detail elsewhere in this text.

The FVPF recommends that assessment for RV occur as part of the routine health history and that it be conducted during standard health assessments, periodic comprehensive health visits, and school and sports physicals. Recommendations also promote assessment during a visit for a new chief complaint and when signs and symptoms raise concerns of possible RV. Assessment should take place in private and with a professional interpreter (not a family member) when indicated. The provider should be aware of and inform his or her adolescent patient of reporting requirements relevant to adolescent RV before inquiring. Past experience in screening for tobacco use and other health-risk behaviors has shown that adolescents are more likely to respond to questions focused on specific behaviors such as "Has your boyfriend ever hit you?" as opposed to more general questions such as "Have you ever been abused?"

Even with effective assessment tools, adolescents may not disclose RV victimization when first asked; therefore, clinicians should routinely ask these questions with their adolescent patients at each health care visit (107,108) and remain alert to clinical red flags that indicate heightened risk for RV, such as an adolescent presenting to the clinic seeking pregnancy testing or prenatal care, or requesting testing for an STI.

Inquiry for RV can take place face-to-face or through written and computer-based surveys. In one study, patients reporting feeling most comfortable with written screening because of the perception that it was more likely to protect their confidentiality and privacy (107). Although computer-based screening may yield more positive screens than face-to-face screening, patients in several studies indicated they preferred discussing these issues in person with their clinician over interacting only with the computer (109,110).

Based on a compilation of published literature and common practice, the Massachusetts Medical Society's Violence Intervention and Prevention Committee (MMS-VIP)has estimated the time required to assess for IPV or RV during a typical primary healthcare visit. MMS-VIP estimates that 85% of the RV assessments will be negative and require only 10 seconds to complete and respond; 14% will be positive but nonurgent or not current and will require approximately 2 minutes to complete a rapid assessment of safety and schedule a follow-up visit to attend specifically to issues of RV; and less than 1% will be both positive and urgent. These few patients, not unlike those with other urgent conditions, will require 10 or more minutes to respond to appropriately (111). These estimates are based on assessing adults for IPV and are likely to change somewhat with the unique requirements of caring for adolescent patients, but still suggest that it should be feasible to incorporate RV assessment into routine care. Incorporating routine inquiry for adolescent RV into other routine screening activities, such as queries about tobacco use and excessive drinking, can make it easier to implement in into routine practice. Since a high correlation exists between these problem behaviors and RV, a positive screen for either one would signal a clinician to assess for RV (112).

ADOLESCENT DISCLOSURE OF RELATIONSHIP VIOLENCE DURING THE HEALTHCARE VISIT

Before initiating inquiry about RV, providers should reinforce to the patient the confidential nature of the interaction and discuss the limits of confidentiality imposed by local and state laws, as well as any reporting requirements that pertain to the adolescent. Providers should also recognize that for contemporary youth today, terms such as "dating" may hold limited meaning and may fail to capture the range and type of relationships that adolescents view as intimate and meaningful (113).

When an adolescent discloses that he or she is or has been the victim of RV, the provider should respond with supportive and empathetic comments such as "I'm sorry this happened," "This is not your fault," "You deserve better," and "I care about you, and about your safety and well-being" (94,114,115).

A danger assessment should be conducted with adolescents who are currently in a violent dating or intimate relationship or who have contact with an ex-partner who has been abusive. This assessment should include evaluation of risks for suicide as well as retaliatory and defensive violence, and the safety, if applicable, of children in the home. A danger assessment tool specifically for adolescents is not currently available; however, an adult-oriented tool developed by Campbell (117) provides a useful starting point and as do recommendations in the *Family Violence Prevention Funds' Child Exposure to Intimate Partner Violence and Adolescent Dating Violence: Guidelines for*

Medical Providers. If there are indications that the young person is in immediate danger, or is at risk of harming him or herself or others, appropriate steps should be taken to ensure the youth's safety. It is important to note that RV victims' assessment of the danger they are in is often inaccurate (116). In a recent study of female homicide victims, only half of 456 women who were killed or almost killed by an intimate partner accurately perceived their risk of being killed by this partner (117).

A safety plan should be developed with the teen prior to the end of the visit, and he or she should be provided with referrals to more comprehensive support services before the patient leaves the healthcare setting (94). Tools such as A Teen's Safety Plan (118) are available to aid providers in this process. The *FVPF's National Consensus Guidelines* also includes a safety planning tool that can be adapted for use with adolescents. As part of this plan, young people should be given telephone numbers and web URLs for national, state, and local IPV, rape crisis, and teen runaway hotlines, as well as the numbers of local shelters . In all cases, teens should first be asked if it is safe to take printed materials before they are given to the patient. All at-risk patients should be given an opportunity to place help and information-seeking calls in a private and confidential setting, and should be advised about ways to keep printed resource information private (so the perpetrator does not find it) once the patient exits the healthcare facility. A list of telephone resources available to teenagers in the United States is contained in Sidebar 34.1 at the end of this chapter; providers should check on local availability and appropriateness prior to their recommendation.

Finally, providers should be aware that assessing for RV in adolescents may also result in revelations of other forms of abuse in the young persons' life. Thus, it is important to be prepared to respond not only to the adolescents' needs in relation to RV, but also to family, school, and community violence as well (113). Resources to help providers in this broader task are available from the AMA (115,119,120).

CONFIDENTIALITY AND LEGAL CONSIDERATIONS FOR HEALTHCARE PROVIDERS

When preparing to incorporate adolescent RV services into practice, providers should first determine how their state defines and classifies adolescent RV. Some states classify RV or dating violence that involves a minor as child abuse. In these cases, mandatory reporting to child protective services is required. Other states have enacted legal exemptions that allow a minor as young as 12 years old to seek a domestic violence (DV) protective order for RV or dating violence without the approval of a parent or guardian.

Providers also should familiarize themselves with reporting requirements for assaultive injuries in their state. In all states, a traumatic injury to a minor inflicted by another person is considered an assaultive injury and must be reported to law enforcement officials. However, some states classify the injuries as child abuse in these circumstances, whereas others may classify them as DV. Typically, the health professional is only required to report that an injury has taken place, or that the minor is suspected of being in danger.

Providers must also consider reporting requirements for statutory rape that may be applicable, for instance, in the case of a young teenage girl with an older partner. Some states may require that some, but not all, consensual sexual activity between minors be reported. For example, in California, sexual intercourse must be reported if one partner is under 16 years of age and the other is age 21 or older (Penal Codes 261.5, 288-c). Adolescents' beliefs about what can and cannot be reported about them if they disclose abuse can have a chilling effect on their willingness to seek help from the professional community. Community workers relay stories of teenager girls delaying receipt of prenatal care and other services out of fear of these requirements (63).

Finally, providers need to know the regulations in their state governing an adolescent's right to seek care without parental consent or notification. Again, states vary in the rights they afford to adolescents in this area. In some states, a minor who discloses dating violence may fall outside these confidentiality protections, and the provider may be required by law to report the abuse to parents and authorities. In cases in which discretion is allowed, the pros and cons of parental notification should be explored with the patient. Although some parents can provide support for a child in a violent dating relationship, in other instances, a young person's disclosure of physical or sexual abuse, or of an unplanned pregnancy, can place the teenager at risk for more abuse, including abuse by a guardian or parent, or of witnessing abuse between family members in reaction to the disclosure (121–125).

The federal Health Insurance Portability and Accountability Act (HIPAA) authorizes healthcare professionals to refuse to release information to a patient's personal representative if the provider believes that the representative has subjected the patient to abuse or neglect, or may do so in the future. Resources to assist providers in making determinations about reporting requirements and assessing policy-level barriers to accessing RV services for adolescents affected by RV are available through the Family Violence Prevention Fund at www.endabuse.org.

CONCLUSION

Approximately 10%–25% of adolescents in the United States experience severe dating violence, and many more report exposure to emotional and verbal abuse in their intimate relationships. The effects of RV during adolescence can be devastating and lifelong, affecting a young person's identity, sense of personal competence and self-mastery, and emerging sexuality. Early RV experience can become the template upon which a young person bases his or her adult intimate relationships.

Adolescent RV is a distinct phenomenon from adult IPV that requires prevention and intervention efforts tailored specifically to the unique characteristics and developmental and situational needs of adolescents. Because many states do not include adolescent RV in their family violence statutes, adolescents are frequently ineligible for RV services, including protective orders. Many adult resources such as shelters do not accept teens, or if they do, inadequately address the particular needs of the teen victim.

Healthcare providers can play an important role in the primary and secondary prevention of RV in their adolescent patients through incorporating routine inquiry and risk assessment, early preventive education, and assistance to violence-affected teens (both victim and perpetrator) in the form of safety planning and linked referrals to appropriate services. Unfortunately, most healthcare providers do not routinely assess their adolescent patients for RV or provide preventive education and referrals. Resources are available that can assist healthcare professionals in incorporating RV assessment, counseling, and referral services for their adolescent patients into routine practice; and new evidence is emerging that points to the usefulness of healthcare-based interventions in

Sidebar 34.1: Resources for Health Care Professionals on Adolescent Relationship Violence

Family Violence Prevention Fund
(www.endabuse.org)
National Consensus Guidelines on Responding to Domestic Violence; Victimization in the Health Care Setting; Screen to End Abuse Training Video; information on mandatory reporting laws by state and HIPAA requirements related to dating violence; Child Exposure to Intimate Partner Violence and Adolescent Dating Violence Assessment tool

Massachusetts Medical Society
(http://www.massmed.org)
Partner Violence: How to Recognize and Treat Victims of Abuse: A guide for Physicians and other Health Care Professionals; Parent TIP Cards on dating violence

The American Bar Association (http://www.abanet.org/publiced/teendating.shtml)
Teen Dating Violence: Prevention Recommendations. Recommendations in the report were developed by teams of teenagers from across the country.

Peter Stringham's web page on youth violence
(http://people.bu.edu/pstring)
Dr. Stringham is a family physician and provides some useful material for parents, youth and professionals related to dating violence and youth violence based on his years of practice in the community

The National Youth Violence Prevention Resource Center (http://www.safeyouth.org)
A clearinghouse of information on youth violence prevention including screening tools, recent research articles, and fact sheets including adolescent dating violence.

Center for the Study and Prevention of Violence
(http://www.colorado.edu/cspv/blueprints)
This site contains information on evidence-based violence prevention interventions. While there are few interventions specific to dating violence, the list grows each year.

National Telephone Resources for Teens
National Domestic Violence Hotline 800-799-SAFE (7233), 800-787-3244 (TTY) or www.ndvh.org
National Teen Dating Abuse Helpline 866-331-9474, 866-331-8453 (TTY), or www.loveisrespect.org

reducing aggression and victimization among young persons.

In general, however, the topic of adolescent RV has been overshadowed by attention to other forms of youth violence, by important efforts to transform provider responses to adult victims of RV, and perhaps by assumptions that adolescent and adult RV are more similar than not. There is still much to understand about the underlying dynamics of adolescent RV and also about what constitutes effective practice in this area. Healthcare professionals, researchers, and policy makers must increase the attention given to adolescent RV, increase or expand developmentally appropriate and effective interventions available for adolescent victim and perpetrators of RV, and develop effective legislation governing the classification, response, and treatment of the same.

Helpful resources for healthcare professionals regarding adolescent dating violence are listed in Sidebar 34.1.

IMPLICATIONS FOR POLICY, PRACTICE, AND RESEARCH

Policy

- State family violence statutes should be modified to accommodate adolescent victims of RV, and to provide adolescents with access to developmentally appropriate and culturally sensitive RV services. In states where child protective service systems are the designated responders to adolescent RV, resources need to be allocated to allow effective responses to RV-involved adolescents.
- Reporting requirements should be examined for the impact they have on adolescents' willingness to seek help for RV, and modified to reduce negative effects without loss of protection.
- The input of young victims and perpetrators of RV, their families, their schools, and their communities should be sought by policy makers about the impact of existing policies and laws on their ability to seek and obtain assistance, and this information should be used to inform future policy-making in these areas.

Practice

- More resources need to be developed that are specific to the needs of the adolescent victim or perpetrator, rather than relying primarily on resources and tools developed for adult populations. Relationship violence is not "one-size-fits-all." The developmental and situational needs of adolescents vary greatly from those of adults and require resources and tools specific to these needs.

- Inadequate attention is paid to identifying and assisting youthful perpetrators of RV. Recognizing that violence is a cycle and that many, if not most, young perpetrators were or are also victims of violence, it is essential that the needs of these youths not be overlooked.

- Significant expansion is needed in the availability of developmentally and culturally appropriate intervention services for adolescents involved in RV such as shelters, community programs, and legal services. Funding needs to be allocated to more widely disseminate evidence-based prevention programs like Safe Dates. Developmentally appropriate services for adolescent RV need to be expanded.

- Medical and nursing schools, residency training programs, and other health professional training settings should include training on adolescent RV, as well as the interconnectedness of different forms of violence.

- Providers' involvement with adolescent RV should not be limited to the exam room. Health professionals can have a substantial impact on local, state, and even national policies related to adolescent RV and should leverage their positions of respect by joining community coalitions and advocating for improved services, laws, and practices.

- Input from victims, perpetrators, and families, as well as from front-line service providers should be sought and incorporated into national, state, and local efforts to improve practice in this area.

Research

- More research is needed on the nature, causes, and prevention of adolescent RV; in particular, research is needed to determine which health-care-based interventions are most effective in preventing or reducing harm from adolescent RV, and to determine the impact of RV assessment and counseling on adolescents' overall well-being and safety.

- In addition to existing epidemiological and intervention research, community-based participatory research approaches are needed that involve adolescents, families, front-line service providers, and communities as equal partners in the construction and conduct of research on the causes and particularly the solutions to adolescent RV. Adolescents, their families, and front-line providers should, as appropriate, be included on review teams for research funding and as members of research teams.

- Finally, consideration must be given to larger cultural factors that promote and even encourage violence among young people in this country, and tacitly or explicitly encourage violent or abusive behavior toward girls or women.

References

1. Saltzman LE, Fanslow JL, McMahon MJ, Shelley GA. *Intimate partner violence surveillance: Uniform definitions and recommended data elements.* Atlanta, GA: Department of Health and Human Services, Centers for Disease Control and Prevention, National Center for Injury Prevention and Control, 1999.

2. Freedner N, Freed L, Yang L, Austin S. Dating violence among gay, lesbian, and bisexual adolescents: Results from a community survey. *J Adolesc Health.* 2002;31:469–474.

3. Spivak H. The role of the pediatrician in youth violence prevention in clinical practice and at the community level. *Pediatrics.* 1999;103(1): 1080–1081.

4. CDC. Youth risk behavior surveillance: United States, 2004. *MMWR Morb Mortal Wkly Rep.* 2005;49 (SS–5):1–94.

5. Betz CL. Teen dating violence: An unrecognized health care need. *J Pediatr Nurs.* 2007;22(6):427–429.

6. Silverman J, Raj A, Mucci L, Hathaway J. Dating violence against adolescent girls and associated substance use, unhealthy weight control, sexual risk behavior, pregnancy, and suicidality. *JAMA.* 2001;286(5):572–579.

7. Coker A, Smith P, McKeown R, King M. Frequency and correlates of intimate partner violence by type: Physical, sexual, and psychological battering. *Am J Public Health.* 2000;90:533–539.

8. Ackard D, Neumark-Sztainer D. Date violence and date rape among adolescents: Associations with disordered eating behaviors and psychological health. *Child Abuse Negl.* 2002;26(5):455–473.

9. Ackard D, Neumark-Sztainer D, Hannan P. Dating violence among a nationally representative sample of adolescent girls and boys: Associations with behavioral and mental health. *J Gend Specif Med.* 2003;6(3):39–48.

10. Halpern CT, Oslak SG, Young ML, et al. Partner violence among adolescents in opposite-sex romantic relationships: Findings from the national longitudinal study of adolescent health. *Am J Public Health.* 2001;91(10):1679–1685.

11. Spencer GA, Bryant SA. Dating violence: A comparison of rural, suburban, and urban teens. *J Adolesc Health.* 2000;27(5):302–305.

12. Malik S, Sorenson SB, Anehensel CS. Community and dating violence among adolescents: Perpetration and victimization. *J Adolesc Health.* 1997;21(5): 291–302.

13. Rickert V, Wiemann C, Vaughn R, White J. Rates and risk factors for sexual violence among an ethnically diverse sample of adolescents. *Arch Pediatr Adolesc Med.* 2004;158(12):1132–1139.

14. Wingood G, DiClemente R, McCree D, et al. Dating violence and sexual health of black adolescent females. *Pediatrics.* 2001;107:72.

15. Rickert V, Wiemann C. Date rape among adolescents and young adults. *J Pediatr Adolesc Gynecol.* 1998;11:167–175.

16. Johnson-Reid M, Bivens L. Foster youth and dating violence. *J Interpers Violence.* 1999;14:1249–1262.

17. Heise L, Ellsberg M, Gottemoeller M. *Ending violence against women.* Baltimore, Maryland: Johns Hopkins University Center for Communications Programs, 1999.

18. Garcia-Moreno C, Jansen H, Ellsberg M, Heise L, Watts C. *WHO multi-country study on women's health and domestic violence against women: Initial results on prevalence, health outcomes, and women's responses.* Geneva, Switzerland: World Health Organization, 2005.

19. Eaton DK, Kann L, Kinchen S, et al. Youth risk behavior surveillance: United States, 2005. *MMWR Morb Mortal Wkly Rep..* 2006;55(SS5):1–108.

20. Bachman R, Saltzman LE. *Violence against women: Estimates from the redesigned survey, National Crime Victimization Survey, special report.* NCJ-154348. US Department of Justice, Office of Justice Programs, Bureau of Justice Statistics; August 1995.

21. Gazmararian JA, Lazorick S, Spitz AM, et al. Prevalence of violence against pregnant women. *JAMA.* 1996;275(24):1915–1920.

22. Weimann C, Agurcia C, Berenson A, et al. Pregnant adolescents: Experiences and behaviors associated with physical assault by an intimate partner. *Matern Child Health J.* 2000(4)2:93–101.

23. Harrykissoon SD, Rickert VI, Wiemann CM. Prevalence and patterns of intimate partner violence among adolescent mothers during the postpartum period. *Arch Pediatr Adolesc Med.* 2002;156: 325–330.

24. Chang JC, Berg C, Saltzman L, Herndon J. Homicide: A leading cause of injury deaths among pregnant and postpartum women in the United States, 1991–1999. *Am J Public Health.* 2005;95(3):471–477.

25. Sousa C. Teen dating violence: The hidden epidemic. *Fam Concil Courts Rev.* 1999;37(3):356–374.

26. Gray H, Foshee V. Adolescent dating violence: Differences between one-sided and mutually violent profiles. *J Interpers Violence.* 1997;12(1):126–141.

27. Molidor C, Tolman R, Kober J. Gender and contextual factors in adolescent dating violence. *Prevention Researcher.* 2000;7(1):1–4.

28. O'Keefe M, Treister L. Victims of dating violence among high school students. Are the predictors different for males and females? *Violence Against Women.* 1998;4(2):195–223.

29. Symons PY, Groer MW, Kepler-Youngblood P, Slater V. Prevalence and predictors of adolescent dating violence. *J Child Adolesc Psychatr Nurs.* 1994;7(3):14–23.

30. Molidor C, Tolman R. Gender and contextual factors in adolescent dating violence. *Violence Against Women.* 1998;4(2):180–194.

31. Sheehan K, Kim L, Gavin J. Urban children's perceptions of violence. *Arch Pediatr Adolesc Med.* 2004;158(1):74077.

32. Arriaga XB, Foshee VA. Adolescent dating violence: Do adolescents follow in their friends' or their parents' footsteps? *J Interpers Violence.* 2004;19(2):162–184.

33. Foshee VA, Bauman KE, Arriaga XB, et al. An evaluation of safe dates, an adolescent dating violence prevention program. *Am J Public Health.* 1998;88(1):45–50.

34. Schwartz M, O'Leary S, Kendziora K. Dating aggression among high school students. *Violence Vict.* 1997;12:295–305.

35. White JW, Koss MP. Courtship violence: Incidence in a national sample of higher education students. *Violence Vict.* 1991;6(4):247–256.

36. HIckman L, Jaycox L, Aronoff J. Dating violence among adolescents: Prevalence, gender distribution, and prevention program effectiveness. *Trauma Violence Abuse.* 2004;5(2):124–143.

37. Koss M, Gidycz C, Wisniewski N. The scope of rape: Incidence and prevalence of sexual aggression and victimization in a national sample of higher education students. *J Consult Clin Psychol.* 1987;55(2):162–170.

38. Muuss R. *Theories of adolescence,* 6th ed. New York: McGraw-Hill Inc, 1996.

39. Carver K, Joyner K, Udry J. National estimates of adolescent romantic relationships. Carolina Population Center, 1999.

40. CDC. Youth risk behavior surveillance: United States, 2003. *MMWR Morb Mortal Wkly Rep.* 2002;49(SS–5):1–94.

41. Wolfe D, Feiring C. Dating violence through the lens of adolescent romantic relationships. *Child Maltreat.* 2000;5:360–363.

42. Foshee V, Benefield T, Ennett S, et al. Longitudinal predictors of serious dating violence victimization during adolescence. *Prev Med.* 2004;39:1007–1016.

43. Roscoe B, Callahan J. Adolescents self-report of violence in families and dating relationships. *Adolescence.* 1983;10:545–563.

44. Roscoe B, Kelsey T. Dating violence among high school students. *Psychology: A Quarterly Journal of Human Behavior.* 1986;23:198–202.

45. Rosewater A. *Promoting prevention targeting teens: An emerging agenda to reduce domestic violence.* San Francisco: Family Violence Prevention Fund, 2002.

46. Ashley O, Foshee V. Adolescent help-seeking for dating violence: Prevalence, sociodemographic correlates, and sources of help. *J Adolesc Health.* 2003;36:25–31.

47. Riggs N, Houry D, Long G, et al. Analysis of 1,076 cases of sexual assault. *Ann Emerg Med.* 2000;35(4):358–362.

48. Foshee V, Fletcher L, MacDougall J, Bangdiwala S. Gender differences in the longitudinal predictors of adolescent dating violence *Prev Med.* 2001;32: 128–141.

49. Baynard V, Cross C, Modecki K. Interpersonal violence in adolescence: Ecological correlates of self-reported victimization. *J Interpers Violence.* 2006;21(10):1314–1332.

50. Anderson D, Harris J. Violence against women: An education program for rural community health workers. *Aust J of Rural Health.* 1997;5:17–21.

51. Foshee VA, Bauman KE, Ennett ST, et al. Assessing the long-term effects of the Safe Dates program and a booster in preventing and reducing adolescent dating violence victimization and perpetration. *Am J Public Health.* 2004;94 (4):619–624.

52. Widom CS. An update on the "cycle of violence." *NIJ Research in Brief.* February 2001.

53. Whitfield CL, Anda RF, Dube SR, Felitti VJ. Violent childhood experiences and the risk of intimate partner violence in adults. *J Interpers Violence.* 2003;18(2):166–185.

54. Banyard V, Cross C, Modecki K. Interpersonal violence in adolescence: Ecological correlates of self-reported victimization. *J Interpers Violence.* 2006;21(10):1314–1332.

55. Wolfe D, Wekerle C, Scott KL, et al. Predicting abuse in adolescent dating relationships over 1 year: The role of child maltreatment and trauma. *J Abnorm Psychol.* 2004;113(3):406–415.

56. O'Hearn H, Margolin G. Men's attitudes condoning marital aggression: A moderator between family of origin abuse and aggression against female partners. *Cognit Ther Res.* 2000;24(2):159–174.

57. Howard A, Riger S, Campbell R, Wasco SM. Counseling services for battered women. *J Interpers Violence.* 2003;18(7):717–734.

58. Gwartney-Gibbs P, Stockard J. Courtship aggression and mixed-sex peer groups. In: Pirog-Good M, Stets J, eds. *Violence in dating relationships: Emerging social issues.* New York, NY: Praeger; 989:185–204.

59. Johnson S, Frattaroli S, Campbell J, et al. I know what love means: Gender based violence in the lives of urban adolescents. *J Womens Health.* 2005;14(2):1249–1262.

60. Heise LL, Garcia-Moreno C. Intimate partner violence. In: Krug E, ed. *World Health Report on violence and health.* Geneva: World Health Organization, 2002.

61. Heise LL, Garcia-Moreno C. Intimate partner violence: The need for primary prevention in the community. *Ann Intern Med.* 2002;136:8.

62. Counts D BJ, Campbell J. *Sanctions and sanctuary.* Boulder, CO: Westview, 1992.

63. Hill A, Horne J, Scott E, Teare C. Protections for child and adult abuse victims fail adolescents. *Youth Law News.* 1999;20(3):1–6.

64. Lewis SF, Fremouw W. Dating violence: A critical review of the literature. *Clin Psychol Rev.* 2001;21(1):105–127.

65. Avery-Leaf S, Cascardi M, O'Leary KD, Cano A. Efficacy of a dating violence prevention program on attitudes justifying aggression. *J Adolesc Health.* 1997;21(1):11–17.

66. Wekerle C, Wolfe DA. Dating violence in mid-adolescence: Theory, significance and emerging prevention initiatives. *Clin Psychol Rev.* 1999; 19(4):435–456.

67. Watson J. High school students' responses to dating. *Violence Vict.* 2001;16(3):339–348.

68. Warshaw C. Identification, assessment and interventions with victims of domestic violence. In: Lee D, Durborow N, Salber P, eds. *Improving the health care response to domestic violence: A resource manual for health care providers.* San Francisco, CA: Family Violence Prevention Fund, 2006.

69. Roberts T, Klein J, Fisher S. Longitudinal effect of intimate partner abuse on high-risk behavior among adolescents. *Arch Pediatr Adolesc Med.* 2003;157(9):875–881.

70. Domino JF. Prior physical and sexual abuse in women with chronic headache: Clinical disorders. *Headache.* 1987(27):310–314.

71. Drossman D, Leserman J, Nachman G, et al. Sexual and physical abuse in women with functional or organic gastrointestinal disorders. *Ann Intern Med.* 1990;113:828–833.

72. McCauley J, Kern DE, Kolodner K, et al. The "battering syndrome": Prevalence and clinical characteristics of domestic violence in primary care internal medicine practices. *Ann Intern Med.* 1995;123:737–746.

73. Petro J, Quann P, Graham W. Wife abuse: The diagnosis and its implications. *JAMA.* 1978; 240(3):240–241.

74. Decker M, Silverman J, Rai A. Dating violence and sexually transmitted disease/HIV testing and diagnosis among adolescent females. *Pediatrics.* 2005;116(2):E272–E276.

75. Coker AL, McKeown RE, Sanderson M, et al. Severe dating violence and quality of life among South Carolina high school students. *Am J Prev Med.* 2000;19(4):220–227.

76. Bullock KA, Schornstein SL. Improving medical care for victims of domestic violence. *Hosp Physician.* September 1998:42–58.

77. Campbell A. Epidemic of women battering: Recognition and intervention by health care professionals. *J Fla Med Assoc.* 1995;82(10):684–686.

78. Campbell DW, Gary FA. Providing effective interventions for African American battered women: Afrocentric perspectives. In: Campbell JC, ed. *Empowering survivors of abuse: Health care for battered women and their children.* Thousand Oaks, CA: Sage;1998:229–240

79. Campbell J. Health consequences of intimate partner violence. *Lancet.* 2002;359:1331–1336.

80. Cokkinides VE, Coker AL, Sanderson M, et al. Physical violence during pregnancy: Maternal complications and birth outcomes. *Obstet Gynecol.* 1999;93(5 Pt 1):661–666.

81. Horon I, Cheng D. Enhanced surveillance for pregnancy-associated mortality: Maryland, 1993–1998. *JAMA.* 2001;285(11):1455–1459.

82. McFarlane J, Campbell JC, Sharps P, Watson K. Abuse during pregnancy and femicide: Urgent implications for women's health. *Obstet Gynecol.* 2002;100(1):27–36.

83. Murphy C, Schei B, Myhr TL, DuMont J. Abuse: A risk factor for low birth weight? A systematic review and meta-analysis. *Child Maltreat.* 2001;164(11):1567–1572.

84. Parker B, McFarlane J, Soeken K. Abuse during pregnancy: Effects on maternal complications and birth weight in adult and teenage women. *Obstet Gynecol.* 1994;84(3):323–328.

85. *Domestic violence and birth control sabotage: A report from the teen parent project.* Chicago, IL: Center for Impact Research, 2000.

86. Hanson M. Characteristics of health behavior in adolescent women reporting and not reporting intimate partner violence: A secondary analytic nursing study. At http://escholarship.bc.edu/dissertations/AAI3134963/. Accessed 11/4/2005.

8.7 Smith PH, White JW, Holland LJ. A longitudinal perspective on dating violence among adolescent and college age women. American J of Public Health, 2003: 93(7): 1104-1109.

88. Women's Law Initiative. Information for teens, At www.womenslaw.org/teens.htm. Accessed 11/04/2008.

89. Foshee V. Gender differences in adolescent dating abuse prevalence, types and injuries. *Health Educ Res.* 1998;11:275–286.

90. Foshee V, Linder G, Bauman K, et al. The safe dates project: Theoretical basis, evaluation design, and selected baseline findings. *Am J Prev Med.* 1996; 12(5 Suppl):39–47.

91. Slaby R. Telephone interview. May 25, 2004.

92. Mentors in violence prevention. At http://www.sportinsociety.org/mvp.html; Accessed 4/23/2005.

93. Love Is Not Abuse. Liz Claiborne, Inc. At http://www.loveisnotabuse.com. Accessed 11/4/2008.

94. *Consensus recommendations on identifying and responding to domestic violence for child and adolescent health.* San Francisco, CA: Family Violence Prevention Fund, 2004.

95. Ramsay J, Richardson J, Carter Y, et al. Should health professionals screen women for domestic violence? Systematic review. *Br J Med.* 2002;325: 314–325.

96. Muelleman RL, Feighny KM. Effects of an emergency department-based advocacy program for battered women on community resource utilization. *Ann Emerg Med.* 1999;33(1):62–66.

97. Borowsky I, Mozayeny S, Stuenkel K, Ireland M. Effects of a primary care based intervention on violence behavior and injury in children. *Pediatrics.* 2004;114:392–399.

98. Stringham P. Domestic violence. *Prim Care.* 1999;26(2):373–384.

99. *Guidelines for Adolescent Preventive Services (GAPS): Recommendations monograph.* Chicago, IL: American Medical Association, 1997.

100. *Bright futures: Guidelines for health supervision of infants, children, and adolescents,* 2nd ed. Arlington, VA: National Center for Education in Maternal and Child Health, 2002.

101. Forceir M, Patel R, Kahn J. Pediatric residents' attitudes and practices regarding adolescent dating violence. *Ambul Pediatr.* 2003;3(6): 317–323.

102. Sugg NK, Inui T. Primary care physicians' response to domestic violence: Opening Pandora's box. *JAMA.* 1992;267(23):3157–3160.

103. Griffith J. Opinions in pediatric and adolescent gynecology: Screening for dating violence: Are we ready to screen? *J Pediatr Adolesc Gynecol.* 2004;17:53–55.

104. Forcier M, Patel R, Kahn J. Pediatric residents' attitudes and practices regarding adolescent dating violence. *Ambul Pediatr.* 2003;3(6):317–323.

105. Garimella RN, Plichta SB, Houseman C, Garzon L. How physicians feel about assisting female victims of intimate-partner violence. *Acad Med.* 2002;77(12):1262–1265.

106. Parsons L, Goodwin MM, Petersen R. Violence against women and reproductive health: Toward defining a role for reproductive health care services. *Matern Child Health J.* 2000;4(2):135–140.

107. Phelan MB. Screening for intimate partner violence in medical settings. *Trauma, Violence Abuse.* 2007;8:199–213.

108. Scheiman L, Zeoli A. Adolescents' experiences of dating and intimate partner violence: "Once is not enough." *J Midwifery Womens Health.* 2003;48(3):226–228.

109. Trautman DE, McCarthy M, Miller N, et al. Intimate partner violence and emergency department screening: Computerized screening versus usual care. *Ann Emerg Med.* 2007;49(4):526–534.

110. McCord-Duncan E, Floyd M, Kemp E, et al. Detecting potential intimate partner violence: Which approach do women want? *Fam Med.* 2006;38(6):416–422.

111. Alpert E, ed. *Partner violence: How to recognize and treat victims of abuse: A guide for physicians and other health care professionals,* 4th ed. Massachusetts Medical Society Committee on Violence, 1998.

112. Gerber M, Ganz M, Lichter E, et al. Adverse health behaviors and the detection of partner violence by clinicians. *Arch Intern Med.* 2005;165(9): 1016–1021.

113. Glass N, Fredland N, Campbell J, et al. Adolescent dating violence: Prevalence, risk factors, health outcomes and implications for clinical practice. *JOGNN.* 2003;32:227–238.

114. Treating dating violence victims: National Youth Violence Prevention Resource Center: www.safeyouth.org/scripts/faq/treatdate.asp. Accessed 5/1/2004.

115. Sege R, Licenziato V, Webb S. Bringing violence prevention into the clinic: The Massachusetts Medical Society Violence Prevention Project. *Am J Prev Med.* (In press.) (Special supplement: training healthcare professionals in youth violence prevention.)

116. Peralta RL, Fleming MF. Screening for intimate partner violence in a primary care setting: The validity of "feeling safe at home" and prevalence results. *J Am Board Fam Pract.* 2003;16(6):525–532.

117. Campbell J, Sheridan D. Domestic violence assessments. In: Jarvis C, ed. *Physical examination and health assessment,* 4th ed. St. Louis, MO: Saunders; 2004:73–82.

118. Kaufhold M. A Teen's Safety Plan. California Medical Training Center. 2003. Available from: http://www.ccfmtc.org/d_violence.asp. Accessed 11/19/2008.

119. Sege R, Flanigan E, Levin-Goodman R, et al. Case study: The American Academy of Pediatrics' Connected Kids program. *Am J Prev Med.* (In press.) (Special supplement: training healthcare professionals in youth violence prevention.)

120. Knox L. *Connecting the dots to prevent youth violence: A training and outreach guide for physicians and other health professionals.* Chicago, IL: American Medical Association, 2002.

121. Foo L, Margolin G. A multivariate investigation of dating aggression. *J Fam Violence.* 1995;10: 351–377.

122. Kalmuss D. The intergenerational transmission of marital aggression. *J Marriage Fam.* 1984; 46(1):11–19.

123. Jackson Y. Review of the book: Protecting children from abuse and neglect. *J Pediatr Psychol.* 1996;22:133–136.

124. O'Keefe M. Predictors of dating violence among high school students. *J Interpers Violence.* 1997;12(4):546–569.

125. Straus MA, Gelles RJ, Steinmetz SK. *Behind closed doors: Violence in the American family.* Garden City, NY: Anchor Press/Doubleday, 1980.

Chapter 35

Intimate Partner Violence Among the Elderly and People with Disabilities

Diana Koin

KEY CONCEPTS

- Intimate partner violence (IPV) is a health problem and criminal justice matter that includes elderly and disabled people, but is seldom recognized in that population.
- Abuse of elders and people with disabilities has the potential of presenting as many different kinds of crimes: assault, neglect, financial abuse, sexual assault, abandonment, and psychological abuse.
- When IPV affects elders and people with disabilities, reporting guidelines for both IPV and elder/dependent adult abuse must be followed.
- Dementia, depression, and chronic disabling health problems increase the risk of IPV among older people.
- Data substantiating incidence of IPV of older people is in its infancy, but suggests that IPV decreases with age.
- Healthcare professionals and the criminal justice system fail to identify IPV in the elderly because they believe it to be a crime of younger people.

Experts in elder/dependent adult abuse and intimate partner violence (IPV) have made significant progress in the last decade in preventing, identifying, and intervening in interpersonal violence. Laws have evolved and become more sophisticated for elder/dependent adult abuse and IPV. Cadres of health professionals and criminal justice experts have become skilled and knowledgeable about these crimes. Despite all of this progress, elder abuse and IPV often remain in separate realms. Social services, health professionals, and the criminal justice system have made excellent progress in both IPV and elder abuse, but the knowledge and skills that have been gained by widespread experience in the field seldom overlap between the two areas.

The case of Emily T., in Sidebar 35.1, represents the pitfalls that deter recognition and intervention of IPV in older or disabled victims. The patient's injuries are attributed to falls and underlying impaired mobility. A victim's silence is mistakenly attributed to either dementia in an elderly patient or cognitive/communication impairment in a disabled person. Thus, healthcare providers miss IPV unless they understand the key factors.

Sidebar 35.1: Case History

Emily T. is 81 years old and has been married for 53 years. When she arrived at the emergency department with a fractured hip, bruises were noted on both arms and she had a black eye. The emergency physician asked about the bruising, but Emily closed her eyes and did not speak. Her husband was at her side. During her hospitalization, staff found that she had no cognitive limitations; she was fully able to make medical decisions for herself. Emily T. successfully underwent surgery for her hip. At the time of discharge when she was to be transferred to a skilled nursing unit for rehabilitation, her husband insisted that she come home and that he "would care for her".

A MULTIFACETED CRIME

Elder abuse and abuse of people with disabilities have multiple manifestations. Physical abuse includes assault, but also extends to encompass such things as inappropriate use of physical restraints or expecting a frail person to perform tasks that place them at great risk for harm.

Neglect is a more complex construct in that it is based on failed responsibility by someone in a position of trust. Typical manifestations of neglect are pressure ulcers, dehydration, and malnutrition/starvation of the victim (1,2). Failure to obtain medical care for an elder or a disabled person who needs to see a doctor, and failure to obtain medical care in a timely fashion are also forms of neglect. Environmental hazards such as inadequate cooling in a heat wave or summer clothing in the midst of winter also constitute neglect or perhaps even physical abuse due to the pain and suffering incurred by the victim.

Sexual assault in the elderly and the disabled is the health issue most likely to go undetected. Older women are embarrassed and hesitant to disclose to family, health providers, or police, particularly if the perpetrator is a family member. Women living in nursing homes are particularly unlikely to come forward because of the multiple hurdles facing their disclosure. Staff often view their reports of assault as paranoid or delusional, and patients with cognitive impairments cannot consistently report the event. Women with disabilities report an 83% incidence of sexual assault (3). Victims are fearful about disclosing their assault. Anecdotal reports have shown that people with disabilities can provide accurate and consistent testimony in court despite communication limitations.

Experts anticipate that within the next decade the greatest transfer of wealth ever seen on Earth will occur as elders die and their assets are inherited. This phenomenon has simultaneously targeted elders as potential victims for criminal predators. Elders are at particular risk for "undue influence," a strategy that entails befriending a lonely elder, diminishing their contact with friends and family, and steadily having assets transferred from the elder to the perpetrators. The elder becomes increasingly trusting of the perpetrator. Isolation thus becomes a high-risk factor for financial abuse as the elder is separated from family, friends, and financial/legal advisors (4). A typical scenario occurs when an older person is "befriended" by a perpetrator who rapidly establishes a relationship but convinces the victim that their family and friends are no longer interested in them. The elder's funds and possessions are the target.

Abandonment takes many forms, but all versions have inherent within them an older or disabled person left in an unsafe situation. Frequently encountered scenarios include elders with dementia left alone while family members work, or caregivers leaving town without adequate food or supervision planned.

Psychological abuse typically consists of threats and intimidation. The abuse is intended to engender control over the person. The most commonly encountered psychological threat is of being "put in a nursing home." Tragically, elderly victims with dementia may not be able to recall the specific content of a threat but only remember the context of fear that accompanies the threat.

Self-neglect is viewed by experts in the field as a special form of elder abuse. Although no perpetrators are involved, self-neglecting elders are vulnerable to abuse and exploitation by others. Key to approaching self-neglect is the ability to determine whether the victim has the capacity to make safe and wise decisions. Thus, self-neglect represents a spectrum of individuals from eccentric individuals opting for an alternative lifestyle to those who are suffering from mental health problems that need treatment. Cognitive and functional assessment provides specific information that will assist healthcare providers in providing appropriate support and treatment. Coordination with social services agencies can offer additional help for elders who are self-neglecting.

POPULATION PROFILE DIFFERENCES

Our society's view of the elderly and of those with disabilities plays an important role in our ability to identify and intervene in abuse and violence in late life. Although society typically defines "elderly" as anyone over the age of 65, dramatic differences exist between the young old (age 65–85) and the oldest old (those over 85). Those over 85 have increased likelihood of health problems, including immobility, dementia, depression, and incontinence. Elderly victims have health issues that need to be incorporated into the intervention plan. A careful assessment of the chronic physical problems is important, with particular attention paid to the ability to perform activities of daily living. If a person has limitations in memory, depression, or their activities of daily living, it places him at greater risk of abuse and violence.

Depression and dementia have been shown to be important risk factors for elder abuse. The work of Dyer and colleagues demonstrated that the prevalence of depression in a population of abused elders was 62% versus 12% in a control population; 51% of the abused cohort was found to be demented versus a control of 30% (5). Other important risk factors include age, race, low-income status, functional impairment, a history of family violence, and recent stressful events (6).

When one looks at the elder abuse literature, surveys document that women are victims of abuse much more frequently than are men. This is true after adjustment for the larger percentage of women in the population over the age of 65. Elderly women are 57.6% of the elderly population, yet 71.4% of physical abuse cases, 63% of financial abuse cases, and 60% of neglect cases are reports of women (7).

EPIDEMIOLOGY AND TYPOLOGY OF VIOLENCE IN LATE LIFE

Abuse of older women is a serious public health problem. Investigation of a population of 91,749 women

aged 50–79, who were subjects in the Women's Health Initiative, provided incidence and prevalence data on abuse and violence among postmenopausal women. Subjects were asked: "Over the past year, were you physically abused by being hit, slapped, pushed, shoved, punched, or threatened with a weapon by a family member or close friend?" Eleven percent of the study participants reported physical abuse at baseline; 5% were abused in a 3-year follow-up. The women studied in this research were described as independent; the study was limited in that it did not include any of the "oldest old" population (8).

Bonomi and colleagues researched IPV in women over the age of 65. In a study of 370 older women, lifetime partner violence prevalence was assessed utilizing five questions from the Behavioral Risk Factor Surveillance System and 10 questions from the Women's Experience with Battering (WEB). Physical abuse, forced intercourse, forced sexual contact, verbal threats, and controlling behavior were identified. They found a prevalence of lifetime partner violence of 26.5%. Forced sex or sexual contact accounted for 39.1% of the study subjects to rate their abuse as severe, whereas threats represented 70.7% (9).

Rennison and Rand (10) attempted to study prevalence and incidence of IPV in three different age cohorts. Because this study includes younger age cohorts than those typically included in elder abuse studies, it is difficult to extrapolate to women over 65, 75, and/or 85. Their study substantiates the fact that young women suffer much higher rates of IPV. The investigation utilized data from the National Crime Victimization Survey. Those aged 12–24 experience IPV at a rate of 12.27%, whereas those 25–54 have a rate of 8.7%. For the over-55 cohort, the rate was only 0.44%.

Lachs' pioneering study has documented the seriousness of these health threats (11). Elders who are physically abused have a threefold increase in mortality when compared to an age and comorbidity controlled population. Surprisingly, the mortality was not secondary to their abuse-induced injuries.

INTIMATE PARTNER VIOLENCE IN ELDERS AND PEOPLE WITH DISABILITIES VERSUS IN YOUNGER PEOPLE

In a study analyzing case studies of elderly women experiencing abuse situations, Penhale focused on gender as a factor (12). Her hypothesis was that if the predominant form of abuse is physical abuse by males toward females, it must be identified so that an intervention can be initiated. Penhale based her proposition on the earlier work of Whittaker (13) that utilized a feminist analysis basing observations on control of power. A cohort of six women were followed for 18 months; the study participants were aged 82–88 at the onset of the study. The types of violence encountered were physical, financial, psychological, and neglect. Interestingly, the abusers were not limited to spouses or spouse surrogates, nor were they all male. All of the victims were found to be dependent on the perpetrator, and all of the victims suffered from isolation, thus indicating possible risk factors for IPV.

Schaffer (14) addressed the issue of isolation and abuse in a study conducted in Australia. She utilized interviews and a telephone survey to investigate the status of 90 women aged 50–78. The project's intent was to identify the needs of older women who were living in isolated situations with partners known to be violent, in the hope that the information would guide public policy development of services. The most important issue identified by the study participants was what they described as "being believed." Other frequently mentioned issues included social support, access to reliable information, appropriate responses from service providers, accurate legal information, and income assistance. Emergency housing was also important to the women studied; they noted the need to be able to access it quickly and to make certain it was appropriate for older women. Women living in rural areas identified special needs that included lack of transport, conservative patriarchal culture, gun ownership, limited medical and social services, poverty, and what Schaffer described as a "small town syndrome" (i.e., fear that the violence in their households would be publicly noticed). Although not an intended part of the research, the women reported affirmation in simply participating in the study and telling their stories.

Profile of the Older Victim

Elder abuse victims have been studied in an attempt to identify a risk profile for those who are particularly vulnerable. The risk factors identified (Table 35.1) include age, prior abuse episodes, dementia, depression, impaired functional ability, and isolation (15). Identification of risk factors is not only important for

Table 35.1 Risk Factors for Elder and Dependent Adult Abuse
Dementia
Depression
Substance abuse
Isolation
History of interpersonal violence
Limitations performing activities of daily living
Behavior issues secondary to dementia
Lack of continuity in medical care

screening, but because addressing and treating factors such as depression, substance abuse, impaired functional status, and isolation can prevent abuse.

Profile of the Offender

Because older and disabled persons often need assistance in performing activities of daily living, they require caregivers. Family members provide the majority of care for people living in the community. However, for those whose care needs exceed reasonable care at home, institutional care is indicated. In settings such as nursing homes, developmental centers, or residential care facilities for the elderly, most of the actual physical care is provided by nursing assistants. Low pay, difficult patient behaviors, long hours with frequent double shifts, and limited training contribute to the risk of aggressive behavior by caregivers (16).

Bonnie Brandl (17) points out that there is significant jeopardy of placing the victim at even greater risk if the crime is dismissed as only "elder abuse secondary to caregiver stress" rather than IPV:

> When professionals do not analyze the potential power imbalances surrounding instances of abuse and instead automatically attribute the violent behavior to caregiver stress, they may unwittingly be doing the following: (1) blaming the victim; (2) colluding with the batterer's excuses; and (3) discouraging the involvement of the justice system.

Understanding the factors that lead a perpetrator to abuse an elder or dependent adult has thus moved away from attributing all crimes to "caregiver stress." Ramsey-Klawsnick's work has described what she terms a "typology of offenders." She based her work on her clinical and forensic experience working with victims and offenders, as well as consulting with criminal justice and social service agencies (18). Ramsey-Klawsnick's perpetrators represent a spectrum of reasons for abuse, varying from "The Overwhelmed" and "The Impaired" in situations where care providers are unable to cope, to "The Narcissistic," "The Domineering/Bullying," and "The Sadistic," where harm is inflicted with increasingly targeted intent.

IS IT INTIMATE PARTNER VIOLENCE OR IS IT ELDER/DEPENDENT ADULT ABUSE?

When abuse of an older or disabled person occurs in the home, it is often helpful to consider whether the crime is elder/dependent abuse, IPV, or both. Intimate partner violence definitions do not exclude older or disabled victims, albeit the focus is more specifically on physical and psychological abuse. A hallmark of both crimes is that they are typically repetitive. Perhaps the greatest limiting factor is that healthcare professionals and the criminal justice system think of IPV as a crime of younger people. This is particularly true when the abuse includes sexual issues.

Elder/dependent adult abuse definitions in the United States are increasingly based on legal definitions. Most states specify elder abuse as a crime in which victims are over the age of 65, and "abuse" may include multiple crimes such as physical abuse, neglect, and financial abuse. The United Nations report on elder abuse noted that definitions vary in different societies. The report defined elder abuse as "a single or repeated act, or lack of appropriate action occurring within any relationship where there is an expectation of trust, which causes harm or distress to an older person" (19). Disabled persons are those individuals who have physical or psychological limitations that jeopardize their ability to care for themselves.

If interpersonal violence occurs to an older or disabled victim in a domestic setting, reporting must follow guidelines for both elder/dependent adult abuse and IPV if the perpetrator of the abuse is known to be a current or former spouse, intimate partner, or cohabitant. Thus, law enforcement and adult protective services may well be notified. If the crime involves institutional care, the cross-reporting should include the ombudsman, using the reporting strategies required by the state where the violence occurs.

One of the important questions prosecutors then consider is whether the crimes should be approached as an elder/dependent adult abuse or domestic violence (DV) case, and that can depend upon the differences in the potential prosecution remedies. In most jurisdictions, the consequences of elder abuse warrant less severe penalties than do those of DV. A recent case of death by starvation of a 36-year-old dependent adult was prosecuted as an elder/dependent adult abuse case (*People v. Grubbs*, Monterey County California). The victim had moved into his brother's home after his mother became too frail to care for him. His adult weight had been 160 pounds; his weight at death was 65 pounds. Although prosecution was successful, the sentences were only a few months of incarceration.

Identifying resources and services for older victims of IPV may be more challenging. Shelters may be unwilling to welcome older or disabled victims, or may not provide appropriate services if the person requires assistance with activities of daily living. Intimate partner violence advocates may not be familiar with working with a population of people with cognitive, communication, or sensory deficits.

IMPLICATIONS FOR POLICY, PRACTICE, AND RESEARCH

Policy

- Community providers of both healthcare services and social services should expand their interdisciplinary teams to include experts in both elder abuse and IPV.
- Specialized elder abuse teams (for financial crimes and death review) should add IPV to their mission and facilitate education for all team members on this topic.

Practice

- Service providers more accustomed to working with younger victims will need special skills as they expand their scope to serve older people. Not only do they need to have a basic understanding of dementia, they will need to be able to screen victims for cognitive and decisional limitations.

- Healthcare professionals and social service providers must be vigilant in identifying financial abuse, and they must also gain skill in understanding the importance of the dynamics of undue influence.

Research

- The greatest priority for understanding interpersonal violence in late life is research to understand why increased mortality occurs among abused elders.

References

1. Lachs M, Pillemer K. Elder abuse. *Lancet.* 2004;364(9441):1263–1272.
2. Dyer C, Connolly M, McFeeley P. The medical forensics of elder abuse and neglect in elder mistreatment. In: Bonnie RJ, Wallace RB, eds. *Abuse, neglect and exploitation in an aging America.* Washington DC: National Academic Press;2002:339–381.
3. Sobsey D, Doe T. Patterns of sexual abuse and assault. *J Sexuality Disabil.* 1991;9(3): 243–359.
4. Quinn M, Tomita S. *Elder abuse and neglect: Causes, diagnosis, intervention strategies.* New York: Springer, 1997.
5. Dyer C. The high prevalence of depression and dementia in elder abuse or neglect. *J Am Geriatr Soc.* 2000;48(2):205–208.
6. Lachs MS. Risk factors for reported elder abuse and neglect: A nine-year observational cohort study. *Gerontologist.* 1997;37(4):469–474.
7. Mouton CP. Intimate partner violence and health status among older women. *Violence Against Women.* 2003;9(12):1465–1477.
8. Mouton CP, Rodabough RJ, Rovi SL, et al. Prevalence and 3-year incidence of abuse among postmenopausal women. *Am J Public Health.* 2004;94(4):605–612.
9. Bonomi A, Anderson M. Intimate partner violence in older women. *Gerontologist.* 2007;47(1):34–41.
10. Rennison CM, Rand MR. Nonlethal intimate partner violence against women: A comparison of three age cohorts. *Violence Against Women.* 2003;9(12):1417–1428.
11. Lachs M, Williams C, O'Brian S. The mortality of elder mistreatment. *JAMA.* 1998;280(5):428–432.
12. Penhale B. Bruises on the soul: Older women, domestic violence and elder abuse. *J Elder Abuse Negl.* 1998;11(1):1–22.
13. Whittaker T. Violence, gender, and elder abuse: Towards a feminist analysis and practice. *J Gend Stud.* 1995;4(1):35–45.
14. Schaffer J. Older and isolated women and domestic violence project. *J Elder Abuse Negl.* 1999;11(1):59–77.
15. Seghal S, Mosqueda L. Elder mistreatment and neglect. In: Ham R, Sloane P, Warshaw G, et al, eds. *Primary care geriatrics: A case-based approach.* St. Louis: Mosby, 2007.
16. Pillemer K, Moore D. Abuse of patients in nursing homes: Findings from a survey of staff. *Gerontologist.* 1989;29:314–320.
17. Brandl B. Power and control: Understanding domestic abuse in later life. *Generations.* 2000;24(2):39–45.
18. Ramsey-Klawsnick H. Elder abuse offenders: A typology. *Generations.* 2000;24(2):17–22.
19. *Abuse of older persons: Recognizing and responding to abuse of older persons in a global context.* United Nations Economic and Social Council, Commission for Social Development, 2002.

Chapter 36

Caring for the Care Provider

Jane Liebschutz

KEY CONCEPTS

- Vicarious traumatization, compassion fatigue, and secondary traumatic stress are related concepts that reflect the negative psychological impact of caring for trauma survivors.
- Opening oneself up to the patient, combined with a sincere desire to alleviate suffering, can make any provider vulnerable to experiencing secondary traumatic stress symptoms.
- A clinician's personal history of trauma exposure may increase his or her vulnerability to secondary traumatic stress symptoms.
- Greater professional experience caring for trauma survivors may protect a provider against experiencing secondary traumatic stress symptoms.
- Providers can improve their resiliency to developing secondary traumatic stress symptoms by discussing cases with colleagues or community-based advocates.

Although caring for survivors of interpersonal violence can enrich a provider's personal and professional satisfaction, it can also cause the clinician distress, variably described in the literature as *compassion fatigue, vicarious traumatization,* and *burnout.* This distress can compromise a provider's personal welfare and effectiveness with patients. This chapter defines these areas of potential difficulty, reports the key published literature, and then addresses ways to prevent and manage them.

EMOTIONAL RESPONSES TO TREATING TRAUMA SURVIVORS

A provider's emotional reactions to treating survivors of interpersonal violence may manifest in several ways (Table 36.1).

Helplessness and Lack of Control

One of the hallmark features of a traumatic event is the sense of helplessness and lack of control it engenders. For example, some survivors of intimate

Table 36.1 Common Reactions to Caring for Survivors of Trauma

Reaction	Manifestation
Helplessness	• Depressive symptoms • Feeling ineffective with patients • Reacting negatively to patients • Thinking of quitting clinical work
Fear	• Recurrent thoughts of threatening situations • Chronic suspicion of others • Sleep disruptions • Physical symptoms • Inability to relax or enjoy pleasurable activities
Anger	• Reacting angrily to patients, staff, colleagues • Feelings of guilt • Decreased self-esteem
Detachment	• Avoiding patients • Avoiding emotional topics during patient encounters • Ignoring clues from patients about trauma • Failing to fulfill social or professional roles • Chronic lateness
Boundary violation and transference	• Taking excessive responsibility for patient • Seeing patient after hours • Doing something out of usual practice pattern (e.g., prescribe medication usually managed by specialist) • Sharing own problems with patient • Patient trying to care for doctor
Use of alcohol or drugs	• Increased use of alcohol • Initiation or use of drugs • Misuse of prescription medication

partner violence (IPV) want to leave an abusive relationship but find themselves unable to make changes despite the availability of counseling, shelters, and other resources. A clinician who has made referrals and counseled the patient at length may then feel helpless when the patient remains in the abusive relationship months or years later. Even if the trauma has passed long ago, the sense of helplessness formed during the trauma may imbue the patient with helplessness in all aspects of her life. The clinician may, in turn, pick up on the patient's helplessness (1). For some patients, suicidal thoughts may result from this sense of helplessness about intrusive memories or persistent abuse. The clinician may begin to agree

subconsciously that death, indeed, would be the only way to terminate memories or abuse, and may not be as aware of signs of possible suicidal attempt. The clinician's sense of helplessness and hopelessness may creep beyond the specific patient encounters and more broadly into the practice of medicine. This can contribute to thoughts about quitting medicine, reacting negatively to all patients, or even experiencing major depression (2).

Fear: Lack of a Sense of Safety in the World

Trauma can shatter one's sense of the world as a safe place. Clinicians who hear stories of human atrocity and violence may begin to wonder about their own safety. The images and emotions of the patient's trauma may become incorporated into the clinician's cognitive schema (3). The clinician may then start to see the world from the viewpoint of the traumatized patient. They may wonder "Am I safe?" "Is my family safe?" Daily life may look like opportunities for predators to attack. This can transform an ability to trust into chronic suspicion of others, and may also intrude into the private world of the clinician. The clinician's heightened sense of vulnerability may interfere with a capacity for relaxation and enjoyment. Chronic fear and intrusive thoughts of the trauma may also disturb sleep and induce chronic symptoms, such as stomach upset or headache (3,4).

A corollary to this sense of fear is a mistrust of others. Some providers suffering from secondary traumatic stress may feel victimized by patients they perceive to be threatening or manipulative (4). This may impede their ability to listen to or empathize with patients, relate to colleagues and staff, and to develop intimacy.

Anger

Trauma can also disrupt one's sense of justice in the world, leading to feelings of anger. The anger can be directed at a variety of targets: the perpetrator, God, political authorities, colleagues, staff members, or even the patient. Acting on anger may disrupt relationships and impede the clinician's effectiveness. Furthermore, acting angrily can perpetuate a sense of loss of control and helplessness. It can also cause feelings of guilt and decreased self-esteem in the clinician.

Detachment

Detachment and emotional numbing are coping responses trauma survivors sometimes utilize when feeling overwhelmed or vulnerable. Providers may also employ these responses, either consciously or unconsciously. They may avoid the known trauma survivor or any emotional closeness or discussion of trauma-related issues. This may render the patient even more isolated and lonely because the person she comes to for help is unable to connect with her. It also may cause the provider to miss important cues and dull his or her enjoyment of the work. Sometimes, this detachment (and other emotions noted earlier) may contribute to impairment of the day-to-day functioning in professional, social, and personal roles, such as missed appointments and chronic lateness (4).

Boundary Violation—Transference

Providers may find their roles transformed as part of their reaction to patients' traumatic experiences. This can come in the form of boundary violation, that is, a disruption in the accepted and expected psychological and social distance between patient and provider (5,6). Providers may take on excessive responsibility for the patient's life in an attempt to rescue the patient from an overwhelming situation. For example, a provider may agree to see a patient after hours, and then be late to pick up his/her own child. Another example is a provider who agrees to prescribe a medication that is usually initiated and managed by another type of provider (e.g., by a psychiatrist or subspecialist) because the patient refuses to see the other provider ("I don't want to see another doctor"). Treating a patient with special care may be particularly helpful and therapeutic for both patient and provider. However, it is not helpful when such treatment disempowers the patient or interferes with the provider's social or professional roles. Sometimes a provider uses the patient to fulfill his own needs generated by caring for traumatized patients. This can involve sharing his own personal problems, or a reaction from the patient to avoid sharing difficult details in order to protect the provider. The psychology literature terms these various role disruptions as *traumatic counter-transference* (1).

Use of Alcohol and Drugs

One reaction to trauma exposure may be increased use of alcohol or drugs (7). As many as half of patients in substance abuse treatment programs suffer from post-traumatic stress disorder (PTSD), and the vast majority have experienced traumatic life events (8–10), many of which predate the development of substance abuse disorders. Therefore, it is not surprising that increased use of alcohol and drugs may be a response to secondary traumatic stress. Studies of disaster relief workers have shown that increased alcohol use was associated with higher PTSD and depressive symptoms (11). In particular, providers who may have personal or family histories of substance misuse are particularly at risk for developing such problems.

SECONDARY TRAUMATIC STRESS

To put together a comprehensive model of these various negative emotional responses, different paradigms (e.g., vicarious traumatization, burnout, compassion fatigue) have been used to describe the negative psychological impact of caring for trauma survivors among mental health professionals. The common element in each paradigm is an empathetic engagement with the patient. That is, in order to be affected by the patient's trauma experience, the provider must open himself up to the suffering of the patient, as well as possess a strong desire to alleviate that suffering. Another component common to these various paradigms is a combination of provider characteristics and practice environment that promote clinician distress. Several schools of psychological thought developed these theories, which can inform approaches to prevention and treatment. For practitioners outside the mental health realm, however, these distinctions are unlikely to be important. Therefore, this chapter uses the term "secondary traumatic stress" to describe the phenomena of vicarious traumatization, compassion fatigue, and traumatic counter-transference.

FIGLEY MODEL

Trauma psychologist Charles Figley created a theoretical model to explain the development of secondary traumatic stress symptoms in the care provider (12). First, the provider must have the ability to empathize with a patient's suffering and the desire to alleviate that suffering. Also necessary is the clinician's exposure to trauma survivors through direct patient contact and discussion of the traumatic experience.

In conjunction with patient exposure, the provider must make an effort to empathize with the patient. This empathic understanding is the key determinant of the patient–provider relationship's therapeutic potential. However, empathy may come at a cost to the practitioner—what Figley terms "compassion stress": the "residue of emotional energy from the empathic response to the client." This stress can be moderated by the practitioner's sense of achievement from offering care to trauma survivors. It can also be reduced by the provider's ability to disengage or distance himself from the patient's misery in between clinical encounters. Figley suggests that this disengagement is also part of the psychological work of the patient, and thus the provider's ability to do so may help the client. Prolonged exposure to trauma survivors may increase secondary traumatic stress. Two other factors, which are provider-specific, can contribute to development of secondary traumatic stress: a personal history of traumatic exposure and life disruption (e.g., family illness, divorce, etc.).

The symptoms of secondary traumatic stress can parallel those of PTSD, and apply mainly to the work environment. Symptoms of secondary traumatic stress include those similar to the *Diagnostic and Statistical Manual of Mental Disorders* (DSM-IV) symptoms for PTSD: reexperiencing the survivor's event, avoidance of reminders of the traumatic event, and persistent arousal. Avoidance may include avoiding the patient(s) altogether, or avoiding engaging with the patient(s) on issues that may relate to the trauma. Overidentification with the client can be another symptom of this secondary traumatic stress syndrome, characterized by idealism, excessive advocacy for the client, and guilt for a perceived failure to provide adequate assistance (13).

EMPIRICAL STUDIES OF TRAUMATIC STRESS AND BURNOUT

Published studies of secondary traumatic stress are limited in a number of ways. One main limitation is the lack of a uniform measurement for secondary traumatic stress. Many existing measures have not been validated against an external standard and examine different domains. They also have not been developed for use in a clinical setting (14–16).

Studies of traumatic stress and compassion fatigue have generally been designed to correlate higher scores on one or more of the just mentioned measures with various risk factors for developing these problems. Unfortunately, the studies do not report an overall prevalence of such symptoms (17–19). Furthermore, many of these studies are not generalizable to non–trauma specialists and non–mental health clinicians due to selection bias. For example, one study compared social workers who were members of the International Society of Traumatic Stress Studies with social workers who were members of the Association of Oncology Social Workers to evaluate the effect of caring for assault survivors on the development of vicarious traumatization (20). The samples were not comparable because the oncology social workers had heavier caseloads and different working environments.

RISK FACTORS FOR DEVELOPING SECONDARY TRAUMATIC STRESS

Despite these methodological problems, the studies do offer some informative results on risk factors for developing symptoms consistent with vicarious traumatization and compassion fatigue, which researchers classify into provider-related factors and practice-related factors. Among provider-related factors, a personal history of trauma is generally an important precondition for developing traumatic stress (12,17,20). However, not all studies show a robust correlation between development of secondary traumatic stress and a personal history of trauma (18). Longer experience in the field was consistently associated with fewer secondary traumatic stress symptoms (19,21). Other factors are personality characteristics that cause individuals to be drawn to certain professions. For example, 47% of the rescue workers (firefighters, emergency personnel) reporting to the scene of the Oklahoma City bombing had a lifetime prevalence of alcohol abuse disorders, but also had a low prevalence of PTSD symptoms after the event (22,23).

Survivor as Provider

Providers with their own traumatic history may be particularly vulnerable to triggering traumatic memories while caring for trauma survivors. The prevalence of prior physical and sexual abuse among healthcare personnel reflects that of the general population. In one study of medical students and faculty, 24% reported some sort of abuse in their lifetime: 13% of respondents reported one form of physical abuse or forced sexual activity by a partner in their adult life, and 15% reported physical or sexual abuse as a child (24). Another study of first-year medical students showed 38% reported a personal history of IPV (25). The prevalence of PTSD among healthcare providers has not been studied. In the general population, 8% of people have a lifetime history of PTSD (26). Those with such histories may benefit from vigilance to self-care, as described later, to cope with the stress of bearing witness to violence in their patients.

Practice setting can also influence risk of developing secondary traumatic stress. This can include the types of patients seen or the organizational set-up of personnel. Among practice setting–related factors, professional supervision was associated with lower distress, as was working in a nonhospital setting (17). In some studies, exposure to more trauma patients showed an increase in distress symptoms and disruption of worldview (17,20). However, in another study, a larger caseload of trauma survivors predicted less vicarious trauma (19). These differences, however, may have reflected different professional statuses among the subjects in that study and not the caseload of trauma survivors.

PREVENTION AND INTERVENTION FOR SECONDARY TRAUMATIC STRESS

To prevent and intervene for secondary traumatic stress, providers and organizations must acknowledge that patient experiences of violence are common and impact one's health. Likewise, it is important for clinicians to realize that identification and management of violence-related issues may impact providers. Some of the mechanisms to prevent or alleviate secondary traumatic stress can be implemented at the individual provider level and others require an organizational approach to the issue. Although the literature on prevention and treatment of secondary traumatic stress syndrome is limited, interventions effective for PTSD patients might also benefit clinicians suffering from secondary traumatic stress.

Individual Level

The first level of protection against distress caused by caring for trauma survivors is for the provider to care for his own basic needs: sleep, nutrition, and health. When a person's physical vulnerability is heightened through sleep deprivation, malnutrition, or illness, the psychological vulnerability for secondary traumatic stress increases. In addition to enhancing physical stamina, exercise is also a useful outlet for reducing psychological stress (27,28).

A second level of protection is to obtain sufficient physical and psychological distance from the source of the traumatic stress (12). Such distance can be obtained through meaningful time away from the work environment, by creating and maintaining other social roles, such as parent, sibling, singer, painter, and the like. Providers who find themselves immersed in work to the exclusion of other important roles may be at particular risk for developing secondary traumatic stress. Vacation time can be helpful for creating distance between patients' problems and the provider's ability to prevent or improve secondary traumatic stress symptoms. Developing spiritual outlets, whether through organized religious communities, visual or performing arts, political activism, or nature may energize a provider and create resilience against negative emotions. Providers should also establish relationships with their own primary care clinicians as first-line evaluators in case secondary traumatic stress should develop.

The third level of protection involves processing the emotions and reactions that surface after bearing witness to trauma survivors, the "compassion stress" coined by Figley (12). This processing can occur through numerous venues, some of which were noted earlier. Sometimes it is important to discuss the specifics of the patient's case or one's reactions to it with colleagues, staff, friends, or family. Discussions with family and friends should be undertaken carefully. First, it is essential to preserve the patient's anonymity. Second, family and friends may carry uninformed ideas about the root causes of violence and its aftermath.

Alliances with other professionals may also be helpful in both preventing and treating secondary traumatic stress. Nonphysicians such as nurses, social workers, community advocates, and crisis counselors can offer support to the patient, as well as specific expertise about surviving violence. A consultation with a mental health professional may be useful to evaluate a patient for comorbid psychiatric problems, as well as to share the burden of care. Not all patients will have access to or attend such consultations. As an alternative or addition to such a referral, a case discussion with mental health colleagues may be particularly useful in devising an approach to future interactions with the patient and to make sense of the feelings engendered. In the mental health literature, this is termed *supervision*, and it has been shown to be important in decreasing traumatic stress symptoms in providers (29). Similarly, involvement in professional development groups, such as those modeled on the method of Michael Balint, may improve clinician satisfaction and effectiveness in communication with patients (30,31). There is no data on the specific effect of Balint groups in preventing symptoms related to caring for survivors of trauma.

Educational programs and skill training in caring for survivors of violence have been shown to improve clinicians' confidence rating in handling these issues with patients, as well as self-efficacy (32,33). The Family Violence Prevention Fund (www.endabuse.org) has online materials for healthcare professionals and can help identify training opportunities in the field.

Entering psychotherapy with a trained mental health professional can play an important role in treating secondary traumatic stress. This differs from a general discussion or consultation with a mental health colleague in that the underlying causes and personal meaning of the symptoms for the provider, not the patient's situation, are the focus of the treatment. Medication may also be part of the treatment for secondary traumatic stress. This should be directed through a primary care or psychiatric clinician trained in the use of psychiatric medication (34). A useful guide to evidence-based treatment of PTSD is the Veterans Administration National Center for PTSD website (http://www.ncptsd.va.gov).

Organizational Level

First and foremost, healthcare organizations should develop plans to minimize the risk of physical danger from violence. Sources of workplace violence can include IPV, stalking, sexual assault, harassment, and physical assault. Compared to other types of workplaces, health services, social services, and nursing facilities have among the highest rates of violence (http://www.osha.gov/Publications/osha3148.pdf). Although the subject of workplace safety is beyond the scope of this chapter, developing systems to prevent violence and to respond to violence quickly

and effectively is a key component in developing a sense of physical safety in healthcare clinicians. Maintaining a violence-free workplace can include keeping a potential perpetrator out of the workplace, responding quickly to any perpetrators who have entered the workplace, and having plans to deal with an incident if it occurs. Depending on the size and structure of the organization, plans for workplace safety can involve professional security personnel, local law enforcement (e.g., restraining order information), and creative organizational changes (e.g., removing employee names from phone and e-mail directories). The Family Violence Prevention Fund website (www.endabuse.org) has a section on specific protections for organizations on security related to IPV.

An organization whose clinicians respond to and deal with survivors of violence can foster an environment in which reactions to patients' violent experiences are expected and built into the structure of the organization. Some individual-level protections, such as professional supervision or use of allied health professionals, may be incorporated into the methods of patient referral and care. For example, hiring an IPV advocate to cover a wide range of clinicians may help provide training, directly service patients, and also be a resource for consultation (case supervision). Routine lecture series (grand rounds, for example) should include information on violence on a yearly basis. Similarly, the workplace should offer routine trainings in caring for survivors of violence.

Diversity in work responsibilities may also be protective. This could include an assorted caseload of trauma survivors (29). It may also include variety in job activities, so that clinicians do not spend all their time in direct care or stressful conditions. Likewise, encouraging vacations and a positive work environment may protect against development of secondary traumatic stress.

If a group of staff members collectively experience an episode of violence (such as occurred when caring for victims of a nightclub fire in Rhode Island in 2003), a hospital may hire a specialist to debrief and work with the providers to avoid development of secondary traumatic stress. Once a provider does develop these symptoms, the workplace should offer services for exposure to trauma or violence or referrals for such services.

A number of psychological measures exist that may be used by supervisors and managers to quantify dimensions of vicarious traumatization and burnout among providers. The Traumatic Stress Institute Belief Scale (TSIBS) is an 80-item self-report questionnaire that measures level of concern about safety, trust, esteem, control, and intimacy (14). A higher score indicates more disruption in function. Little has been published about its psychometric properties in peer-reviewed literature. The Compassion Fatigue Self-Test for psychotherapists (CFST) assesses the degree of secondary traumatization, along with a measure of burn-out (15). The Maslach Burnout Inventory measures three different items: level of being mentally and emotionally overextended and exhausted by one's work; level of detachment from one's patients; and level of enjoyment of competence and success in a job working with people (inversely related to burnout) (16).

CONCLUSION

Providers who treat survivors of violence are at risk for developing symptoms of secondary traumatic stress. This may occur as a result of predisposing factors, such as a personal history of violence, lack of social or structural support in the workplace, and lack of experience in dealing with trauma survivors. Symptoms can be prevented through developing balance in both work and personal life, processing emotions engendered by caring for patients, and workplace structures that support caring for trauma survivors.

IMPLICATIONS FOR POLICY, PRACTICE, AND RESEARCH

Policy

- Medical workplace organizations should make available mental health clinicians or advocates to consult on trauma cases.
- Medical and mental health organization should provide yearly training sessions on treating trauma survivors; the curriculum should include the impact on clinicians.
- Healthcare organizations should encourage clinicians to take vacations and care for themselves, as a way to protect against development of secondary traumatic stress.

Practice

- Clinicians treating trauma survivors should develop networks of colleagues, including allied health professionals and community advocates, to consult on management or emotional reaction to difficult patients.
- To prevent secondary traumatic stress, clinicians treating trauma survivors should build self-care activities into their routine, such as exercise, hobbies, and spiritual activities.

Research

- Researchers should develop uniform definitions and measures of secondary traumatic stress.

References

1. Collins S, Long A. Working with the psychological effects of trauma: Consequences for mental health-care workers: A literature review. *J Psychiatr Ment Health Nurs.* 2003;10(4):417–424.
2. Saxe GN, Liebschutz JM, Edwardson E, Frankel R. Bearing witness: The effect of caring for survivors of violence on health care providers. In: Liebschutz JM, Frayne SM, Saxe GN, eds. *Violence against women: A physician's guide to identification and management.* Philadelphia: American College of Physicians Press;2003:157–168.
3. McCann L, Pearlman LA. Vicarious traumatization: A framework for understanding the psychological effects of working with victims. *J Trauma Stress.* 1990;3:195–206.
4. Herman J. *Trauma and recovery.* New York: Basic Books, 1992.
5. Linklater D, MacDougall S. Boundary issues. What do they mean for family physicians? *Can Fam Physician.* 1993;39:2569–2573.
6. Butterfield MI, Frayne SM. Boundary issues in the management of patients with previous victimization. In: Liebschutz JM, Frayne SM, Saxe GN, eds. *Violence against women: A physician's guide to identification and management.* Philadelphia: American College of Physicians;2003:253–261.
7. Kilpatrick DG, Acierno R, Resnick HS, et al. A 2-year longitudinal analysis of the relationships between violent assault and substance use in women. *J Consult Clin Psychol.* 1997;65(5): 834–847.
8. Liebschutz J, Savetsky JB, Saitz R, et al. The relationship between sexual and physical abuse and substance abuse consequences. *J Subst Abuse Treat.* 2002;22(3):121–128.

9. Reynolds M, Mezey G, Chapman M, et al. Co-morbid post-traumatic stress disorder in a substance misusing clinical population. *Drug Alcohol Depend.* 2005;77(3):251–258.

10. Mills KL, Lynskey M, Teesson M, et al. Post-traumatic stress disorder among people with heroin dependence in the Australian treatment outcome study (ATOS): Prevalence and correlates. *Drug Alcohol Depend.* 2005;77(3):243–249.

11. Palm KM, Polusny MA, Follette VM. Vicarious traumatization: Potential hazards and interventions for disaster and trauma workers. *Prehosp Disaster Med.* 2004;19(1):73–78.

12. Figley CR. Compassion fatigue: Psychotherapists' chronic lack of self care. *J Clin Psychol.* 2002;58(11):1433–1441.

13. Muhlberger C. Vicarious traumatization. *Parsons Child and Family Center.* 2004;1(1):1.

14. Pearlman L. Psychometric review of TSI Belief Scale, Revision L. In: Stamm BH, ed. *Measurement of stress, trauma and adaptation.* Lutherville, MD: Sidran Press;1995:415–417.

15. Jenkins SR, Baird S. Secondary traumatic stress and vicarious trauma: A validational study. *J Trauma Stress.* 2002;15(5):423–432.

16. Maslach C, Jackson SE. The measurement of experienced burnout. *J Occupation Behav.* 1981;2:99–113.

17. Pearlman L, Mac Ian P. Vicarious traumatization: An empirical study of the effects of trauma work on trauma therapists. *Prof Psychol Res Pract.* 1995;26(6):558–565.

18. Schauben L, Frazier P. Vicarious trauma: The effects on female counselors of working with sexual violence survivors. *Psychol Women Q.* 1995;19:49–54.

19. Baird S, Jenkins SR. Vicarious traumatization, secondary traumatic stress, and burnout in sexual assault and domestic violence agency staff. *Violence Vict.* 2003;18(1):71–86.

20. Cunningham M. Impact of trauma work on social work clinicians: Empirical findings. *Soc Work.* 2003;48(4):451–459.

21. Eidelson RJ, D'Alessio GR, Eidelson JI. The impact of September 11 on psychologists. *Prof Psychol Res Pract.* 2003 2003;34(2):144–150.

22. North CS, Tivis L, McMillen JC, et al. Coping, functioning, and adjustment of rescue workers after the Oklahoma City bombing. *J Trauma Stress.* 2002;15(3):171–175.

23. North CS, Tivis L, McMillen JC, et al. Psychiatric disorders in rescue workers after the Oklahoma City bombing. *Am J Psychiatry.* 2002;159(5): 857–859.

24. deLahunta EA, Tulsky AA. Personal exposure of faculty and medical students to family violence. *JAMA.* 1996;275(24):1903–1906.

25. Cullinane PM, Alpert EJ, Freund KM. First-year medical students' knowledge of, attitudes toward, and personal histories of family violence [see comments]. *Acad Med.* 1997;72(1):48–50.

26. Kessler RC, Sonnega A, Bromet E, et al. Posttraumatic stress disorder in the National Comorbidity Survey. *Arch Gen Psychiatry.* 1995;52:1048–1060.

27. Hurwitz EL, Morgenstern H, Chiao C. Effects of recreational physical activity and back exercises on low back pain and psychological distress: Findings from the UCLA Low Back Pain Study. *Am J Public Health.* 2005;95(10):1817–1824.

28. King AC, Baumann K, O'Sullivan P, et al. Effects of moderate-intensity exercise on physiological, behavioral, and emotional responses to family caregiving: A randomized controlled trial. *J Gerontol Biol Sci Med Sci.* 2002;57(1):M26–M36.

29. Pearlman L, Saakvitne K. *Trauma and the therapist: Countertransference and vicarious traumatization in psychotherapy with incest survivors.* New York: WW Norton and Company, 1995.

30. Balint M. *The doctor, his patient, and the illness.* New York: International Universities Press, 1957.

31. Margalit AP, Glick SM, Benbassat J, Cohen A. Effect of a biopsychosocial approach on patient satisfaction and patterns of care. *J Gen Intern Med.* 2004; 19(5 Pt 2):485–491.

32. Hamberger LK. Domestic partner abuse: Expanding paradigms for understanding and intervention. *Violence Vict.* 1994;9(2):91–94.

33. Elliott L, Nerney M, Jones T, Friedmann P. Barriers to universal screening for domestic violence. *J Gen Intern Med.* 1998;13(Suppl 1):121.

34. Foa EB, Keane TM, Friedman MJ, eds. *Effective treatments for PTSD.* The Expert Consensus Guideline Series. New York: Guilford Publications, 2000.

Index

Note: Endnotes are indicated by n after the page number. Figures or tables are indicated by *f* or *t* after the page number, respectively.